CANCER MANAGEMENT IN MAN

Biological Response Modifiers, Chemotherapy,
Antibiotics, Hyperthermia, Supporting Measures

Cancer Growth and Progression

SERIES EDITOR: HANS E. KAISER

Department of Pathology, University of Maryland, Baltimore, Md, U.S.A.

Scientific Advisors:

Kenneth W. Brunson / Harvey A. Gilbert / Ronald H. Goldfarb / Alfred L. Goldson / Elizier Gorelik / Anton Gregl / Ronald B. Herberman / James F. Holland / Ernst H. Krokowski [†] / Arthur S. Levine / Annabel G. Liebelt / Lance A. Liotta / Seoras D. Morrison / Takao Ohnuma / Richard L. Schilsky / Harold L. Stewart / Jerome A. Urban / Elizabeth K. Weisburger / Paul V. Woolley

Cancer Management in Man

Biological Response Modifiers, Chemotherapy, Antibiotics, Hyperthermia, Supporting Measures

Edited by

PAUL V. WOOLLEY
Division of Oncology
Vincent T. Lombardi Cancer Research Center
Georgetown University School of Medicine
Washington, D.C., U.S.A.

Springer-Science+Business Media, B.V.

Library of Congress Cataloging in Publication Data

Cancer management in man : biological response modifiers,
  chemotherapy, antibiotics, hyperthermia, supporting measures /
  edited by Paul V. Woolley.
      p.   cm. -- (Cancer growth and progression ; 10)
    Includes index.
    ISBN 978-94-010-6983-0   ISBN 978-94-009-1095-9 (eBook)
    DOI 10.1007/978-94-009-1095-9

    1. Cancer--Treatment--Congresses. 2. Biological response
  modifiers--Therapeutic use--Congresses. 3. Cancer--Immunotherapy-
  -Congresses. 4. Cancer--Chemotherapy--Congresses. 5. Cancer-
  -Adjuvant treatment--Congresses.   I. Woolley, Paul V. II. Series:
  Cancer growth and progression ; v. 10.
    [DNLM: 1. Antineoplastic Agents. 2. Neoplasms--drug therapy.]
  RC270.8.C362 1989
  616.99'406--dc19
  DNLM/DLC
    for Library of Congress   88-23018
                                                           CIP
  ISBN 978-94-010-6983-0

Published by Kluwer Academic Publishers,
P.O. Box 17, 3300 AA Dordrecht, The Netherlands.

Kluwer Academic Publishers incorporates
the publishing programmes of
Martinus Nijhoff, Dr W. Junk, D. Reidel, and MTP Press.

Sold and distributed in the U.S.A. and Canada
by Kluwer Academic Publishers,
101 Philip Drive, Norwell, MA 02061, U.S.A.

In all other countries, sold and distributed
by Kluwer Academic Publishers Group,
P.O. Box 322, 3300 AH Dordrecht, The Netherlands.

Cover design by Jos Vrolijk.

INTRODUCTION

This volume, the last in this series on cancer growth and progression, is a companion volume to Volume IX and further explores established and novel approaches for the therapy of patients with malignant neoplasms. The strategies reflected in these volumes are direct extrapolations from the basic science of cancer biology, growth and progression described in earlier volumes of this series. Some approaches are directed towards the eradication or modification of the properties of heterogeneous malignant tumor cells at various stages of tumor progression, while other approaches are directed towards modification of the host antitumor defense systems, e.g., enhancement of host antitumor immune reactivity.

The chapters reviewing immunotherapy and biological response modifiers in cancer treatment indicate how advances in the basic science of cancer biology and tumor immunology (see Volumes I–IV) have been rapidly extended to clinical strategies for therapy of human neoplasms. Indeed, these new approaches may yield effective modalities for cancer treatment with a high margin of safety and efficacy with the capacity to overcome conventional drug resistance and tumor heterogeneity. Additional approaches towards cancer treatment, as well as advances in conventional treatment are also reviewed in this volume and include: transcatheter management, antifolates, purine metabolites, alkylating agents, platinum compounds, nitrosoureas, triazine and hydrazine derivatives, anthracycline antibiotics, actinomycin and other antitumor antibiotics.

Moreover, the current status of plant-derived vinca alkaloids and non-alkaloid natural products is summarized. Advances in hyperthermia and additional approaches for the therapy of malignancies are also presented.

The volume continues with chapters on bone marrow transplantation as well as hematologic and nutritional support for the cancer patient. Blood pressure in the cancer patient, therapy for nausea and vomiting as well as pain are discussed. The last chapter is devoted to the problems of the terminally ill, including evaluations of the burden relatives and friends of the cancer patient have to bear.

It is clear that important advances in the basic science of cancer growth and progression (reviewed in Volumes I–IV of this series) coupled with an understanding of cancer in man as compared to other species (Volume V), and an understanding of the etiology of cancer in man (Volume VI), local invasion and spread of cancer in man (Volume VII), and patterns of metastasis/dissemination in man (Volume VIII) are all essential features for the formulation of new advances in cancer management for human neoplasms. The recent and substantial advances in cancer management reviewed in this volume, and in Volume IX, indicate the rapid and expanding progress that will continue to emerge from this continuum of basic sciences, preclinical studies in therapy and diagnosis models in animals, and ultimate extrapolation to the management of cancer in man.

Series Editor   Volume Editor
Hans E. Kaiser   Paul V. Woolley

TABLE OF CONTENTS

Inspiration and encouragement for this wide ranging project on cancer distribution and dissemination from a comparative biological and clinical point of view, was given by my late friend E. H. Krokowski.

Those engaged on the project included 252 scientists, listed as contributors, volume editors and scientific advisors, and a dedicated staff. Special assistance was furnished by J. P. Dickson, J. A. Feulner, and I. Theloe.

I. Bauer, D. L. Fisher, S. Fleishman, K. Joshi, A. M. Lewis, J. Taylor and K. E. Yinug have provided additional assistance.

The firm support of the publisher, especially B. F. Commandeur, is deeply appreciated. The support of the University of Maryland throughout the preparation of the series is acknowledged.

To the completion of this undertaking my wife, Charlotte Kaiser, has devoted her unslagging energy and invaluable support.

CONTRIBUTORS

David L. ANTON, PhD.
Beth Israel Hospital
Harvard Medical School
330 Brookline Avenue
Boston, MA 02215, USA
Current address:
E.I. Du Pont De Nemours & Company
Wilmington, Delaware 19898, USA

Nicolas BACHUR, M.D.
Maryland Cancer Center
University of Maryland Hospital
22 S. Greene Street
Baltimore, MD 21201, USA

William BECHTEL, M.D.
M.D. Anderson Hospital and Tumor Institute
6723 Bertner Avenue
Houston, Texas 77030, USA

Dwight B. BROCK, Ph.D.
Epidemiology, Demography & Biometry Program
National Institute on Aging
7550 Wisconsin Ave
Bethesda, MD 20892, USA

C. Humberto CARRASCO, M.D.
M.D. Anderson Hospital and Tumor Institute
6723 Bertner Avenue
Houston, TX 77030, USA

Mickey C. CASTLE, Ph.D.
Department of Pharmacology
Eastern Virginia Medical School
P.O. Box 1980
Norfolk, VA 23501, USA

Chulsip CHARNSANGAVEJ, M.D.
M.D. Anderson Hospital and Tumor Institute
6723 Bertner Avenue
Houston, TX 77030, USA

Germaine CORNÉLISSEN, M.D.
Chronobiology Laboratories
Department of Laboratory Medicine and Pathology
University of Minnesota
Minneapolis, Minnesota 55455, USA

Lilian DELMONTE, D.Sc.
Biomedical Communication Consultant
440 East 62nd Street
Apt. 7E
New York, NY 10021, USA
formerly Memorial Sloan Kettering Cancer Center
New York, New York

Mark W. DEWHIRST, DVM, Ph.D.
Medical Center
Duke University
Durham, NC 27710, USA

Peter B. FARMER, Ph.D.
MRC Toxicology Unit Medical Research Council Laboratories
Woodmansterne Road
Carshalton, Surrey SM5 4EF, UK

DAN J. FOLEY, M.S.
Epidemiology, Demography & Biometry Program National
   Institute on Aging
7550 Wisconsin Avenue
Bethesda, MD 20892, USA

Robert M. FRANK, R.Ph.
Department of Pharmacy
Mount Sinai School of Medicine at The Mount Sinai Hospital
The Mount Sinai Medical Center of the City University
   of New York
One Gustave L. Levy Place
New York, NY 10029, USA

Paul A. FRIEDMAN, M.D.
Beth Israel Hospital
Harvard Medical School
330 Brookline Avenue
Boston, MA 02215, USA
Current address:
Merck Sharp & Dohme Research Laboratories
Division of Merck & Co.
West Point, PA 19486, USA

Robert M. FRIEDMAN, M.D.
Department of Pathology
Uniformed Services University of the Health Sciences
4301 Jones Bridge Road
Bethesda, MD 20814, USA

Erna HALBERG, B.S.
Health Sciences Center
University of Minnesota
Minneapolis, Monnesota 55455, USA

Francine HALBERG, M.D.
Department of Radiation Oncology
University of California
San Francisco, California 94115, USA

Franz HALBERG, M.D.
Chronobiology Laboratories
Department of Laboratory Medicine and
   Pathology, University of Minnesota
Minneapolis, MN 55455, USA

Julia HALBERG, B.A., M.S., M.P.H., M.D.
St. Paul-Ramsey Medical Center
St. Paul, Minnesota 55101, USA

Thomas HODGSON, Ph.D.
National Center for Health Statistics
3700 East West Highway
Hyattsville, MD 20782, USA

Hans E. KAISER, D.Sc.
Department of Pathology
University of Maryland, School of Medicine
10 S. Pine Street
Baltimore, MD 21201, USA

David G.I. KINGSTON, Ph.D.
Department of Chemistry, College of Arts and Sciences
Virginia Polytechnic Institute and State University
Blacksburg, VA 24061, USA

Dahlia V. KIRKPATRICK, M.D.
Pediatric Oncology, Department of Pediatrics
Tulane University Medical School
New Orleans, LO 70112, USA

M. LANE, M.D.
Baylor College of Medicine
One Baylor Plaza, Houston, TX 77030, USA

John LASZLO, M.D.
American Cancer Society, Inc.
3340 Peachtree Road, N.E.
Atlanta Georgia 30026, USA

Charles L. LITTERST, M.D.
National Cancer Institute
National Institutes of Health
Bethesda, MD 20891, USA

V. Sol Lucas, Jr., B.S. Pharm., R.Ph.
Burroughs Wellcome Company
Research Triangle Park
NC 27709, USA

Garrett R. LYNCH, M.D.
Baylor College of Medicine
Medical Oncology, Ben Taub General Hospital
Houston, TX 77030, USA

Hartmut MAIER-GERBER, M.D.
Langensteinbacherhoehe
7510 Karlsbad b. Karlsruhe, FRG

Madhavan G. NAIR, Ph.D.
Department of Biochemistry
University of South Alabama
Mobile, AL 36688, USA

Binh T. NGUYEN, Ph.D.
Department of Pharmacy
University of California, School of Pharmacy
San Francisco, CA 94143, USA

Takao OHNUMA, M.D., Ph.D.
Department of Neoplastic Diseases
The Mount Sinai Medical Center of the City University of
    New York
One Gustave L. Levy Place
New York, NY 10029, USA

Robert K. Oldham, M.D.
BTI Biological Therapy Institute
Riverside Drive
Franklin TN 37064, USA

John C. PHARES, M.D.
Hematology and Oncology
Naval Hospital
Bethesda, MD 20814, USA

Garth POWIS, D.phil.
Division of Developmental Oncology Research
Mayo Clinic
Rochester, MN 55905, USA

Eddie REED, Ph.D.
National Cancer Institute
National Institutes of Health
Bethesda, MD 20892, USA

Wolfgang SADÉE, Ph.D.
Department of Pharmacy
University of California, School of Pharmacy
San Francisco, CA, 94143, USA

Sidney WALLACE, M.D.
Department of Diagnostic Radiology
The University of Texas, System Cancer Center
M.D. Anderson Hospital & Tumor Institute
6723 Bertner Ave., Houston, TX 77030, USA

Derry E.V. WILMAN, Ph.D.
Institute of Cancer Research
Cancer Research Campaign Laboratory, Clifton Avenue
Sutton, Surrey, England, UK

Paul V. WOOLLEY, M.D.
Division of Oncology
Vincent T. Lombardi Cancer Research Center
Georgetown University School of Medicine
3800 Reservoir Road, N.W.
Washington DC, 20007, USA

1

BIOLOGICAL RESPONSE MODIFIERS

ROBERT K. OLDHAM

ABSTRACT

Biotherapy represents a new modality of cancer treatment. It utilizes biologicals and biological response modifiers. Many of these substances are of 'natural' origin eminating from mammalian cells as physiologic mediators of immune response and as substances active in the regulation of growth and maturation. With the advent of molecular biological techniques, hybridoma technology and computer applications, it is now possible to prepare these biological substances in highly purified form and in large quantities for use as medicinals. The expertise required to apply these biotherapeutic approaches to the treatment of cancer often involves the use of immunological and/or molecular biological capabilities. Because of the rather specialized expertise needed to understand and apply these substances as anticancer approaches, those individuals with expertise in the application of chemotherapy to patients with cancer are not necessarily well prepared for the translation of biotherapy to the clinic. Biotherapeutic approaches are broad and involve a whole range of physiological responses inherent in cancer biology. The approaches needed to bring these biotherapeutic capabilities to the clinic need to be considered carefully and the use of new techniques and new methods of application should be encouraged so as not to inhibit these potentially powerful anticancer approaches. As natural mediators, many biologicals have much less inherent toxicity than the drugs previously used in systemic cancer therapy. Therefore, the systems for translating these substances from the laboratory to the clinic should be restructured for the rapid translation of biotherapy to the patient.

INTRODUCTION

Biologicals could encompass any substance of biological origin but generally represent the products of the mammalian genome. With modern techniques of genetic engineering the mammalian genome represents the new 'medicine cabinet'. Biological response modifiers (BRM) are agents and approaches whose mechanisms of action involve the individual's own biological responses. Biologicals and BRM can act in several ways in the biotherapy of cancer:

(a) augment the host's defenses by administering cells, natural biologicals or the synthetic derivatives thereof as effectors or mediators (direct or indirect) of an antitumor response;

(b) increase the individual's antitumor responses through augmentation and/or restoration or effector mechanisms and/or decrease a component of the host's reaction that may be deleterious;

(c) augment the individual's responses using modified tumor cells or vaccines to stimulate a greater response by the individual or increase tumor cell sensitivity to an existing response;

(d) decrease transformation and/or increase differentiation (maturation) of tumor cells;

(e) increase the ability of the host to tolerate damage by cytotoxic modalities of cancer treatment.

While several of these approaches involve the augmentation of biological responses, an understanding of the biological properties of immune response molecules, growth and maturation factors and other biological substances will assist in the development of specific molecular entities which can have direct actions on biological responses and/or on tumor cells. Thus, one can visualize the development of biological approaches with response modifying as well as direct cytolytic, cytostatic, or maturational effects on tumor cells.

It is clear that the mechanisms are now available for the development of biotherapy. To put these approaches into clinical practice it is important to dispel a historical dogma of immunotherapy. Biotherapy can have activity on clinically apparent disease, and the testing is not restricted to situations where the tumor cell mass is imperceptible (38). Thus, the clinical trial designs for biotherapy can be similar to those used previously for other modalities of cancer treatment, as long as one is sensitive to the need to measure both pharmacokinetics and the biological responses affected by these approaches (34). Thus, testing is continuing for the interferons, lymphokines/cytokines, growth and maturation factors, monoclonal antibodies and immunoconjugates thereof, vaccines and cellular therapy.

HISTORICAL PERSPECTIVES

Given the variability of cancer's clinical presentation, it is not surprising that randomized trials of nonspecific and specific immunotherapy, as translated from animal models, have not been uniformly successful in cancer treatment (21, 22). Naturally occurring cancers arise in a particular organ from one cell or a few cells under some carcinogenic stimulus. In humans, these initial foci of cancer cells may grow over very long periods of time (from 1% to 10% of the human life span) before there is any clinical evidence of the disease. Dissemination of cells from initial focus may occur at any time during the development of the primary tumor. Thus, growth and metastasis occur over months to years, allowing complex biological interactions to take place.

By contrast, experimentally induced cancer is an artificial situation. The tumor cells injected into young, normal ani-

1

P.V. Woolley (ed.), Cancer management in Man: Biological Response Modifiers, Chemotherapy, Antibiotics, Hyperthermia, Supporting Measures
© 1989. Kluwer Academic Publishers, Dordrecht.

mals, thereby circumventing the influences of environmental or genetic factors which may be operative in the natural host during tumor development, and the injection represents a single instantaneous point source for a defined tumor load which has been manipulated *in vitro*. Regardless of whether that tumor load is 10^1 or 10^8 cells, it is being placed artificially into a single site and allowed to grow and metastasize from that selected single site. Thus, these transplantable cancers are not analogous to clinical cancer.

The modern era of cancer treatment began in the 1950s with the recognition that most cancers were systemic problem. It became obvious that lymphatic and blood-borne metastases often occurred simultaneously with local growth and regional spread. The early success of alkylating agents in the systemic treatment of lymphoma prompted a massive search for drugs which might have cytolytic or cytostatic effects on cancer cells. There is now widespread recognition that drugs in cancer treatment can effectively palliate and sometimes cure. The development of three modalities (surgery, radiotherapy and chemotherapy) and their subsequent integration into what is now multimodal cancer treatment have been recently summarized (8).

In the last 5 years, we have reached a plateau in cancer treatment. New surgical techniques and new methods of radiotherapy are being developed but these two modalities are useful mainly in the local and regional cancer treatment. Chemotherapy continues to evolve, with new drugs and new combinations of drugs being developed for cancer treatment. There has been continued slow progress in the treatment of highly replicative and drug sensitive malignancies over the last 10 to 15 years. It is now apparent that further progress with chemotherapy will probably depend on a greater understanding of the metabolic processes of cancer cells and the differences between these and normal cells. In addition, there are the problems of selectivity of action and drug delivery. Clearly, cancer cells are more like than unlike normal cells with respect to sensitivity to current chemotherapeutic agents. There is little evidence of selectivity in the delivery or effects of anticancer drugs. Many chemotherapeutic agents are highly cytolytic, but the problems of normal tissue toxicity, drug delivery, and tumor cell resistance remain (8, 18). Thus, cancer remains a systemic problem which requires further systemic approaches for more effective treatment.

The scientific base is now firm for the establishment of biotherapy as the fourth modality of cancer treatment. Historically, there was an attempt to establish immunotherapy in this role. While immunotherapeutic effects were reproducible under selected experimental conditions, it was not strikingly effective in animals bearing palpable tumors. Given the observation that immunotherapy was more effective with smaller tumor burdens, investigators began to study both 'specific' and 'nonspecific' immunotherapy as treatment for minimal residual disease. Although it became widely accepted that the treatment of animals with minimal residual disease was analogous to the postsurgical treatment of cancer in humans, this analogy was often stretched to the limit. Immunotherapy in young and normal animals was often begun on the day (or 1–2 days) of the tumor transplant using a transplant of a very small number of tumor cells (one to 1000) into a single site. In many of these studies and in studies where the tumor was surgically resected and no

evident disease remained, the effects of immunotherapy were reasonably reproducible and were most beneficial when the tumor mass was $< 10^6$ cells.

These experimental results developed into the dogma that immunological manipulation or immunotherapy could work only when the tumor cells mass was imperceptible (38). This posed real problems for the immunotherapy of human malignancies since the tumor cell mass is at least two orders of magnitude greater than 10^6 cells at clinical diagnosis. Even in the postsurgical adjuvant setting, the timing of most recurrences would seem to indicate that larger numbers of cells were probably present (although clinically imperceptible) than immunotherapy would likely have been able to cure.

Despite the obvious difficulties with the experimental results in animal tumor models, clinicians began immunotherapy trials in the 1970s. Initial, small nonrandomized trials would often be reported as being positive. Larger, randomized, controlled studies were done to confirm or deny the efficacy of a particular immunotherapeutic regimen in a particular cancer. While some of the controlled studies were positive, most yielded marginal or negative results. Thus, the negative attitude of most clinicians toward immunotherapy by the end of the 1970s (51).

Why did immunotherapy fail to establish itself as a major modality for cancer treatment? An important factor was the lack of definition and purity of the reagents for immunotherapy. Many of the nonspecific approaches involved the use of complex chemicals, bacteria, viruses, and poorly defined extracts in an attempt to 'stimulate' the immune response without any molecular definition as to the actual stimulating entities (such as tumor-associated antigens) which might have been involved in the treatment. Given the lack of analogy between model systems and man, the poorly characterized reagents and the problems of variability in experimental procedures, the lack of efficacy was hardly surprising.

Biological control mechanisms should be envisioned on a much broader basis than the immune system. While immunotherapy remains a subcategory of biotherapy, there are numerous additional possibilites for the control of cancer. Growth and differentiation factors, the use of synthetically derived molecular analogs, and the pharmacologic exploitation of biological molecules now involves a much broader range of approaches than those previously considered as immunotherapy.

There were specific developments that led to biotherapy becoming the fourth modality of cancer therapy (37). First, advances in molecular biology have given scientists the capability to clone individual genes and thereby produce significant quantities of highly purified products of the mammalian genome for analysis. Unlike extracted and purified biological molecules, which were available only in small quantities in semi-purified mixtures, the products of cloned genes have a level of purity on a par with drugs and can be analyzed alone or in combination as to their effects in cancer biology. In addition, recent progress in nucleic acid sequencing and translation, protein sequencing and synthesis, the isolation and purification of biological products and mass cell culture, has given us the opportunity to alter proteins at the nucleotide of amino acid levels to manipulate and optimize their biological activity.

A second major technical advance was the discovery of hybridomas. A major limitation for the use of antibodies was the inability to make high-titer specific antisera and to define these preparations on a molecular basis. Immunoglobulin reagents can now be produced with the same level of molecular purity as cloned gene products and drugs. These monoclonal antibodies are powerful tools in the isolation and purification of tumor-associated antigens, lymphokines/cytokines and other biological molecules which can be used in biological therapy. The advances in molecular biology and hybridoma technology have eclipsed previous techniques for the discovery and purification of biological molecules.

Technological advances in equipment and computers have been critically important for isolating and purifying biological molecules. We now have the capability to construct nucleotide or amino acid sequence to fit any biological message that we are able to decipher. While this synthetic capability is currently limited to smaller genes and gene products, the techniques are rapidly becoming available where analysis and construction of nucleotide sequences will occur in an automated way, making enormously complex molecules possible to synthesize and manufacture.

DETECTION OF BIOLOGICAL ACTIVITY IN PRECLINICAL MODELS

Central to the identification of biotherapy that might be useful in clinical oncology is the recognition that, in the main, the challenge in humans is the eradication of metastases. In this regard, two important facts must be kept in mind: First, metastases can result from different subpopulations of cells that reside within the primary neoplasm (12), which may explain the fact that cells residing within a metastasis can be antigenically distinct from those that predominate in the parental tumor (2, 11, 30), and from other metastases (2, 50). The implications of such findings as they relate to the outcome of specific immunotherapy are obvious. Second, normal animals are not comparable to animals or humans bearing autochthonous neoplasms (30). Specific or nonspecific defects may exist in animals and in humans that lead to the development of their autochthonous tumors. Corrections of such defects may require a totally different form of biotherapy than that required to assist the normal host in controlling an implanted cancer.

SCREENING CRITERIA

Theoretically, an ideal procedure for screening should employ a system of sequential and progressively more demanding studies designed to select a maximum number of effective agents.

The term screening denotes a series of sequential assays through which many agents are tested for therapeutic potential. For some BRM, a general screening procedure may be inappropriate. For example, the activity of a monoclonal antibody with antitumor specificity would not be detected by use of the general activity screen. The design of a general screening system for biological therapy has been reviewed (13, 31). Such a step-by-step approach to the screening of

potential BRM has been designed to define their effects on T-cell, B-cell, NK cell, and macrophage functions. A progressive sequence *in vitro* to *in vivo* allows the variables of dose, schedule, route, duration and maintenance of activity, adjuvanticity, and synergistic potential to be explored in an orderly fashion.

EFFICACY TESTING

The preclinical evaluation of biotherapy requires the *in vivo* testing of these agents in relevant model systems. The importance of the use of primary hosts with autochthonous tumors for investigating approaches that show preliminary therapeutic potential in transplantable animal tumor models cannot be overemphasized. Although this concept has been frequently discussed, the ability to obtain significant numbers of primary hosts in a reasonable time after initiation of a tumor by chemical or physical carcinogens remains a problem. Spontaneous neoplasms (of unknown cause) arise in rodents, but the use of these tumors as models is currently not practical.

The UV radiation carcinogenesis model developed by Kripke and co-workers (27, 28), has been useful in screening. In this system, chronic exposure of mice to UV radiation results in the development of single or multiple skin neoplasms. These tumors are antigenic, and most are rejected when transplanted into normal, synergeneic recipients. However, the tumors grow progressively in immunologically deficient recipients or in synergeneic mice that have been exposed to low-dose, nontumorigenic UV radiation. The immune response of UV-irradiated mice to a variety of exogenous antigens is normal, suggesting that suppressor cells with selectivity for antigens expressed on autochthonous UV radiation-induced tumors exist.

An ideal carcinogen-induced tumor system would be one in which the carcinogen is easily administered, has a short latent period, is not highly toxic, and is capable of reproducibly inducing palpable primary tumors that metastasize in a high percentage of rodents. The induction of mammary tumors in rats by IV injections of single-dose N-nitroso-N-methylurea appears to be a suitable carcinogen-induced tumor system with many of these characteristics and is being used as a second model in this screening process (29).

SCREENING EVALUATION

Screening programs for chemotherapeutic agents were initiated in the mid-1950's and attempts have been made to randomly examine thousands of compounds for antitumor activity. Such large screening programs are empirically rather than rationally based and are no longer appropriate (1). The biotherapy screen should confirm, standardize, and extend previous laboratory observations in a valid, systematic, and interpretable way to provide a vehicle for the translation of data to the clinical reality.

Whether induced or transplantable animal tumor systems are valid models for testing therapeutic modalities for human cancer has been a controversial issue (21, 22). In patients, therapy successful for one type of tumor may not be successful for another type or even for another patient with the same histologic type of cancer. Unlike the model systems where treatment can be given with precise timing relative to the metastatic phase of an implanted tumor or injected tumor cells, cancer diagnosis is generally late in humans, and micrometastases and often macrometastases have become established before treatment can be initiated. Thus, screening programs can only provide tentative indications on agents/approaches of interest. The testing of biotherapy in an involving, controlled system may help eliminate arbitrary decisions on the use of a given biological approach and ultimately may contribute to the development of novel approaches for the treatment of disseminated cancer.

BIOTHERAPY: SPECIFIC AGENTS AND APPROACHES

Nonspecific immunomodulators: Since the early 1900's, immunotherapy with bacterial or viral products has been utilized with the hope of 'nonspecifically' stimulating the host's immune response (38). These agents have been useful as adjuvants and as nonspecific stimulants in animal tumor models. However, human trials have been disappointing. Clearly, in the animal tumor models, specific requirements for immune stimulation are much better defined. It may be possible that purified components of bacterial cell walls, fungi, purified viruses, or specific chemicals (Table 1) will lead to the development of more effective adjuvants or stimulants of the immune response for use in association with tumor associated antigens and synthetic peptide vaccines for active specific immunotherapy or immunoprophylaxis. The use of purified derivative of bacterial components such as muramyl di- (or tri-) peptide packaged in liposomes as a method to stimulate macrophages to greater anticancer activity is an approach of greater promise.

Active specific immunotherapy. There has been a substantial effort to actively immunize autochthonous or synergeneic hosts with irradiated or chemically modified tumor cells in an attempt to use active specific immunotherapy (39). Inherent to this approach is the assumption that tumor cells express immunogenic tumor associated antigens (TAA). Treatment of tumor cells with a variety of unrelated agents such as irradiation, mitomycin, lipophilic agents, neuraminidase, viruses, or admixtures of cells with bacterial adjuvants have produced nontumorigenic tumor cell preparations that are immunogenic upon injection into synergeneic hosts.

Recently, a reevaluation of the procedures of active specific immunotherapy using BCG-tumor cell ('antigens') vaccines has been undertaken using a synergeneic hepatocarcinoma in an inbred strain of guinea pigs. Investigations of several variables of vaccine preparation, such as a ratio of organisms to viable, metabolically active tumor cells, the procedures of cryobiologic preservation, and the irradiation attenuation of cells, have resulted in the development of an optimal nontumorigenic BCG-tumor cell vaccine, as well as an effective regimen for the treatment of both micrometastatic and limited macrometastatic disease (19, 20).

The nature of the anatomic alteration in metastatic nodules that accompanies active specific immunotherapy was

Table 1. Biologicals and biological response modifiers.

Lymphokines and cytokines

Antigrowth factors	Migration inhibitory
Chalones	factor (MIF)
Colony-stimulating factor	Maturation factors
(CSF)	T-cell growth factor
Growth factors (transform-	[TCGF-interleukin 2
ing growth factor-TSF)	(IL-2)]
Lymphocyte activation factor	Interleukin 3 (IL-3)
[LAF-interleukin 1(IL-1)]	T-cell replacing factor
Lymphotoxin (LT)	(TRF)
Macrophage activation	Thymocyte mitogenic
factor (MAF)	factor (TMF)
Macrophage chemotactic	Transfer factor
factor	B-cell growth factor
	(BCGF)
	Tumor necrosis factor
	(TNF)

Monoclonal antibodies

Monoclonal antibodies to	Antitumor antibody (including
growth promoting factors	antibody fragments and/or
Anti-T-cell and anti-T-	conjugates with drugs, toxins,
suppressor cell antibodies	and isotopes)

Antigens

Tumor-associated antigens	Vaccines

Effector cells

Macrophages	T-cell cytotoxic clones
NK cells	Lymphokine activated cells

Miscellaneous approaches

Allogeneic immunization	Plasmapheresis and *ex vivo*
Bone marrow transplantation	treatments (activation columns
and reconstruction	and immunoabsorbents)
Viral oncolysates of cells	

Immunomodulator and/or immunostimulating agents

Alkyl lysophospholipids	Levan
(ALP)	Muramyldipeptide (MDP)
Azimexon	Malic anhydide-divinyl
BCG	ether (MVE-2)
Bestatin	Mixed bacterial vaccines
Brucella abortus	N-137
Corynebacterium parvum	Nocardia rubra cell wall
Cimetidine	skeleton
Sodium diethylithio-	Picibanil (OK 432)
carbamate (DTC)	Prostaglandin inhibitors
Endotoxin	(aspirin, indomethacin)
Glucan	Staphage lysate (SPL)
'Immune' RNAs	Thiobendazole
Therafectin	Tilorones
Krestin	Tuftsin
Lentinan	

Interferons and interferon inducers

Interferons	Brucella abortus
Poly IC–LC	Viruses
Tilorones	

Thymosins

Thymosin alpha-1	Other thymic factors
Thymosin fraction 5	

explored further by use of a specific monoclonal antibody as a probe to assess vascular permeability within these tumor models (24, 25). Immunohistologic analysis of antibody distribution showed that significantly more antibody accumulated in tumors from vaccinated animals than in comparable tumors from untreated guinea pigs. Insufficient attention has been given to the possibility that the anatomic characteristics of tumor foci restricted drug or host interactions, thus protecting tumors not only from immunotherapy but from other forms of treatment as well (18).

The regulation of the blood supply to neoplastic tissue may be different from that of the host tissues invaded by the tumor. This biologic state of the tumor metastatic nodule contributes to the fact that blood-borne substances, such as chemotherapeutic agents, monoclonal antibodies, and immune effector cells, would encounter this vascular barrier, thus limiting their access to all portions of the tumors. Such vascular barriers may provide an environment in which some tumor cells survive blood-borne chemotherapeutic and biologic agents. In this respect, solid tumor nodules may serve as 'pharmacologic sanctuaries', allowing even drug-sensitive tumor cells to continue to grow (18).

Hanna and co-workers (20), demonstrated that strategically timed chemotherapy *subsequent* to immunotherapy can effectively double the number of survivors attainable with immunotherapy alone. Furthermore, it has been shown that the synergistic effects obtained by combining immunotherapy with chemotherapy are not drug-specific. These results suggest a new basis for active specific immunotherapy in the treatment of solid tumors. Inflammatory disruption of anatomic barriers of metastatic nodules combined with strategically administered chemotherapy or biological therapy may prove to be useful in the design of future clinical trials in man.

Another approach might involve the delivery of lymphokines/cytokines such as tumor necrosis factor, lymphotoxins, macrophage cytotoxic factors, and activated complexes (such as those generated by plasma perfusion over protein A columns) to the tumor and its vascular bed. The delivery of these substances to tumor nodules might increase the vascular permeability and increase the access of antibody, immunoconjugates, drugs, and activated cells to the cancer cells (18).

A major limitation of active-specific immunotherapy has been the availability of purified tumor antigens. As presently established, the necessity of adhering to a strict protocol for whole-cell vaccine preparations (which may differ among different tumors) constitutes a major limitation in adapting this procedure for the clinic. While the present vaccine preparations must contain viable, nontumorigenic cells prepared from individual tumors, it is possible that in the future monoclonal antibody-defined purified tumor antigens would be available for large-scale immunizations. With these, a procedure can be visualized which would include antigen purification and characterization followed by genetic engineering of the antigen for vaccine production. Alternatively, synthetic peptide sequences of the active portion of tumor associated antigens may prove useful in the near future. Even the combining site of antibody to TAA has recently been suggested as a potential vaccine. All of these technologies are at hand and specific preparations will soon be available for clinical evaluation.

Thymic factors. It has been known for years that thymic extracts have biological activity on cells in the immune system (17). Thymosin fraction 5 and thymosin alpha-1 have received the most attention in the laboratory and the clinic. Thymosin fraction 5 is an extract containing a variety of thymic polypeptides, and alpha-1 is a synthetic polypeptide component present in many thymic extracts. Components of thymic preparations have been shown to enhance and suppress immune responses in both intact and thymectomized animals. Many investigators have reported that the thymosins can correct selected immunodeficiency states, both natural and laboratory-induced. There have also been reports that thymic factors can augment suppressed or depressed T-cell responses in patients with cancer. Studies are in progress with thymosin fraction 5 and with alpha-1 to determine their efficacies in patients with cancer. Studies in preclinical screening have demonstrated stimulation of T-cell activity (48), but clinical studies have not shown striking effects (9, 47, 48).

Interferons. Interferons are small, biologically active proteins with antiviral, antiproliferative and immunomodulatory activities. Each interferon has distinctive capabilities in altering a variety of immunological and other biological responses. As a class, the interferons appear to have some growth-regulating capacity in that antiproliferative effects are measurable with *in vitro* assays and in animal model systems. The relative efficacy of the mixtures of natural interferons that occur after virus stimulation as compared to the cloned interferons remains to be precisely determined. Because there may be > 20 interferon molecules (and hundreds of recombinant hybrids thereof) and because attempts have already begun at recombining the different molecules into mixtures of interferon and because of efforts are underway altering individual interferon molecules in specific ways, the range of biological activities of the interferons as antiviral agents, as immunomodulating agents and as antiproliferative agents may be very broad (35).

In addition to antiviral and antiproliferative activity, the interferons have profound effects on the immune system. Relatively low doses will enhance antibody formation and lymphocyte blastogenesis, while higher doses will inhibit both of these functions. Low to moderate doses may inhibit delayed hypersensitivity while enhancing macrophage phagocytosis and cytotoxicity, natural killer (NK) activity, and surface antigen expression. Interferons prolong and inhibit cell division, in both transformed and normal cells. In addition, interferon stimulates the induction of several intracellular enzyme systems with resultant profound effect on macromolecular activities and protein synthesis. All of these functions have been documented in murine systems, but complete dose-response effects for all types of interferons in these cellular activities have not been thoroughly investigated in either mouse or man. The alpha interferons have been most extensively tested but it would appear that beta and gamma interferon have similar effects, but relative potency may vary.

With respect to cancer therapeutics, it is still unclear whether the interferons work primarily by their antiproliferative activity or through alterations of immune responses. Most of the current evidence with lymphoma supports a direct antiproliferative effect in that higher doses induce more responses and patients failing in lower doses can be reinduced to respond to higher doses (5, 16, 49). What is clear from the current preclinical and clinical studies is that the interferons have antitumor activity even in bulky drug resistant cancers (46, 47). Clinical activity has been seen most reproducibly with a variety of lymphomas, but response in many other tumor types have been seen (36, 37). The best dose, schedule, route of administration, and type of interferon needs to be determined by further efficacy studies, and the use of interferon in combination with other anticancer agents is just beginning (34).

Lymphokines and cytokines. Many of the biologicals which will be tested in biotherapy are cell products (cytokines), lymphocytes products (lymphokines) or direct cytotoxic factors of activated lymphocytes (lymphotoxins) or macrophages (cytotoxins) (38). The lymphokines have a specific ability to regulate certain components of the immune response, which may be useful in altering the growth and metastasis of cancer in man. For example, it is possible that certain lymphokines may augment the ability of T-cells to respond to tumor-associated antigens, and others may induce higher responsiveness with respect to B-cell activity in cancer patients. Additionally, lymphokines which decrease suppressor functions may be useful in enhancing immune responses through a lessening of suppressive effects. Another specific use of lymphokines may be in the pharmacologic regulation of tumors of the lymphoid system. While many of these tumors are considered to be generally unresponsive to normal growth-controlling mechanisms mediated by lymphokines, it is possible that large quantities of pure lymphokines administered as medicinals or the use of certain molecular analogs of these naturally occurring lymphokines may be useful in the treatment of lymphoid malignancies. This concept has recently been extended to other cancers in that *in vitro* observations now suggest an antiproliferative activity of the interferons in many solid tumors. A major question exists on how to maximize the use of these substances. Their antiproliferative effects might be maximized by testing the tumor cells of each patient to 'custom tailor' the treatment rather than giving these biologicals as general treatment in the method used for anticancer drugs (42, 44).

Interleukin 1 (IL-1), originally known as lymphocyte activating factor, is a macrophage-derived cytokine that was identified originally as a result of its nonspecific enhancing effect on murine thymocyte proliferation. Both IL-1 and viable macrophages are necessary for the initial step in activation of interleukin 2 (IL-2). Cloning of IL-1 and Il-2 has made large quantities of highly purified materials available for further studies.

Clinical studies with IL-2 have been oriented around *in vitro* cell production protocols and/or induction or maintenance of antitumor T-cell effects *in vivo* (6, 36). The reports of Rosenburg using IL-2 to activate peripheral blood cells has stimulated much interest. These activated cells are generally more active against cancer cells than normal cells although their lineage (T-cell, NK-cell, LAK cells, etc.) is not clear. This approach though expensive and cumbersome, illustrates the rapidity with which developments in biotherapy are occurring (42, 44).

A lymphotoxic product of antigen mitogen-stimulated leukocytes was the first lymphotoxin described. Lymphotoxin may be the principle effector of delayed hypersensitivity and, although conflicting data have been reported, may

also be involved in the cytotoxic reactions of T-cell-mediated lysis and NK or K-cell lysis. Depending upon the type of tumor cell involved, the *in vitro* effect of lymphotoxin may be either cytolytic or cytostatic. Mouse tumor cells are frequently killed by homologous and heterologous lymphotoxins, whereas in other species, reversible inhibition of tumor cell proliferation is more common.

Human lymphotoxin has been produced from peripheral blood lymphocytes or tonsillar lymphocytes by stimulation with phytohemagglutinin or concanavalin A, and it has been harvested from supernatants of lymphoblastoid cell lines which constitutively produce small amounts of lymphotoxins (45). Isolation of human lymphotoxin for *in vivo* studies is complicated by the coproduction of at least five major species and several subspecies which result from the association with other components and by the subsequent spontaneous degradation to lower molecular weight forms. The recent purification and cloning of tumor necrosis factor (TNF) a lymphotoxin like molecule will resolve the molecular heterogenity issue as it did for the alpha interferons and will make available sufficient material for clinical evaluation. Clinical trials with TNF are now underway in Japan and the US with early reports of direct anticancer activity and some considerable toxicity.

Combined treatments with lymphotoxin, local or systemically administered, with other antitumor agents may be more valuable than lymphotoxin alone. What may be important is the ability of lymphotoxin to inhibit chemical and radiation-induced neoplastic transformation (10). Lymphotoxin used as an adjunct to chemotherapy may permit higher levels of effective but potentially carcinogenic agents to be used with less risk of producing a second malignancy.

Lymphotoxin antitumor activity may be potentiated when it is given with other lymphokines such as macrophage-activating factor TNF interferon, and IL-2. Lymphotoxin directly inhibits the growth of some tumor cells and also renders these cells more susceptible to NK-mediated lysis. Since interferon enhances the activity of NK cells, lymphotoxin and interferon given together or in sequence may result in more NK-mediated killing than that obtainable with either agent alone. There is now evidence that the combined use of various lymphokines may give enhanced antiproliferative effects (Oldham, R.K., unpublished observations). Selective assays for lymphokine antiproliferative cocktails may prove useful in tailoring such preparations for individual patients. (42).

More than 100 biological molecules have already been described and named as lymphokines. Clearly, several biologicals such as the interferons, lymphotoxins, TNF macrophage-activating factor, IL-1, IL-2, and IL-3 are now available and under evaluation as antitumor agents since each, through its own distinct mechanism, may contribute to tumor control. Such studies require quantities of material sufficiently pure to exclude contributions by other factors and permit definitive evaluation of each lymphokine/cytokine. Larger-scale studies will require standardized preparations, in quantities best obtained through genetic engineering, with the use of sensitive and rapid assay procedures to monitor production, purification, bioavailability.

Monoclonal antibody. The advent of hybridoma technology in the late 1970's has made available an important tool for the production of monoclonal antibodies for therapeutic trials (4). Hybridoma/monoclonal antibody technology has revolutionized studies with antibody across the whole field of immunology. These reagents can now be produced in huge quantities, in highly purified form, and in high titer, making available specific reagents of a type never possible with heteroantisera. These antibodies have already proven useful in purifying lymphokines/cytokines and in defining and isolating tumor associated antigens. As such, these monoclonal antibodies will undoubtedly define a whole new range of antigens on the cell surfaces, which will improve our understanding of cell differentiation and of cancer biology. Major problems in understanding the biology of the cancer cell have been the difficulties of isolating, purifying, and characterizing tumor-associated antigens. The use of monoclonal antibody technology will better define the neoplastic cell surface and identify its differences from the normal counterpart, will be of value in cancer diagnosis and histopathologic classification, and will be useful in the imaging of tumor cell masses and in the therapy of cancer (14, 16, 23, 24, 32, 37, 41, 43, 46). Finally, antibody may be a useful reagent in treating certain immune deficiencies and in altering immune responses. The removal of T-cells from bone marrow to improve bone marrow transplantation techniques is an example of using antibody as a BRM (32).

In spite of encouraging data for the use of antibody and especially immunoconjugates as targeting agents, the heterogeneity of cancer is an important consideration. If one uses a single antibody or a combination of a few antibodies that cover only a portion of the tumor cells and, if that preparation does not eliminate the true replicating cell population (stem cell) from the tumor population present in the patient, eventual outgrowth of viable cells and perhaps resistant cells will be inevitable. Therefore, it seems logical to proceed with attempts to type human tumors and to deliver toxic substances to them utilizing 'cocktails' of antibodies sufficient to cover all the tumor cells known to exist in each patient. This type of approach may require a considerable amount of testing for each patient and a 'typing' of one or more tumors from each patient. Such approaches may be much more custom tailored than is easily approachable through the product development paradigm which has been used with some success in the development of new cancer drugs. If indeed, the spectrum of human tumor heterogeneity is great, the possibility of the ideal antibody conjugated to the ideal toxic agent may not be achievable.

The difficulties in preparing antibodies and immunoconjugates, for clinical use, are obvious and these approaches will be complex and time consuming. Initially, it will be important to deliver unconjugated antibody in a way to better understand its biodistribution, pharmacokinetics and clinical effects. Then, we should proceed to the delivery of immunoconjugates in a way as to best learn what their clinical effect might be. Testing of this sort is now underway and investigators and patients alike can anticipate an improvement in the selective delivery of toxic agents to the cancer cell in the near future.

PERSPECTIVES

What should we expect from biotherapy in this decade? At the onset, it is clear that we now have much more powerful tools for improving cancer therapy in the future. We now have the techniques to decipher the major problems in cancer biology down to the genetic level. The development of these techniques, along with the recognition that biotherapy can provide increased specificity in cancer treatment, supports the belief that new and highly effective approaches are coming. As with the other three modalities, biotherapy should not stand alone. It provides an additional technique which may work most effectively in combination with surgery or radiotherapy to decrease the local and regional tumor or with chemotherapy to reduce the systemic tumor burden. It may work very effectively with radioisotopes specifically to the tumor site or with traditional chemotherapy with respect to enhancing the specificity of drug delivery.

The use of biotherapy is at an early stage. It is already clear that highly purified biologicals can be effective in patients with clinically apparent tumors. Clinical studies with alpha interferon and IL-2 have now demonstrated the responsiveness of drug-resistant lymphoma, melanoma, and renal carcinoma. These results, along with the early clinical results using monoclonal antibody, confirm the concept that we need not think of biotherapy as a tool that can be used only in patients with undetectable and minimal tumor burdens. While this modality may work best with minimal tumor burdens, a situation which is also true for chemotherapy, biotherapy can be useful as a single modality in clinically apparent disease. It may be even more effective in multimodality treatment regimens. Biotherapy offers the hope for selective treatments in ways that should significantly enhance the therapeutic toxic ratio and lessen the problem of nonspecific toxicity, a major impediment to the development of more effective anticancer treatment. The 1980s will provide new opportunities to pursue new approaches in cancer treatment. Given these new techniques and new approaches, we must now begin to redesign many of the mechanisms for the development and testing of new anticancer agents (33). It may well be possible that specifically tailored treatment will require biotherapy to be developed much more individually as compared to the historical development of therapy for broad disease categories. We must be prepared to change and adapt to the challenges and opportunities afforded by biotherapy (37).

REFERENCES

1. Alexander P: Back to the drawing board: The need for more realistic model systems for immunotherapy. *Cancer* 40:469, 1977
2. Baldwin RW: Relevant animal models for immunotherapy. *Cancer Immunol Immunother* 1:97, 1976
3. Bernhard MI, Foon KA, Oeltmann TN, Key ME, Hwang KM, Clark GC, Christensen WL, Hoyer LC, Hanna MG Jr. Oldham RK: Guinea pig line 10 hepatocarcinoma model: Characterization of monoclonal antibody and *in vivo* effect of unconjugated antibody and antibody conjugated to diphtheria toxin A chain. *Cancer Res* 43:4420, 1983
4. Boss BD, Langman R, Trowbridge I, Dulbecco R. (eds) *Monoclonal Antibodies and Cancer*. Academic Press, 1983
5. Bunn PA, Foon KA, Ihde DC, Longo DL, Eddy J, Winker CF, Veach SR, Zeffren J, Sherwin SA, Oldham RK: Recombinant leukocyte A interferon: An active agent in advanced cutaneous T-cell lymphomas. *Annals of Int Med* 101:484, 1984
6. Cheever MA, Greenberg PD, Fefer A: Potential for specific cancer therapy with immune T lymphocytes. *J Biol Resp Modif* 3:113, 1984
7. De Vita VT: Progress in cancer management: Keynote address. *Cancer* 51:2401, 1983

8. De Vita VT: The relationship between tumor mass and resistance to chemotherapy: implication for surgical adjuvant treatment of cancer. *Cancer* 51:1209, 1983

9. Dillman RO, Beauregard JC, Mendelsohn J. *et al:* Phase I trials of thymosin fraction 5 and thymosin alpha-1. *J Biol Resp Modif* 1:35, 1982

10. Evans CH: Lymphotoxin-an immunologic hormone with anticarcinogenic and antitumor activity. *Cancer Immunol Immunother* 12:181, 1982

11. Fidler IJ, Gersten DM, Budman MB: Characterization *in vivo* and *in vitro* of tumor cells selected for resistance to syngeneic lymphocyte-mediated cytotoxicity. *Cancer Res* 36:3160, 1976

12. Fidler IJ, Gersten DM, Hart IR: The biology of cancer invasion and metastasis. *Adv Cancer Res* 28:149, 1978

13. Fidler IJ, Berendt M, Oldham RK: The rationale for and design of screening assays for the assessment of biological response modifiers for cancer treatment. *J Biol Resp Modif* 1:15, 1982

14. Foon KA, Bernhard MI, Oldham RK: Monoclonal antibody therapy: assessment by animal tumor models. *J Biol Resp Modif* 1:277, 1982

15. Foon KA, Schroff R, Bunn PA, Mayer D, Abrams PG, Fer MF, Ochs J, Bottino G, Sherwin SA, Carlo DJ, Herberman RB, Oldham RK: Effects of monoclonal antibody therapy in patients with chronic lymphocytic leukemia. *Blood* 64:1085, 1984

16. Foon KA, Sherwin SA, Abrams PG, Longo DL, Fer MF, Stevenson HC, Ochs JJ, Bottino GC, Schoenberger CS, Zeffren J, Jaffe E, Oldham RK: Treatment of advanced non-Hodgkin's lymphoma with recombinant leukocyte A interferon. *New England J of Med* 311:1148, 1984

17. Goldstein AL, and Chirigos MA: In: *Progress in Cancer Research and Therapy*, Vol. 20, pp. 1-324, Raven Press, New York, 1982

18. Hanna MG Jr, Key ME, Oldham RK: Biology of cancer therapy: Some new insights into adjuvant treatment of metastatic solid tumors. *J Biol Resp Modif* 4:295, 1983

19. Hanna MG Jr, Brandhorst JS, Peters LC: Active specific immunotherapy of residual micrometastasis: an evaluation of sources, doses and ratios of BCG with tumor cells. *Cancer Immunol Immunother* 7:165, 1979

20. Hanna MG Jr, Key ME: Immunotherapy of metastases enhances subsequent chemotherapy. *Science* 217:367, 1982

21. Herberman RB, Counterpoint: Animal tumor models and their relevance to human tumor immunology. *J Biol Resp Modif* 2:39, 1982

22. Hewitt HB: Animal tumor models and their relevance to human tumor immunology. *J Biol Resp Modif* 1:107, 1982

23. Hwang KM, Foon KA, Cheung PH, Pearson JW, Oldham RK: Selective antitumor effect on L-10 hepatocarcinoma cells of a potent immunoconjugate composed of the A chain of abrin and a monoclonal antibody to a hepatome-associated antigen. *Cancer Res* 44:4578, 1984

24. Key ME, Bernhard MI, Hoyer LC, Foon KA, Oldham RK, and Hanna MG JR: Guinea pig 10 hepatocarcinoma model for monoclonal antibody serotherapy: *In vivo* localization of a monoclonal antibody in normal and malignant tissues. *J Immunol* 139:1451, 1983

25. Key ME, Brandhorst JS, Hanna MC Jr: Synergistic effects of active specific immunotherapy and chemotherapy in guinea pigs with disseminated cancer. *J Immunol* 130:2987, 1983

26. Kirkwood JM, Ernstoff MS: Interferon in the treatment of human cancer. *J Clin Oncol* 2:336, 1984

27. Kripke ML, Fisher MS: Immunologic parameters of ultraviolet carcinogenesis. *J Natl Cancer Inst* 57:211, 1976

28. Kripke ML, Lofgreen JS, Beard J, Jessup JM, Fisher MS: *In vivo* immune responses of mice during carcinogenesis by ultraviolet irradiation. *J Natl Cancer Inst* 59:1227, 1977

29. McCormick DL, Adamowski CB, Fiks A, Moon RC: Lifetime dose-response relationships for mammary tumor induction by a single administration of N-methyl-N-nitrosourea. *Cancer Res* 41:1690, 1981

30. Miller FR, Heppner GH: Immunologic heterogenicity of tumor cell subpopulations from a single mouse mammary tumor. *J Natl Cancer Inst* 63:1457, 1979

31. Oldham RK: Biological response modifier program *J Biol Resp Modif* 1:81, 1982

32. Oldham RK: Monoclonal antibodies in cancer therapy. *J of Clin Onc* 1:582, 1983

33. Oldham RK: Biologicals: New horizons in pharmaceutical development. *J Biol Resp Modif* 2:199, 1983

34. Oldham RK: Biologicals and biological response modifiers: New strategies for clinical trials. In: *Interferon IV,* edited by Finter NB, Oldham RK. Amsterdam Elsevier Biomedical Press, 1984

35. Oldham RK: In: *Interferon VI.* edited by Burke D, Cantrell K, Gresser I, De Maeyer E, Landy M, Revel M, Vilcek J. New York Academic Press, 1984

36. Oldham RK (ed.): *In vivo* effects of Interleukin 2. *J Biol Resp Modif* 3:455, 1984

37. Oldham RK: Biologicals and biological response modifiers: The fourth modality of cancer treatment. *Cancer Treat Rep* 68:221, 1984

38. Oldham RK, and Smalley RV: Immunotherapy: The old and the new. *J Biol Resp Modif* 2:1, 1983

39. Oldham RK and Smalley RV: The role of interferon in the treatment of cancer. In: *Interferon: Research, Clinical Application and Regulatory Consideration*, edited by Zoon KT, Noguchi PC, Liu TY, pp. 191-205. *Elsevier Science Publishing*, 1984

40. Oldham RK, Thurman GB, Talmadge JE, Stevenson HC, Foon KA: Lymphokines, monoclonal antibodies and other biological response modifiers in the treatment of cancer. *Cancer* 54:2795, 1984

41. Oldham RK, Foon KA, Morgan AC, Woodhouse CS, Schroff RW, Abrams PG, Fer M, Schoenberger CS, Farrell M, Kimball E, Sherwin SA: Monoclonal antibody therapy of malignant melanoma: *In vivo* localization in cutaneous metastasis after intravenous administration. *J Clin Onc* 2:1235, 1984

42. Oldham RK: The role of biological response modifiers in the therapy of cancer: An overview. Natural Immunity Symposium (Hawaii), 1985

43. Oldham RK, Abrams P: *Monoclonal Antibody Therapy of Solid Tumors*. Dordrecht Martinus Nijhoff Publishers, 1985

44. Oldham RK: Biological response modifiers, In: Introduction, Torrence, PF, (eds.) *Biological Response Modifiers*, edited by Torrence PF. Academic Press, New York, 1984

45. Rosenau W: Lymphotoxin: properties, role and mode of action. *Int J Immunopharm* 3:1, 1981

46. Sherwin SA, Knost JA, Fein S, Abrams PG, Foon KA, Ochs JJ, Schoenberger CS, Maluish AE, Oldham RK: A multiple dose Phase I trial of recombinant leukocyte A interferon in cancer patients. *JAMA* 248:2461, 1982

47. Smalley RV, Oldham RK: Biological response modifiers: preclinical evaluation and clinical activity. *CRC Crit Rev in Oncol Hemat* 1:259, 1984

48. Smalley RV, Talmadge JA, Oldham RK, Thurman GB: The thymosins: preclinical and clinical studies with fraction V and alpha-1. *Cancer Treat Rev* 11:69, 1984

49. Stevenson HC, Ochs JJ, Halverson L, Oldham RK, Sherwin SA, Foon KA: Recombinant alpha interferon in retreatment of two patients with pulmonary lymphoma, Dramatic responses with resolution of pulmonary complications. *Am J Med* 77:355, 1984

50. Sugarbaker EV, Cohen AM: Altered antigenicity of spontaneous pulmonary metastases from an antigenic murine sarcoma. *Surgery* 73:155, 1972

51. Terry MD, Rosenberg SA (eds.): *Immunotherapy of Cancer*, pp. 1-398. Excerpta Medica, New York, 1982

UPDATED REFERENCE

Oldham RK (ed.): *Principals of Cancer Biotherapy*. New York, Raven Press, 502 pp., 1987

2

ANTITUMOR EFFECTS OF INTERFERONS*

ROBERT M. FRIEDMAN and ROBERT K. OLDHAM

ANTITUMOR EFFECTS OF INTERFERONS IN ANIMAL SYSTEMS

Numerous studies have been reported, examining the effects of Interferons (IFNs) on tumors of different type and histology in various animal systems. Both IFNs and IFN inducers have been used to study inhibitory effects on virus, chemical and radiation induced tumors as well as transplantable and spontaneous tumors. These have been reviewed extensively elsewhere (2, 33, 83)

The findings that IFNs could inhibit the multiplication of oncogenic viruses as well as nononcogenic viruses led to the discovery that IFN preparations could also inhibit cell transformation and tumor production caused by these oncogenic viruses. In animals inoculated with polyoma, Rous sarcoma or Shope fibroma viruses, tumors were inhibited and animal survival increased if IFN treatment was prior to virus inoculation. In contrast, in mice inoculated with Friend and Rauscher leukemia viruses, it was necessary to continue IFN treatment after viral infection in order to inhibit the various manifestations of these leukemias (33). Since virus multiplication occurs throughout the course of these diseases, continued repression of virus multiplication by IFN may have been necessary for inhibition of evolution of the disease.

In order to examine the possibility that IFNs might be inhibiting multiplication of the tumor cells themselves or might be enhancing tumor-cell rejection in the host, Gresser and his associates (34, 35, 38) studied the growth of inoculated tumors in several strains of mice. These tumors developed from transplanted tumor cells and not from transformation of host cells by virus. Less success was usually attained in the treatment of solid transplantable tumors than in the treatment of ascites tumors. IFN therapy was most effective when the tumor inoculum was low; once the tumor was well established regression did not occur (33). However, IFN treatment inhibited the development of both the subcutaneous nodules of the Lewis lung carcinoma at the site of transplantation and the development of pulmonary metastases from the transplant (37).

Another approach that has been employed to study direct effects of IFN on tumor growth has been to use immunosuppressed hosts. Gresser and Bourali-Maury (1973) (37a) found that treating mice with anti-lymphocyte serum or X-irradiation did not alter IFN's inhibitory effect on transplantable tumors. Additionally, in another study, the development of tumors from transplanted HeLa cells and xenografts of human breast cancers in nude mice was markedly suppressed by human IFN (87). These studies suggest the possibility that the inhibitory activity of IFN against a tumor may result from a direct antigrowth action on the tumor cells themselves, bypassing the immune response of the host.

There have not been many reports on the antitumor effects of gamma IFN, mainly due to the lack of availability until recently of sufficient quantities of gamma IFN preparations to carry out significant studies. There are several reports indicating that in the treatment of certain tumors, the antitumor activity of gamma IFN was more potent per antiviral unit of IFN than the alpha or beta preparations (18, 31, 74); however, due to the presence of many lymphokines in these gamma IFN preparations, conclusions cannot yet be made concerning the antitumor activities of this form of IFN.

Another important area of investigation concerns the use of IFN in conjunction with other antitumor agents to determine whether the effects are additive, synergistic or antagonistic. In one study, IFN treatment inhibited murine leukemia only after the number of tumor cells was first reduced by treatment with 1,3-bis (2-chloroethyl)-1-nitrosourea (16). Direct injections of IFN followed by poly-rI:poly-rC after several hours, led to a synergistic inhibitory effect on autochthonous Moloney murine sarcoma virus-induced tumors (83) while, IFN and cyclophosphamide were reported to have additive effects on increasing survival after diagnosis of lymphoma in AKR mice (41).

POSSIBLE BASES OF ANTITUMOR ACTIVITIES OF INTERFERONS

Several hypotheses have been proposed attempting to explain the antitumor effects of IFNs. These include: (1) inhibition of tumor virus replication and cell transformation by virus; (2) inhibition of tumor development through primary effects on the immune system of the host; and, (3) direct inhibition of proliferation of the tumor cell itself.

Inhibition of virus replication

Interferon treatment results in a marked decrease in the production of oncogenic viruses and in the efficiency of cell

---

* The opinions or assertions contained herein are the private views of the authors and should not be construed as official or necessarily reflecting the views of the Uniformed Services University of the Health Sciences or Department of Defense.

9

P.V. Woolley (ed.), Cancer management in Man: Biological Response Modifiers, Chemotherapy, Antibiotics, Hyperthermia, Supporting Measures
© 1989. Kluwer Academic Publishers, Dordrecht.

transformation by virus. IFNs were thought to inhibit tumor viruses through the same mechanism as that involved in the inhibition of other viruses. However, for the inhibition of both the DNA and RNA tumor viruses that have been studied extensively, the mechanism of IFN action appears to be complex. For the SV40 system, treating cells with IFN at various times relative to virus infection yields different results. These different effects have been reviewed (25, 72). If IFN was added to cells prior to SV40 infection, virus production and T-antigen synthesis were inhibited. It has been suggested that these effects resulted from IFN blocking the transcription of SV40 DNA molecules by the cell RNA polymerase (58). The findings that infection of these cells with SV40 DNA instead of intact virions overcame the antiviral effect of IFN suggested that IFN was also inhibiting SV40 uncoating (95) and probably thus early transcription (9). Addition of IFN to cell during the early phase of SV40 infection (before viral DNA synthesis) failed to inhibit production of SV40 early RNA. In contrast, IFN addition during the late phase of the virus lytic cycle resulted in inhibition of viral protein synthesis at the level of translation in the absence of inhibition of viral mRNA synthesis or significant inhibition of host cell protein synthesis (72). Data from studies on the effect of IFN on SV40-transformed cells indicate that transcription and translation of the T-antigen are not sensitive to IFN in SV40-transformed cells, although T-antigen production is sensitive during the late phase of the SV40 lytic cycle. The very interesting question as to why a single viral gene may be sensitive to IFN in certain phases of virus growth and resistant in others, remains to be elucidated.

Similar to the situation with SV40-transformed cells, IFN treatment of cells chronically infected with C-type leukemia viruses resulted in no inhibition of viral RNA or protein synthesis (6, 27, 29, 71). RNA tumor viruses are, however, sensitive to IFN and it appears that IFN acts at a late stage of virus maturation. In some systems, IFN treatment resulted in marked inhibition of virus release while in others, particle production appeared normal; however, the released virus was deficient in infectivity (25). The data suggest that IFN may be inhibiting these viruses by altering the membrane through which these viruses are exported out of the cell (14, 26) and/or by altering cellular or viral protein(s) necessary for proper maturation of the virus particle (13, 60, 70).

Studies with cells infected with an adeno-SV40 hybrid virus which contains a combination of an IFN-sensitive (SV40 virus) and an IFN-insensitive (adenovirus) genome have yielded interesting findings. In simultaneous infection of cells with both complete viruses the sensitivity of adenovirus or SV40 T-antigen production was characteristic of infection with either virus separately. In contrast, in cells infected with an SV40-adenovirus hybrid, production of both T-antigens was as resistant as adenovirus T-antigen production in infection with adenovirus alone (67).

There is evidence that the SV40 genome is covalently linked to the adenovirus genome in the hybrid or to cellular DNA in SV40-transformed cells. The mRNA produced by the integrated SV40 genome contains host sequence, and the mRNA of the hybrid contains both adenovirus and SV40 sequences. The resistance to IFN treatment of SV40 T-antigen production directed by an integrated viral genome

may indicate that the primary sequence in the mRNA that specifies the viral protein does not determine sensitivity to IFN. Other sites on the genome such as those concerned with initiation or control of genetic expression may then be the loci of IFN action. This may also explain the lack of IFN-induced inhibition or murine RNA tumor virus protein production in chronically infected cells where the proviral DNA is integrated into host DNA.

In experimental systems with virally induced tumors, such as hamsters inoculated with polyoma virus or chickens infected with Rous sarcoma virus, IFN most likely inhibited development of tumors by inhibiting virus multiplication and/or an early virus-dependent step involved in cell transformation. It is unlikely, however, that the antiviral activities of IFNs are responsible for inhibition of tumors which are apparently not virus-induced, or tumors in which virus replication is not involved in the progression of development. One possibility is that IFN inhibits replication of the tumor cell itself. IFN may also have effects on the host's capacity for tumor rejection. For example, the demonstration that leukemia L1210 cells, that were resistant to the cell growth inhibition activity of IFN *in vitro*, could be inhibited *in vivo* suggested that the antitumor effect of IFN in these mice was not a result of direct inhibition of tumor cell multiplication (40).

Effects of interferons on the immune system

IFNs have inhibitory as well as stimulatory effects on many different immunological reactions. These have been reviewed (30, 33, 77, 79, 83). IFN treatment appears to affect all of the cells of the immune system and thus, influences many humoral and cellular aspects of the immune system.

IFNs were shown to exert a dosage and time dependent effect on antibody response. Administration of high titers of alpha and beta IFNs to mice after immunization with sheep red blood cells (SRC) resulted in suppression of plaque-forming cell (PFC) response; however, lower doses of alpha or beta IFN resulted in enhancement of the PFC response to SRBC (8). When mice were treated with IFN 4–48 hrs before sensitization with SRBC, the PFC response was greatly suppressed.

If treatment was 58–72 hrs after sensitization with SRBC, the PFC response was enhanced (79). Gamma IFN was also shown to have a dosage regulatory effect on antibody production and the immunosuppressive activity of gamma IFN was substantially more potent on the basis of antiviral titer than that of alpha or beta IFN (80, 91).

Interferons also exert an immunoregulatory effect on the IgE system. Treatment of spleen cells from sensitized animals with interferon resulted in a decreased ability to transfer cutaneous anaphylaxis. Interferon was also found to increase the release of histamine from basophils after exposure to ragweed antigen or to anti-IgE antibodies. The addition of infectious or inactivated viruses to human leukocyte cultures facilitated histamine release, when the cultures were subsequently exposed to anti-IgE. There was a temporal relationship between the augmentation of histamine release and the induction of interferon in the cultures. It is in this context that interferon has been ascribed a potential role in the development of asthma during upper respiratory tract infections. Additionally, the interferons may serve to induce other cofactors associated with the reagenic response, such as the IgE binding factors (44).

Many of the observed effects of interferon on the cellular immune system may stem from interferon-induced changes in membrane-associated antigens and receptors on lymphoid cell types. These changes may be analogous to other interferon-induced changes in the cell surface (26). Interferon has been demonstrated to augment *in vitro* the expression of histocompatibility antigens on murine thymocytes and splenic lymphocytes. Substantially higher concentrations were required to induce Ia and Lyt 1, 2, and 3 antigens on thymocytes. No increase in theta antigen was observed upon treatment with alpha and beta interferon preparations. Gamma interferon-containing preparations were found to induce histocompatability antigens at significantly lower concentrations of interferon. Similarly, the induction of Ia and Lyt antigens, as well as theta antigen, was inducible. Interferon-enhanced IgG Fc receptor binding by murine macrophages has also been demonstrated. As was observed for the induction of thymocyte membrane antigens, gamma interferon preparations were found to be considerably more efficacious (by approximately 33-fold) in the induction of FcR (30).

Evidence from studies of the murine system also suggest a role of activated macrophages in the direct destruction of tumor cells (77). Several types of macrophage activities have been shown to be affected by IFNs. Administration of IFN resulted in increase of macrophage activation, measured by macrophage spreading, and in enhanced phagocytosis of carbon particles by macrophages (77, 79). Macrophages can also be induced by IFNs to be tumoricidal. Addition of IFN to cultures of macrophages and leukemia cells induced the resting macrophages to inhibit the growth of the leukemia cells and this action was reversed by addition of prostaglandins E1 and E2 and hydrocortisone (79).

A role for interferons in the regulation of cell-mediated immunity has been recognized for some time; however, the specific mechanisms by which interferons exert their varied effects are from being elucidated. One of the earliest recognized and most striking effects of interferon on cell-mediated immune responses *in vivo* was the demonstration that interferon inducers or interferon-rich culture supernatants significantly delayed the rejection of skin grafts across major or minor histocompatibility differences in mice. It was subsequently demonstrated that administration of interferon inducers or interferon-rich preparations to mice previously sensitized with picryl chloride or sheep erythrocytes resulted in inhibition of delayed type hypersensitivity (ear or footpad swelling) upon challenge with the sensitizing antigen. Interferon not only inhibited the delayed type hypersensitivity reaction upon challenge, but also depressed sensitization when administered prior to the sensitizing injection. Tilorone (an interferon inducer in mice) administration inhibited the cell-mediated response to a number of intracellular parasites as well as to sheep erythrocytes. As there are many examples of depressed cell-mediated immunity following virus infection, these findings strongly implicated interferons as suppressive agents. The timing of administration of interferon was found to be critical with regard to the modulation of delayed hypersensitivity. As was observed for

the modulation of antibody synthesis (see above), administration of interferon prior to sensitization with antigen led to a depression of the cell-mediated response; however, when administered after the sensitizing antigen, an augmentation could be demonstrated. The dosage of antigen was also critical, so that interferon-induced enhancement of the cell-mediated response occurred only when suboptimal or non-sensitizing doses of antigen were used (30).

Interferons have also been shown to modulate a number of *in vitro* responses felt to reflect *in vivo* cell-mediated immunity. Interferon depressed the proliferative responses of lymphocytes to the T cell mitogen, phytohemagglutinin (PHA), or to an allogeneic stimulus. Subsequently, it was demonstrated that the T cell response to concanavalin A (Con A) was also depressed by *in vitro* exposure to interferon and that *in vivo* administration of interferon led to the depression of proliferation in response to PHA or Con A *in vitro*. Interferon mediates the suppression exhibited by Con A-induced human suppressor cells, including the response of normal lymphocytes to Con A. Taken collectively, these findings suggest that interferons can exert on T lymphocytes a strong antiproliferative effect analogous to that observed for B lymphocytes (see above). It is interesting to note that exogenous interferon enhanced or depressed the production of lymphokines by Con A-stimulated human leukocytes, depending on the concentration of interferon added to the cultures. Since the manifestations of delayed type hypersensitivity are closely associated with the production of lymphokines, this provides an underlying mechanism for the observed effect of interferon on delayed type hypersensitivity responses *in vivo* and *in vitro* (30).

One possible mechanism by which IFNs might contribute to the inhibition of tumor growth is by activation of cells that are cytotoxic to tumors. Lindahl *et al.* (54) demonstrated that IFN could enhance the specific cytotoxicity of sensitized murine T lymphocytes but had no effect on normal lymphocytes, although there are several reports that longer incubation times resulted in lysis or inhibition of growth of target cells (7, 15, 86). Another mechanism of mononuclear cell killing that might play a role in antitumor defense is antibody-dependent, cell-mediated cytotoxicity (ADCC) which is mediated by killer (K) cells; IFNs have been shown to enhance ADCC *in vitro* (42, 43). All types of IFN have also been shown to be potent activators or natural killer (NK) cell cytotoxicity *in vivo* and *in vitro* (80). It is interesting to note that NK cells challenged with cells carrying foreign antigens produce alpha IFN (89).

In addition, various preparations of interferon have been shown to augment the generation of cytotoxic lymphocytes (CTL) and killer cells (K cells) associated with antibody-dependent cell cytotoxicity. These findings led investigators to hypothesize that interferons provide an essential signal in the generation of cytolytic effector cells; however, the precise role of interferons in the generation of CTLs and the requirement for additional cytokine signals is not yet understood (reviewed in ref. 30).

Natural killer (NK) cells comprise a heterogenous subpopulation of lymphoid cells that possess spontaneous cytolytic activity both *in vivo* and *in vitro* against a variety of cellular targets. No previous sensitization with the target cell is required for their lytic activity. They exist in man, mouse, and a wide variety of other species and are felt to form the cellular basis for nonspecific host resistance to tumors as well as to intracellular infectious agents. NK cells were originally recognized by their characteristic ability to lyse a broad range of tumor cells *in vitro*; however, other studies have since extended the lytic reactivity of NK cells to include virus-infected, as well as certain normal cells, such as hematopoietic bone marrow cells. In this regard, it has been suggested that NK cells may play a role not only in surveillance and resistance against neoplasia and viral disease, but also in the control of normal development of hematopoietic cells.

The participation of interferons as modulators of NK cell activity has been recognized for approximately seven years during which time a large number of reports have demonstrated for murine and human systems that the *in vivo* and *in vitro* administration of interferons or interferon inducers resulted in a 2- to 10-fold augmentation of NK cell activity. Interferons also induce differentiation of the pre-NK cells to fully cytolytic forms.

The effect of interferons on NK target cells presents a curious paradox. Several investigators have demonstrated that interferon treatment of the target cells decrease their sensitivity to NK cell cytolysis in a dose-dependent fashion. Under optimal conditions, this inhibition of cytotoxicity can be greater than 99% (30).

It is important to note that although under certain experimental conditions IFNs interact with macrophages and lymphocytes, but it is not known if the same effects are observed under natural conditions of tumor growth in the host. Along these lines, Gresser and Bourali-Maury (1973) found that IFN was still effective in inhibiting tumor growth in mice whose lymphocyte and macrophage activities had been depressed by X-irradiation, anti-lymphocyte serum, or silica; however, it is possible that depression of lymphocyte and/or macrophage functions was not complete or that another cell population involved in antitumor activities was not affected by X-irradiation, antilymphocyte serum or silica. Additionally, in studies with athymic "nude" mice, human IFN was able to suppress the development of human breast tumors leading the investigators to conclude that IFN was exerting a direct effect on cell proliferation (87).

With the wide variety of effects that IFNs have on most aspects of the immune system, it is possible that at least part of IFN's antitumor activity is mediated through the immune response. However, studies on the antitumor action of IFNs have not yet provided any unequivocal instance of the immune response being responsible for slowing the growth of a cancer.

Inhibition of cell proliferation

With the demonstrations that purified molecules of IFN can inhibit both virus replication and cell multiplication (39, 49) it is well established that IFNs can inhibit the growth of a wide range of cell types. The sensitivities of cells to the growth inhibitory effects of IFNs range from very sensitive to resistant and the same cell type can show varying sensitivities under varying assay conditions: growth of colonies in agar is more sensitive than growth on a solid support; and sparsely seeded culture appear to be more sensitive than the same cells seeded at high densities (87).

There seems to be conflicting evidence about whether tumor cells are more sensitive to the growth inhibitory effects of IFNs than are normal cells. The multiplication of HeLa cells was shown to be inhibited to a greater extent than that of human fibroblasts (25); similarly, the inhibition of the multiplication of human osteosarcoma cells was greater than that of nontumor cells (85). In contrast, the multiplication of retrovirus carrier cells (5), or of X-ray transformed cells (10) derived from C3H fibroblasts was less inhibited by IFN than that of nontransformed cells. Moreover, in the comparison of normal human mammary epithelial cells to breast cancer cells, or 3T3 cells to SV40-transformed 3T3 cells, the normal cells were at least as sensitive to the growth inhibitory effects as the respective transformed cells (4). Thus, many different cell types, both normal and malignant appear to be affected by IFNs *in vitro*. There are some studies that suggest similar effects *in vivo*. IFNs can inhibit the multiplication of tumor cells as well as normal cells in animals (36); inhibit the multiplication of allogenic lymphocytes and syngeneic bone marrow cells, when these were transformed into irradiated mice (12); and, inhibit liver cell regeneration in partially hepatectomized mice (24). It should be noted, however, that the dosages of IFN used in these studies were much higher than those needed to inhibit tumor cell growth.

There are many possible sites at which IFNs can act to inhibit the complex process of cell multiplication. Different approaches are being used to examine aspects of control of cell growth and what effects IFNs have on these processes: (i) examination of IFNs' effects on the cell cycle; (ii) study of cellular functions that may be involved in control of cell growth or cellular parameters that are altered in malignant cells; and, (iii) determination of whether any of the molecular mechanisms thought to be implicated in IFN's antiviral activities play any role in the antiproliferative activities of IFN.

Interferons and the cell cycle

The effects of IFNs on cell cycles of both asynchronously dividing cells and synchronized cultures have been examined (87). The available data suggests that IFNs do not arrest cells in one phase of the cell cycle. IFN treatment reduces the rate of entry into S phase and also increases the duration of the G_1 and $S + G_2$ phases (3). Thus, the increased length of cell cycle time observed in IFN-treated cultures (17) is probably due to the extension of these phases.

Quiescent cells that can be stimulated to divided synchronously by mitogens provide an excellent system to study the events in G_1 which are crucial to the initiation of DNA synthesis and what effects IFNs have on these activities. The events that occur after stimulation of these cells with mitogens, but preceding DNA synthesis, can be divided into 'early' and 'late' categories. Early events occur within minutes after mitogen stimulation and are not dependent on cellular protein synthesis. These events include changes in intracellular cAMP levels and increased uptake of ions, nucleotides, and sugars. Late events, that occur hours after mitogen stimulation, are protein synthesis dependent and include secondary increases in sugar and ion uptake and an increase in the activities of certain enzymes. One of these enzymes, orinthine decarboxylase (ODC), catalyzes the first rate limiting step in the synthesis of polyamines, that are involved in the regulation of various cellular reactions, including transcription and translation. Increases in ODC activity are associated with the proliferative response of cells in culture, in tumors and also with tumor promotion (46).

Addition of IFN to quiescent Swiss 3T3 cells at the time of mitogen stimulation had no effect on the early increase in uptake of ions, nucleosides or sugars; however, IFN treatment showed a differential effect on protein synthesis-dependent events: induction of ODC activity was inhibited while the second phase of stimulation of 2-deoxy glucose uptake was not affected. These results were observed with serum, with a combination of growth factors, or with a tumor promoter serving as the mitogen (81, 82). Similar findings were recently reported on the inhibitory effect of IFN on the induction of S-adenosyl-L-methionine decarboxylase, another enzyme involved in polyamine biosynthesis (53). Thus, it appears that there is a common IFN-sensitive step involved in the stimulation of DNA synthesis by serum, tumor promoters or growth factors. Further evidence suggesting an IFN-sensitive step crucial to DNA synthesis is derived from the examination of two clones isolated from Swiss 3T3 cells with differential sensitivities to both antiviral and antiproliferative activities of IFNs. One clone was more sensitive to IFN in terms of inhibition of cell division, DNA synthesis, and induction of ODC activity when IFN was added at the time of serum stimulation. Additionally, under the same conditions, NIH 3T3 cells which were sensitive to the antiviral effect of IFN against murine leukemia virus exhibited no inhibition of cell division, DNA synthesis, or ODC induction (19). One argument against ODC induction being the crucial step involved in the stimulation of DNA synthesis is that the inhibition of ODC synthesis in human embryo skin fibroblasts did not result in the inhibition of DNA synthesis upon stimulation from quiescence. This suggested that the pool of polyamines in these cells was sufficient for one further cycle of replication (46). There is now strong evidence to indicate that inhibition of DNA synthesis caused by IFN is not dependent on the inhibition of ODC activation that is also caused by IFN. Concomitant inhibition of DNA synthesis and of activation of the enzyme was observed only when polypeptide hormones were used as stimulants; cholera toxin-stimulated DNA synthesis was inhibited by IFN toxin-stimulated ODC activation was not (53). These results indicate that a poor correlation exists between the activation of ODC and DNA synthesis in quiescent 3T3 cells that are stimulated to proliferate. Thus, ODC induction may not be the critical step in DNA synthesis inhibition caused by IFN; however, the role it plays in the cell growth inhibition caused by IFN treatment is not yet clearly understood.

Effects of interferons on other cellular parameters
Information concerning the many varied effects of IFNs on cell structure and function is increasing rapidly. [For reviews see (33, 83, 87)] IFN treatment of cells results in significant alterations of the cell surface including increased expression of histocompatibility antigens (54); increased net negative charge on the cell surface (49); decreased thymidine uptake (11); and alteration in the density of the plasma membrane (14). Alterations in the cell membrane resulting from IFN treatment most likely play a role in the IFN-induced inhibition of murine leukemia viruses discussed earlier. Additionally, SV40 transformed cells that normally produce and

release plasminogen activator (PA) seem to accumulate PA at the plasma membrane after IFN treatment (76). It is possible that IFN might alter the cell surface in a manner that prevents particle shedding in one system of C-type virus particles and in another, of PA. Since cell to cell contact plays a role in cell growth regulation, alteration induced in the plasma membrane by IFN treatment could well cause alterations in cell DNA synthesis and growth.

A direct negative effect on cell growth would, of course, be an ideal mechanism of action for an antitumor substance. In many respects IFNs would seem to be negative growth control factors. Thus, they are an unusual class of biological substances, since almost all growth factors that have been studied stimulate cell synthesis. It is likely that many of the 'toxic' effects observed in IFN therapy, such as leukopenia, thrombocytopenia and hair loss, are indeed extensions of the growth inhibitory properties of IFN. Another structure that has been studied is the cytoskeleton. Changes in the cytoskeleton, which is composed of microtubules, microfilaments (actin and myosin) and the cytoplasmic matrix, have been observed in conjunction with transformation. It is not yet clear, however, whether these changes are a cause or result of transformation. What relationship exists between IFNs and the cell's cytoskeleton has been and is being examined mainly by following the effects of agents that alter the cytoskeleton on the various activities of IFNs. For example, drugs such as colchicine, that disrupt the cytoskeleton inhibit the development of the antiviral action of IFN, while compounds such as sodium butyrate, which has been reported to promote cytoskeletal organization, appear to enhance IFN action (87).

The antiviral activities of IFNs were shown to be potentiated by dibutyryl cAMP (28). Additionally, it was reported that IFN-treated cells contained increased levels of cAMP (56, 92). Since it appeared that increased levels of cAMP might be involved with inhibiting cell growth rates of several systems (73), it was thought that membrane adenylate cyclase activities might play a role in the antiproliferative response to IFNs. It was, however, shown recently that more time of treatment with IFN was necessary for alteration of cAMP levels than for detection of cell growth inhibition (88). Additionally, growth of Schwann cells, human keratinocytes, and human mammary epithelial cells is stimulated by both cholera toxin and cAMP analogues (87). Thus, the relationship between IFNs and cAMP appears to be complex. It is also interesting that cyclic GMP levels are also increased after IFN treatment (88) and reduced levels of cGMP are found in proliferating cells (59).

Interferons and oncogene expression
The level of expression of *oncs* appears to be related to malignant transformation, and to cellular differentiation and growth (52, 90). It is possible that the effects of IFNs on differentiation and growth involve a regulatory activity of IFNs on *onc* expression; therefore, the inhibitory effects of IFNs on the growth of some tumors may be linked to a decrease in *onc* expression. This might occur in cancers where oncogenesis is related to increased production of an *onc*-specified product. Therefore, a change in the expression of *oncs* could be an important mechanism in carcinogenesis. There are two basic mechanisms for *onc*-induced transformation: an alteration in an *onc* product, or an increase in

its production. In some cancers, therefore, a decrease in *onc* expression could result in reversion to an untransformed state. Such a modulation in *onc* expression may be induced by a potent biological response modifier such as an IFN. The current rationale for the use of IFN in the therapy of cancers is their cell growth inhibitory activity; however, IFNs do not have a consistent, selective effect on transformed cell growth. On the other hand, a regulatory effect of IFNs on *onc* expression might result in a selective effect on the growth of tumors, the etiology of which is related to an increase in *onc* expression.

During the course of studies involving treatment with IFN of RS485 cells, an NIH 3T3 line transformed by a human c-Ha-*ras* oncogene, there was phenotypic reversion of a portion of the previously transformed RS485 cells. The revertant RS485 cells were morphologically similar to NIH 3T3 cells, had a low saturation density in culture, and did not form colonies in soft agar or tumors in nude mice. While the revertants retained the transfecting c-Ha-*ras* DNA, they produced significantly decreased amounts of the c-Ha-*ras*-specified gene product, p21, and c-Ha-*ras* mRNA, than did RS485 cells (75).

Correlation of antiviral and antiproliferative activities of interferons

Several specific proteins that are induced in IFN-treated cells and which are most likely involved in the antiviral activities of IFN, have been identified [for reviews see (1, 72)]. One of these proteins is the oligoadenylate synthetase which polymerizes ATP into pppA2' p5'A2'p5'A . . . oli-gomers (chains of adnylic residues linked by 2'5' phosphodiester bonds) that, in turn, activate an endoribonuclease (RNase F). Another is a phosphokinase which phosphorylates the initiation factor eIF2 (21).

Are these proteins, in any way, involved in the cell growth inhibitory activities of IFN? In one report, mouse embryonal carcinoma stem cells which were insensitive to the antiviral and antiproliferative effects of IFN did not demonstrate RNaseF induction after IFN treatment. After differentiation, RNaseF was induced and growth of these cells was inhibited (51); however, many changes occur within a cell upon differentiation and it is difficult to assign responsibility for acquired sensitivity to any one of these changes.

The role of the $(2'5')A_n$ synthetase in these antiproliferative effects has been studied by examining the effects of 2'5' oligo adenosine directly on cells (45, 68, 93). The dephosphorylated timer, that can apparently pass through the cell membrane, has also been shown to inhibit DNA synthesis in lymphocytes stimulated by lectins (48). The induction of these proteins in NIH 3T3 cells after IFN treatment was studied. These cells were sensitive to the antiviral effects of IFN against murine leukemia virus; however, IFN treatment resulted in no antiviral activity against a lytic virus such as encephalomyocarditis virus, and no inhibition of cell division, induction of ODC activity, or DNA synthesis (19). Both $(2'-5')A_n$ synthetase and kinase activities were induced in these cells after IFN treatment and only the endonuclease ordinarily activated by 2'5' oligo adenosine appeared to be absent. These results suggest that kinase activity is not sufficient for cell growth inhibition, and also suggest a pos-

Table 1. Interferon preparations used for clinical trials.

Interferon	Purity	Comments
Alpha		
Natural (Cantell) (10–25 subtypes)	Impure, semipure, highly pure	Less pure in trials before 1982
Recombinant α_2	Highly pure	*E. coli*-produced, position-2 arginine, position-44 deletion
Recombinant A	Highly pure	*E. coli*-produced, position-23 lysine, position-44 deletion
Recombinant D or α_1	Highly pure	*E. coli*-produced, 29 amino acid variation from A
Lymphoblastoid (6–10 subtypes)	Semipure, highly pure	From cultured lymphoma cells or from hamsters
Beta		
Natural	Semipure	From fibroblasts or SV-40 transformed cells
Recombinant β_1	Highly pure	Position-17 cysteine
Recombinant β_{ser}	Highly pure	Position-17 serine
Gamma		
Natural	Impure, semipure	Less pure in earlier trials
Recombinant γ_1	Highly pure	*E. coli*-produced, probably different from natural γ

sible role of the 2'5' oligo activated pathway in the antiproliferative activities of IFN (20).

In one system the antiviral action of interferons has been clearly disassociated from its antiproliferative effect (87).

CLINICAL STUDIES

Modern cancer therapy began during the 10-year period between the mid-1940s to mid-1950s, when it was recognized that most human tumors are, at diagnosis, systemic problems requiring systemic treatment. The first reports of favorable clinical responses to certain drugs that have cytolytic or cytostatic effects on cancer cells stimulated a massive search for more and better chemotherapeutic agents. Of more than half a million compounds tested as possible anticancer agents over the past four decades, only some 40 have reached the clinic; of those, perhaps about 10 may be regarded as moderately effective, the others as only marginally effective. With all clinically available chemotherapy, moreover, dose-limiting normal tissue toxicity, inadequate drug delivery to tumors, and tumor resistance to drugs are major problems (61).

In recent years, another systemic approach to the treatment of cancer – biotherapy has attracted increasing attention (62). Although the use of biologic or synthetic co pounds to modulate the body's responses to cancer was investigated in the 1960s, interest became intense only in the late 1970s. The major reasons included technical advances in molecular biology and recombinant DNA technology, the advent of hybridoma technology and improvements in computer applications.

Among all biologicals with known or potential systemic activity against human cancer, the interferons may be regarded as prototypes. They were the first lymphokines and cytokines to be clearly identified and the first anticancer agents to be genetically engineered to be clinically available at modest cost, in highly purified form and in large quantity.

Interferons have been used in hundreds of patients with various neoplasms (61, 63).

In clinical trials, the preponderance of available data relates to alpha interferon – the impure Cantell, the relatively pure lymphoblastoid, and the highly pure recombinant forms (Table 1). Much of the data comes from phase I, or toxicity, studies not designed to measure therapeutic efficacy.

With those limitations in mind, we can draw some preliminary conclusions about interferon therapy for human cancer. One is that the Cantell, lymphoblastoid and recombinant alpha interferons are similar, both quantitatively and qualitatively, in their toxicity, antitumor efficacy, and other biologic effects. Second, objectively defined antitumor responses in phase I alpha interferon trials (most involving lymphoma, myeloma, Kaposi's sarcoma, melanoma, and renal cancer) have been observed in about 10% of patients. That value may not seem impressive, but it does compare favorably with an average response rate of 1% to 2% in phase I trials or recently developed chemotherapeutic agents (61). We should also note that in phase I alpha interferon studies there have been very few responses in patients with tumors of the colon, lung, or lower genitourinary system (Table 2).

A third impression, suggested by increased response rates with higher alpha interferon doses, is that interferons may produce their acute antitumor effect by a direct cytostatic action, rather than an indirect immunomodulatory mechanism. Finally, very preliminary clinical experience with beta and gamma interferons indicates that the beta type produces response rates and response patterns similar to those obtained with alpha interferon and that the gamma type may not be much more potent against cancer than the other two types. In view of the preclinical data suggesting gamma interferon's strong immunomodulatory and antiproliferative activities, that last findings is particularly disappointing if borne out by future results.

During the 1970s, Scandinavian and U.S. investigators studied the effects of natural alpha interferon – primarily the

Table 2. Solid tumors: interferon results summary – 1985.

Tumor	Dosage (MU/wk)	Number evaluated	Complete or partial response (%)	Assessment
Colon	1–300	> 150	< 5	No effect
With 5-FU	5–50	> 30	5–10	No effect over 5-Fu alone
Gastric	10–20	14	0	No effect
Lung				
Non-small-cell	1–200		< 5	No effect
Small-cell	1–500		0–10	No effect as single agent
Ovary	10–400	> 100	0–20	Possible palliative effect
Uterine cervix	50–150	18	0	No effect
Melanoma	1–500	> 300	5–15	Visceral disease responses < 10% (comparable to those with dacarbazine); addition of cimetidine not effective

Cantell preparation – in patients with multiple myeloma, non-Hodgkin lymphoma, renal cell carcinoma, and breast cancer. In patients with osteosarcoma initial analysis, based on comparison with historical controls, indicated that interferon treatment added to surgery was beneficial. In a randomized study of an interferon-treated group in comparison to a chemotherapy-treated and a nontreated group, all three groups did better than historical controls yet did not differ significantly among themselves. Recent trials involving small numbers of patients with advanced disease have indicated no benefit in osteosarcoma.

Studies by Merigan showed that Cantell alpha interferon administered over a longer period at 1–3 Million Units (MU) per day induced intolerable fatigue, malaise, and weight loss. In more recent phase I trials, with alpha interferon obtained by a process similar to Cantell's, the maximally tolerated dose was about 18 MU/m per day with two different products, and the single maximal tolerated dose was 60 MU/m for a third. Aside from the major dose-limiting effects, natural alpha interferon preparations sometimes produced mild hepatic toxicity (elevated serum glutamic-oxaloacetic transaminase) and myelosuppression (reduce neutrophil and lymphocyte counts). As for clinical efficacy, trials reported on polyacrylamide gel electrophoresis there are real constitutional differences among Cantell alpha interferon products; nevertheless, toxicity and clinical efficacy have been reasonably comparable.

As for clinical efficacy, trials reported in the early 1980s added hairy cell leukemia, chronic myeloid leukemia, juvenile laryngeal papillomatosis, and bladder papillomatosis to the list of conditions responsive to natural alpha interferon.

Altogether, most clinical trials with impure alpha interferon preparations evaluated doses of 3 to 10 MU per day administered intramuscularly or subcutaneously for 28 to 35 days. Serum levels reached 1 to 300 U/ml within four to six hours, with measurable activity still present at 24 hours. The major immunologic effect noted was increased natural killer cell activity. A 3 MU dose initially augmented NK cell cytotoxicity (24–48 hr after administration), with a fall to baseline 7 to 10 days later in spite of continued treatment.

Lymphoblastoid and recombinant alpha interferons have been studied in a number of phase I and phase II trials. Tolerable doses of lymphoblastoid preparation ranged for 15 to 30 MU/m (administered intramuscularly twice a day for seven days, intramuscularly three times a week for five days by a six hour infusion). Other recent studies showed that recombinant clone A alpha interferon was tolerable at 25 to 50 MU/m (intramuscularly three times a week), and recombinant alpha-2, at 20 to 30 MU/m (intravenously or intramuscularly daily for five days every three weeks). As with the impure alpha interferon products, fever, chills, anorexia, weight loss, and fatigue were the major dose-limiting effects. Chronic dosing at moderate and higher levels with the purer alpha interferon products also first boosted, then suppressed NK cell cytotoxicity.

Objectively defined clinical responses to either lymphoblastoid or recombinant alpha interferon have been noted in patients with hairy cell leukemia, myeloma, non-Hodgkin's lymphoma, renal cell carcinoma, Kaposi's sarcoma, malignant glioma and breast cancer. The pattern of antitumor activity resembles that seen with impure alpha interferon.

However, high doses (30 MU/m) of recombinant clone A alpha interferon were needed to obtain responses in melanoma, and breast cancer has been less responsive to the purer alpha interferon products than to the Cantell interferon preparation. A major overall finding with lymphoblastoid and recombinant alpha interferons is that higher doses lead to increased response rates. This dose response effect has been seen in patients with Kaposi sarcoma, renal cell carcinoma, lymphoma, and malignant melanoma.

For any given tumor type, issues such as optimal dose, schedule, route of administration, and alpha subtype are still unresolved. The most impressive results have been seen in selected hematologic malignancies (Table 3). Among solid tumors, there are also encouraging preliminary results, but most of the common solid tumors have been quite unresponsive.

Table 3. Hematologic malignancies: summary of responses to alpha interferon.

Tumor type	Response rate (%)
Multiple myeloma	18–27
Chronic lymphocytic leukemia	0–77
Hairy-cell leukemia	80
Low-grade lymphoma	38–73
High-grade lymphoma	0–10
Kaposi sarcoma	25–40
Chronic myelogenous leukemia	88

Adapted from Bonnem EM, Spiegel RJ: *J Biol Response Modif* 3: 580, 1984

Phase II trials in acute myelogenous leukemia documented that alpha interferon reduced levels of circulating tumor cells, but it did not produce prolonged remission. Similar results were obtained in patients with chronic lymphocytic leukemia. In both chronic myelogenous leukemia and hairy cell leukemia, however, complete clinical response rates on the order of 75% or better have been reported; treatment resulted in generally excellent (but not always complete) clearing of leukemia cells from peripheral blood and bone marrow, and patients have remained in remission for periods of more than one year.

Almost as encouraging are the results in non-Hodgkin's lymphoma patients. Aggressive tumors in this category have been relatively unresponsive, but about 50% of indolent, favorable histology, low grade tumors (e.g., nodular, poorly differentiated lymphocytic lymphomas) and intermediate grade tumors (e.g., diffuse, poorly differentiated lymphocytic lymphomas) have responded. The responses were more often partial than complete, and the median duration of response has been little more than six to eight months. Many of the treated patients had bulky advanced disease that were progressive and drug and radiation resistant.

In a recently reported phase II trial of recombinant alpha interferon in previously treated patients with relapsing non-Hodgkin's lymphoma, 13 of 24 patients with low grade tumors had objective responses, four of which histologically confirmed as complete; two of six patients with intermediate grade lymphoma also responded (one completely), whereas only one partial response was seen in seven patients with high-grade tumors. Patients whose responses ceased with low dose maintenance interferon could be reinduced to respond with higher doses (4) was given to sustain responses (4).

In solid tumors, phase II trials with Cantell, lymphoblastoid, or recombinant alpha interferon have demonstrated overall (complete and partial) response rates of about 15–40% in patients renal cancer, melanoma and Kaposi's sarcoma. In patients, with renal cancer, Cantell or recombinant alpha interferon induced significant responses in 15–25%. Approximately the same rates (20–30%) were seen when patients with melanoma were treated with recombinant alpha interferon; some responses occurred in patients with visceral disease, and some were complete. Recombinant alpha interferon also induced partial or complete responses in patients with Kaposi sarcoma, the highest overall rated being 41%. Breast cancer response rates have fallen with further testing. Two studies using a 3 MU/m per day of natural alpha interferon found antitumor activity in about 25% of patients, whereas later studies, using lymphoblastoid or recombinant alpha interferon, found less or no such activity (Table 4). Other common solid tumors have been almost uniformly unresponsive to alpha interferon treatment.

Studies with recombinant beta and gamma interferons are only beginning so less can be said about their biologic effects and antitumor efficacy. Early studies with partially purified nonrecombinant beta and gamma preparations, however, showed that both types were inactivated after intramuscular injection and the half-lives were very brief (78). Results to date with recombinant preparations confirm the need for an intravenous route of administration, but the relative merits of prolonged infusion versus repetitive dosing remain to be determined (22).

In summary, it is clear that the interferons are promising agents for the treatment of human cancer. Their clinical activity has been seen most reproducibly in a variety of hematologic malignancies, but the responses of other tumor types have also been observed. Further studies must resolve the issues of appropriate dose, schedule, route of administration, and interferon type. It is also unclear whether interferons work primarily by direct antiproliferative activity or indirectly by altering immune responses. Most of the available evidence – especially that from lymphoma studies, supports the view that a direct antiproliferative effect is responsible, since higher interferon doses induce more responses than lower doses and patients failing at lower doses respond at higher doses.

Perhaps the most important finding in preclinical and clinical interferon studies is that these biologicals have antitumor activity even in advanced, bulky cancer that are resistant to drugs or radiation (6–8).

REFERENCES

1. Bagloini G: Interferon-induced enzymatic activities and their role in the antiviral state. *Cell* 17: 255, 1979
2. Balkwill FR: Antitumor effects of interferons in animals. In: *Interferons in vivo and clinical studies*, edited by Finter, NB Oldham, RK pp. 23–46. Elsevier, Amsterdam, 1985
3. Balkwill FR, Taylor-Papadimitriou J: Interferon affects both G_1 and $S + G_2$ in cells stimulated from quiescence to growth. *Nature (London)* 274: 789, 1978
4. Balkwill FR, Watling D, Taylor-Papadimitriou J: Inhibition by lymphoblastoid interferon of growth of cells derived from the human breast. *Int J Cancer* 22: 258, 1978
5. Billiau A: Sensitivity of oncornavirus-carrier lines to the antiviral and growth inhibitory properties of interferon. In: *Proc Symp Clin Use of Interferon*. pp. 105–112. Zagreb, Yugoslavia. 1975

Table 4. Breast cancer: interferon results summary – 1985.

Interferon type	Dosage (MU/wk)	Number entered	Number evaluated	Complete or partial response
Alpha				
Leukocyte	21–63	17	6	6
Leukocyte	21–63	26	23	5
Recombinant	18–172	9	9	0
Lymphoblast	11–700	11	11	0
Recombinant	150	19	17	0
Recombinant	6–150	14	14	2
Recombinant	14	11	11	0
Lymphoblast	1.5–9	37	29	1
Recombinant	21–350	23	23	1
Recombinant	6	7	7	0
Recombinant	250	7	7	0
Recombinant	70	10	7	2
Recombinant	140–350	15	12	2
Lymphoblast	30	18	15	0
Recombinant	9–50 (total dose)	30	30	2
Lymphoblast	0.5 (total dose)	20	19	1
Lymphoblast	30 (total dose)	17	10	0
Beta				
Fibroblast	9–18	4	4	0
Fibroblast	42	9	9	0

Adapted from Laszlo *et al: J Biol Response Mod* 6: 206–210, 1986

6. Billiau A: Hermans H, Allen PT, DeMaeyer-Guinard J, DeSomer P: Trapping of oncornavirus particles at the surface of Interferon-treated cells. *Virology* 73:537, 1976

7. Borecky L, Lackovic V, Waschke K: Immunological implications of interferon production in leukocytes. In: pp. 745–754. *Symposium on Developmental Aspects of Antibody Formation and Structure,* Prague and Slapy, 1969

8. Braun W, Levy HB: Interferon preparations as modifiers of immune responses. *Proc Soc Exp Biol Med* 141:769, 1972

9. Brennan MB, Stark GR: Interferon pretreatment inhibits simian virus 40 replication by blocking the onset of early transcription. *Cell* 33::811, 1983

10. Brouty-Boye D, Gresser I, Baldwin C: Decreased sensitivity to interferon associated with *in vitro* transformation of X-ray-transformed cells. *Int J Cancer* 24:261, 1979

11. Brouty-Boye D, and Tovey MG: Inhibition by interferon of thymidine uptake in chemostat culture of L_{1210} cells *in vitro*. *Intervirology* 9:243, 1977

11a. Cantell K: Why is interferon not in clinical use today? In: *Interferon I* (I. Gresser I (ed.). New York, Academic Press, pp. 1–28, 1979

12. Cerottini JC, Brunner KT, Lindahl P, Gresser I: Inhibitory effect of interferon preparations and inducers on the multiplications of transplanted allogenic spleen cells and syngenic bone marrow cells. *Nature New Biol* 242::152, 1973

13. Chang, EH, and Friedman RM: A large glycoprotein of Moloney leukemia virus derived from interferon-treated cells. *Biochem Biophys Res Commun* 77:392, 1977

14. Chang EH, Jay FT, Friedman RM: Physical, morphological and biochemical alterations in membranes of AKR cells after interferon treatment. *Proc Natl Acad Sci USA* 75: 1859, 1978

15. Chernyakhovskaya IY, Slavina EG, Svet-Moldavsky GJ: Antitumor effect of lymphoid cells activated by interferon. *Nature* 228:71, 1970

16. Chirigos MA, Pearson JA: Cure of murine leukemia with drug and interferon treatment. *J Natl Cancer Inst* 51:1367, 1973

17. Collyn-d'Hooghe M, Brouty-Boye D, Malaise EP, Gresser I: Interferon and cell division XII prolongation by interferon of the intermitotic time of mouse mammary tumor cells *in vitro*. *Exp Cell Res* 105:73, 1977

18. Crane JL Jr, Glasgow LA, Kerr ER, Youngner JS: Inhibition of murine osteogenic sarcoma by treatment with type I or type II interferon. *J Natl Cancer Inst* 61:871, 1978

19. Czarniecki CW, Sreevalsan T, Friedman RM, Panet A: Dissociation of interferon effects on murine leukemia virus and encephalomyocarditis in mouse cells *J Virol* 37:827, 1981

20. Epstein DA, Czarniecki CW, Jacobsen J, Friedman RM, Panet A: A mouse cell line which is unprotected by interferon against lytic virus infection, lacks ribonuclease F activity. *Eur J Biochem* 118:9, 1981

21. Farrell PJ, Broeze RJ, Lengyel P: Accumulation of an mRNA and protein interferon treated Ehrlich ascites cells. *Nature* 279:523, 1979

22. Foon KA, Sherwin SA, Abrams PG, Longo DL, Fer MF, Stevenson HC, Ochs JJ, Bottino GC, Schoenberger CS, Zeffren J, Jaffe E, Oldham RK: Treatment of advanced non-Hodgkin's lymphoma with recombinant leukocyte A interferon. *New Engl J Med* 311:1148, 1984

23. Foon KA, Sherwin SA, Abrams PG, Holmes P, Maluish AE, Oldham RK, Herberman RB: A phase I trial of recombinant gamma interferon in patients with cancer. *Ca Immun Immunother*, 1985

24. Frayssinet C, Gresser I, Tovey M., Lindahl P: Inhibitory effect of patent interferon preparations on liver regeneration. *Nature (London)* 245:146, 1973

25. Friedman, RM: Antiviral activities of interferons. *Bact Rev* 41:543, 1977

26. Friedman RM: Interferons: interactions with cell surfaces. In: *Interferon I* Edited by Gresser I, pp. 53–73. Academic Press, New York, 1979

27. Friedman RM, Chang EH, Ramseur JM, Meyers MW: Interferon-directed inhibition of chronic murine leukemia virus production in cell cultures: lack of effect on intracellular viral markers. *J Virol* 16:569, 1975

28. Friedman RM, Pastan I: Interferon and cyclic-3'5'-adenosine monophosphate: potentiation of antiviral activity. *Biochem Biophys Res Commun* 36:735, 1969

29. Friedman RM, Ramseur JM: Inhibition of murine leukemia virus production in chronically infected AKR cells: a novel effect of interferon. *Proc Natl Acad Sci USA* 71:3542, 1974

30. Friedman RM, Vogel SN: Interferons with special emphasis on the immune system. *Adv in Immunol* 34:97, 1983

31. Glasgow LA, Crane JL Jr, Kerr ER, Youngner JS: Antitumor activity of interferon against murine osteogenic sarcoma *in vivo* and *in vitro*. *Cancer Treat Rep* 62, 1881, 1978

32. Greenberg HB, Pollard RB, Lutwick LI, Gregory PB, Robinson WS, Merigan TC: Human leukocyte interferon and hepatitis B virus infection. *New Engl J Med* 295:517, 1976

33. Gresser I: Antitumor effects of interferon. In: *Cancer — A Comprehensive treatise,* edited by Becker EF, Vol. 5, PP. 521–571. Plenum Press, New York, 1977

34. Gresser I, Bourali C: Exogenous interferon and inducers of interferon in the treatment of Balb/c mice inoculated with RC19 tumor cells. *Nature* 223:844, 1969

35. Gresser I, Bourali C: Development of newborn mice during prolonged treatment with interferon. *Eur J Cancer* 6:553, 1970

36. Gresser I, Bourali C: Antitumor effects of interferon preparations in mice. *J Natl Cancer Inst* 45:365, 1970

37. Gresser I, Bourali C: Inhibition by interferon preparations of a solid malignant tumor & pulmonary metastases in mice. *Nature New Biol* 236:78, 1972

37a. Gresser I and Bouraly-Maury C: Antitumor effect of interferon in lymphocyte and macrophage depressed mice. *Proc Soc Exp Biol and Med* 144: 144:898, 1973

38. Gresser I, Bourali C, Levy JP: Increased survival in mice inoculated with tumor cells and treated with interferon preparations. *Proc Natl Acad Sci USA* 63:51, 1969

39. Gresser I, De Maeyer-Guignard J, Tovey MG, De Maeyer E: Electrophoretically pure mouse interferon exerts multiple biological effects. *Proc Natl Acad Sci USA* 76:5308 1979

40. Gresser I, Maury C, Brouty-Boye D: On the mechanisms of the antitumor effect of interferon in mice. *Nature* 239:167, 1972

41. Gresser I, Maury C, Tovey MG: Efficacy of combined interferon-cyclophosphamide therapy after diagnosis of lymphoma in AKR mice. *Eur J Cancer* 14:97, 1978

42. Herberman RB, Djeu JY, Ortaldo JR, Holden HT, West WH, Bonnard GD: Role of interferon in augmentation of natural and antibody-dependent cell-mediated cytotoxicity. *Cancer Treat Rep* 62:1893, 1978

43. Herberman RB, Ortaldo JR, Bonnard GD: Augmentation by interferon of human natural and antibody mediated cytotoxicity. *Nature (London)* 277:221, 1979

44. Hooks JJ, Moulsopoulos HM, Notkins AL: The role of interferon in immediate hypersensitivity & autoimmune diseases. *Ann NY Acad Sci* 350:21, 1980

45. Hovenessian AG, Wood J, Meurs E, Montagnier K: Increased nuclease activity in cells treated with pppA2'p5'A2'-p5A. *Proc Natl Acad Sci USA* 76:3261, 1979

46. Janne J, Pogo H, and Raina A: Polyamines in rapid growth and cancer. *Biochem Biophys Acta* 473:241, 1978

47. Jordan GW, Fried RP, Merigan TC: Administration of human leukocyte interferon in herpes zoster I safety, circulating antiviral activity and host responses to infection. *J Infect Dis* 130:56, 1974

48. Kimchi A, Shure H, Revel M: Regulation of lymphocyte mitogenesis by 2'5'-oligoisoadenylate. *Nature* 282:849, 1979

49. Knight E Jr, Korant BD: Fibroblast interferon induces synthesis of 4 proteins in human fibroblast cells. *Biochem Biophys Res Commun* 74:707, 1977

50. Kohn LD, Friedman RM, Holmes JM, Lee G: Use of thyrotropin and cholera toxin to probe the mechanism by which interferon initiates its antiviral activity. *Proc Natl Acad Sci USA* 73:3695, 1976

51. Krause F, Silverman RH, Jacobsen H, Leisy SA, Samid D, Chang EH, Friedman RM: Regulations of ppp(A2'p)mR-dependent RNase levels during interferon treatment and cell differentiation. *Cur J Biochem* 146:611, 1985

52. Land H, Parada LF, Weinberg RA: Cellular oncogenes and multistep carcinogenesis. *Science* 22:771, 1983

53. Lee E, Sreevalsan T: Interferon as an inhibitor of polyamine enzymes. In: *Advances in Polyamine Research,* Vol. III, edited by Vincenzo Zappia. Raven Press, New York, 1981

54. Lindahl P, Leary P, Gresser I: Enhancement by interferon of the specific cytotoxicity of sensitized lymphocytes. *Proc Natl Acad Sci USA* 69:721, 1972

55. Lindahl P, Leary P, Gresser I: Enhancement by interferon of the expression of cell surface antigens on murine leukemia L$_{1210}$ cells. *Proc Natl Acad Sci USA* 70:2785, 1973

56. Meldolesi MT, Friedman RM, Kohn LD: An interferon-induced increase in cyclic AMP precedes the establishment of the antiviral state. *Biochem Biophys Res Commun* 79:239, 1977

57. Merigan TC, Sikora K, Breeden JH, Levy R, Rosenberg SA: Preliminary observations on the effect of human leukocyte interferon on non-Hodgkin's lymphoma. *New Engl J Med* 299:1449, 1978

58. Metz DH, Levin MJ, Oxman MN: Mechanism of interferon action: further evidence for transcription as the primary site of action in SV40 infection. *J Gen Virol* 32:227, 1976

59. Miller Z, Lovelace E, Gallo M, Pastan I: Cyclic guanosine monophosphate and cellular growth. *Science* 190:1213, 1975

60. Naso RB, Yeong-Huei CW, Edbauer CA: Antiretroviral effect of interferon: proposed mechanism. *J Interferon Res* 2:75, 1982

61. Oldham RK, Smalley RV: The role of interferon in the treatment of cancer. In: *Interferon: Research, Clinical, Application, and Regulatory Consideration* edited by Zoon KC, Noguchi PC, Lui TY, pp. 191–205. *Elsevier Science Publishing,* 1984

62. Oldham RK: Biologicals and biological response modifiers: The fourth modality of cancer treatment. *Cancer Treat Rep* 68:221, 1984

63. Oldham RK: Biologicals and biological response modifiers: New strategies for clinical trials. In: *Interferons, IV,* edited by Finter NB., Oldham RK, pp. 235–249. *Elsevier Science Publishers B.V.* 1985

64. Oldham RK: Interferon: A model for future biologicals. In: *Interferon VI,* edited by Burke D, Cantell K, Gresser I, DeMaeyer E, Landy M, Revel A, Vilcek J, pp. 127–143. Academic Press, 1985

65. Oldham RK: Biologicals for cancer treatment: Interferons. *Hospital Practice,* December, 1985

66. Oldham RK: Biological response modifiers, In: *Biological Response Modifiers,* edited by Torrence PF. Academic Press, 1985

67. Oxman MM, Rowe WP, and Black PH: Studies of adenovirus-SV$_{40}$ hybrids VI differential effects of interferon on SV40 virus, adenovirus and adenovirus-SV40 hybrids viruses. *Proc Natl Acad Sci USA* 57:941, 1967

68. Panet A, Czarniecki CW, Falk H, Friedman RM: Effect of 2'5'-oligoadenylic acid on a mouse cell line partially resistant to interferon. *Virology* 114:567, 1981

69. Paucker K, Cantell K, Henle W: Quantitative studies on viral interference in suspended L-cells. III Effect of interfering viruses and interferon on the growth rate of cells. *Virology* 17:324, 1962

70. Pitha PM, Fernie B, Maldarelli F, Hattman T, Wivel NA: Effect of interferon on mouse leukemia virus (MuLV) V. Abnormal proteins in virions of Rauscher MuLV produced in the presence of interferon. *J Gen Virol* 46:97, 1980

71. Pitha PM, Rowe WP, Oxman MM: Effect of interferons on exogenous, endogenous and chronic murine leukemia virus infection. *Virology* 70:324, 1976

72. Revel M: Molecular mechanisms involved in the antiviral effects of interferon. In: *Interferon I'* edited by Gresser I, pp. 101–163. Academic Press, New York, 1979

73. Rozengurt E: Synergistic stimulation of DNA synthesis by cyclic AMP derivatives and growth factors in mouse 3T3 cells. In: *Surface of Normal and Malignant Cells'* edited by Hynes RO, pp. 323–343. John Wiley, 1979

74. Salvin SB, Youngner JS, Nishio J, Neta R: Tumor suppression by a lymphokine released into circulation of mice with delayed hypersensitivity. *J Natl Cancer Inst* 55:1233, 1975

75. Samid D, Chang EH, Friedman RM: Biochemical correlates of phenotypic reversion in interferon-treated mouse cells transformed by a human oncogene. *Biochem Biophys Res Comm* 126:509, 1984

76. Schroeder EW, Chou IN, Jäken S, Black P: Interferon inhibits the release of plasminogen activator from SV3T3 cells. *Nature* 276:828, 1978

77. Schultz RM: Macrophage activation by interferons. In: *Lymphokine Reports,* Vol. I, edited by Pick E. Academic Press, New York, 1980

78. Sherwin SA, Knost JA, Fein S, Abrams PG, Foon KA, Ochs JJ, Schoenberger C, Maluish AE, Oldham RK: A multiple dose Phase I trial of recombinant leukocyte A interferon in cancer patients. *J Am Med Assoc* 248:2461, 1982

79. Sonnenfeld G: Modulation of immunity by interferon. In: *Lymphokine Reports,* Vol.I, edited by Pick E. Academic Press, New York, 1980

80. Sonnenfeld G, Mandel AD, Merigan TC: Time and dosage-dependence of immunoenhancement by murine type II interferon preparation. *Cell Immunol* 34:193, 1977

81. Sreevalsan T, Rozengurt E, Taylor-Papadimitriou J, Burchell J: Differential effect of interferon on DNA synthesis, 2 deoxyglucose uptake and orithine decarboxylase activity in 3T3 cells stimulated by polypeptide growth factors and tumor promoters. *J Cell Physiol* 104:1, 1979

82. Sreevalsan T, Taylor-Papadimitriou J, Rozengurt E: Differential effect of interferon on DNA synthesis, 2 deoxyglucose uptake and ornithine decarboxylase activity in 3T3 cells stimulated by polypeptide growth factors and tumor promoters. *J Cell Physiol* 104:1, 1980

83. Stewart II WE: *The Interferon System,* edited by Stewart II WE, Springer-Verlag. Wien, New York, 1979

84. Strander H: Interferons: antineoplastic drugs? *Blut* 35:277, 1977

85. Strander H, Einhorn S: Effect of human leukocyte interferon on the growth of human osteosarcoma cells in tissue culture. *Int J Cancer* 19:468, 1977

86. Svet-Moldavsky GJ, Chernyakhovskaya IY: Interferon and the interactions of allogenic normal and immune lymphocyte with L-cells. *Int J Cancer* 19:468, 1967

87. Taylor-Papadimitriou J: Effect of interferons on cell growth and function. *Nature* 215:1299, 1980

88. Tovey MG, Rochette-Egly C, Castagna M: Antiviral activity induced by culturing lymphocytes with tumor-derived or virus-transformed cells. Enhancement of human natural killer cell activity by interferon and antagonistic inhibition of susceptibility of target cells lysis. *Proc Natl Acad Sci USA* 76:3890, 1979

89. Trinchieri G, Santoli D: Retroviruses as mutagens: insertion and excision of a non-transforming provirus alter expression of a resident transforming provirus. *J Exp Med* 147:1314, 1978

90. Varmus HE, Quintnell N, Orgiz S: Immunosuppressive effects of lymphocyte (Type II) and leukocyte. *Cell* 26:23, 1981

91. Virelizier JL, Chan EL, Allison AC: (Type I) interferon on primary antibody responses *in vivo* and *in vitro. Clin Exp Immunol* 30:299, 1977

92. Weber JM, Stewart RB: Interaction of interferon with cells: limited heterologous reactivity or chick and mouse interferon. *J Gen Virol* 28:363, 1975

93. Williams BRG, Kerr IM: Inhibition of protein synthesis by 2'5'-linked adenine oligonucleotides in intact cells. *Nature* 282:88, 1978
94. Wood JN, Hovanessian AG: Interferon enhances 2'-5' A synthetase in embroyonal carcinoma cells. *Nature* 282:74, 1979
95. Yamamoto K, Yamaguchi N, Oda K: Mechanisms of interferon-induced inhibition of early Simian virus 40 (SV_{40}) functions. *Virology* 68:58, 1975

POSTSCRIPT

Hematopoietic growth factors could be of great importance in the treatment of neoplastic diseases following aplasiogenic chemotherapy and bone marrow transplantation (11). Genetic engineering techniques permit large scale production of substances produced during the immune response which may have therapeutic value for the modification of biologic response to cancer (8). The role of contact inhibition and cell shape was nil in the malignant fibrosarcoma line HT1080. Treatment of HT1080 cells with low concentration of human fibroblast interferon (less than 40 units/ml) restored shape-dependent proliferation but had little effect on normal cells. Subantiproliferative doses of interferon restored contact-inhibited proliferation control to malignant cells previously lacking it (10).

Recombinant DNA technology is able to produce large amounts of several interferons (20). Gamma-interferon is perhaps stronger in boosting immune recognition and rejection of tumor cells than alpha and beta interferons (2). Immunomodulators in clinical medicine, cancer and acquired immunodeficiency syndrome alike were reviewed by Fauchi and co-workers (5). It is unexplained why only a small proportion of patients show an objective response to interferon (3; see also 9, 23, 18, 21, 6, 17). Antigen-nonspecific suppressor factors may have an important physiological role in regulating immune responses and cell division in general (1). Antiproliferative effects of interferon alfa 2b were seen *in vitro* and *in vivo*. This interferon showed as a single agent maximum tumor cell colony reduction when used in high concentrations with continued cell exposure. Combined with doxorubicin clinical responses in patients with ovarian, cervical, colorectal and pancreatic carcinoma and one case of lymphoma were observed (24). The role of interferon in cancer therapy lies in the combination with other agents as the 4th arm of cancer therapy (7). Interferon can be a potent inducer of various degrees of transformation, differentiation, and proliferation in different subsets of normal and malignant B cells (16, see also 15). Endogenous production of tumor necrosis factor in normal mice and human cancer patients by interferons and other cytokines combined with biological response modifiers of bacterial origin was investigated by Satoh (19). Interferons preferentially inhibit the chemotaxis of transformed and tumor-derived cell lines when compared to control fibroblasts (12). Objective tumor effects in Japan have been observed in renal cell carcinoma, brain tumor, multiple myeloma, malignant lymphoma, adult T cell leukemia, chronic lymphocytic leukemia, chronic myelogenous leukemia and by local injections in skin cancer such as malignant melanoma and cutaneous lymphoma (13). The inducing agents of interferons include viruses, bacteria, bacterial products, polymers, low molecular weight compounds, and antigens or mitogens. Interferon gamma employed alone and in combination with interferon alpha may dramatically increase interferons activity (22). Toxicity of interferons exhibits fever, chills, myalgias, arthragias, and headache with some variation according to type of interferon, route of administration, schedule and dose. The most important nonacute symptom is fatigue (14). Clinical immunology exhibits three active developments namely immunopharmacology of immunosuppressive drugs; clinical use of the alpha-beta and gamma interferons and interleukin-2; and monoclonal antibody applications in marrow transplantations and antitumor therapy (4).

POSTSCRIPT REFERENCES

1. Aune TM: Role and function of antigen nonspecific suppressor factors. CRC Crit Rev Immunol 7(2):93, 1987
2. Boiron M: Interferons in hemato-cancerology. Nouv Rev Fr Hematol 291(1):49, 1987
3. Boiron M: Future developments in interferon therapy. Int J Cancer (Suppl) 1:41, 1987
4. Fahey JL, Sarna G, Gale RP, Seeger R: Immune interventions in disease (published erratum appears in Ann Intern Med 1987 106(6):783). Ann Intern Med 106(2):257, 1987
5. Fauci AS, Rosenberg SA, Sherwin SA et al: NIH conference. Immunomodulators in clinical medicine. Ann Intern Med 106(3):421, 1987
6. Figlin RA: Biotherapy with interferon in solid tumors. Oncol Nurs Forum 14(6 Suppl):23, 1987
7. Goldstein D, Laszlo J: The role of interferon in cancer therapy: a current perspective. CA 38(5):258, 1988
8. Guillou PJ: Potential impact of immunobiotechnology on cancer therapy. Br J Surg 74(8):705, 1987
9. Kirchner H: The interferon system as an integral part of the defense system against infections. Antiviral Res 6(1):1, 1986
10. Kulesh DA, Greene JJ: Shape-dependent regulation of proliferation in normal and malignant human cells and its alteration by interferon. Cancer Res 46(6):2793, 1986
11. Lindemann A, Oster W, Herrmann F, Mertelsmann R: Cytokines in tumor therapy. Arzneimittelforsch 38(3A):466, 1988
12. Melchiori A, Allavene G, Bohm J et al: Interference inhibit chemotaxis of transformed cells and their invasion of a reconstituted basement membrane. Anticancer Res 7(3 Pt B):475, 1987
13. Ohno R: Clinical studies on interferon in cancer therapy in Japan. Gan To Kagaku Ryoho 143(5 Pt 1):1194, 1987
14. Quesada JR, Talpam M, Rios A et al: Clinical toxicity of interferons in cancer patients: a review. J Clin Oncol 4(2):234, 1986
15. Rios A, Stringfellow DA, Fitzpatrick Fa et al: Phase I study of 2-amino-5-bromo-6-phenyl-4(3H)-pyrimidinone (ABPP): an oral interferon inducer, in cancer patients. J Biol Response Mod 5(4):330, 1986
16. Robert KH, Juliusson G, Einhorn S et al: Activation of malignant B-lymphocytes: pathophysiologic and clinical importance. Scand J Haematol 37(5):363, 1986.
17. Roth MS, Foon KA: Biotherapy with interferon in hematologic malignancies. Oncol Nurs Forum 14(6 Suppl):16, 1987
18. Sager R: Genetic suppression of tumor formation: a new frontier in cancer research. Cancer Res 46(4 Pt 1):1573, 1986
19. Satoh M, Inagawa H, Shimada Y et al: Endogenous production of tumor necrosis factor in normal mice and human cancer patients by interferons and other cytokines combined with biological response modifiers of bacterial origin. J Biol Response Mod 6(5):512, 1987
20. Schneider FJ: The interferon system. A review of biological principles and clinical uses. Z Gesamte Inn Med 41(22):613, 1986
21. Stahel RA: Current status and perspectives in the treatment of tumor with biological substances. Ther Umsch 45(6):358, 1988
22. Stanton GJ, Weigent DA, Fleischmann WR Jr et al: Interferon review. Invet Radiol 22(3):259, 1987
23. Strander H: Interferon treatment of human neoplasia. Adv Cancer Res 46:1, 1986
24. Welander CE: Overview of preclinical and clinical studies of interferon alfa-2b in combination with cytotoxic drugs. Invest New Drugs 5 Suppl:547, 1987.

3

TRANSCATHETER MANAGEMENT OF NEOPLAMS

C. HUMBERTO CARRASCO, SIDNEY WALLACE, CHUSILP CHARNSANGAVEJ
and W. BECHTEL

The development of percutaneous angiographic techniques has made possible selective catheterization of most clinically important vascular territories in the human body. The interventional radiologist has integrated these techniques with others derived from established surgical procedures for a more aggressive approach to the management of the cancer patient. Our ability to gain access to neoplasms by either direct punctures or through vascular catherizations, to establish the nature and extent of the disease, and to assess its response to therapy have been greatly augmented by developments in the various imaging modalities, particularly image intensification, ultrasound and computed tomography. Vascular occlusions and infusions, and percutaneous drainage procedures have now become the province of the interventional radiologist.

INTRA-ARTERIAL INFUSION CHEMOTHERAPY

The therapeutic activity of an antineoplastic agent is related in part to its concentration at the target organ which is determined by dosage, schedule, metabolic processes, and route of administration. The responses achieved by most chemotherapeutic agents have been accomplished by their intravenous administration, however, higher drug concentrations at the target organ may be achieved by the intra-arterial route. At the present, two major modes of intra-arterial administration of chemotherapeutic agents are available and consist of isolation perfusion and infusion techniques. Isolation perfusion chemotherapy (5, 46, 3, 4, 1) is usually performed by surgical cannulation of vessels and maintenance of circulation through an extracorporeal pump oxygenator. The chemotherapeutic agent is administered into the isolated artery and the venous outflow is recirculated, thus minimizing the systemic escape of the drug. This technique permits the use of very large doses of chemotherapeutic agents which would otherwise be lethal. During intra-arterial infusion chemotherapy there is no recirculation of the venous effluent via an extracorporeal circuit and variable amounts of the drug, not taken up by the infused tissues during the first pass, reach the systemic circulation.

Intra-arterial infusion of chemotherapeutic agents was introduced in 1950 when Klopp et al. (73) and Bierman et al. (11) independently reported their experiences with the arterial administration of nitrogen mustard in the manage-

ment of various neoplasms. They observed profound tissue changes within the territory supplied by the infused artery that had not been noted following the intravenous administration of the drug. Their experience also suggested greater therapeutic efficacy and a decreased systemic toxicity when this drug was administered intra-arterially as opposed to intravenously.

The rationale for intra-arterial infusion is to expose a given neoplasm to a higher concentration of a chemotherapeutic agent than that achieved by its intravenous administration in order to obtain a greater therapeutic effect in a limited anatomic area. The cytotoxic effect of a given chemotherapeutic agent is not only concentration time dependent but also varies according to its total body clearance, its metabolic alterations, its intratumoral disposition, and the intrinsic sensitivity of the tumor to the drug. A linear physiologically based pharmacokinetic model was used by Chen and Gross (22) to study drug delivery characteristics of chemotherapeutic agents after intra-arterial and intravenous infusion. This model confirms that intra-arterial infusion produces higher local tissue levels and a reduction in the systemic drug availability. The increase in local drug concentration depends largely on the blood flow rate through the infused artery and the rate of drug elimination by the rest of the body, whereas the reduction in systemic drug delivery is dependent on the ability of the infused region to eliminate the drug. Ensminger et al (36) discovered that hepatic extraction of 5-fluoro 2'-deoxyuridine (floxuridine) was in the order of 94% to 99% and that of 5-fluorouracil was 19% to 51% after a single pass through the liver following hepatic artery infusion. During hepatic artery infusion, the systemic levels of floxuridine were 25% and those of 5-fluorouracil were 60% of corresponding systemic concentrations with peripheral venous infusion. Hepatic extraction was also demonstrated for doxorubicin (adriamycin) which had an extraction ratio of 45% to 50% depending on the dosage of the drug administered. The systemic levels of adriamycin during hepatic arterial infusion were 25% lower than the corresponding systemic levels with peripheral venous infusion (41). Similar observations were made by Kelsen et al. (72) with hepatic arterial infusion of cis-diamminedichloroplatinum (cisplatin) in dogs which yielded a coefficient of extraction of 72% to 97%. Therefore, hepatic arterial infusion should have greater advantage over the intravenous route in the management of hepatic neoplasms at least with relation to the use of floxuridine, 5-fluorouracil, adriamycin and cisplatin.

Jaffe et al. (59) demonstrated consistently elevated cisplatin concentrations in the local vein as opposed to a

From The Department of Diagnostic Radiology, The University of Texas, M.D. Anderson Hospital and Tumor Institute.

21

P.V. Woolley (ed.), Cancer management in Man: Biological Response Modifiers, Chemotherapy, Antibiotics, Hyperthermia, Supporting Measures
© 1989. Kluwer Academic Publishers, Dordrecht.

peripheral vein during arterial infusion of this agent for the management of patients with osteosarcoma. Concentrations of cisplatin in the neoplasms were directly related to the number of arterial infusions. A direct relationship between the neoplastic concentrations of cisplatin and degree of tumor destruction was also noted.

In the attempt to increase the efficacy of intra-arterial infusion chemotherapy, various techniques aimed at reducing the blood flow through the infused territory have been attempted. Theoretically, by decreasing the rate of blood flow there is an increase in the concentration of the infused agent and concomitantly a decrease in the transit time results in prolongation of the tissue contact time. Tourniquets have been applied to the abdomen and extremities during intra-arterial infusion chemotherapy in order to achieve this effect (13, 14, 15, 16) Anderson *et al.* (5) by combining intra-arterial infusion of 14C labelled 5-fluorouracil with temporary vascular occlusion using a double lumen balloon· catheter in the external iliac artery of a dog increased the local tissue concentration of this drug by 7 to 9 times when compared to intra-arterial infusion alone. The tissue levels of 5-fluorouracil were 30 to 50 times greater than those obtained by the intravenous administration. Wright *et al.* (137) using a percutaneous approach combined arterial balloon occlusion infusion of floxuridine with recirculation of the venous effluent with the aid of a pump oxygenator and achieved local tissue levels 27 times greater than those obtained by arterial balloon occlusion infusion alone.

TRANSCATHETER EMBOLIZATION

Therapeutic embolization has been in use for over 50 years (48), it was initially employed in the management of arteriovenous fistulas (122, 78) and malformations (84, 85), particularly of those occurring in the brain. With the development of percutaneous transcatheter techniques, the uses of embolization were extended to the control of hemorrhage (112) in various regions of the body and devascularization of tumors prior to surgery in order to minimize intraoperative blood loss. The changes observed in neoplasms following surgical arterial ligation and the occasional iatrogenic arterial occlusion occurring during catheterization for infusion chemotherapy led to the realization that occlusion could be an effective tool in the local control of neoplasms. (132) Devascularization is a general term which includes surgical arterial ligation, catheter induced arterial injury, drug induced arteritis, as well as transcatheter embolization. The goal of tumor embolization is to apply superselective catheterization techniques for vascular occlusion in order to achieve maximal tumor necrosis with minimal normal tissue infarction.

Arterial embolization can result in central or peripheral occlusion depending on the size of the embolic particles employed and, therefore, on the caliber of the vessels occluded. Central embolization, analogous to surgical ligation, consists of occlusion of an artery maintaining its peripheral branches patent. Reconstitution of the peripheral branches then occurs immediately, in most vascular territories, through a different route. This technique is used to redistribute blood flow to a single vessel where a given neoplasm is supplied by more than one artery. In this man-

ner, only one catheter is employed for effective infusion of the entire neoplasm (23). Central embolization is also performed to protect a vascular territory not involved by tumor from the effects of chemotherapeutic agents or embolic materials injected proximally to its origin (46, 76). In most vascular territories tissue infarction does not occur secondary to central embolization. The purpose of peripheral embolization in tumor management is the production of ischemic necrosis of the neoplasms in question. Small particles, usually measuring less than 0.5 mm in diameter are employed for this purpose.

The choice of embolic materials will depend on their availability, ease of use, their effectiveness as occluding agents and on whether central or peripheral embolization is desired. Although a large number of embolization materials is available, the most commonly ones used at UT M.D. Anderson Hospital and Tumor Institute are absorbable gelatin foam (Gelfoam) polyvinyl alcohol foam (Ivalon) (46), dehydrated ethanol and stainless steel coils (25, 132). These materials have been used in over 1000 procedures with minimal complications.

HEPATIC NEOPLASMS

The liver is one of the major organs most commonly involved by metastatic neoplasms that usually originate in the alimentary tract. The extent of the hepatic metastases and the functional state of the residual normal hepatic parenchyma appear to be the most important factors influencing the course of the disease and the duration of survival (63). A median survival time of 75 days for patients with untreated hepatic metastases from a variety of primary neoplasms was reported by Jaffe and colleagues (63). Other authors reported median survival times of 4.2 months (136) and 13 months (17) for patients with untreated hepatic metastases from colorectal carcinomas. The prognosis for primary hepatic neoplasms is similar to that of metastatic disease (9). Rarely, hepatic neoplasms are localized and thus amenable to surgical resection (41). In unresectable disease, alternative modes of treatment such as systemic chemotherapy (110) and surgical dearterialization of the liver have been used with limited success (3, 97, 121). Hepatic artery infusion chemotherapy and hepatic artery embolization are also being used in an effort to control the local progression of the disease and prolong the survival of patients with hepatic neoplasms.

HEPATIC ARTERY INFUSION CHEMOTHERAPY

Since hepatic neoplasms derive most of their blood supply from the hepatic artery (14, 50, 119) while the normal liver parenchyma receives only 25%, these tumors are exposed to relatively higher concentrations of the agents infused intra-arterially. Hepatic neoplasms refractory to systemic chemotherapy may respond to arterial infusion of the same agent dosage (6). Hepatic inactivation of some of the cytotoxic agents infused (49) may also lessen the systemic toxic side effects. Increased tumor response rates have been reported with hepatic artery infusion of some chemotherapeutic agents with prolongation of the median survival time in the

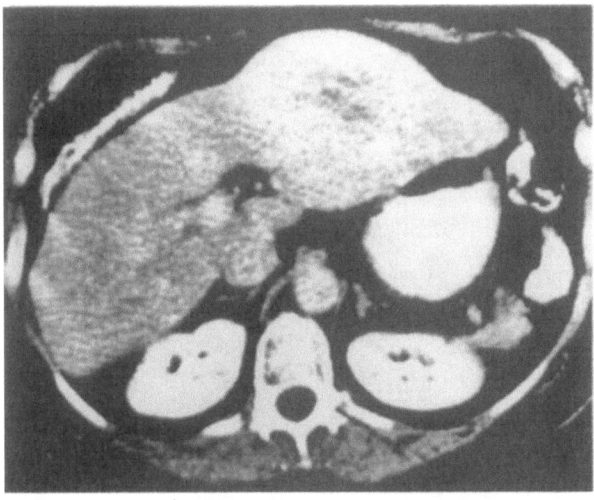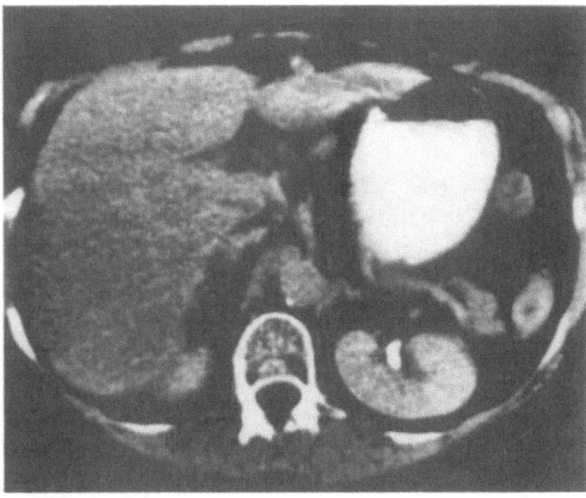

Figure 1. Hepatocellular carcinoma. A. Computed tomography demonstrates a large tumor in the left lobe of the liver. B. Following three courses of hepatic artery infusion chemotherapy there was complete resolution of the mass. Biopsies at laparotomy failed to demonstrate viable tumor.

responders (41, 99, 103, 104). A response rate of 43.4% with a median overall survival of 11 months was observed in a group of 55 patients with metastatic colorectal carcinoma confined to the liver treated with floxuridine and mitomycin C by hepatic arterial infusion. The median survival in patients with intentional or inadvertent arterial occlusion was prolonged to 15 months as opposed to 8 months for those with an intact arterial tree (105). In a group of 12 patients with hepatocellular carcinoma treated with intra-arterial floxuridine, adriamycin and mitomycin C there were seven partial and one complete remissions (Figure 1). A prolongation of the median survival time (14 months) was also observed in patients with hepatic arterial occlusion when compared to those patients without it (6 months) (106).

Several chemotherapeutic agents are used for infusion into the hepatic artery. Floxuridine, mitomycin C and cis-platin are used for metastases from colorectal carcinomas. These agents in combination with adriamycin are also used to treat primary hepatic neoplasms and various metastatic neoplasms. Cisplatin is used to treat hepatic metastases from melanoma and breast carcinoma. Other agents used for hepatic artery infusion include 5-fluorouracil, vincristine, dacarbazine, and streptozotocin.

HEPATIC ARTERY EMBOLIZATION

Markowitz in 1952 (89) suggested hepatic artery ligation as a possible method of treating neoplasms. Following hepatic artery ligation, Gelin and associates (45) demonstrated a 90% decrease in tumor blood flow and a 35% to 40% decrease of flow in the normal liver parenchyma. Variable

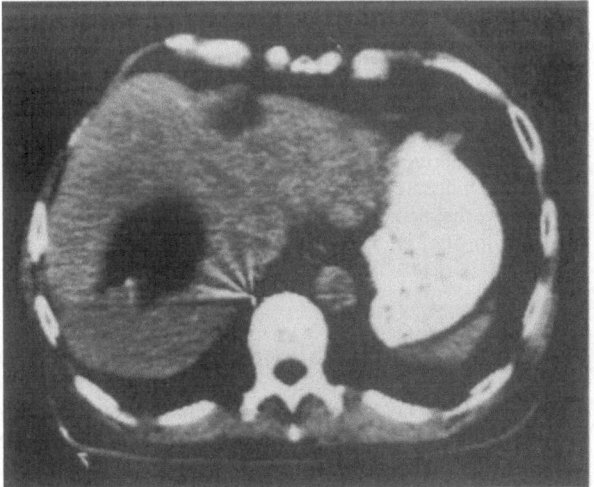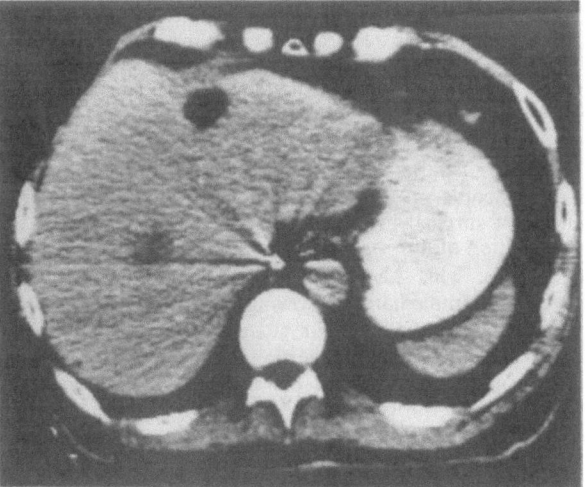

Figure 2. Metastatic carcinoid. A. Computed tomography demonstrates two metastatic foci in the liver. B. Partial remission of the hepatic metastases following hepatic artery embolization.

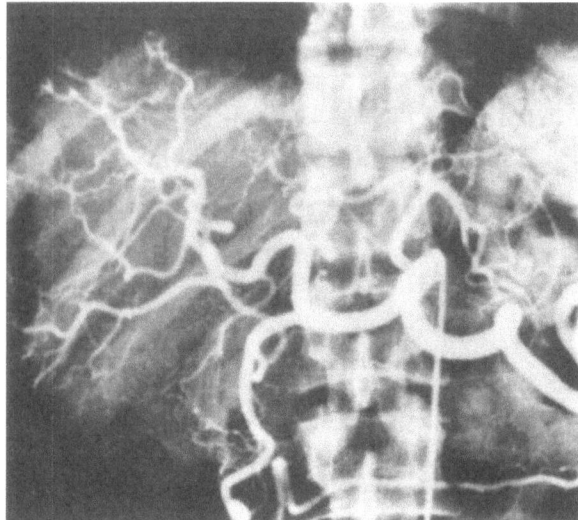

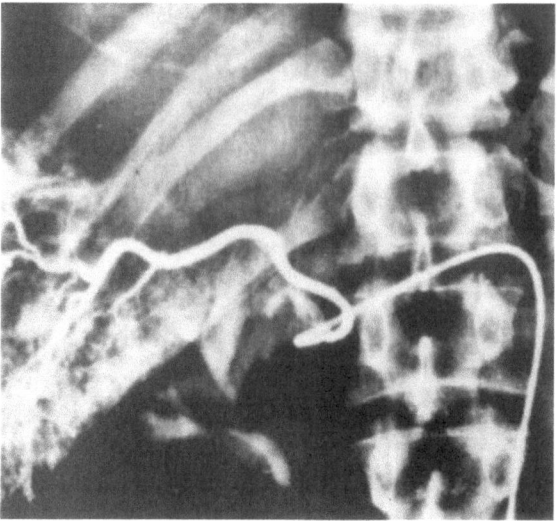

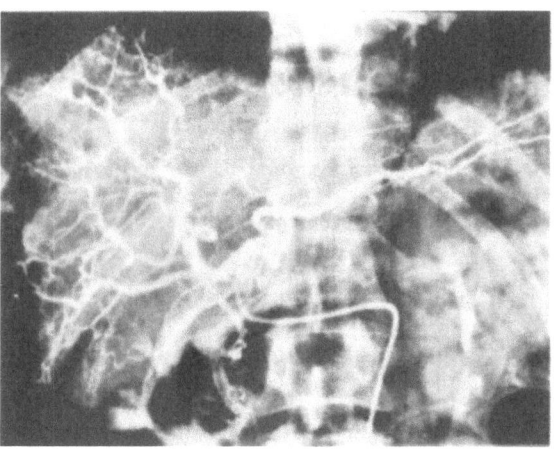

Figure 3. Hepatic artery embolization for redistribution. A. Celiac arteriogram. Note accessory right hepatic artery arising from the gastroduodenal artery. B. Catheterization of the accessory right hepatic artery prior to its occlusion with a stainless steel coil. C. Proper hepatic arteriogram. Reconstitution of the embolized artery has occurred through intrahepatic collaterals.

results of hepatic artery ligation in the management of hepatic neoplasms have been reported (74, 7, 91, 37) but the effects of surgical ligation are usually short-lived since reconstitution of flow occurs through intra- and extra-hepatic collaterals. This phenomenon is demonstratable angiographically immediately following central occlusion of any part of the hepatic arterial system and forms the basis for redistribution of flow in the presence of aberrant hepatic arteries (23). Occlusion of the more peripheral branches through embolization with fine particles has a longer lasting effect and causes varying degrees of necrosis of hepatic neoplasms by depriving them of their blood supply. The normal liver parenchyma is protected from infarction by reason of its dual blood supply.

The collateral circulation that develops after occlusion of any portion of the hepatic arterial system will determine, at

least in part, the degree of necrosis of hepatic neoplasms. The more peripheral the occlusion, the less effective the collateral circulation, and therefore, the greater the tumor necrosis. It is also possible that some neoplasms are more sensitive to ischemia than others. Complete necrosis of hepatic neoplasms does not usually occur following the initial hepatic embolization and therefore, the procedure must be performed periodically. Initially, embolizations are spaced approximately one month apart, and depending on the response, subsequent procedures are performed at longer intervals. A median survival time of 11.5 months after the first hepatic artery embolization in patients with hepatic neoplasms in whom other forms of therapy, including hepatic artery infusion chemotherapy, had failed has been reported previously (24).

When portal hypertension with secondary ascites and esophageal varices occur due to arterio-portal shunting in some hepatic neoplasms, particularly hepatomas, hepatic artery embolization may decrease the shunt and reverse the hepatofugal flow in the portal vein. Resolution of the symptoms of portal hypertension may occur subsequently.

In cases of hormone-secreting hepatic tumors such as metastases from neuroendocrine tumors, hepatic artery embolization will decrease the tumor's production of pharmacologically active substances. Patients with the carcinoid syndrome whose clinical symptomatology is usually determined by the hepatic metastases will experience relief of their symptoms for variable periods of time (Figure 2). (2, 20, 86, 109)

HEPATIC ARTERY REDISTRIBUTION

The classic sequence of the common hepatic artery originating from the celiac artery and continuing as the proper hepatic artery which then divides into right, middle and left hepatic arteries only occurs in 55% of the population (92). In the remainder, aberrant hepatic arteries arising from the left gastric artery and the superior mesenteric artery pose an obstacle to effective arterial infusion of chemotherapeutic agents. In order to infuse the entire liver through a single catheter it is necessary to occlude the aberrant vessels. Central embolization of an aberrant hepatic artery is readily achieved with stainless steel coils which will lead to immediate reconstitution of its territory through intrahepatic collaterals arising from the still patent celiacal hepatic artery (23) (Figure 3).

RENAL CELL CARCINOMA

The treatment for primary renal cell carcinoma confined to the renal capsule (Stage I) is radical nephrectomy (111). Renal artery embolization as a therapeutic modality was first suggested by Lalli *et al.* in 1969 (77) and it is now utilized prior to surgery in cases of large neoplasms in order to facilitate resection and decrease operative blood loss (134) (Figure 4). It has been reported that over 50% of a group of patients with Stage I neoplasms measuring over 6.5 cm in diameter were found to have lymph node metastases (54) and it is possible that these may benefit from a possible immunologic response against the neoplasm following pre-operative renal infarction.

Patients with metastatic disease at the time of their initial presentation pose a therapeutic dilemma. Chemotherapy, radiation therapy and hormonal manipulation have generally been of no value in prolonging survival nor causing regression of metastases in patients with renal cell carcinoma. Based on the initial work of Almgard *et al.* (4) who reported stabilization of metastases in several of their patients with renal adenocarcinomas following renal artery embolization, a protocol involving renal infarction, nephrectomy, and hormonal therapy was established at UT M.D. Anderson Hospital and Tumor Institute. Evaluation of the first 100 cases with long term follow-up demonstrated

an overall response rate (including those patients showing a complete or partial response or prolonged stabilization) of 28% (128). The median survival time for the responding patients was over 30 months with one-third surviving 5 years. The overall survival rates for this group of patients do not represent an improvement when compared to historical controls treated at UT M.D. Anderson Hospital and Tumor Institute by nephrectomy and hormonal-chemotherapeutic protocols without renal embolization. However, in patients with only pulmonary metastases a significant increase in the survival rates was observed in comparison to controls treated by nephrectomy alone. This improvement in the survival rates was almost entirely due to those patients with only pulmonary parenchymal metastases. The median survival time of patients with metastases confined to the lung parenchyma was twice as high (18 versus 9 months) that of patients with hilar mediastinal lymphadenopathy or pleural effusion (with or without parenchymal metastases).

The apparent clinical benefit of renal embolization and nephrectomy in some patients with pulmonary parenchymal metastases from renal cell carcinoma continues to be an empiric observation. It has been suggested that immunological factors play a role based on the assumption that infarction of the neoplasm may release or uncover tumor antigens thereby triggering an antineoplastic response (20).

Our current management of patients who present with pulmonary parenchymal metastases include transcatheter embolization of the primary tumor with Gelfoam and stainless steel coils followed by radical nephrectomy approximately 1 week later. Following nephrectomy, these patients are treated with medroxyprogesterone acetate (Depro-Provera) 400 mg intramuscularly twice weekly as long as there is no progression of their disease. Patients with metastases to sites other than the pulmonary parenchyma alone do not appear to benefit from infarction and nephrectomy and are,

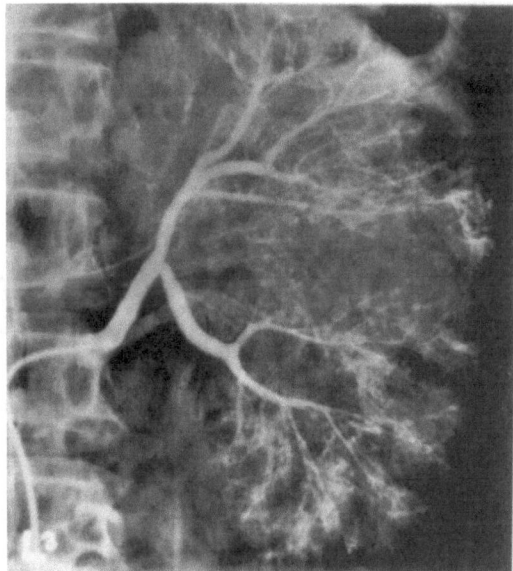 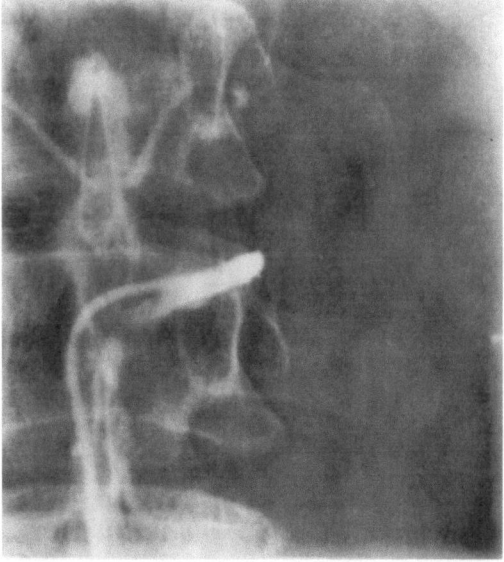

Figure 4. Renal cell carcinoma. A. Left arteriogram. Diffuse neoplastic infiltration of the kidney with tumor vessels extending into the renal vein. An additional left renal artery is faintly opacified. B. Complete occlusion of the renal artery following embolization with dehydrated ethanol.

therefore, offered experimental protocols that include renal embolization with BCG, and infarction and nephrectomy followed by daily injections of human leukocyte interferon.

PELVIC NEOPLASMS

Pelvic neoplasms often undergo extensive local growth prior to metastasizing and local recurrence following primary treatment modalities is a frequent occurrence. In such cases, these neoplasms are unsuitable for extirpative surgery or radiation therapy but are amenable to arterial infusion chemotherapy.

The majority of pelvic neoplasms managed by intra-arterial infusion chemotherapy receive their blood supply from branches of both internal iliac arteries, thus requiring simultaneous catheterization of each one of these vessels for infusion. The local concentration of the infused chemo-therapeutic agents can be augmented by central emboliza-tion of the superior and inferior gluteal arteries (Figure 5). These two vessels, after giving origin to a variable number of pelvic visceral branches, exit from the pelvis to supply the tissues of the buttocks and posterior aspect of the proximal thighs. Since these two vessels usually account for over half of the blood flow derived from the internal iliac arteries, their occlusion will prevent infusion of tissues not usually compromised by pelvic neoplasms while at the same time increasing the concentration of the drug in the area of interest. Occlusion of both gluteal arteries can be accom-plished with stainless steel coils and Gelfoam fragments. Reconstitution of their peripheral branches occurs usually through collateral circulation arising from the fourth lum-bar artery, the superficial iliac circumflex artery and bran-ches of the deep femoral artery. The pelvic blood flow derived from each internal iliac artery is then estimated by radionuclide angiography utilizing 99 mTc macroaggre-gated albumin and the dose of the chemotherapeutic agents

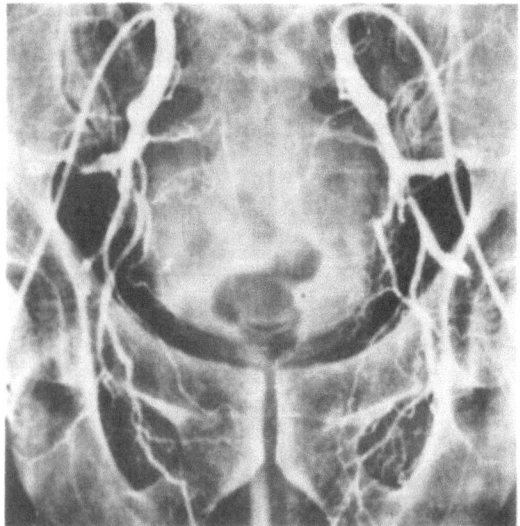

Figure 5. Occlusion of both superior and inferior gluteal arteries with steel coils. Bilateral internal iliac angiography prior to infusion chemotherapy demonstrates flow limited to the pelvic cavity.

to be infused is fractionated between the two infusion cath-eters accordingly. Bilateral internal iliac artery infusion chemotherapy for pelvic neoplasms is usually performed at monthly intervals for three courses following which the infusions are spaced at longer intervals depending on the response or the suitability of other modes of treatment following remission.

CARCINOMA OF THE UTERINE CERVIX

The treatment of patients with squamous cell carcinoma of the uterine cervix varies according to the extent of their disease. Surgical resection or radiation therapy are usually employed in those patients with Stage I and II tumors (131). Patients with locally advanced (Stage III and IV) disease are usually treated solely by radiation therapy because of the difficulty of ensuring adequate surgical margins and the high incidence of pelvic and para-aortic lymph node metastases which contraindicate primary surgery (13, 131). Neverthe-less, persistence or local recurrence of disease continues to be a major problem and is often associated with intractable pain, bleeding, foul discharge and fistulas. In these patients palliation has been difficult to achieve by systemic chemo-therapy. During the past three decades arterial infusion of chemotherapeutic agents has been utilized to increase the local concentration of drugs but responses have been gener-ally poor and of short duration.

In 1952 Cromer *et al.* (32) reported on the intra-aortic injection of nitrogen mustard in 16 patients with carcinoma of the cervix and vagina. They observed regression of the local disease in 8 patients and a reduction in the size of the pelvic tumor in 4 patients. Krakoff and Sullivan (75) using the percutaneous approach, also found some objective bene-fit in 3 of a group of 6 patients with carcinoma of the cervix following the intra-aortic injection of nitrogen mustard. Sullivan *et al.* (124) used surgically implanted catheters into the internal iliac arteries for the infusion of methotrexate and noted total or partial tumor regression in all 4 of their evaluable patients with carcinoma of the cervix. Hulka and Bise (53) also infused chemotherapeutic agents (5-fluoroura-cil, floxuridine or methotrexate) selectively into the internal iliac arteries of a group of 13 patients with carcinoma of the cervix and vagina. These investigators observed a complete remission in four patients with Stage III and IV disease who also underwent irradiation following chemotherapy. Mor-row *et al.* (94) employed intra-arterial infusion of bleomycin in 20 patients with carcinoma of the cervix without a signifi-cant response rate. Libshitz *et al.* (81) using intra-aortic methotrexate alone or in combination with vincristine ob-served tumor regression in 3 of 14 patients with a mean survival time of 13 months compared to 7.9 months for the nonresponders. Their 3 patients who experienced objective tumor response had all received combination methotrexate and vincristine. None of their patients treated with metho-trexate alone had tumor regression. Swenerton *et al.* (130) used intra-aortic or common iliac artery infusions of com-bination vincristine, bleomycin and mitomycin C in 20 pa-tients with carcinoma of the cervix. There were no complete responders and only three patients experienced partial re-sponses which were generally short lived. In a study perfor-med at UT M.D. Anderson Hospital and Tumor Institute, cisplatin was selectively infused into the internal iliac arteries of 9 patients with cervical carcinoma. A partial remission was observed in 3 patients with a mean survival of 13 months compared to 7 months for the nonresponders (18).

In an attempt to lower the local recurrence rate and improve the response rates to chemotherapy of Stage III and IV patients, a study consisting of intravenous administration of vincristine (2 mg) with intra-arterial infusion of mitomycin C ($10\,mg/m^2$), bleomycin ($20\text{--}40\,mg.m^2$) and cisplatinum ($100\text{--}110\,mg/m^2$) is being performed at UT M.D. Anderson Hospital and Tumor Institute. Three courses spaced three weeks apart are given via percutaneously placed catheters into each internal iliac artery. The initial results of this study are encouraging; 30 out of 41 evaluable patients without previous therapy were considered responders (Figure 6) and 7 patients had stable disease. All of these 37 patients underwent subsequent external irradiation and 24 patients (59%) remain free of disease at a median follow-up of 8 months (range 1–31 months). Thirteen of the 41 patients relapsed at a median of 5 months and their median survival time after relapse was only 3 months. The median length of follow-up in this group of patients is still short and the impact of this therapeutic modality on survival and local recurrence is as yet unknown. An identical drug regimen was employed in 17 patients with recurrent disease following primary radiation with an overall response rate of 41%. However, partial responses (29%) were of short duration and did not lead to a significant prolongation of the patients' survival (69).

CARCINOMA OF THE URINARY BLADDER

A variety of forms of local therapy are employed in the treatment of patients with carcinoma of the urinary bladder in stages O and A. The treatment of invasive carcinoma (Stages B and C) usually consists of a combination of radiation therapy and radical excision (66). Surgical therapy or irradiation are of no value in patients with advanced disease (Stage D–D_2). Different chemotherapeutic agents administered via the intravenous or the intra-arterial routes have been employed in patients with unresectable bladder carcinomas. In 1961, Byron *et al.* (15) reported on their experience with intra-arterial infusion of several antineoplastic agents in a group of patients with various malignancies. No responses were observed in their two patients with bladder carcinomas. Ogata *et al.* (101) noted various degrees of antitumor effect in all of their 33 patients treated with mitomycin C via surgically placed catheters into the internal iliac arteries. Nevin *et al.* (98) utilizing a similar technique infused 5-fluorouracil into each internal iliac artery. A complete response in 9 of a group of 15 patients undergoing infusion chemotherapy followed by radiation therapy was reported. A partial response occurred in 5 patients and only one patient failed to respond. No worthwhile response was demonstrated in another group of patients with recurrent bladder disease after radiation therapy nor in those patients with squamous cell carcinomas.

With the introduction of newer agents and techniques for the percutaneous approach to catheter placement, various therapeutic modalities were investigated at UT M.D. Anderson Hospital and Tumor Institute. In a group of 18 patients with advanced carcinoma of the bladder (Stage D_1–D_2) cisplatin was infused into each internal iliac artery at a dose of $80\text{--}120\,mg/m^2$ over a 24 hr period. The infusions in three of the 18 patients were performed after surgery or radiation therapy had eliminated all measurable traces of the disease and were therefore considered as adjuvant

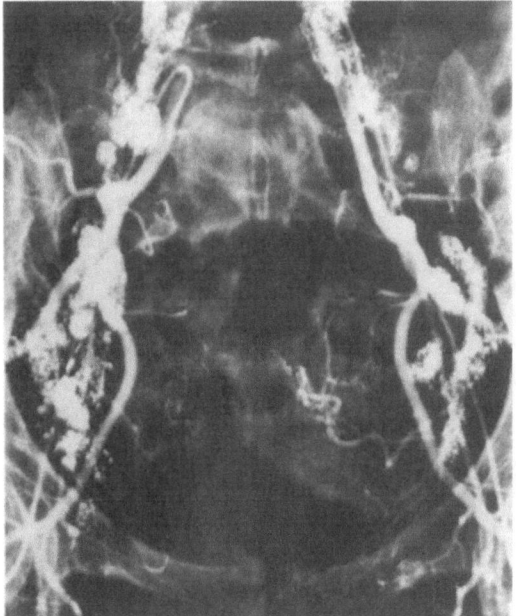

Figure 6. Carcinoma of the uterine cervix. Bilateral internal iliac angiography. A. large hypervascular pelvic tumor. B. Marked improvement following arterial infusion chemotherapy.

therapy. In the remaining 15 patients, there were 6 complete responses, 3 partial responses and 6 failures. The overall response rate was 60 percent (9 of 15 patients) with a median survival of 75 weeks. Pelvic pain in 12 of 15 patients and hematuria in 8 of 10 patients were adequately controlled (135).

In another group of 29 patients, 5-fluorouracil was administered intra-arterially during the intravenous infusion of adriamycin and mitomycin C. Seventeen (58%) of the 29 patients achieved an objective response. Twelve of the 20 patients with transitional cell carcinomas responded. All four patients with adenocarcinomas and one patient with adenocarcinomatous transformation responded to the infusion chemotherapy. No response was observed in the three patients with squamous transformation of transitional cell carcinoma nor in the single patient with a spindle cell variant neoplasm (83).

A third group consisting of 28 patients with unresectable bladder carcinomas who had no evidence of distant visceral metastases were managed with intravenous and intra-arterial CISCA (cytoxan, adriamycin and cisplatin) chemotherapy. For intra-arterial CISCA, only cisplatin was administered intra-arterially; cytoxan and adriamycin were infused via the intravenous route. All patients had locally advanced disease with or without nodal metastases. These patients either had unresectable tumor at presentation (26 patients) or had failed initial therapy consisting of cystectomy or irradiation (2 patients). The tumors were of bladder origin in 26 patients and of ureteral origin in 2 patients. All but two patients received a combination of intra-arterial and intravenous CISCA chemotherapy. Those patients with only locally advanced disease received three courses of intra-arterial CISCA spaced one month apart. Patients with nodal

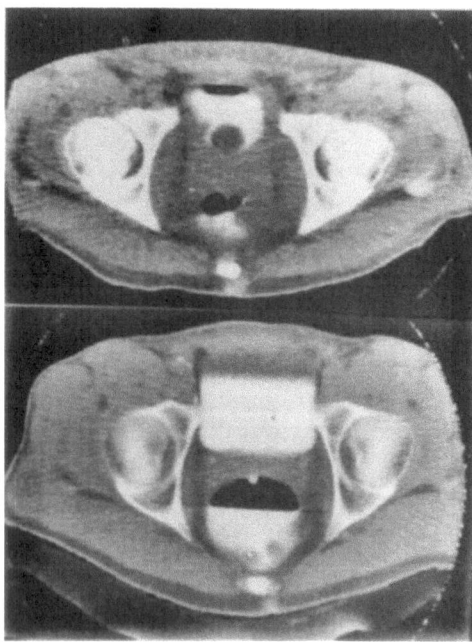

Figure 7. Carcinoma of the urinary bladder. **A** Computed tomography demonstrates a large neoplasm about the right lateral and posterior aspects of the bladder. **B.** Complete remission following bilateral internal iliac artery infusion chemotherapy.

metastases received their initial chemotherapy intravenously followed by intra-arterial CISCA if an objective response was achieved. The doses for intra-arterial CISCA consisted of cytoxan 650 mg/m^2, adriamycin 50–60 mg/m^2 and cisplatin 100 mg/m^2. A complete remission occurred in 11 patients (39%) with a median duration of remission 49 weeks (range 25–108 weeks) (Figure 7). In seven (25%) additional patients an objective regression of tumor occurred. Ten patients (36%) failed to respond. A significant improvement in the survival rate was documented for the complete responders but there was no difference in the survival rates between those patients achieving an objective response and the nonresponders (82).

OSTEOSARCOMA

For many years, radical surgery has been the principal mode of therapy for primary osteosarcomas. The overall survival rate for patients with osteosarcoma employing this therapeutic modality is around 20% (43). Radiologic evidence of pulmonary metastases occurs at a median of 8.5 months following potentially curative surgery (64, 88) and patients usually die within six months after detection of pulmonary metastases (129).

The fatal outcome of most osteosarcoma patients following surgery led to the use of radiation therapy for local control (16, 65, 80) in an effort to spare patients likely to develop pulmonary metastases unnecessary mutilation. It was also believed that radiation might change tumor cell viability and prevent implantation of cells dislodged during surgery. However, this approach yielded survival rates comparable to those achieved by surgery alone (43) and so radiation therapy was discarded as a primary treatment modality.

Chemotherapeutic agents were also utilized in an attempt to improve on the results obtained by surgery alone. Initially, the agents used yielded far from ideal results (39, 47, 123, 125). However, more recently, response rates in the order of 35 to 40 % have been obtained using methotrexate (57, 58), adriamycin (30), cisplatin (100) and cytoxan (107). Their administration alone or in combination has led to eradication of established metastases, destruction of primary tumors and prolongation of disease-free survival. The fact that osteosarcoma is microscopically disseminated at the time of diagnosis, as evidenced by the rapid onset of clinically evident pulmonary metastases soon after amputation, has led to the administration of adjuvant chemotherapy following surgery (28, 126).

Advances achieved with chemotherapy led to the search for alternative methods to treat the primary tumor short of amputation the most significant of which has been limb salvage (60, 107, 114). Preoperative chemotherapy was also used initially in an attempt to contain the primary tumor while awaiting the production of a customized endoprosthesis for limb salvage surgery (87, 116). Subsequently, preoperative chemotherapy and delayed surgery were employed with the intent to treat the primary tumor and identify an effective chemotherapeutic agent for adjuvant therapy based on the degree of tumor necrosis (86, 114, 115). Rosen *et al.* (115) using methotrexate, adriamycin, bleomycin, cytoxan and actinomycin achieved an overall disease-free rate of 72%.

Intra-arterial infusion chemotherapy was performed in order to increase the exposure of the primary osteosarcoma to the antineoplastic agents and thus attempt to improve on the results obtained by their systemic administration. Akaoshi *et al.* (1) used mitomycin C, 5-fluorouracil and methotrexate by continuous intra-arterial infusion for 8 to 48 days followed by surgery and bronchial artery infusion in 14 patients with osteosarcoma. Metastases occurred in 60% of patients during the first year. The projected 5-year survival rate was 44% in those patients in whom the infusion lasted longer than 3 weeks compared to 26% for those who received shorter infusions. Eilber *et al.* (35) using the intra-arterial infusions of adriamycin followed by radiation therapy in 36 patients, observed tumor cell necrosis in over 80% of the resected specimens. In more than half of the specimens, 90 to 100% destruction of the neoplasm was noted. Jaffe *et al.* (60) observed between 90 to 100% tumor destruction in 3 of 5 patients who underwent intra-arterial infusion of adriamycin and systemic methotrexate. In another report, Jaffe *et al.* (61) noted one partial and three complete responses among nine patients who underwent intra-arterial infusion of methotrexate as part of a randomized study. No responses occurred in the six patients who recieved intravenous methotrexate.

Preoperative intra-arterial cisplatin is currently being administered to patients with localized osteosarcomas at UT M.D. Anderson Hospital and Tumor Institute. A response rate of 66% was achieved in 18 patients treated with intra-arterial cisplatin; there were nine complete and three partial responses (62) (Figure 8). The results were determined by clinical, angiographic and histologic parameters (needle biopsy, amputation, and local resection). Increased tumor destruction was found to be a function of the number of infusions (three or more), high cisplatin concentration within the neoplasms, and tumor subtype (osteoblastic). In contrast, decreased tumor destruction was associated with less than four infusions, smaller concentrations and the telangiectatic subtype (59).

In another group of 40 evaluated adult patients, ten (25%) showed 100% tumor necrosis and 13 (32.5%) showed 90% to 99% necrosis in the resected specimens. Twenty-four (60%) of the 40 adult patients underwent limb salvage surgery, whereas 16 (40%) required amputation because of early disease progression (two patients), size or location of tumor (nine patients), or inappropriately placed biopsy (five patients). Only six of the 24 patients who underwent limb salvage surgery were considered candidates for this procedure at presentation. Therefore, preoperative chemotherapy increased the number of patients in whom the extremities could be preserved. The overall two-year survival rate projected according to the Kaplan–Meier life-table analysis was 82% with a continuous disease-free survival rate of 60%. The most important predictor of prolonged, continuous disease-free survival was the degree of response to preoperative chemotherapy. Patients with at least 90% tumor necrosis had a three-year rate of 85%, compared with 30% for those with less than 90% tumor necrosis (116).

In summary, systemic methotrexate, adriamycin, cisplatin, mitomycin C, and 5-fluorouracil are effective in the treatment of the primary tumor in osteosarcoma, with

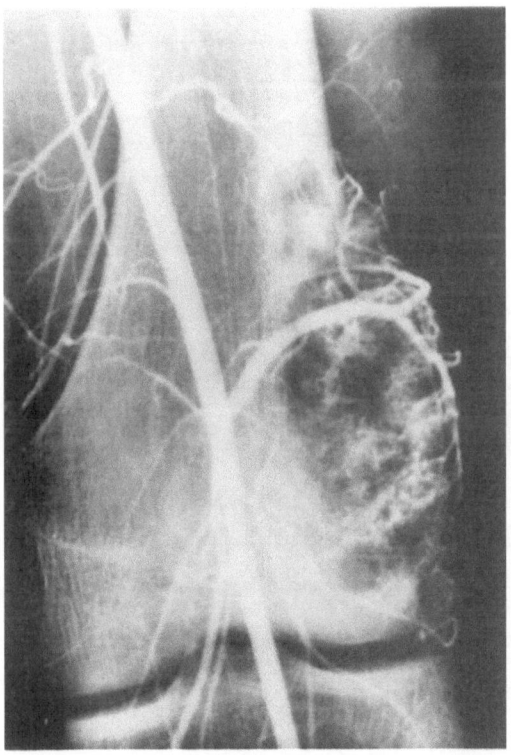
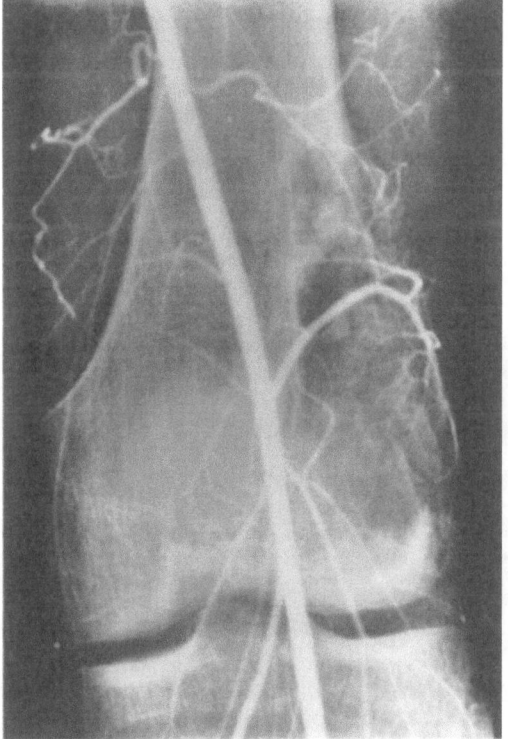

Figure 8. Femoral osteosarcoma. Superficial femoral arteriography. A. Hypervascular neoplasm prior to arterial infusion chemotherapy. B. Decreased vascularity of the tumor consistent with response to intra-arterial chemotherapy.

methotrexate appearing to be the most efficacious yielding response rates of up to 80% (117). In contrast to the intravenous administration, the intra-arterial route delivers high tumoricidal concentrations to the primary tumor. The response rates to intra-arterially administered adriamycin and irradiation (135) were higher than those achieved by its intravenous infusion (118). With cisplatin, the responses were increased from approximately 20% to 50% for its systemic administration (20, 37, 39, 95, 132) to approximately 66% for its intra-arterial infusion (111). The intra-arterial administration of methotrexate did not prove to be more effective than the systemic route which yielded comparable and even superior results (50, 62, 117). Intra-arterial adriamycin and cisplatin infusions may be complicated by skin and subcutaneous tissue reactions. Skin reactions secondary to cisplatin usually consist of erythema and brawny induration, however, those caused by adriamycin may lead to sloughing and ulceration.

EMBOLIZATION OF SKELETAL NEOPLASMS

Embolization of skeletal neoplasms was initially performed as an adjunct to surgical resection for hypervascular tumors in order to decrease operative blood loss (73, 97, 104). Subsequently, this technique was used for palliation of pain caused by skeletal metastases (68) and later it was extended to the management of patients with certain benign bone tumors who had failed other therapeutic modalities (67).

Bone metastases from renal carcinoma are frequently hypervascular which can influence their surgical manage-

ment. When a pathological fracture occurs, internal fixation is usually indicated to relieve pain and to allow the patient to remain ambulatory. Surgical excision and prosthetic replacement may be considered in cases of solitary lesions located in accessible sites (90). However, surgical intervention is often complicated by excessive blood loss which can be avoided in the majority of cases by preoperative embolization (69, 77). In six of eight patients managed in this manner at UT M.D. Anderson Hospital and Tumor Institute the estimated operative blood loss averaged 550 ml. In the two remaining patients, embolization was inadequate and blood losses were 3800 ml and 7000 ml respectively (69). Radiation therapy, at times in conjunction with hormonal and chemotherapeutic agents, is usually the primary modality employed in palliation of pain due to skeletal metastases. Embolization is performed when the patient fails to respond to conventional treatment (25, 69, 128) (Figure 9). In a group of 21 patients with bone metastases treated in this manner, mild to marked pain relief lasting from one to seven months occurred in all patients (25).

Embolization has been performed in the management of unresectable giant cells tumors and aneurysmal bone cysts after failure of other modes of therapy or as a primary treatment modality (31, 64, 67, 84). Twelve patients with giant cell tumor and/or aneurysmal bone cyst were treated by arterial embolization at UT M.D. Anderson Hospital and Tumor Institute (18, 64). The tumor were located in the sacrum in four patients, sacrum and lumbar spine in two patients, sacrum and ilium in one patient, ilium only in two patients and in one patient each in the thoracic spine (T–10), the lumbar spine (L–4) and the humerus. All patients had

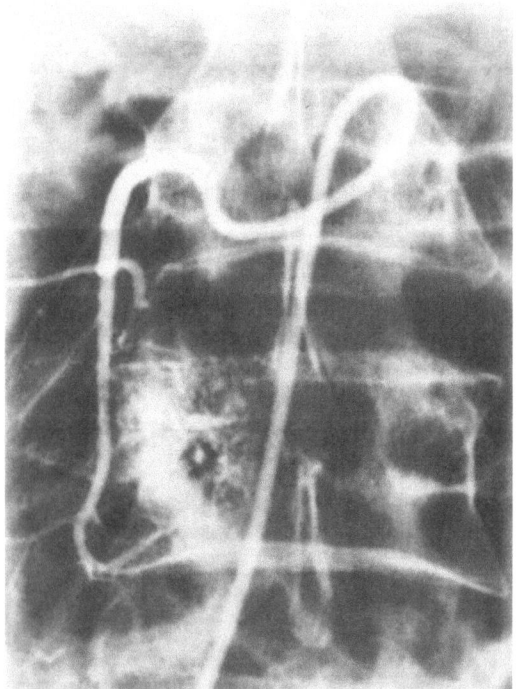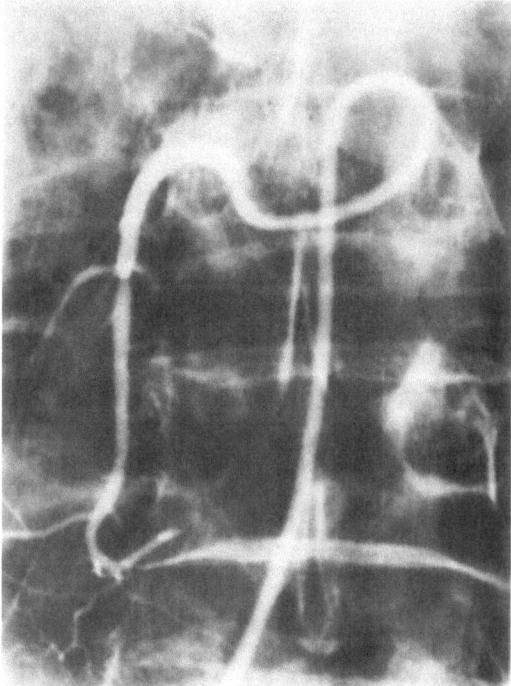

Figure 9. Skeletal metastases from renal cell carcinoma. A. Lumbar angiography. Hypervascular metastases at the L–3 vertebral body. B. Post embolization arteriogram demonstrates adequate occlusion of the lumbar artery supplying the tumor. The patient experienced marked pain relief following embolization.

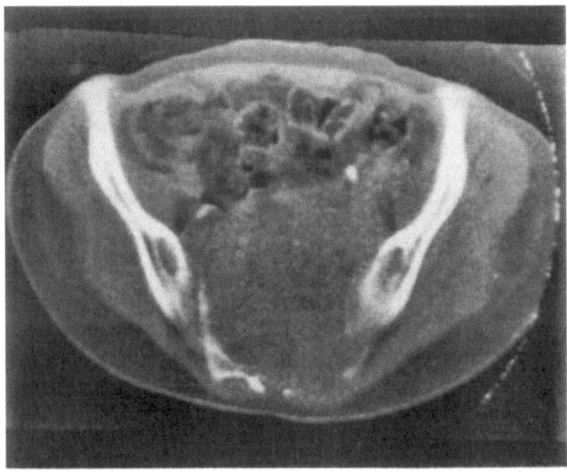 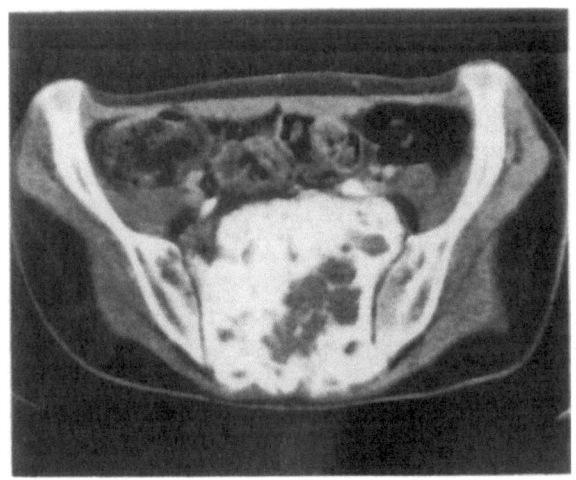

Figure 10. Giant cell tumor. A. Computed tomography demonstrates a large lytic and expansile tumor destroying the sacrum. B. Following arterial infusion of cisplatin and bilateral internal iliac embolization there is healing of the tumor.

some degree of pain as the initial symptom. Five of the 12 patients had failed to respond to both chemotherapy and irradiation. Two additional patients had had chemotherapy alone and all had some form of surgery. Seven of the 12 patients experienced significant pain relief but radiographic features of healing (calcium deposition within the tumor and decrease in size of the soft tissue mass) were observed in only six patients (Figure 10). These seven patients had excellent clinical response lasting 14 to 55 months.

REFERENCES

1. Akahoshi Y, Takeuchi S, Chen S, et al: The results of surgical treatment combined with intra-arterial infusion of anti-cancer agents in osteosarcoma. *Clin Orthopaed* 120: 103, 1976
2. Allison DJ, Modlin IM, Jenkins WJ; Treatment of carcinoid liver metastases by hepatic artery embolisation. *Lancet* 2: 1323, 1977
3. Almersjo O, Bengmark S, Rudenstam CM, et al: Evaluation of hepatic dearterialization in primary and secondary cancer of the liver. *Am J Surg* 124: 5, 1972
4. Almgard LE, Fernstrom I, Haverling M, et al: Treatment of renal adenocarcinoma by embolic occlusion of the renal circulation. *Br J Urol* 45: 474, 1973
5. Anderson JH, Gianturco C, Wallace S: Experimental transcatheter intra-arterial infusion-occlusion chemotherapy. *Invest Radiol* 16: 496, 1981
6. Ansfield FJ, Ramirez G, Skibba JL, et al: Intrahepatic arterial infusion with 5-fluorouracil. *Cancer* 28: 1147, 1971
7. Aune S, Schistad G: Carcinoid liver metastases treated with hepatic dearterialization. *Am J Surg* 123: 715, 1972
8. Baum ES, Gaynon P, Greenberg L, et al: Phase II trial of cisplatin in refractory childhood cancer: Children's cancer study group report. *Cancer Treat Rep* 65: 815, 1981
9. Bengmark S, Hafstrom L: The natural history of primary and secondary malignant tumors of the liver. I. The prognosis for patients with hepatic metastases from colonic and rectal carcinoma by laparotomy. *Cancer* 23: 198, 1969
10. Benjamin RJ, Chuang VP, Wallace S, et al: Preoperative chemotherapy for osteosarcoma (abstract C–675) *ASCO* 1: 174, 1982

11. Bierman HR, Byron RL, Miller ER, Shimkin MB: Effects of intra-arterial administration of nitrogen mustard. *Amer J Med* 8: 535, 1950
12. Bowers TA, Murray JA, Charnsangavej C, Soo C-S, Chuang VP, Wallace S: Bone metastases from renal carcinoma. *J Bone Joint Surg* 64–A: 749, 1982
13. Brady L: Radiotherapy treatment of cervical cancer. In: *Gynecologic Oncology*, edited by McGowan L, New York, Appleton-Century-Crofts, 1978 pp. 224–225
14. Breedis C, Young G: The blood supply of neoplasms in the liver. *am J Pathol* 30: 969, 1954
15. Byron RL, Perez FM, Yonemoto RH, Bierman HR, Gildenhorn HL, Kelly KH: Left brachial arterial catheterization for chemotherapy in advanced intra-abdominal malignant neoplasms. *Surg Gyn Obstet* 112: 689, 1961
16. Cade S: Osteogenic sarcoma: A study based on 113 pts. *JR Coll Surg Edinb* 1: 79, 1955
17. Cady B, Monson DO, Swinton NW: Survival of patients after colonic resection of carcinoma with simultaneous liver metastases. *Surg Gyn Obstet* 131: 697, 1970
18. Carlson JA Jr, Freedman RS, Wallace S, et al: Intra-arterial cisplatinum in the management of squamous cell carcinoma of the uterine cervix. *Gynecol Oncol* 12: 92, 1981
19. Carpenter PR, Ewing JW, Cook AJ, Kuster AH: Angiographic assessment and control of potential operative hemorrhage with pathologic fractures secondary to metastasis. *Clin Orthop* 123: 6, 1977
20. Carrasco CH, Chuang VP, Wallace S: Apudomas metastatic to the liver: Treatment by hepatic artery embolization. *Radiology* 149: 79, 1983
21. Channon GM, Williams LA: Giant cell tumor of the ischium treated by embolisation and resection. A case report. *J Bone Joint Surg (Br)* 64: 164, 1982
22. Chen H-SG, Gross JF. Intra-arterial infusion of anticancer drugs: Theoretic aspects of drug delivery and review of responses. *Cancer Treat Rep* 64: 31, 1980
23. Chuang VP, Wallace S: Hepatic arterial redistribution for intra-arterial infusion of hepatic neoplasms. *Radiology* 135: 295, 1980
24. Chuang VP, Wallace S: Hepatic artery embolization in the treatment of hepatic neoplasms. *Radiology* 140: 51, 1981
25. Chuang VP, Soo CS, Wallace S: Ivalon embolization in abdominal neoplasms. *AJR* 136: 729, 1981
26. Chuang VP, Soo CS, Wallace S, Benjamin RS: Arterial occlu-

sion. Management of giant cell tumor and aneurysmal bone cyst. *AJR* 136: 1127, 1981

27. Chuang VP, Wallace S, Swansen D, et al: Arterial occlusion in the management of pain from metastatic renal carcinoma. *Radiology* 133: 611, 1979

28. Cortes EP, Necheles TF, Holland JF, Glidewell O: Adriamycin (ADR) alone versus ADR and high dose methotrexate-citrovorum factor rescue (HDM-CFR) as adjuvant to operable primary osteosarcoma. A randomized study by Cancer and Leukemic Group B (CALGB). *Proc Am Assoc Cancer Res* 20: 412, 1979

29. Cortes EP, Holland JF, Wang JJ, et al: Doxorubicin in disseminated osteosarcoma. *JAMA* 221: 1132, 1972

30. Cortes EP, Holland JF, Wang JJ, et al: Amputation and adriamycin in primary osteosarcoma. *N Engl J Med* 291: 998, 1974

31. Creech O Jr, Krementz ET, Ryan RF, Winblad JN: Chemotherapy of cancer: regional perfusion utilizing an extracorporeal circuit. *Ann Surg* 148: 616, 1958

32. Cromer JK, Bateman JC, Berry GN, Kennelly JM, Klopp CT, Platt LI: Use of intra-arterial nitrogen mustard therapy in the treatment of cervical and vaginal cancer. *Am J Obstet Gynecol* 63: 538, 1952

33. Dick HM, Bigliani LU, Michelsen WJ, Johnston AD, Stinchfield FE: Adjuvant arterial embolization in the treatment of benign primary bone tumors in children. *Clin Orthop* 139: 133, 1979

34. Eftekhari F, Wallace S, Chuang VP, et al: Intra-arterial management of giant cell tumors of the spine in children. *Pediatr Radiol* 12: 289, 1982

35. Eilber FR, Grant T, Morton DL. Adjuvant therapy for osteosarcoma: Pre-operative treatment. *Cancer Treat Rep* 62: 213, 1978

36. Ensminger W, Rosowsky A, Raso V, et al: A clinical-pharmacological evaluation of hepatic arterial infusions of 5-fluoro-2'-deoxyuridine and 5-fluorouracil. *Cancer Res* 38: 3784, 1978

37. Evans JT: Hepatic artery ligation in hepatic metastases from colon and rectal malignancies. *Dis Colon Rectum* 22: 370, 1979

38. Feldman F, Casarella WJ, Dick HM, Hollander BA: Selective intra-arterial embolization of bone tumors. *AJR* 123: 130, 1975

39. Finkelstein J, Hittle RE, Hammond UD: Evaluation of high dose cyclophosphamide regimen in childhood tumors. *Cancer* 23, 1239, 1969

40. Fortner JG, Maclean BJ, Kim DK, et al: The seventies evolution in liver surgery for cancer. *Cancer* 47: 2162, 1981

41. Fortuny IE, Theologides A, Kennedy BJ: Hepatic arterial infusion for liver metastases from colon cancer: Comparison of mitomycin C (NCS–26980) and 5-fluorouracil (NCS–19893). *Cancer Chemotherapy Rep* 59: 401, 1975

42. Freeman AI, Ettinger LJ, Brecher ML: *Cis*-dichloro-diammineplatinum II in childhood cancer. *Cancer Treat Rep* 63: 1615, 1979

43. Friedman MA, Carter SK: The therapy of osteogenic sarcoma: Current status and thoughts for the future. *J Surg Oncol* 4: 482, 1972

44. Garmick MB, Ensminger WB, Israel M: A clinical-pharmacological evaluation of hepatic arterial infusion of adriamycin. *Cancer Res* 39: 4105, 1979

45. Gelin LE, Lewis DH, Nilsson L: Liver blood flow in man during abdominal surgery. II. The effect of hepatic artery occlusion on the blood flow through metastatic tumor nodules. *Acta Hepatosplenol* 15: 21, 1968

46. Granmayeh M, Wallace S, Schwarten D: Transcatheter occlusion of the gastroduodenal artery. *Radiology* 131: 59, 1979

47. Greesbeck HP, Cudmore JTP: Evaluation of 5-fluorouracil (5–FU) in surgical practice. *Am Surg* 29: 638, 1963

48. Hamby WA, Gardner WJ: Treatment of pulsating exophthalmus. *Arch Surg* 27: 676, 1933

49. Hashimoto Y: Fundamental investigations on local chemotherapy for liver cancer. *Arch Jpn Chir* 47: 302, 1978

50. Healey JE, Sheena KS: Vascular patterns in metastatic liver tumors. *Surg Forum* 14: 121, 1963

51. Hilal SK, Michelsen JW: Therapeutic percutaneous embolization for extra-axial vascular lesions of the head, neck, and spine. *J Neurosurg* 43: 275, 1975

52. Hitchcock CR, Bascom J, Strobel CJ, Mueller GF, Shepard R, Haglin J: Selective intra-arterial perfusion of total abdominal viscera for cancer. *Surg Gyn Obstet* 111: 484, 1960

53. Hulka JF, Bisel HF: Combined intra-arterial chemotherapy and radiation treatment for advanced cervical carcinoma. *Am J Obstet Gynecol* 91: 486, 1965

54. Hulten L, Rosencrantz M, Seeman T, et al: Occurrence and localization of lymph node metastases in renal carcinoma. A lymphographic and histopathological investigation in connection with nephrectomy. *Scand J Urol Nephrol* 3: 129, 1969

55. Hurley JD, Wall T, Worteman LW, Schulte WG: Experiences with pelvic perfusion for carcinoma. *Arch Surg* 83: 111, 1961

56. Huvos AG, Rosen G, Marcove RC: Primary osteogenic sarcoma. Pathologic aspects in 20 patients after treatment with chemotherapy, *en bloc* resection and prosthetic bone replacement. *Arch Pathol Lab Med* 101: 14, 1977

57. Jaffe N: Osteogenic sarcoma. State of the art with high-dose methotrexate treatment. *Clin Orthopaed* 120: 95, 1976

58. Jaffe N, Link M, Traggis D, et al: The role of high dose methrotrexate in osteogenic sarcoma: Sarcomas of soft tissue and bone in childhood. *NCI Monogr* 56: 2101, 1981

59. Jaffe N, Knapp J, Chuang VP, et al: Osteosarcoma: Intra-arterial treatment of the primary tumor with *cis*-diamminedichloroplatinum II (CDP). Angiographic, pathologic and pharmacologic studies. *Cancer* 51: 402, 1983

60. Jaffe N, Watts H, Fellows KE, Vawter C: Local *en bloc* resection for limb preservation. *Cancer Treat Rep* 62: 217, 1978

61. Jaffe N, Prudich J, Knapp J, et al: Osteosarcoma: treatment of the primary tumor with intra-arterial high dose methotrexate (MTX-CF): Pharmacokinetic, clinical, radiographic and pathologic studies. (abstract C–409). *AACR* 22: 195, 1981

62. Jaffe N, Bowman R, Wang Y-M, et al: Chemotherapy for primary osteosarcoma by intra-arterial infusion. Review of the literature and comparison with results achieved by the intravenous route. *Cancer Bull* 36: 37, 1984

63. Jaffee BM, Donegan WL, Watson F, et al: Factors influencing survival in patients with untreated hepatic metastases. *Surg Gyn Obstet* 127: 1, 1968

64. Jeffree CM, Price CHG, Sessons HA: The metastatic patterns of osteosarcoma *Br J Cancer* 32: 87, 1975

65. Jenkin RDT, Allt WEC, Fitzpatrick PJ: Osteosarcoma: an assessment of management with particular reference to primary irradiation and selective delayed amputation. *Cancer* 30: 393, 1972

66. Johnson DE: Surgery for carcinoma of the urinary bladder. *Cancer Treat Rev* 1: 271, 1974

67. Karakousis CP, Kanter PM, Lopez R, Moore R, Holyoke ED: Modes of regional chemotherapy. *J Surg Res* 26: 134, 1979

68. Karakousis CP, Rao U, Holtermann OA, Kanter PM, Holyoke ED: Tourniquet infusion chemotherapy in extremities with malignant lesions. *Surg Gyn Obstet* 149: 481, 1979

69. Kavanagh JJ Jr: Regional chemotherapeutic approaches to the management of pelvic malignancies. *Cancer Bull* 36: 52, 1984

70. Kay JA: The role of perfusion therapy in malignant melanomas. *Canad Med Ass J* 99: 11, 1968

71. Keller FS, Rosch J, Bird CB: Percutaneous embolization of bony pelvic neoplasms with tissue adhesive. *Radiology* 147: 21, 1983

72. Kelsen DP, Hoffman J, Alcock N, et al: Pharmacokinetics of cisplatin regional hepatic infusions. *Am J Clin Oncol (CCT)* 5: 173, 1982

73. Klopp CT, Alford TC, Bateman J, Berry GN, Winship T: Fractionated intra-arterial cancer chemotherapy with methyl bis amine hydrochloride; a preliminary report. *Ann Surg* 132: 811, 1950

74. Kondahl G, Funding J: Hepatic artery ligation in primary and secondary hepatic cancer. *Acta Chir Scand* 138: 289, 1972

75. Krakoff IH, Sullivan RD: Intra-arterial nitrogen mustard in the treatment of pelvic cancer. *Ann Int Med* 48: 839, 1958

76. Kuribayashi S, Phillips DA, Harrington DP, et al: Therapeutic embolization of the gastroduodenal artery in hepatic artery infusion chemotherapy. *AJR* 137: 1169, 1981

77. Lalli AF, Peterson N, Bookstein J: Roentgen guided infarction of kidneys and lungs. Potential therapeutic technique. *Radiology* 93: 434, 1969

78. Lang ER, Bucy PC: Treatment of carotid-cavernous fistula by muscle embolization alone: The Brooks method. *J Neurosurg* 22: 387, 1965

79. Lawrence W Jr, Kuehn P, Masle ET, Miller DG: An abdominal tourniquet for regional chemotherapy. *J Surg Res* 1: 142, 1961

80. Lee ES, Mackenzie DH: Osteosarcoma: A study of the value of preoperative megavoltage radiotherapy. *Br J Surg* 51: 252, 1964

81. Libshitz S, Railsback LD, Buchsbaum HJ: Intraarterial pelvic infusion chemotherapy in advanced gynecologic cancer. *Obstet Gynecol* 52: 476, 1978

82. Logothetis CJ, Samuels ML, Selig DE, Wallace S, Johnson DE: Combined intravenous and intra-arterial cytoxan, adriamycin, and cisplatin (CISCA) in the management of select patients with invasive urothelial tumors. *Cancer Treat Rep* 69: 33, 1985

83. Logothetis CJ, Samuels ML, Wallace S, et al: Management of pelvic complications of malignant urothelial tumors with combined intra-arterial and IV chemotherapy. *Cancer Treat Rep* 66: 1501, 1982

84. Luessenhop AJ, Spence WT: Artificial embolization of cerebral arteries: Report of use in a case of arteriovenous malformation. *JAMA* 172: 1153, 1960

85. Luessenhop AJ, Kachmann R, Selvin W, Farrero AA: Clinical evaluation of artificial embolism in the management of large cerebral arteriovenous malformations. *J Neurosurg* 23: 400, 1965

86. Lunderquist A, Ericsson M, Nobin A, Sanden G: Gelfoam powder embolization of the hepatic artery in liver metastases of carcinoid tumors. *Radiologe* 22: 65, 1982

87. Marcove RC: *En bloc* resection for osteogenic sarcoma. *Can J Surg* 20: 521, 1977

88. Marcove RC, Mike V, Hajek JV, et al: Osteogenic sarcoma in childhood. *N.Y. State J Med* 71: 855, 1971

89. Markowitz J: The hepatic artery. *Surg Gyn Obstet* 95: 644, 1952

90. McBride C: Advanced melanoma of the extremities. Treatment by isolation-perfusion with a triple drug combination. *Arch Surg* 101: 122, 1970

91. McDermott WV, Hensle TW: Metastatic carcinoid to the liver treated by hepatic dearterialization. *Ann Surg* 180: 305, 1974

92. Michels NA: Newer anatomy of the liver and its variant blood supply and collateral circulation. *Am J Surg* 112: 337, 1966

93. Miller DG, Lawrence W Jr, Kim M, Dorencamp D, Randall HT: Midtorso occlusion for regional cancer chemotherapy. *Cancer Chemotherapy Rep* 18: 43, 1962

94. Morrow CP, DiSaia PJ, Mangan CF, Lagasse LD: Continuous pelvic arterial infusion with bleomycin for squamous carcinoma of the cervix recurrent after radiation therapy. *Cancer Treat Rep* 61: 1403, 1977

95. Morton DL, Eilber FR, Townsend CN Jr, Grant TT, Mirra J, Weisenburger TH: Limb salvage from a multidisciplinary treatment approach for skeletal and soft tissue sarcomas of the extremity. *Ann Surg* 184: 268, 1976

96. Murphy WA, Strecker WB, Schoenecker PL: Transcatheter embolization therapy of an ischial aneurysmal bone cyst. *J Bone Joint Surg (Br)* 64: 166, 1982

97. Murray-Lyon IM, Parson VA, Blendis LM, et al: Treatment of secondary hepatic tumours by ligation of hepatic artery and infusion of cytotoxic drugs. *Lancet* 2: 172, 1970

98. Nevin JE, Hoffman AA: Use of arterial infusion of 5-fluorouracil either alone or in combination with supervoltage radiation as a treatment for carcinoma of the prostate and bladder. *Am J Surg* 130: 544, 1975

99. Oberfield RA, McCaffrey JA, Polio J, et al: Prolonged and continuous percutaneous intraarterial hepatic infusion chemotherapy in advanced metastatic liver adenocarcinoma from colorectal primary. *Cancer* 44: 414, 1979

100. Ochs JJ, Freeman AI, Douglass HO, Higby DJ, Mindell R, Sinks T: Cis-dichloro-diammineplatinum (II) in advanced osteogenic sarcoma. *Cancer Treat Rep* 62: 239, 1978

101. Ogata J, Migita N, Nakamura T: Treatment of carcinoma of the bladder by infusion of the anticancer agent (mitomycin C) via the internal iliac artery. *J Urol* 110: 667, 1973

102. Parrish FF, Murray JA: Surgical treatment for secondary neoplastic fractures. A retrospective study of ninety-six patients. *J Bone Joint Surg* 52a: 665, 1970

103. Patt YZ, Mavligit GM, Chuang VP, et al: Percutaneous hepatic arterial infusion (HAI) of mitomycin C and floxuridine (FUDR): An effective treatment for metastatic colorectal carcinoma in the liver. *Cancer* 46: 261, 1980

104. Patt YZ, Bedikian AY, Chuang VP, et al: New approaches to the treatment of Duke's C colorectal carcinoma and metastatic colorectal carcinoma confined to the liver. In: edited by Stroehlein J, Romsdahl MM. pp. 391–403. *Gastrointestinal Cancer*, New York, Raven Press, 1981

105. Patt YZ, Chuang VP, Wallace S, Hersh EM, Freireich EJ, Mavligit GM: The palliative role of hepatic arterial infusion and arterial occlusion in colorectal carcinoma metastatic to the liver. *Lancet* 1: 349, 1981

106. Patt YZ, Chuang VP, Wallace S, Benjamin RS, Fuqua R, Mavligit GM: Hepatic arterial chemotherapy and occlusion for palliation of primary hepatocellular and unknown primary neoplasms in the liver. *Cancer* 51: 1359, 1983

107. Pinkel D. Cyclophosphamide in children with cancer. *Cancer* 15: 42, 1969

108. Pratt CB, Hayes A, Green AA, et al: Pharmacokinetic evaluation of cisplatin in children with malignant solid tumors: A Phase II study. *Cancer Treat Rep* 65: 1021, 1981

109. Pueyo I, Jimenez JR, Hernandez J, et al: Carcinoid syndrome treated by hepatic embolization. *AJR* 131: 511, 1978

110. Rapoport AH, Burleson RL: Survival of patients treated with systemic fluorouracil for hepatic metastases. *Surg Gyn Obstet* 130: 773, 1970

111. Robson CJ: Radical nephrectomy for renal cell carcinoma. *J Urol* 89: 37, 1968

112. Rosch J, Dotter CT, Brown MJ: Selective arterial embolization: A new method for control of acute gastrointestinal bleeding. *Radiology* 102: 303, 1972

113. Rosen G, Nirenberg H, Caparros B. et al: Cisplatin in metastatic osteogenic sarcoma. In: *Cisplatin: Current Status and New Developments* edited by Prestayko AW, Crooke ST, Carter SK, pp. 465–475. Academic Press, New York, 1980

114. Rosen G, Marcove RC, Caparros B, Nirenberg A, Kosloff C, Huvos AG: Primary osteogenic sarcoma. The rationale for preoperative chemotherapy and delayed surgery. *Cancer* 43: 2163, 1979

115. Rosen G, Caparros B, Huvos A, et al: Preoperative chemotherapy for osteogenic osteosarcoma: Selection of postoperative adjuvant chemotherapy based on the response of the primary tumor to preoperative chemotherapy. *Cancer* 49:

1221, 1982

116. Rosen G, Murphy ML, Huvos AG, et al Chemotherapy, *en bloc* resection and prosthetic bone replacement in the treatment of osteogenic sarcoma. *Cancer* 37: 1, 1976

117. Rosen G, Nirenberg A, Juergens H, et al: Response of primary osteogenic sarcoma to single agent therapy with high-dose methotrexate with citrovorum factor rescue. In: *Current Chemotherapy and Infectious Disease*, edited by Nelson JD, Grassi C, pp. 1633–1635. *Proc 11th ICC and 19th ICAAC*, vol 2, Washington DC: The American Society Microbiology, 1980

118. Rosen G, Caparros B, Nirenberg A, et al: Cisplatinum (DDP)–Adriamycin (ADR) combination chemotherapy (CT) in evaluable osteogenic sarcoma (OS). (abstract C–672). *ASCO* 1: 173, 1982

119. Segall HN: An experimental anatomical investigation of the blood and bile channels of the liver. *Surg Gyn Obstet* 37: 152, 1923

120. Soo C-S, Chuang VP, Wallace S, Charnsangavej C: Interventional angiography in the treatment of metastases. *Radiol Clin North Am* 20: 591, 1982

121. Sparks FC, Mosher MB, Hallaner WG, et al: Hepatic artery ligation and postoperative chemotherapy for hepatic metastases: Clinical and pathophysiological results. *Cancer* 35: 1074, 1975

122. Speakman TJ: Internal occlusion of a carotid cavernous fistula. *J Neurosurg* 21: 303, 1964

123. Sullivan MP, Sutow WW, Taylor G: L–phenylalanine mustard as treatment for osteogenic sarcoma in children *J. Pediatr.* 63: 227, 1963

124. Sullivan RD, Wood AM, Clifford P, et al: Continuous intraarterial methotrexate with simultaneous, intermittent, intramuscular citrovorum factor therapy in carcinoma of the cervix. *Cancer Chemother Rep* 8: 1, 1960

125. Sutow WW: Evaluation of dosage schedules of mitomycin C (NCS–26980) in children. *Cancer Chemother Rep* 55: 285, 1971

126. Sutow WW, Sullivan MP, Wilbur JR, Cangir A: A study of adjuvant chemotherapy in osteogenic sarcoma. *J Clin Pharmacol* 7: 530, 1975

127. Swanson DA: The current immunologic status of renal carcinoma. *Cancer Bull* 31: 36, 1979

128. Swanson DA, Johnson DE, von Eschenbach AC, Chuang VP, Wallace S: Angioinfarction plus nephrectomy for metastatic renal cell carcinoma. An update. *J Urol* 130: 449, 1983

129. Sweetnam R, Knowelden J, Seddon H: Bone sarcoma: Treatment of irradiation, amputation or a combination of the two. *Br Med J* 2: 363, 1971

130. Swenerton KD, Evers JA, White GW, Boyes DA: Intermittent pelvic infusion with vincristine, bleomycin, and mitomycin C for advanced recurrent carcinoma of the cervix. *Cancer Treat Rep* 63: 1379, 1979

131. Van Nagell JR, Donaldson ES, Gay EC: Evaluation and treatment of patients with invasive cervical cancer. *Surg Clin NA* 58: 67, 1978

132. Wallace S, Gianturco C, Anderson JH, et al: Therapeutic vascular occlusion utilizing steel coil technique: Clinical applications. *Am J Roentgenol* 127: 381, 1976

133. Wallace S, Granmayeh M, deSantos LA, et al: Arterial occlusion of pelvic bone tumors. *Cancer* 43: 322, 1979

134. Wallace S, Chuang VP, Swanson D, et al: Embolization of renal carcinoma: experience with 100 patients. *Radiology* 138: 563, 1981

135. Wallace S, Chuang VP, Samuels M, Johnson D: Transcatheter intraarterial infusion of chemotherapy in advanced bladder cancer. *Cancer* 49: 640, 1982

136. Watkins E Jr, Khaazei AE, Nahra KS: Surgical basis for arterial infusion chemotherapy of disseminated carcinoma of the liver. *Surg Gyn Obstet* 130: 581, 1970

137. Wright KC, Charnsangavej A, Wallace S, Chuang VP, Savaraj N: Regional isolation-perfusion: An experimental percutaneous approach tested and compared to arterial occlusion-infusion. *Cardiovasc Interven Rad* 7: 294, 1984

POSTSCRIPT

Transcatheter management of certain neoplasms, either as arterial infusion (chemotherapy) or as embolization, has been done with a number of organs, especially the liver, and with primary or metastatic tumors as well. Advantages and disadvantages of Lipiodol-Transcatheter arterial embolization in diagnosis and treatment of hepatocellular carcinoma were outlined by Shimotsuma *et al.* (2) and Shimamura *et al.* (1). Transarterial embolization or infusion in regard to unresectable liver cancer were discussed by Taniguchi *et al.* (3). Infusion chemotherapy of primary neoplasms is especially known from Japan with its high incidence of liver cancer (see chapter 6/Vol. VI) or in metastatic cancer to the liver. Embolization is used in patients with primary and metastatic cancer: Primary tumors and their treatment were described and metastatic ones such as islet cell tumors metastatic to the liver or from colorectal cancer. Other recent studies dealt with combined treatment for primary and metastatic neoplasms and complications. Some papers were more of technical nature or reported experimental work.

POSTSCRIPT REFERENCES

1. Shimamura Y, Ishii M, Shima Y, et al.: Advantages and disadvantages of L-TAE in diagnosis and treatment of hepatocellular carcinoma. *Gan To Kagaku Ryoho* 15(8 Pt 2):2535, 1988

2. Shimotsuma M, Taniguchi H, Sawai K, et al.: Cytofluorometric and histopathological studies on non-cancerous liver lesions after lipiodol-transcatheter arterial embolization. *Gan To Kagaku Ryoho* 15(8 Pt 2):2460, 1988

3. Taniguchi H, Shioaki Y, Itoh A, et al.: Trans-arterial embolization or transcatheter infusion of anti-cancer drugs suspended in a lipid contrast medium against unresectable metastatic liver cancer. *Gan To Kagaku Ryoho* 15(8 Pt 2):2568, 1988

4

ANTIFOLATES

M.G. NAIR

INTRODUCTION

By definition, folate antagonists are compounds which are capable of interfering with tetrahydrofolate utilization. The source of folic acid (1) in man is exogenous. All biologically relevant coenzymatic forms of folic acid possess a tetrahydropteridine ring system (11). Folic acid is converted to 5,6,7,8-tetrahydrofolic acid by a stepwise reduction mediated by the key enzyme dihydrofolate reductase (EC 1.5.1.3). The stereochemistry of the enzymatic reduction of folic acid to its tetrahydroderivative was investigated by Charlton and Young (19), and they defined the absolute configuration at C-6 of this derivative as (S). The (S) configuration at C-6 of tetrahydrofolic acid is usually referred to as the 'natural configuration'. This stereochemical assignment was in agreement with that proposed by Fontecilla-Camps et al. (44) by X-ray crystallography.

In contrast to the enzymatic reduction, the chemical reduction of folic acid results in the formation of d,l-L-tetrahydrofolic acid, which is a mixture of diastereomers. The individual diastereomers are l-L-tetrahydrofolic acid and d-L-tetrahydrofolic acid. The former compound is the natural isomer of tetrahydrofolic acid having the (S) configuration at C-6 and the later is the unnatural isomer (79). All known folate cofactors, which take part in the biochemical reactions catalyzed by folate dependent enzymes have the natural configuration at C-6. The crystal and molecular structure of folic acid dihydrate has been determined by Mastropaolo and Camerman (86) by X-ray diffraction and found that it is an extended conformation with the pteridine ring in the keto form. The pteridine ring and the phenyl ring interact in a stacking manner, and the investigators speculated that this type of interaction is suggestive of the type of association these rings could form in a complex of folic acid,

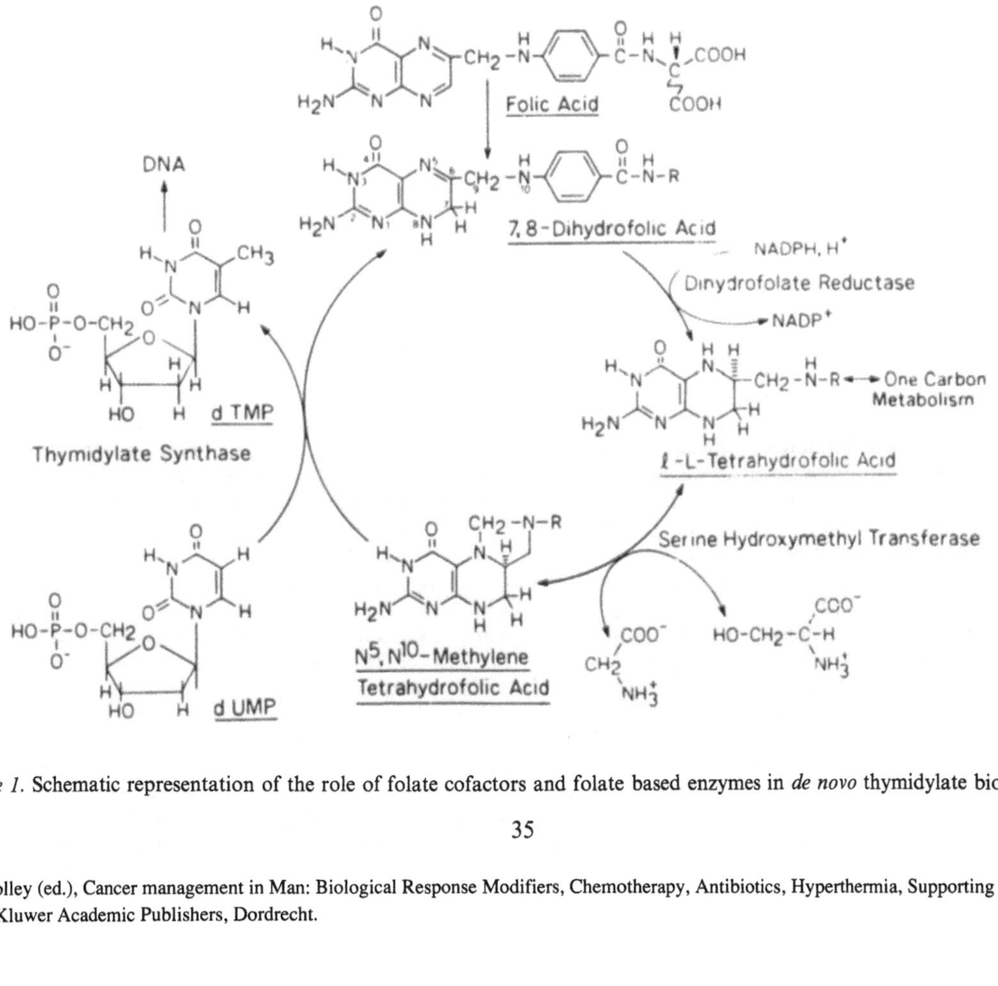

Figure 1. Schematic representation of the role of folate cofactors and folate based enzymes in *de novo* thymidylate biosynthesis.

35

P.V. Woolley (ed.), Cancer management in Man: Biological Response Modifiers, Chemotherapy, Antibiotics, Hyperthermia, Supporting Measures
© 1989. Kluwer Academic Publishers, Dordrecht.

Table 1. Enzymatic reactions.

1.	Dihydrofolic acid + NADPH + H^+	$\xrightarrow{\text{dihydrofolate reductase}}$	Tetrahydrofolic acid + $NADP^+$
2.	Serine + tetrahydrofolic acid	$\xrightarrow{\text{Serine hydroxymethyl transferase}}$	N^5, N^{10}-methylene tetrahydrofolic acid + glycine
3.	N^5, N^{10}-methylene tetrahydrofolic acid + dUMP	$\xrightarrow{\text{Thymidylate synthase}}$	Dihydrofolic acid + dTMP
4.	N^5, N^{10}-methylene tetrahydrofolic acid + NADH + H^+	$\xrightarrow{\text{Methylene tetrahydrofolate reductase}}$	N^5-methyl tetrahydrofolic acid + NAD^+
5.	N^5, N^{10}-methylene tetrahydrofolic acid + $NADP^+$	$\xrightarrow{\text{Methylene tetrahydrofolate dehydrogenase}}$	N^5, N^{10}-methenyl tetrahydrofolic acid + NADPH + H^+
6.	Glycinamide ribo-nucleotide (GAR) + N^5, N^{10}-methenyl-tetrahydrofolic acid + H_2O	$\xrightarrow{\text{GAR-transformylase}}$	N-formyl glycinamide ribo-nucleotide + tetrahydrofolate
7.	Aminoimidazole carboxamide ribo-nucleotide + N^{10}-formyl-tetrahydro folate	$\xrightarrow{\text{AICAR-transformylase}}$	5-formamido imidazole-4-carboxamide ribonucleotide + tetrahydrofolic acid
8.	Homocystein + N^5-methyl-tetrahydro-folic acid	$\xrightarrow{\text{Methionine synthetase}}$	Methionine + tetrahydrofolic acid
9.	N-formimino glutamic acid + tetrahydro-folic acid	$\xrightarrow{\text{Glutamate-formimino transferase}}$	N^5-formimino tetrahydrofolic acid + glutamic acid
10.	Formimino glycine + tetrahydrofolic acid	$\xrightarrow{\text{Glycine-formimino transferase}}$	N^5-formimino tetrahydrofolic acid + glycine
11.	Tetrahydrofolate + Formic acid + ATP	$\xrightarrow{\text{Tetrahydrofolate formylase}}$	N^{10}-formyl tetrahydrofolate + ADP + Pi

NADPH and dihydrofolate reductase. The enzymatic reduction product of 7,8-dihydrofolic acid (*l*-L-tetrahydrofolic acid) serves as a common precursor of all biologically active coenzymatic forms of folic acid. The metabolic fate of dihydrofolic acid as well as it's regeneration *in vivo* is depicted diagrammatically in Figure 1. An outline of the major enzymatic reactions in which folate coenzymes are involved is presented in Table 1. The presence of 7,8-dihydrofolic acid in the cell is the result of its formation as a co-product in the reaction catalyzed by the enzyme thymidylate synthase (EC 2.1.1.45). Dihydrofolate thus generated can become active only if it is reduced to the tetrahydro derivative by dihydrofolate reductase. Tetrahydrofolic acid, as its N^5, N^{10}-methylene derivative plays a unique role in the *de novo* biosynthesis of DNA, by providing the required methylene unit for the conversion of deoxyuridylic acid (dUMP) to thymidylic acid (dTMP). This thymidine nucleotide (dTMP) is required exclusively for the biosynthesis of DNA and hence cell division. Three folate dependent enzymes are directly involved in the conversion of dUMP to dTMP. They are:

(1) *Dihydrofolate reductase:* This enzyme catalyzes the

reduction of dihydrofolate to tetrahydrofolate (reaction 1, Table 1).

(2) *Serine hydroxymethyl transferase,* which catalyzes the transfer of the methylene unit from serine to tetrahydrofolate, with the formation of N^5, N^{10}-methylene tetrahydrofolate and glycine (reaction 2, Table 1).

(3) *Thymidylate synthase:* This enzyme facilitates the transfer of a methylene unit from N^5, N^{10}-methylene tetrahydrofolate to the 5-position of deoxy uridylate (reaction 3, Table 1).

In addition to the unique metabolic role of tetrahydrofolate in *de novo* DNA biosynthesis, it also functions as a key intermediate in all other one carbon transfer reactions. Various derivatives of tetrahydrofolate function as one carbon carriers in many metabolic processes.

The one carbon fragment is carried in a covalent linkage either at N^5, N^{10}, or as a cyclic unit between N^5 and N^{10} of the tetrahydrofolate molecule. The one carbon unit is carried over these positions in various oxidation states of carbon. The partial structures of these derivatives are shown in Table 2 together with a statement of the function of each of these compounds. Examination of this table reveals that

Table 2. Partial structures in various oxidation states of carbon.

Name	Structure	Function
ℓ −L−Tetrahydrofolic acid		Starting material for all folate coenzymes
N⁵−Methyl Tetrahydrofolic acid		Methylation reactions (Methionine biosynthesis; methylation of indolethylamines etc.)
N⁵, N¹⁰−Methylene Tetrahydrofolic acid		dTMP−biosynthesis; Amino acid interconversion
N⁵−Formyl Tetrahydrofolic acid		Growth factor (Citrovorum factor). Reactive intermediate in the interconversion of folate Coenzymes
N¹⁰−Formyl Tetrahydrofolic acid		Purine biosynthesis (C₂ and C₈ of Purine ring)
N⁵−Formimino Tetrahydrofolate		Histidine degradation; Purine biosynthesis

apart from its participation in the synthesis of thymidylic acid, tetrahydrofolate has other important functions as well; such as its role in amino acid interconversion; purine biosynthesis; RNA biosynthesis; histidine degradation; protein synthesis and the formation of methionine. Participation of a folate derivative has been implicated in the biosynthesis of heme. This compound, presumably a folyl-polyglutamate apparently functions as an activator of uroporphyrinogen-I synthase (112). It has been shown that 5-methyl tetrahydrofolic acid can also function as a methyl donor in the methylation of indolethylamines (82). Although, it is well recognized that the folate cofactor used in the GAR-transformylase reaction is N⁵,N¹⁰-methenyl tetrahydrofolate, Benkovic has shown that reaction no. 6 as written in Table 1, requires a second enzyme which is a trifunctional protein, and the true folate cofactor for the GAR-transformylase reaction is L(−)-10-formyl tetrahydrofolate; which is the hydrolysis product of L(+)-5,10-methenyl tetrahydrofolate (134). Historically, the transformylase assay was carried out with a mixture of diastereomers. Therefore, the utilization of L(−)-10-formyl tetrahydrofolate was not previously recognized because L-(+)-10-formyl-tetrahydrofolate is an excellent competitive inhibitor of GAR transformylase.

These observations, taken together clearly indicate that tetrahydrofolate is a vitamin which has a central role in many important biochemical processes and any interference with its utilization *in vivo* might lead to profound biological consequences. Natural folates have complex structures, and they are widely distributed. The complexity of their structures arises from the fact that at least three states of reduction can occur in the pyrazine ring, and six different one carbon substituents can be present at N⁵, N¹⁰ or both of these positions of the folate framework. Each of these derivatives can exist as their respective poly-γ-glutamates with the glutamyl chain length varying anywhere from two to eight (4). The structures of the naturally occurring folate derivatives are shown in Figure 2. During absorption of the vitamin, the polyglutamates are broken down to their respective monoglutamates by the enzyme pteroyl-γ-glutamyl carboxy peptidase (2, 110); also known as 'conjugase'. Evidence has been presented by Butterworth, Baugh and Krumdieck (16) that synthetic poly-γ-glutamates are converted to the monoglutamate form in man shortly after oral ingestion. Folates are circulated in the plasma after they are bound to the folate binding proteins as suggested by Colman and Herbert (23) and Waxman (141). These bound folates are accessible to the active, carrier mediated cell transport system. It has been shown by Huennekens and Henderson (65) that transport of folate compounds into mammalian cells is an active process, which requires energy, carrier mediated and saturable. These cells possess two transport systems, one specific for folic acid itself, and the other for reduced natural folates. Neithammer and Jackson (105) have shown that in human lymphocytes uptake of folic acid and natural reduced folates occurred by separate pathways. These two distinct transport systems are responsible for the influx of folate derivatives to mammalian cell lines.

FOLATE BASED ENZYMES AS TARGETS FOR CANCER CHEMOTHERAPY

The central role of tetrahydrofolate in DNA synthesis, and its importance as a target of cancer chemotherapy has been

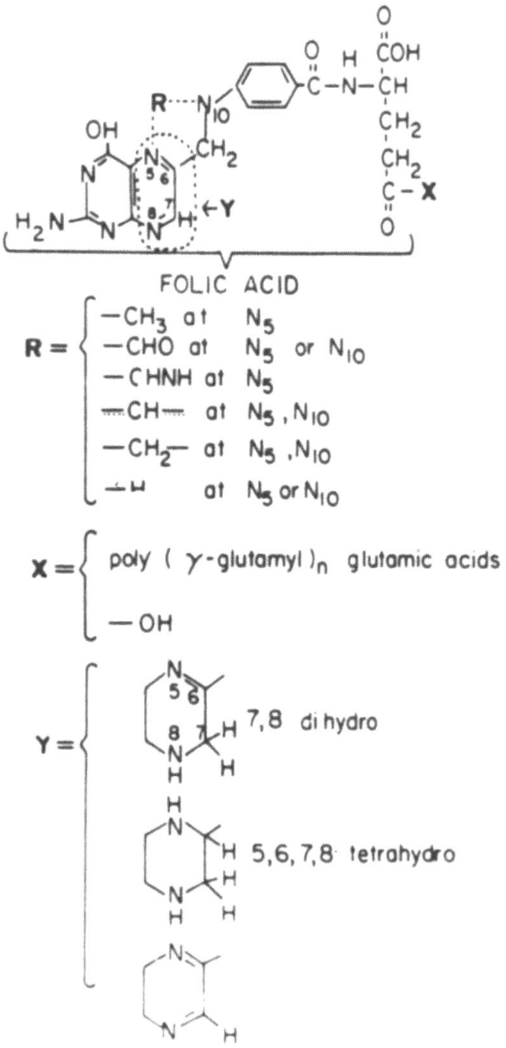

Figure 2. Schematic representations of the theoretical structures of the folates. Adapted from Baugh and Krumdieck: *Annal NY Acad Sci* 186:7–28, 1971.

widely recognized. Any situation which interferes with the formation of tetrahydrofolate will have an adverse effect on the synthesis of purines and pyrimidines which are required for the synthesis of DNA and hence cell division. The enzyme which catalyzes the reduction of dihydrofolate to tetrahydrofolate is dihydrofolate reductase. Therefore, it is not surprising to note that the majority of attempts to block cell division, were targeted primarily at the inhibition of this enzyme.

Another important folate based enzyme, which has been a target for cancer chemotherapy is thymidylate synthase. The inhibition of this enzyme specifically blocks the biosynthesis of a single nucleotide (dTMP) which is exclusively required for DNA synthesis. Inhibitors of both dihydrofolate reductase and thymidylate synthase, are currently used as well known anticancer drugs.

The third enzyme which is a potential target for cancer chemotherapy is serine hydroxymethyl transferase. This enzyme catalyzes the formation of the key intermediate

N^5,N^{10}-methylene tetrahydrofolate, which is a specific coenzyme for the reaction catalyzed by thymidylate synthase. However, this coenzyme can also be formed by the alternate pathways which are shown below.

(a) Tetrahydrofolate + formaldehyde $\xrightarrow{\text{non-enzymatic}}$ N^5,N^{10}-methylene tetrahydrofolate

(b) N^5,N^{10},methenyl tetrahydrofolate + NADPH + H$^+$ $\xrightarrow{\text{dehydrogenase}}$ N^5,N^{10}-methylene tetrahydrofolate + NADP$^+$

It should be noted that N^5,N^{10}-methenyl tetrahydrofolate is formed by the action of cyclohydrolase on N^{10}-formyl tetrahydrofolate which, in turn, originates from tetrahydrofolate and formic acid or via N^5-formyl tetrahydrofolate.

Because of the availability of these alternate pathways, very selective inhibition of serine hydroxymethyl transferase may not contribute to a dramatic reduction of dTMP synthesis. Perhaps, this theoretical consideration might have been the reason for the lack of enthusiasm which prevailed regarding the development of specific inhibitors of this enzyme. However, it should be recognized that a precise understanding of the relative contribution of each of these pathways to the overall production of N^5,N^{10}-methylene tetrahydrofolate is required before any meaningful conclusions regarding this approach in blocking cell division can be derived. At this writing a specific and powerful inhibitor of serine hydroxymethyl transferase, which is useful for the chemotherapy of cancer has not been developed.

Since a majority of folate coenzyme derivatives are interconvertible *in vivo*, at least from a theoretical standpoint, most of the folate based enzymes are potential targets for cancer chemotherapy. Therefore, in addition to the three enzymes mentioned above, two additional enzymes which are directly involved in the *de novo* synthesis of purine nucleotides have to be pointed out. They are GAR-transformylase and AICAR transformylase (Table 1). Specific inhibition of any one of these enzymes, should effectively block DNA and RNA biosynthesis.

Inhibitors of dihydrofolate reductase

Mechanism of action, toxicity and clinical use

The most widely used anticancer drug, which is an inhibitor of DHFR is methotrexate. It is one of the most powerful inhibitors of this enzyme; and this inhibition has been described in the literature using various terms such as noncompetitive (8) pseudo irreversible, and stoichiometric. These descriptions are used to convey the message that one molecule of MTX binds tightly to one molecule of the enzyme, and at pH 6 there is no dissociation of the enzyme inhibitor complex. At the physiological pH and higher, reversible competitive kinetics are observed.

There are only two known sources of dihydrofolic acid in man. They are (1) the dietary source, and (2) the availability of dihydrofolate as a coproduct of the reaction catalyzed by thymidylate synthase. In growing tissues the demand for DNA is high, and one molecule of dihydrofolate is formed for every molecule of thymidylate synthesized. To keep the folate pool functioning at normal levels, dihydrofolate must be reduced to tetrahydrofolate by DHFR and NADPH

(Figure 1). During MTX treatment, DHFR is inhibited and consequently a large fraction of the various folate coenzymes of one carbon metabolism is channeled to 'inert' dihydrofolate. The result is a complete blockade of one carbon metabolism. These observations have been documented. The incorporation of 14-C formate in to the purines is blocked up to 90% in animals receiving MTX (132, 133). Methotrexate also inhibits *de novo* purine biosynthesis in bone marrow cells *in vitro* (138) and Ehrlich ascites cells *in vivo* (119). The incorporation of labeled amino acids into protein in *Escherichia coli* extracts is drastically inhibited by MTX, perhaps due to the scarcity of methionine or N-formyl methionine (41). Williams and co-workers (145) reported the inhibition of ^{14}C formate incorporation into protein of L1210 lymphoma in mice as well as the protein of spleen and liver of these animals. The incorporation of ^{14}C into DNA thymine is drastically reduced in ascites cells by MTX (120). Methotrexate has also been shown to block the degradation of histidine at the formiminotransferase level, which results in increased excretion of formiminoglutamic acid in the urine of patients receiving this drug (13). These results clearly indicate that all major routes to one carbon metabolism are effectively blocked by MTX. This remarkable effect of MTX on one carbon metabolism has a profound influence on rapidly proliferating cells. In most cells, the leading cause of cell death is inhibition of thymidylate synthesis (117) and consequently MTX kills cells in the S phase. In addition, MTX also inhibits the syntheses of purines, RNA and proteins. Therefore, MTX also slows the entry of cells into the S phase. Because of the broader and more general inhibition of MTX on one carbon metabolism it is unable to accomplish an ideal thymineless death.

Borsa and Whitmore (12) observed that the cytotoxicity of MTX was enhanced in certain cultured cell lines when they were exposed to purines in absence of thymine. In certain other systems the cytotoxicity of MTX actually decreased when the cells were exposed to purines, indicating the antipurine effect of the drug. A combination of thymidine and deoxy adenosine could completely reverse the cytotoxicity of MTX in a variety of experimental systems. From these results, it would appear that the cytotoxicity of MTX is due to the depletion of both purine and pyrimidine nucleotides.

Methotrexate is most effective against those tumors with a high growth fraction where the demand for DNA is very high. Therefore, it is not surprising that MTX is curative to Burkitt's lymphoma and choriocarcinoma, both of which have doubling time of less than two days. On the contrary, MTX is not as effective in the treatment of those tumors such as lung and colon cancer which have a doubling time of 3 months. Due to these reasons, MTX toxicity will be more pronounced, and confined to those tissues which have a relatively high growth fraction (135). These include gastrointestinal mucosa, bone marrow and hair follicles. Bone marrow depression, gastrointestinal bleeding and hair loss are very common toxic symptoms in patients receiving MTX chemotherapy. A 72 hr plasma concentration of the drug at 10^{-7} M or above has been associated with high toxicity. Renal toxicity has been observed due to precipitation of the drug in the kidney. The major component of the precipitated material was shown to be 7-hydroxymethotrexate (69). The renal status of the patients has to be carefully monitored, and proper hydration and alkalinization of the urine is necessary to enhance drug clearance. The toxic effect of MTX on bone marrow is manifested as leukopenia and thrombocytopenia. It is absolutely necessary to monitor the leukocyte and platelet counts periodically. Ulceration and bleeding of the intestinal tract and damage to the buccal mucosa are common consequences of methotrexate toxicity. Methotrexate is known to produce hepatotoxicity, and frequent measurements of hepatic enzymes are of clinical value. Other toxic symptoms include alopecia, anorexia, nausea, skin rashes and osteoporosis. Encephalopathy, neurotoxicity, and meningeal irritation have been observed as toxic side effects of intrathecal administration of MTX (142).

Another closely related potent inhibitor of DHFR is aminopterin (**2**). Both aminopterin and methotrexate (**3**) were synthesized by Seeger *et al.*, in 1947 and 1949, respectively (123, 124). Methotrexate is widely used in the treatment of many solid tumor and hematologic malignancies. Major clinical uses of methotrexate are in the treatment of choriocarcinoma, carcinomas of the head and neck, acute lymphocytic leukemia, cancer of the cervix and breast cancer. In the early 1960s, it was reported by Hertz *et al.* (60, 61), that methotrexate was able to produce permanent remission of choriocarcinoma in women. Burkitt *et al.* (15) and Bertino (6) reported the remarkable success of treating Burkitt's lymphoma with methotrexate and reported that 20% of the survivors were free of the disease for up to six years in some series.

In 1966, Burchenal (14a) reported that patients suffering from acute leukemia can be treated with MTX, which produced long-term remissions beyond five years in 65% of 132 cases. In the remission maintenance phase of anti-leukemic therapy intrathecal methotrexate is frequently used (when tumor cells infiltrate into the central nervous system in leukemia patients). The first example of a cure of cancer was achieved with the use of MTX in the treatment of gestational choriocarcinoma of women (60). Methotrexate is also being used to achieve objective responses in patients with epidermoid carcinoma of the cervix, lung cancer and other solid tumors (5). Bitran and co-workers (10) reported a 50% response rate in the treatment of non-small cell bronchogenic carcinoma with a combination of cyclophosphamide, doxorubicin, methotrexate and procarbazine. Methotrexate has also been used in the treatment of advanced gastric cancer (14). A chemotherapy regimen consisting of cisplatin, bleomycin and methotrexate was used for the treatment of advanced squamous cell carcinoma of the head and neck. In this regimen, all evaluable patients had significant reduction ($> 50\%$) of measurable tumor. Complete regression was noted in 27% of patients (43). Methotrexate is still the single drug of choice for the treatment of meningeal leukemia. In spite of this documented success of MTX as a widely used anticancer drug, the toxicity of the drug, particularly to normal proliferating tissues, is a major problem associated with its clinical use.

In order to minimize the toxicity of methotrexate certain rescue techniques have been developed and clinically used with varying degrees of success. The use of high dose methotrexate followed by leucovorin is the most frequently used method to improve the chemotherapeutic index of MTX. Leucovorin is the trivial name for N^5-formyl tetrahydrofolic acid. This compound is also known as citrovorum factor (CF) or folinic acid. The rationale for the design of this rescue technique was based on the assumption that citrovorum factor (CF) does not compete with MTX, at the sites of action of the latter. While MTX is a very powerful inhibitor of DHFR, CF has practically no effect on this enzyme at the levels used, but is a folate coenzyme intermediate which can be interconverted to those coenzyme derivatives, the formation of which are inhibited by MTX. Other methods to alleviate the toxicity of MTX was examined by Kisliuk and co-workers (81) using animal models. They showed that an ip injection of a *L. casei* dihydrofolate reductase preparation into rats and mice given a single dose of MTX caused a marked lowering of free MTX in the blood. Alternatives to CF such as *dl*,L-5-methyl tetrahydrofolate, *d,l*-L-5-methylene tetrahydrofolate and *l*,L-5,10-methylene tetrahydrofolate were effective MTX antagonists. It was interesting to note that *d*,L-5,10-methylene tetrahydrofolate was completely inert.

The design of another rescue technique has the following biochemical rationale. As discussed earlier CF can be metabolized to N^5,N^{10}-methenyl tetrahydrofolate and N^{10}-formyl tetrahydrofolate. These two compounds are necessary for the *de novo* synthesis of purines. It can also be metabolized to N^5,N^{10}-methylene tetrahydrofolate which is the coenzyme needed for *de novo* thymidylate biosynthesis. Since MTX blocks both purine and dTMP biosynthesis, it was hypothesized that a more selective rescue can be accomplished by providing thymidine rather than CF. The end result would be to preserve the antipurine effect of MTX and to bypass the block of MTX on thymidylate synthesis. If, for instance, some tumors are more sensitive to an antipurine effect, a thymidine rescue will be more selective than a CF rescue (64).

Sirotnak and co-workers (126) provided a pharmacologic perspective of high dose MTX therapy with CF in murine tumor models and showed that the uptake of MTX at these levels (800 mg/kg) showed saturation kinetics and the drug persisted much longer in the tumor cells than in the small intestine. The effect of delayed CF on drug levels was the same in tumor cells and small intestine, but much more CF was required to initiate recovery of DNA synthesis in tumor cells. A schedule employing 24 mg/kg of CF sc, 16 hr after 400 mg/kg MTX sc, gave a two-log tumor cell kill and prevented lethal toxicity in most animals.

In the clinical treatment of certain neoplasms high dose methotrexate therapy with CF rescue has been used to improve the therapeutic index of MTX treatment (7, 52, 53). Djerassi and co-workers, developed the use of high-dose pulse methotrexate with citrovorum factor during the course of their studies in childhood acute leukemia (36) lymphosarcoma (37) and primary carcinoma of the lung (35). Although there are conflicting reports about the efficacy of such treatments (125), it has been shown by Djerassi *et al.* (34) that administration in continuous infusion of massive doses of CF reduced potentially lethal toxicity of MTX in several patients with different carcinoma. These results are summarized in Table 3.

Incidence of drug related deaths secondary to high dose methotrexate and CF administration was reported in 498 treated patients. Wide variation in the percentage of fatal toxicities from investigator to investigator was observed with a range of 0–29% (139). As Djerassi notes, the main difficulty with this method is unpredictable toxicity and even in 'good risk' individuals with normal renal function catastrophic side effects may develop.

Results of a study at Memorial Sloan-Kettering Cancer Center (115) has shown that the treatment of metastatic osteogenic sarcoma with high dose methotrexate and leucovorin rescue can be successful only if it is administered in 'exactly the way that experience has dictated objective responses will occur'. A major breakthrough in the chemo therapy of osteogenic sarcoma was reported in 1972 by Jaffe and Paed (71). A threshold dose of 300 mg/kg was initially suggested below which there was no response. Rosen and Nirenberg (115) reported a 40% complete response rate of osteogenic sarcoma to single-agent, high dose methotrexate with leucovorin rescue. The overall partial and complete response was 68%. With more than 5 years experience in treating 200 patients with evaluable disease with approximately 5000 high dose methotrexate treatments, the effective dose of MTX was found to be 8 g/m² in fully grown adoles-

Table 3. Massive CF for potentially lethal MTX-toxicity. Data from Djerassi *et al.*: *Cancer Treat Rep* 61: 749–750, 1977.

Patient No.	Diagnosis	MTX dose (g)	Day of MTX toxicity	Toxic signs	CF	Status
1	Glioma	50	4	Throat and mouth ulcers, skin rash, and jaundice	3 g/1 day	Improved in 24 hr; recovered
2	Carcinoma, lung	30	4	Skin rash and throat and mouth ulcers	3 g/1 day	Improved in 36 hr; cleared in 4 days
3	Carcinoma, lung	18	5	Skin rash, trachial irritation, mucosal ulcers, and jaundice	2 g/1 day	Improved in 48 hr; recovered
5	Hepatoma	12	4	Skin rash and throat and mouth ulcers	1 g/1 day	Improved in 24 hr; recovered
6	Carcinoma, lung	24	5	Mucosal ulcers	4 g/2 days	Improved in 48 hr; recovered
7	Carcinoma, colon	6	2	Skin rash and mouth ulcers	8 g/2 days	Improved in 48 hr; recovered
8	Glioma	24	7	Skin rash and mucosal ulcer	4 g/1 day	Improved in 36 hr; recovered
9	Lymphosarcoma	3 2	4 5	Skin rash and mucosal ulcer	4 g/2 days	Improved in 48 hr; recovered
10	Lymphosarcoma	1.2	4	Skin rash	3 g/1 day	Improved in 24 hr; recovered

cents and $12 g/m^2$ in younger children. The serum levels of MTX should be monitored and leucovorin should be continued until serum MTX level falls below $10^{-7} M$. A 72-hr serum MTX level of $10^{-7} M$ can be potentially toxic. The alkalinization of the urine for the first 24 hr is beneficial to prevent renal toxicity. Under a carefully monitored treatment schedule, these investigators found that high dose MTX with CF rescue is extremely effective in the treatment of osteogenic sarcoma. However, effective chemotherapy of osteogenic sarcoma is difficult to perform, and should not be attempted by those who are not well experienced in the use of high dose MTX with CF rescue.

Several attempts to direct MTX more specifically to target tumor cells have appeared recently. These include, conjugation of the drug with macromolecules of varying specificity such as tumor specific antigens, liposomes and polyamino acids (118). For example, MTX polylysine complex readily penetrate the resistant tumor cells which are deficient in the transport of the drug. It is hoped that the proper selection and use of such conjugates will result in a more favorable chemotherapeutic index of MTX in the treatment of various forms of human cancers.

Metabolism of methotrexate

As a protective measure, mammals usually metabolize ingested foreign substances to compounds, with reduced biological activity, and to structures which permits their easy excretion from the body. The potent folate antagonists aminopterin (2), and MTX (3) were thought to be exceptions to this general phenomenon, because virtually almost all administered drug could be recovered unchanged from urine and feces (45, 59). However, Oliverio and Loo (108) reported that the 3′,5′-dichloro analogue of MTX (DCM) underwent metabolic alteration *in vivo*, and the metabolite of this folate antagonists could be recovered from the urine. In a subsequent paper (84), the structure of this metabolite was disclosed to be 7-hydroxy-DCM. On close examination (72), it was found that not only the dichloro analogue, but also the parent drugs aminopterin and methotrexate, including several other derivatives could be converted to their respective 7-hydroxy derivative in several mammalian species. In rabbit liver, the oxidizing activity was found to be due to aldehyde oxidase. During high-dose MTX therapy, significant amounts of 7-hydroxymethotrexate are eliminated in the urine of humans (69). Conversion of methotrexate to 4-amino-4-deoxy-N^{10}-methyl pteroic acid by intestinal bacteria has been observed in mice. Similar metabolic conversion of MTX in man has not yet been demonstrated. It appears that the metabolism of methotrexate is species specific, and dose dependent, and some of the metabolic pathways of the drug has been overlooked by previous workers due to these reasons.

Although studies in man and certain animals indicated that MTX may, in large part, be recovered as unaltered drug within 24 hr, a minor proportion of the drug was retained in tissues for long periods. The major fraction of this material, having half-life of about 3 months may be recovered from the liver. Significant proportions of the long half-life MTX may also be recovered from the intestine, stomach, and kidneys (107). It was postulated that the long half-life MTX

was actually the proportion of the drug which is bound to dihydrofolate reductase in an irreversible manner, and the drug persists in the cell during its entire lifetime.

The first report on the nature of the long half-life MTX in mammalian tissues emerged from our laboratories (3). Preliminary work tentatively identified two MTX conjugates in red blood cells from a leukemic patient undergoing MTX therapy as the poly-γ-glutamates of MTX having two and three glutamate residues respectively. Additional experiments in rats using tritiated MTX, led to the isolation and characterization of the di- and triglutamates of MTX ($MTXG_1$ and $MTXG_2$) from the tissues of these animals. The unequivocal structural characterization of these metabolites were subsequently accomplished by the unambiguous chemical syntheses of all potential poly-γ-glutamates of MTX, and comparing these synthetic samples with the natural metabolites (95). Subsequent to our work, various investigators have confirmed the formation of the poly-γ-glutamyl metabolites of MTX in tissues of various mammalian species, including man. The structures (21) of these metabolites are shown in Figure 7.

In order to assess the role of this newly discovered polyglutamates to the overall antitumor activity of MTX, evaluation of the biological activity of the metabolites themselves were undertaken. The relative potencies of these analogs in inhibiting the growth of *S. faecium* decreased, as the chain length of the glutamate residues increased (95). It was not known at that time whether the decreased potency was due to the inability of these compounds to penetrate the bacterial wall as efficiently as MTX or their decreased ability to inhibit DHFR. Subsequently, other investigators (68, 70) established that MTX conjugates with a chain length of up to six glutamate moieties were equally powerful as the parent drug in inhibiting DHFR from various sources *in vitro*. The diglutamate showed activity equal to MTX in increasing the survival time of mice bearing L1210 leukemia.

Kisliuk and co-workers (78) found that the polyglutamates of MTX are potent inhibitors of thymidylate synthase derived from several different sources. The triglutamate (MTX G_2) inhibited *L. casei* thymidylate synthase by 50% at $2 \times 10^{-7} M$. This metabolite was 100 times more inhibitory to the *E. coli* enzyme than MTX. Therefore, at least in this instance, a definite additional role of these metabolites to the overall chemotherapeutic effectiveness of MTX became apparent. Cheng and co-workers (21) investigated the effects of various folate and MTX analogues on human thymidylate synthase activity and found that increasing the number of gamma glutamyl residues increased their respective binding affinities towards the enzyme. The other two widely speculated roles of these metabolites with regard to their contribution to cytotoxicity are (1) the greater persistence of these metabolites in the cells, and (2) differential synthesis of the polyglutamates in tumor versus normal proliferative tissues. The greater persistence of these metabolites in the cells may be due to their slower efflux rate, especially with those having longer chain length compared to the efflux rate of MTX. Differential synthesis may be attributed to the enhanced synthesis of the metabolites in the tumor and/or the synthesis of longer chain length metabolites in the tumor versus normal tissues. At any rate, there is a growing consensus among investigators that polyglutamation of MTX has a significant role in the chemotherapeutic effectiveness of this drug.

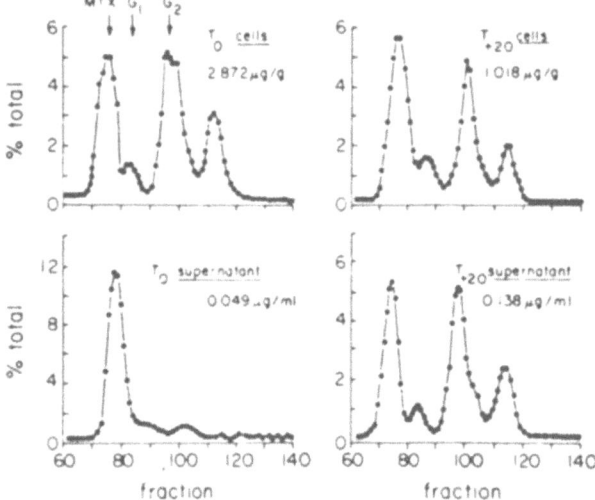

Figure 3. Radioactive elution profiles after DEAE-Sephadex chromatography of heat-treated cellular or supernatant extracts, with *D. pneumoniae* dihydrofolate reductase added to the cell suspension. The vertical axis is total drug, which was 2.872 μg/g wet weight for T_0 cells, 1.018 g/g for T_{+20} cells, after 20 min at 37°; 0.049 μg/ml for T_0 supernatant, 0.138 μg/g for T_{+20} supernatant, after 20 min at 37°. The net intracellular decrease shown equals the net extracellular accumulation. (L1210 cells). Adapted from Poser, Sirotnak and Chello: *Biochem Pharmacol* 29:2701–2704, 1980.

With regard to the synthesis of the polyglutamates it appears that the same synthetase is involved in the polyglutamation of both MTX and natural folates. Whitehead and Rosenblat (144) using mutant Chinese hamster ovary cells, which lack folypolyglutamate synthetase activity showed that these cells are incapable of synthesizing MTX-polyglutamates. While folate polyglutamates having up to eight glutamate residues are readily formed, metabolites of MTX having more than four glutamate residues are formed only in small quantities at higher doses. Thus, the formation of only MTX G_5 has been recognized. One explanation for this different pattern of metabolism by MTX, compared to the natural folates, may be due to the fact that the DHFR bound MTX and its glutamate conjugates are not substrates for the synthetase. Some evidence to support this hypothesis are at hand. MTX resistant baby hamster kidney cells having high levels of DHFR were also shown to require higher concentrations of MTX compared to the sensitive cells for polyglutamate synthesis to occur, indicating that DHFR bound MTX is a poor substrate for the synthetase.

The synthesis of MTX polyglutamates in L1210 murine leukemia cells was reported by Whitehead (143). Jacobs and co-workers (68) found that the diglutamate of methotrexate was accumulated in human liver during MTX therapy. Like the folate cofactors, MTX is metabolized *in vitro* to their polygamma glutamates of varying chain length in murine tissues and tumors (113, 114). Various investigators have speculated that like folate, MTX polyglutamates are indeed storage forms of the drug and they efflux from the cell at a slower rate than free MTX (24, 31, 143). They rationalized that those tissues which are capable of enhanced conversion of MTX to polyglutamates will also have a higher persist-

ence of this drug. Poser, Sirotnak and Chello (113) in an elegant study demonstrated that $MTXG_1$, $MTXG_2$ and $MTXG_3$ efflux from L1210 cells at the same rate as MTX itself (Figure 3). Earlier workers, were unable to detect the efflux of these compounds because the extracellular efflux medium they used contained the enzyme conjugase, which apparently hydrolysed the effluxed polyglutamates to MTX, before they could be detected. To prevent the effluxed polyglutamates from being hydrolyzed by conjugate, Sirotnak added hydrofolate reductase to the medium; thereby trapping the effluxed compounds. Dihydrofolate reductase bound MTX polyglutamates are very poor substrates of the hydrolytic enzyme, conjugate. (Pteroylglutamyl-γ-glutamyl hydrolase). In a subsequent study Sirotnak also found that polyglutamate synthesis in L1210 cells is dose and time dependent, and he detected the formation of MTX polyglutamates of higher chain lengths of up to five glutamate residues, when tumor-bearing mice were treated with [^{3}H]MTX at doses ranging from 3 mg to 400 mg/kg. Under these conditions, no detectable amounts of pentaglutamates were found in the small intestine of the same animal. The formation of a metabolite of still higher chain length with six glutamate residues to an appreciable extent was observed in these tumor-bearing animals at a dose of 12 mg/kg after 16 and 24 hrs. Again, no hexaglutamate was detected in the drug limiting small intestine. These experiments indicated for the first time that tumor specificity in the formation of MTX polyglutamates exists, and it may contribute to the overall therapeutic responsiveness and toxicity of MTX.

Investigations by Goldman (55) revealed that a portion of intracellular MTX in excess to that bound to DHFR may play a critical role in the chemotherapeutic activity of the drug. Although the membrane transport parameters do not appear to affect the rate of decline of intracellular MTX or MTX polyglutamates *in vivo*, they do affect the intracellular concentration of the drug achieved, and thereby influence the synthesis of these metabolites (48). Therefore, it is conceivable that other factors being the same, those tissues or tumors which are able to transport MTX at a faster rate will invariably contain a larger fraction of the drug in the polyglutamate form. As free MTX decline within the cell, the polyglutamates replace the monoglutamate on DHFR and from a relatively stable pool of antifolates above the enzyme binding capacity (49, 116).

The greater persistence of MTX at pharmacologically effective levels in tumor versus normal proliferative tissue has indeed been associated with the selective action of this drug (129). In order to determine the pharmacologic importance of MTX-polyglutamates, Jolivet and co-workers (74) examined the formation, retention, and effect of these metabolites in cultured human breast cancer cells. The two cell lines MCF-7 and ZR-75-B converted MTX to polyglutamates in a dose and time-dependent fashion (Figures 4A and B). All of the MTX G_4 and 47 and 38% of MTX G_3 remained in MCF-7 and ZR-75-B cells respectively and could be identified in the cytosol after 24 hr in drug free medium. These polyglutamates which were retained in the cell lines in excess of DHFR binding capacity led to inhibition of thymidylate and loss of cell viability after removal of extracellular MTX. Although MTX polyglutamates of shorter chain lengths efflux from the cells at the same rate as MTX, those with higher chain lengths are effluxed at a slower rate, thereby partially contributing to the overall retention of the

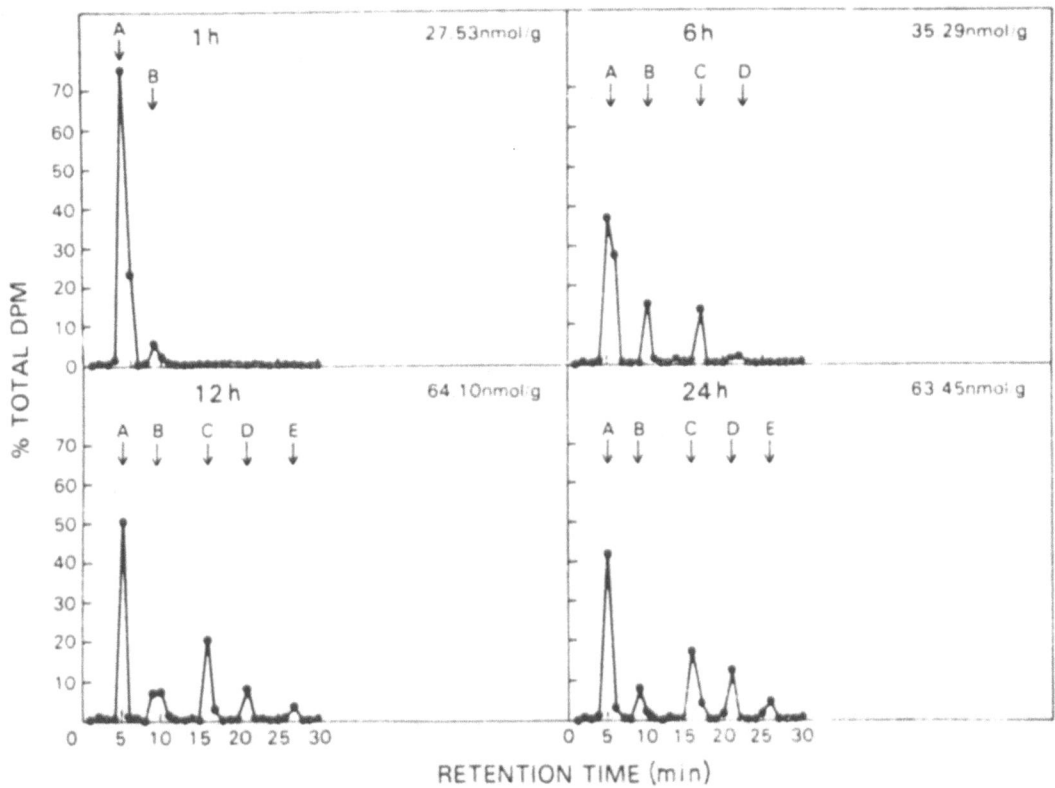

Figure 4A. Time course of MTXPG formation in MCF-7 cells. After 1-, 6-, 12-, and 24-hr incubations with $2 M [^3H]MTX$, cell extracts were chromatographed by HPLC. Peaks A to E represent, respectively, $4-NH_2-10-CH_3-PteGlu_1$ (MTX) to $4-NH_2-10-CH_3-PteGlu_5$. The total amount of intracellular drug in nanomoles per gram of cell protein is given at each time point (70). Data from Jolivet *et al.*: *J Clin Invest* 70:351–360, 1982.

drug in certain tissues. Such prolonged retention of the drug in a non-effluxable form, combined with the differential synthesis of these metabolites is undoubtedly related to the overall therapeutic index of methotrexate. The exact contribution of MTX polyglutamates of varying chain length to the cytotoxicity of MTX is not precisely known at this writing. A great deal of research has to be done to unravel the biological role of these metabolites, and to exploit such results in a practical way to the development of more effective antifolates. One appealing area would be the development of powerful inhibitors of DHFR, capable of enhanced polyglutamation in the tumor, compared to MTX. If such compounds have better chemotherapeutic indices than MTX, further research along these lines might produce very selective antifolates. It may be possible to predict (25) the efficacy of MTX therapy by measuring the extent of MTX-polyglutamate formation in the tumor versus normal tissues of patients undergoing MTX therapy.

Transport and resistance

Transport of MTX to tumor cells plays a very important role in the therapeutic effectiveness of this drug (129). The transport parameters do govern the absolute levels of intracellular MTX, which, in turn, influences the cytotoxicity

of the drug by various mechanisms (48). Defective transport of MTX has been associated with MTX-resistance in certain tumor cells (127). Due to these reasons, investigations regarding the transport of MTX to tumor cells continues to be an active area of current research.

The uptake of natural folates and folate analogues to mammalian cells has been studied by various investigators; and these were reviewed by Goldman (54). Transport of folate compounds in to cultured L1210 murine leukemia cells is an active process requiring energy, is carried mediated and saturable. Two separate transport systems are known to mediate the transport process. One of these is specific for folic acid, and the other one for reduced folates such as 5-methyl tetrahydrofolate. These two systems are readily distinguished. For example, the reduced folate pathway is sensitive to sulfhydryl inhibitors. The uptake of 5-methyltetrahydrofolate is competitively inhibited by MTX and vice versa; but neither compounds inhibit the uptake of folate (65). Using newly synthesized folate analogues, Hornbeak and Nair (63) confirmed the existence of two transport systems in HeLa cells, one specific for folic acid, and the other one for MTX. In human lymphocytes the uptake of folic acid and natural reduced folates occurred by separate pathways, and MTX shared the transport system of the latter (27). Folate analogue transport by isolated murine intestinal epithelial cells was examined by Chello and co-

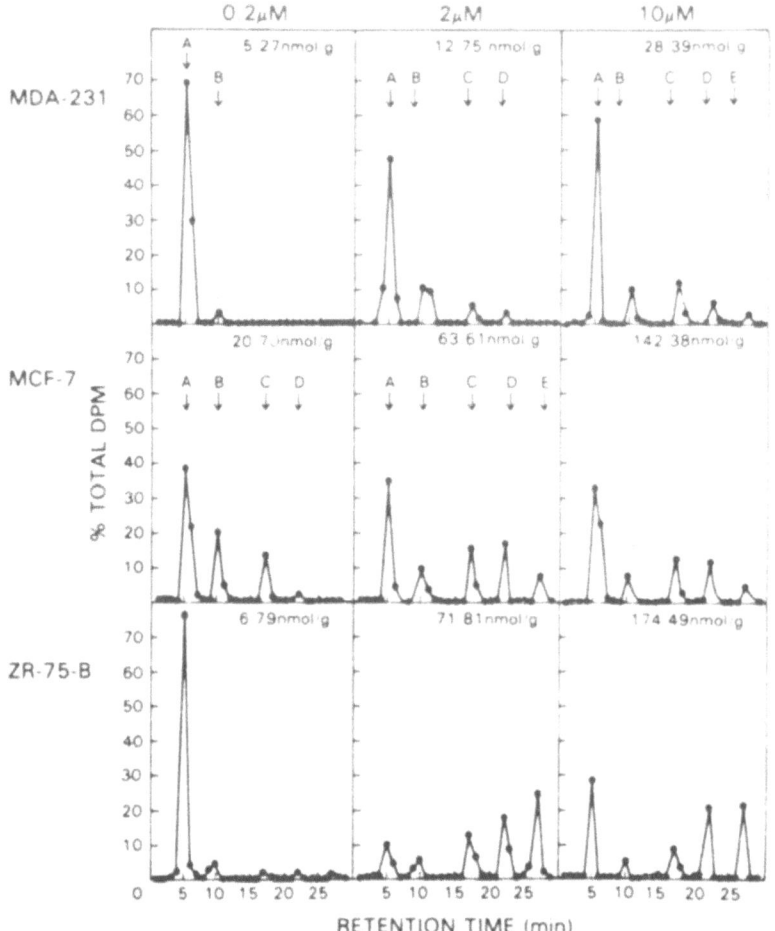

Figure 4B. Dose-response of MTXPG formation in human breast cancer cells. 24-hr incubations with either 0.2, 2, or 10 M [³H]MTX were done in the MDA-231, MCF-7, and ZR-75-B cells, following which cell extracts were chromatographed by HPLC. Peaks A to E represent, respectively, 4-NH₂-10-CH₃-PteGlu₁ (MTX) to 4-NH₂-10-CH₃-Pte-Glu₅. The total amount of intracellular drug in nanomoles per gram of cell protein is given at each time point (132). Data from Jolivet *et al.*: J Clin Invest *70:351–360, 1982.*

workers (20). Suspensions of these cells transported MTX and exhibited Michaelis–Menton saturation kinetics. The influx of the drug was competitively inhibited by natural folates. The transport system exhibited structural specificity for substituents at the 10 position of the folate molecule. The data supported the notion of carried-mediated transport of MTX and other folate analogues.

Several MTX-resistant tumor cells have a defective transport system for influx of the drug. Therefore, it is appealing to consider the possibility of developing powerful antifolates which are capable of being transported by the folic acid transport system for the treatment of transport defective MTX-resistant tumors. Correlations of structure activity relationships with regard to the relative ability of various folate analogues to be transported by each of these transport systems will be very useful in the design of such compounds in the future (62). One such analogue is 10-Oxa aminopterin (99) which was shown to be able to compete with the transport of folic acid in HeLa cells (63). Since MTX shares the same transport system with CF (92), the clinical use of an

antifolate which can be transported through the folic acid transport system in high doses in combination with citrovorum factor (CF) might permit a selective rescue of the host cells, while preserving the antitumor activity of the drug towards the resistant tumor cells.

In spite of the extremely potent anticancer activity of MTX, the clinical usefulness of this drug is limited to a certain extent due to drug resistance. Tumors may acquire resistance as treatment progresses; or some tumors may be inherently resistant to MTX (58). There are several mechanisms by which tumors may accrue resistance to methotrexate: (a) increased levels of dihydrofolate reductase, (b) structural alterations of this target enzyme, (c) restricted uptake of the drug and (d) inactivation of the drug by the resistant cells (5, 17). Methotrexate resistance, which is associated with an elevation of the target enzyme, has been shown to be due to amplification of the gene coding for DHFR. This gene amplification may occur within a single chromosome, producing an expanded homogeniously staining region containing multiple copies of the DHFR gene.

Resistance acquired through such a mechanism is stable and can be passed to both daughter cells during mitosis However, gene amplification on the double minute chromosome is unstable in the absence of the selecting agent (9, 40, 106, 122).

High elevation of the target enzyme DHFR is very common in resistant cells, and they always tend to maintain zone-free enzyme in excess of the binding capacity of the drug (57). In a methotrexate resistant strain of S180 cells (AT/300) the synthesis of DHFR actually represents 6 to 7 percent of the soluble protein synthesis (1). In certain MTX resistant cell lines the rate of DHFR synthesis may be 200–250 fold greater than the sensitive parental line. Domin, Cheng, and Hakala (40) isolated the DHFR from a methotrexate resistant subline of human KB cells, having high levels of this enzyme. They demonstrated that the human KB/MTX enzyme is different from the mouse S180 AT/300 DHFR in its isoelectric point, turnover number, and K_i for MTX. From these studies, they pointed out that extrapolation of enzyme data from other mammalian sources to human enzyme is not warranted. Although, acquired MTX resistance has resulted in the marked elevation of both DHFR and thymidylate synthase (EC 2.1.1.45) in certain bacteria, concurrent elevation of folate dependent enzymes other than DHFR has not been encountered in the mammalian system. Unstable MTX-resistance was observed by Curt and co-workers (26) in human small cell carcinoma. This cell line displayed amplification of the DHFR gene and a large number of double minute chromosomes. Progressive loss of drug resistance was observed when these cells underwent serial passage in tissue culture. This loss of resistance was in association with loss of double minute chromosomes and a decline in dihydrofolate reductase levels.

In order to overcome MTX-resistance due to defective transport of the drug Ryser and Shen (118) investigated the use of a conjugate of MTX with poly(L-lysine). MTX and [³H] MTX were conjugated through a carbodiimide catalyzed reaction to a 70 000 molecular weight poly(L-lysine) in molar ratios of approximately 13 to 1. The MTX conjugate, was transported at a much faster rate in both transport proficient and deficient Chinese hamster ovary cells. The 100-fold difference in drug concentration needed to inhibit the mutant cells and their corresponding wild type was totally abolished by exposing the resistant cells to MTX-Poly(Lys). Since the MTX conjugate did not inhibit DHFR, these authors concluded that, after being transported to the resistant cell lines, the conjugate is hydrolyzed to release the free drug within the cell. The possible delivery of MTX to resistant cells in the form of macromolecular complexes to overcome resistance is an area of active investigation at the present time.

Analogues of methotrexate

In spite of the fact that a large number of aminopterin analogues were synthesized and evaluated, methotrexate continues to enjoy the reputation as one of the very best inhibitors of DHFR. At this writing, it can be stated with some degree of confidence that no further improvement in the inhibitory potency towards DHFR can be expected from close analogues of MTX. Such improvements, if at all possible will in all likelihood result in more toxic compounds.

However, in contrast to the inhibition of DHFR, there are other biological and pharmacological parameters, which might be exploited for the development of analogues with better chemotherapeutic indices than MTX. Some of the parameters include differences in the rate of influx and efflux; polyglutamation, metabolic activation and deactivation of these analogues in the tumor versus normal proliferative tissues. For example, if an analogue which is equally potent as MTX in inhibiting DHFR can be selectively accumulated in the tumor compared to normal intestinal epithelium or bone marrow either by enhanced transport or polyglutamation; it might exhibit a definite therapeutic advantage over MTX.

The transport characteristics of MTX-analogues were shown to be sensitive to structural changes at the C^9,N^{10}-bridge region (128). Several close analogues of aminopterin with structural changes at the C^9,N^{10}-region were synthesized and evaluated using several biochemical and pharmacological test systems (Figure 5). Some of these compounds are N^{10}-propargyl aminopterin **4** (111) N^{10}-cyanomethylaminopterin **5** (94) 10-deaza aminopterin **6**; 10-ethyl-10-deaza aminopterin **7** (32, 33) 10-thio aminopterin (100) 10-oxa aminopterin (91, 99) 11-thiohomoaminopterin (98) and 11-oxa homoaminopterin (97). One of these analogues, 10-deaza aminopterin **6**, exhibited very interesting biological activity. With regard to its inhibition of DHFR and inhibition of growth of *Streptococcus faecium* and *Lactobacillus casei* 10-DA was classified as one of the most potent antifolates (32). The *in vivo* antitumor activity of 10-DA has been shown to be superior to MTX in mice against three of five ascites tumors and two of three solid tumors (130). When 10-DA was compared with MTX at the optimum dose of 12 mg/kg, the increase in the life span of animals bearing a variety of murine ascites tumors was significantly greater in all cases examined and were outstanding in Ehrlich carcinoma, Taper liver tumor and sarcoma 180 (Table 4). Sirotnak has also shown that when given orally 10-DA was twice as potent as MTX against L1210 leukemia at 6 mg/kg. 10-DA had a greater accumulation in tumor, but the persistence was similar for both drugs in drug limiting normal intestinal epithelium. The influx of both MTX and 10-DA was mediated by the same

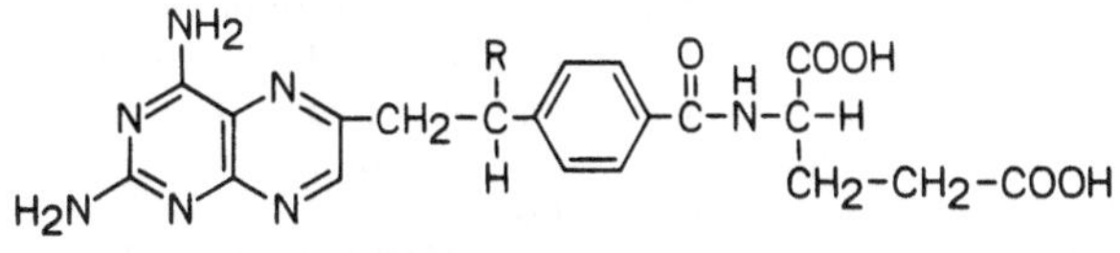

2. R = H
3. R = −CH₃
4. R = −CH₂−C≡CH
5. R = −CH₂−C≡N

6. R = −H
7. R = −CH₂−CH₃

Figure 5. Structures of promising analogues of methotrexate.

Table 4. Relative efficacy of sc administered methotrexate and 10-deaza-aminopterin against a variety of murine ascites tumors. Data from Sirotnak *et al.: Cancer treat Rep* 62: 1047–1051, 1977.

Tumor	Drug	No. of mice*	Dose† (mg/ kg)	MST ± SD (days)	ILS (%)	Average weight‡ (g)
L1210	–	5 × 4	–	6.7 ± 0.8	–	23.1 ± 0.6
	Methotrexate	5 × 2	3	11.5 ± 1.1	71.8	22.8 ± 0.9
		5 × 2	6	14.4 ± 0.8	114.9	22.6 ± 1.9
		5 × 3	9	15.8 ± 0.9	136.0	23.0 ± 1.5
		5 × 3	12	16.7 ± 1.1	149.8	22.2 ± 1.8
		5 × 4	18	15.8 ± 1.9	136.0	18.3 ± 2.4
	10-Deaza-aminopterin	5 × 4	3	13.8 ± 0.7	106.2	22.5 ± 1.7
		5 × 2	6	15.2 ± 1.5	127.0	23.1 ± 2.1
		5 × 3	9	17.9 ± 0.8	167.8	21.5 ± 2.3
		5 × 3	12	18.2 ± 1.3	171.6	20.3 ± 2.3
		5 × 2	18	17.9 ± 1.6	167.8	17.2 ± 2.7
Sarcoma 180	–	5 × 3	–	12.1 ± 1.1	–	28.4 ± 2.7
	Methotrexate	5 × 2	3	11.7 ± 1.7	0	26.2 ± 2.0
		5 × 3	6	15.2 ± 0.9	24.9	29.0 ± 3.1
		5 × 3	9	18.3 ± 2.0	51.3	29.4 ± 2.8
		5 × 3	12	19.8 ± 1.8	64.0	27.2 ± 3.2
		5 × 2	18	19.4 ± 2.7	60.6	19.6 ± 4.1
	10-Deaza-aminopterin	5 × 2	3	15.7 ± 1.1	28.7	26.0 ± 2.2
		5 × 3	6	21.2 ± 1.7	74.8	28.6 ± 1.9
		5 × 4	9	27.2 ± 0.9	124.3	27.2 ± 2.6
		5 × 3	12	> 31.4 ± 2.5	> 159.6§	24.6 ± 2.9
		5 × 2	18	22.1 ± 2.4	84.0	16.8 ± 3.2
P815 plasmacytoma	–	5 × 2	–	8.8 ± 0.9	–	22.4 ± 1.2
	Methotrexate	5 × 2	6	15.4 1.1	75.0	23.4 ± 0.6
		5 × 2	9	17.6 ± 1.6	100.3	22.7 ± 1.7
		5 × 2	12	18.4 ± 1.3	109.1	22.2 ± 0.9
	10-Deaza-aminopterin	5 × 2	6	18.2 ± 1.3	107.5	23.1 ± 0.8
		5 × 2	9	19.0 ± 0.9	116.3	22.4 ± 1.3
		5 × 2	12	19.2 ± 1.2	118.4	19.6 ± 1.8
Ehrlich ascites	–	5 × 2	–	17.2 ± 2.1	–	31.2 ± 1.9
	Methotrexate	5 × 2	6	19.8 ± 2.3	15.1	31.0 ± 2.8
		5 × 2	9	20.8 ± 3.0	20.9	30.4 ± 3.4
		5 × 2	12	20.2 ± 1.9	17.0	29.6 ± 3.2
	10-Deaza-aminopterin	5 × 2	6	23.2 ± 1.8	34.8	30.6 ± 2.4
		5 × 2	9	27.2 ± 2.2	58.1	32.0 ± 4.1
		5 × 2	12	28.2 ± 2.9	64.0	26.6 ± 3.1
Taper liver	–	5 × 2	–	14.2 ± 2.2	–	32.4 ± 1.8
	Methotrexate	5 × 2	6	19.7 ± 2.3	39.0	29.3 ± 2.7
		5 × 2	9	20.6 ± 2.8	44.8	29.7 ± 4.3
		5 × 3	12	20.2 ± 3.1	41.6	30.4 ± 3.8
	10-Deaza-aminopterin	5 × 3	12	26.1 ± 2.9	84.2	29.5 ± 4.8

* No. of mice in each experiment × No. of experiments.
† Given as a single sc injection.
‡ Initial weight = 20 g.
§ Two 60-day survivors.

carrier mechanism and 10-DA showed a greater affinity for the tumor carrier. The differences in the antitumor activities of these drugs can be attributed in part to the differences in their membrane transport to various tissues. The contribution of polyglutamation to antitumor activity, if any, should await further investigations.

Further structural modifications of 10-DA have led to the development of a still better antitumor agent (33). This antifolate, 10-deaza-10-ethyl aminopterin was much superior to 10-DA and exhibited a wide spectrum of anti-

tumor activity in mice. The K_i for the inhibition of L1210 DHFR by compound **7** was 0.0028 nM compared to a K_i of 0.0032 nM for MTX. This ethyl derivative was transported better to L1210 cells in culture than MTX. The Km for the influx of these compounds in this system were 0.89 and 3.42 μM respectively. Finally, the antitumor effects of 10-deaza-10-ethyl aminopterin (**7**), and MTX were determined in mice bearing L1210 leukemia. At the LD_{10} dosages, **7** was considerably more potent than 10-DA, which is itself more potent than MTX. These authors concluded that 'significant improvement in anticancer potential among antifolates can be achieved via modification of their cellular transport and *in vivo* distribution properties. The alterations in lipophilic character about the C^9,N^{10}-bridge region of the folate skeleton were conductive to an improvement in rates of influx into tumor cells versus drug-limiting intestinal epithelium'. Both 10-Deaza aminopterin **6** and its ethyl analogue **7** are undergoing clinical trials at Memorial Sloan-Kettering Cancer Center (131) and it is too early to evaluate their clinical utility. It is hoped that these analogues will offer a greater therapeutic advantage over MTX.

2-Amino-4-oxy antifolates which are not inhibitors of DHFR

According to the definition, a folate antagonist is a compound which is capable of interfering with tetrahydrofolate utilization. Since a large number of folate based coenzymes play a significant role in cellular metabolism, it is conceivable that a powerful inhibitor of any one of these enzymes, can be a potent antifolate. Our discussions on Folate Antagonists belonging to this category will be restricted to those compounds, which are structural analogues of the vitamin folic acid.

As discussed earlier, several MTX-resistant tumors have high levels of dihydrofolate reductase. Rather than developing more powerful inhibitors of DHFR, Friedkin and co-workers (46, 47) were intrigued with the possibility of exploiting high levels of dihydrofolate reductase in resistant cells to convert dihydro analogues of folic acid to lethal tetrahydro derivatives. If a synthetic substrate of DHFR can be enzymatically reduced to its tetrahydro derivative *in vivo*, and if the resulting product is capable of inhibiting a folate dependent enzyme that is crucial to DNA biosynthesis such as thymidylate synthase (EC 2.1.1.45); selective toxicity in the chemotherapy of those cancers that are resistant to MTX can be achieved with varying degrees of success (46, 93). This hypothesis was first subjected to experimental test when DeGraw and co-workers synthesized homofolic acid (**8**) (29). The 7,8-dihydro derivative of homofolic acid served as an excellent substrate of dihydrofolate reductase. This enzymatic reduction product, 1-L-tetrahydrohomofolic acid was shown to be a potent inhibitor of *E. coli* thymidylate synthase (56). However, it was a growth factor for *S. faecium* and *L. casei*. When 7,8-dihydrohomofolate was reduced catalytically to the tetrahydro derivative; the resulting mixture of diastereomers exhibited powerful antifolate activity. This activity was later traced to be due to the "unnatural" diastereomer (80). Homofolic acid **8**, its 7,8-dihydro derivative, and the catalytic reduction product *d,l*-L-tetrahydrohomofolic acid showed *in vivo* antitumor activity in the L1210 murine tumor system (87, 90). These compounds exhibited superior activity against the MTX-resistant tumor line than the sensitive one. A derivative of homofolic acid, *d,l*-L-5-methyl-tetrahydrohomofolate (compound **20**) showed activity against P288 leukemia, Lewis lung carcinoma and B16 melanocarcinoma (77). Because of the alkyl substitution at N^5, compound **20** is chemically more stable than *d,l*-L-tetrahydrohomofolic acid. This compound is presently undergoing Phase 1 clinical trial at the Sidney Farber Cancer Institute in Boston.

The actual mechanism of the cytotoxic action of various homofolate derivatives is not clear. None of the compounds showed potent inhibition of any one of the folate dependent enzymes *in vitro*. There are evidences, however, that various homofolate derivatives inhibit different systems at different sites. The inhibitory effect of *d,l*-L-tetrahydrohomofolate on L1210 serine hydroxymethyl transferase, as well as 5,10-methenyl tetrahydrofolate cyclohydrolase has been documented (77). There is no question, however, that homofolate derivatives interfere with folate metabolism. For example, the toxicity to rhesus monkeys as a result of intravenous administration of the sodium salt of this drug such as anorexia, diarrhea, leukopenia, reticulocytopenia and impaired renal function can be completely reversed by concurrent administration of tetrahydrofolate. Livingston, Crawford and Friedkin (83) have shown that tetrahydrohomofolate does not exert its cytotoxicity by inhibiting either DHFR or thymidylate synthase in MTX-resistant mouse leukemia cells. There is a distinct possibility that these compounds may be metabolized *in vivo* to an antimetabolite which is responsible for their cytotoxicity. Such a metabolite may be a poly-γ-glutamate with a specified chain length (Structure **19**). The 5-methyl derivative of *d,l*-L-tetrahydrohomofolate (**20**) is considerably less toxic to mice than the parent compound at 800–1600 mg/kg. This observation has been confirmed, also in dogs and monkeys. 5-methyl tetrahydrohomofolate is a substrate of cobalamin methyl transferase from mammalian cells. However, this enzyme in intact animals apparently does not metabolize large amounts of this compound. Studies by El-Dareer and co-workers (42) have shown that no appreciable metabolism of this drug occurred in the bodies of mice, dogs or monkeys. Because of the great interest in homofolate derivatives, three reviews have appeared on this subject, and the readers are referred to these reviews for additional details (77, 78, 79). Subsequent to the synthesis and biological evaluation of homofolate derivatives, several 2-amino-4-oxy antifolates were reported from a few laboratories. These compounds are (Figure 6):

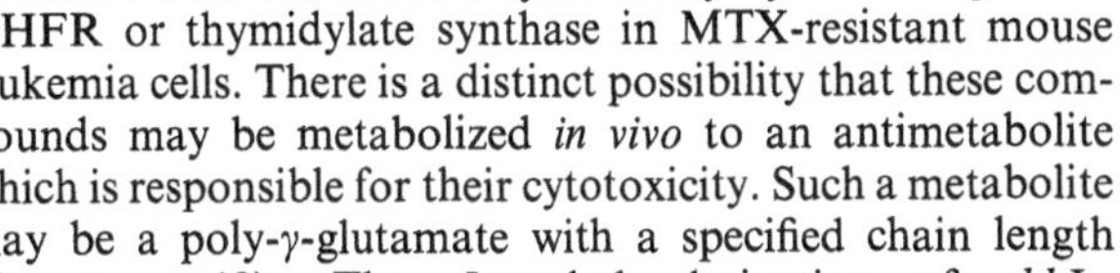

8. X = N; n = 2; Y = -NH
9. X = N; n = 1; Y = S
10. X = N; n = 1; Y = O
11. X = N; n = 2; Y = O
12. X = N; n = 2; Y = S
13. X = -CH; n = 1; Y = -NH

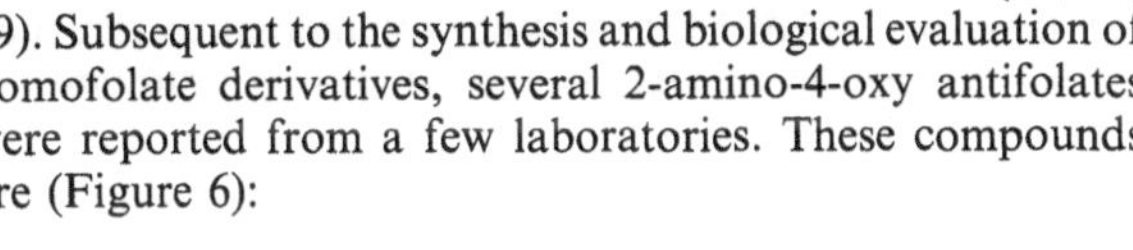

14. R = -CH2-C≡C-H
15. R = -CH2-C≡N
16. R = -CH2-◁
17. R = -CH2-C≡C-CH3

Figure 6. Several 2-amino-4-oxy-antifolates.

(a)   11-Oxahomofolic acid (**11**) and its reduced derivatives (98)
(b)   11-Thiohomofolic acid (**12**) and its reduced derivatives (96)
(c)   Isofolic acid (101)
(d)   10-Thiofolic acid (**9**) (100)
(e)   10-Oxafolic acid (**10**) (99)
(f)   8-Deazafolic acid (**13**) (31)
(g)   10-Deazafolic acid (136)
(h)   5,8-Dideaza-N^{10}-Propargyl folic acid (**14**) (75)
(i)   5,8-Dideaza-N^{10}-cyanomethyl folic acid (**15**) (94)

None of the antifolates mentioned above is a potent inhibitor of DHFR *in vitro*. 11-Oxahomofolic acid (**11**) after chemical reduction to its 7,8-dihydro derivative serves a substrate for *L. casei* DHFR, exhibiting a rate of $> 50\%$ of that of the natural substrate. The enzymatically reduced *l*-L-tetrahydro-11-oxahomofolate showed antifolate activity against both MTX sensitive and MTX resistant strains of *L. casei* and *S. faecium*. The catalytically reduced *d,l*-L-tetrahydro-11-oxahomofolate was 5–10 times more inhibitory than the enzymatic reduction product for both *S. faecium* and *L. casei*. 7,8-dihydro-11-oxahomofolate also served as a substrate for DHFR derived from human KB/6b cell lines. This enzymatic reduction product, however, showed only weak cytotoxicity against human KBP and human KB/6b cell lines in culture (38). Similar investigations were carried out with 11-thiohomofolate and its reduced derivatives. Again, it was observed that the tetrahydro derivative possessing the 'unnatural' configuration at C^6 was more active than the natural isomer.

Another example of a 4-oxy antifolate which showed significant activity in the L1210 system is 8-deazafolic acid (**13**). It is a poor inhibitor of *L. casei* DHFR or thymidylate synthase; or L-1210 DHFR. Other folate analogues which are not inhibitors of DHFR but exhibiting antifolate activity in the microbial system include isofolic acid, (*dl*)-5,8-dideaza-tetrahydrofolate (28); 10-deazafolic acid, 10-oxafolic acid, and 10-thiofolic acid. Some of these analogs were not tested in the mammalian system.

Antifolates which are inhibitors of thymidylate synthase and GAR transformylase

As pointed out earlier, specific inhibitors of thymidylate synthase which are generated *in vivo* by the bioreduction of synthetic substrates of DHFR will have definite advantages in the chemotherapy of those tumors which are overproducers of DHFR. Although this approach is very appealing, the development of such analogues is dependent on the activities of more than one enzyme. Another attractive approach is to develop very specific and potent inhibitors of thymidylate synthase. Several powerful inhibitors of this enzyme such as 5-fluorodeoxy uridine are already available, and a few of them are in clinical use. These inhibitors are analogues of the substrate, deoxy urilylate monophosphate, and they need to be activated by enzymes which are not involved in *de novo* thymidylate biosynthesis, such as thymidine kinase and they frequently get incorporated in biological macromolecules. Such factors seriously limit the clinical usefulness of these compounds.

If, on the other hand, potent inhibitors of thymidylate synthase which are analogues of the coenzyme can be developed, the problems of the need for activation as well as the toxicities associated with the incorporation of the inhibitors to biological macromolecules such as RNA can be eliminated. The reasons are: (a) the independence of coenzyme analogues to metabolic activation; (b) the improbability of the coenzyme analogues becoming incorporated into RNA; (c) a coenzyme analogue which is a specific inhibitor of thymidylate synthase, but not an inhibitor of DHFR will have practically no adverse effect on purine metabolism or other one carbon metabolism pathways; and (d) the metabolic block is confined to the synthesis of only dTMP, which is an obligatory intermediate in *de novo* DNA biosynthesis. In addition to these advantages, these compounds may be expected to have potential use in the chemotherapy of MTX-resistant tumors. Based on these arguments, there have been numerous attempts to develop specific inhibitors of thymidylate synthase of the coenzyme class. The synthesis and biological evaluation of a number of folate and homofolate analogues were carried out during the past two decades. However, with the exception of tetrahydrohomofolate, no other analogue showed any potent inhibition of thymidylate synthase. It was observed by Scanlon et al. (121) and McCuen and Sirotnak (85) that certain 2,4-diamino quinazolines were reasonable inhibitors of thymidylate synthase. In the 2-amino-4-hydroxy-5,8-dideazafolates (4-oxy quinazoline series) it was demonstrated (18) that a methyl group introduced in the 5-position impairs the inhibition, but the same substituent at the tenth position enhances it. As part of a systematic attempt in modifying the structure of 5,8-dideazafolic acid to develop more powerful inhibitors of thymidylate synthase, Jones and co-workers (75) introduced a propargyl substituent at the N^{10}-position of the parent compound. The resulting N^{10}-propargyl-5,8-dideazafolic acid (**14**) exhibited outstanding inhibition of thymidylate synthase derived from L1210 cells with a K_i of 1 nM. The actual mechanism by which **14** inhibits the enzyme is not clear. Presumably, this inhibition which is competitive with respect to N^5,N^{10}-methylene tetrahydrofolate is due to the fact that **14** is a transition state analogue of the coenzyme and that the propargyl substitution at the N^{10}-position increases the affinity of this drug towards the catalytic site of the enzyme. This quinazoline analogue, which is also known as CB-3717 or PDDF showed excellent activity in causing long-term survival of mice inoculated with L1210 cells (Figure 8). It was also active against MTX-resistant L-1210 leukemia (high reductase) in mice.

FURTHER RESEARCH

The key question – how and why a particular drug may kill tumor cells more selectively than the normal cells – has to be answered clearly and completely before a cure for cancer can be found. It is known that certain antifolates show tumor specificity because they are selectively retained in the tumor, either by enhanced transport to or metabolism within these cells. Differential metabolism of antifolates such as polyglutamate synthesis in the tumor versus normal proliferative tissues is known to occur in a variety of tumors; and the contribution of this differential metabolism to the overall chemotherapeutic efficacy of the drug needs to be unravelled. Analogues of MTX which are capable of enhanced

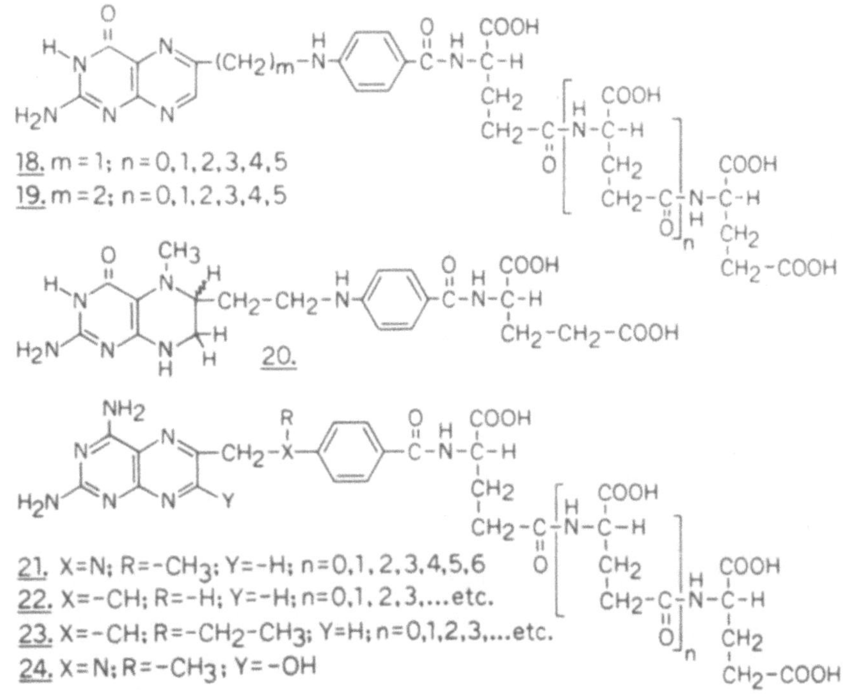

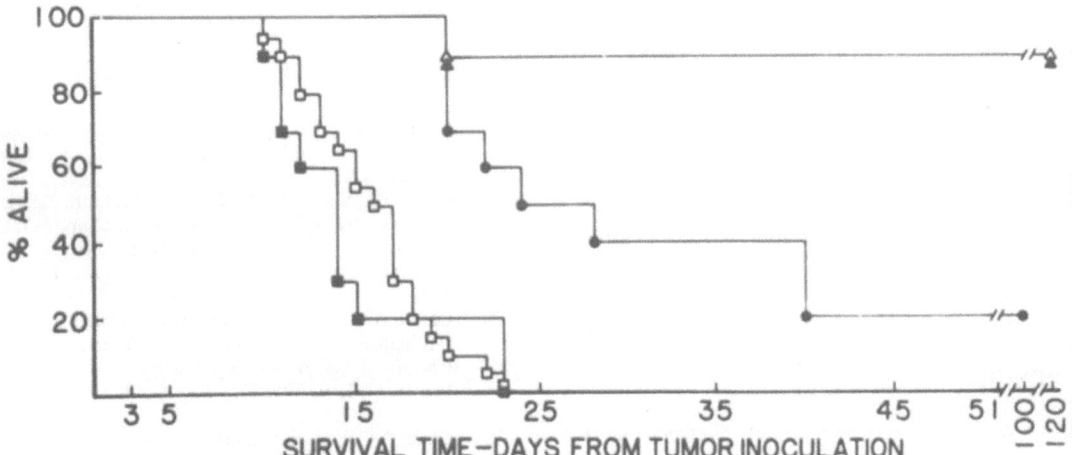

Figure 7. The structures of various poly-γ-glutamates of folic acid; homofoloic acid; methotrexate, 10-deaza aminopterin; 10-deaza-10-ethyl aminopterin; the experimental drug N^5-methyl-tetrahydrohomofolate (**20**) and 7-thydroxymethotrexate [(**24**); $n = 0$].

polyglutamation may have significant advantages over methotrexate in the treatment of those tumors which are overproducers of polyglutamates. In high dose methotrexate therapy a significant amount of MTX is metabolized to its 7-hydroxy derivative and is often precipitated in the kidney of patients. The biochemical details of the formation of this metabolite as well as its metabolic fate including polyglutamation *in vivo* has to be studied in detail.

As noted previously, the chemotherapeutic index of an antifolate can be significantly improved if the drug can be selectively transported to, retained or activated in the tumor. Many tumors have shown a specificity for the C^9,N^{10}-bridge region of various antifolates for transport influx. A detailed understanding of the relationships among the structures of the antifolates and their interaction with the tumor cell transport receptors will lead to the design of better drugs which are capable of enhanced transport to the tumor cells. Structural modifications at the glutamate moiety of various

Figure 8. Survival of L1210-bearing mice injected with CB 3717. ■, No treatment (10 animals)-MTX control; □, no treatment (20 animals)-CB 3717 control. (Animals were injected with 20 mM NaHCO₃ buffer 0.4 ml daily × 5 days); ●, MTX 3 mg/kg daily × 5 (10 animals); ▲, CB 3717 125 mg/kg daily × 5 (10 animals). Survivals from these treatments were identical, hence the data points are superimposed. △, CB 3717 200 mg/kg daily × 5 (10 animals). The difference in the survival of quinazoline- and MTX-treated animals is highly significant, $P < 0.001$ using the log rank test [45]. Adapted from Jones *et al.*: *Eur J Cancer* 17:11–19, 1981.

2,4-diamino folate analogues with a view to enhance polyglutamation in the tumor, may be beneficial in the development of more selective drugs. One might expect that such compounds will be concentrated and retained more in the tumor than the normal tissues. The biochemical reasons of the ability of certain tumors to preferentially synthesize polyglutamates of antifolates such as MTX and its close analogues should be unravelled. Is it due to enhanced activity of the polyglutamate synthetase or decreased activity of 'conjugase' in the tumor compared to normal proliferative tissues? In this regard, design of antifolates which are either better substrates of the polyglutamate synthetase or inhibitors of conjugase may prove to be beneficial. In the case of 10-deaza-10-ethyl aminopterin (**7**), which is a superior antitumor agent compared to MTX or 10-DA, future investigations such as its transport characteristics and polyglutamation *in vivo* should be studied. Results from such studies, can then be utilized for the design of better antitumor agents. The biochemical and pharmacological properties of 10-deazoaminopterin metabolites should be studied in detail both *in vivo* and *in vitro*.

Investigations pertaining to the development of synthetic substrates of dihydrofolate reductase should be continued for the accessibility of 4-oxy antifolates which are capable of exhibiting selective toxicity against MTX-resistant (high reductase) tumors by virtue of the lethal synthesis mechanism. Finally a second generation of N^{10}-propargyl-5,8-dideazafolic acid (**14**), (CB3717) and DDATHE having more desirable biochemical and pharmacological disposition should be synthesized and evaluated. The exciting new lead provided by **14** and DDATHE should be thoroughly exploited for the development of more successful antifolates, which are inhibitors of thymidylate synthase and GAR-transmylase.

ABBREVIATIONS USED

MTX, Methotrexate; $MTXG_1$, methotrexate monoglutamate having two glutamate moieties; $MTXG_2$, methotrexate diglutamate residues, . . . , etc. CF, Citrovorum factor, also known as leucovorin or folinic acid. DHFR, dihydrofolate reductase; TS, thymidylate synthase. 10-DA,10-deazaaminopterin.

ACKNOWLEDGEMENTS

Work reported from the author's laboratory was supported by Grants CA-27101, and CA-32687 from the National Cancer Institute, NSDHHS.

REFERENCES

1. Alt PW, Kellems RE, Schimke RT: Synthesis and degradation of folate reductase in sensitive and methotrexate resistant lines of S-180 cells. *J Biol Chem* 251:3063, 1976
2. Baugh CM, Krumdieck CL, Baker HJ, Butterworth CE: Absorption of folic acid poly-γ-glutamates in dogs. *J Nutrition* 105:80, 1975
3. Baugh CM, Krumdieck CL, Nair MG: Polygammaglutamyl metabolites of methotrexate. *Biochem Biophys Res Comm* 52:27, 1973
4. Baugh CM, Krumdieck CL: Naturally occurring folates. *Ann NY Acad Sci* 186:7, 1971
5. Bertino JR: In: *Antineoplastic and Immunosuppressive Agents, Part II*, edited by Sartorelli AC, Johns DG, p. 468. Springer-Verlag, Berlin, 1975
6. Bertino JR, Johns DG: Folate antagonists. *Ann Rev Med* 28:27, 1967
7. Bertino JR: Rescue techniques in cancer chemotherapy: use of leucovorin and other rescue agents after methotrexate treatment. *Semin Oncol* 4:203, 1977
8. Bertino JR, Booth BA, Cashmore A, Bieber AL, Sartorelli AC: Studies of the inhibition of dihydrofolate reductase by folate antagonists. *J Biol Chem* 239:479, 1964
9. Biedler JL, Spengler BA: Metaphase chromosome anomaly: association with drug resistance and cell specific products. *Science* 191:185, 1976
10. Bitran JD, Desser RK, DeMeester TR et al.: Cyclophosphamide, adriamycin, methotrexate and procarbazine (CAMP)-effective four drug combination chemotherapy for metastatic non-oat cell bronchogenic carcinoma. *Cancer Treatment Reports* 60:1225, 1976
11. Blakley RL: *The Biochemistry of Folic Acid and Related Pteridines*. North Holland, Amsterdam, 1969
12. Borsa J, Whitmore GF: Cell killing studies on the mode of action of methotrexate on L-cells *in vitro*. *Cancer Res* 29:737, 1969
13. Broquist HP: Evidence for the excretion of formimino glutamic acid following folic acid antagonist therapy in acute leukemia. *J Amer Chem Soc* 78:6205, 1956
14. Bruckner HW, Lokich JJ, Stablein DM: Studies of Baker's antifol, methotrexate, razoxane in advanced gastric cancer: a gastrointestinal tumor study group report. *Cancer Treat Reports* 66:1713, 1982
14a. Burchenal JH, Murphy ML: Long-term survivors in acute leukemia. *Cancer Res* 25:1491–94, 1965
15. Burkitt D, Hult MSR, Wright DH: The African lymphoma. Preliminary observations on response to therapy. *Cancer* 18:399, 1965
16. Butterworth CE, Baugh CM, Krumdieck CL: A study of folate absorption and metabolism in man utilizing ^{14}C labeled polyglutamates synthesized by the solid phase method. *J Clin Invest* 48:1131, 1969
17. Calabresi P, Parks RE Jr. In: *The Pharmacological Basis of Therapeutics*, 5th edn, edited by Goodman LS, Gillman A, pp. 1268. McMillan, New York, 1975
18. Calvert AH, Jones TR, Dady PJ, Sztabert GB, Paine RM, Taylor GA, Harrap KR: Quinazoline antifolates with dual biochemical loci of action. Biochemical and biological studies directed towards overcoming methotrexate resistance. *Europ J Cancer* 16:713, 1980
19. Charlton PA, Young DW: Stereochemistry of reduction of folic acid using dihydrofolate reductase. *JCS Chem Comm* 20:922, 1979.
20. Chello PL, Sirotnak FM, Dorick DM, Gura J: Folate analog transport by isolated murine intestinal epithelial cells. In: *Chemistry and Biology of Pteridines*, edited by Kisliuk RL, Brown GM, p. 521. Elsevier North Holland, Inc., New York, 1979
21. Cheng YC, Szeto DW, Dolnick BT: Human thymidylate synthetase. Action of folate and methotrexate analogues. In: *Chemistry and Biology of Pteridines*, edited by Kisliuk RL, Brown GM, p. 395. Elsevier, North Holland, New York, 1979
22. Cheng YC, Dutschman GE, Starnes MC, Fisher MH, Nanavati NT, Nair MG: Activity of the new antifolate N^{10}-propargyl-5,8-dideazafolate and its polyglutamates against dihydrofolate reductase, human thymidylate synthase, and KB cells containing different levels of dihydrofolate reductase. *Cancer Res* 45:598, 1985
23. Colman N, Herbert V: Kinetic and chromatographic evidence for heterogeneity of the high affinity folate binding proteins in serum. In: *Chemistry and Biology of Pteridines*, edited by Kisliuk RL, Brown GM, p. 525. Elsevier, North

Holland, New York, 1979

24. Covey JM: Polyglutamate derivatives of folic acid coenzymes and methotrexate. *Life Sciences* 26:655, 1980
25. Curt G, Jolivet J, Carney D, Bailey BD, Chabner BA: Methotrexate (MTX) resistance in cultured human small cell lung cancer (SCLC). *AACR Proc* 23:9, 1982
26. Curt GA, Carney DN, Cowan KH, Jolivet J, Bailey BD, Drake JC, Kao-shan CS, Minna JD, Chabner BA: Unstable methotrexate resistance in human small cell carcinoma associated with double minute chromosomes. *New Engl J Med* 308:199, 1983
27. Das KC, Hoffbrand AV: Studies of folate uptake by phytochaemagglutinin-stimulated lymphocytes. *Brit J Haematol* 19:203, 1970
28. DeGraw JI, Goodman L, Weinstein B, Baker BR: Potential anticancer agents. LXIX. Tetrahydroquinazoline analogues of tetrahydrofolic acid. IV. The synthesis of 5,8-dideaza-5,6,7,8-tetrahydroaminopterin. *J Org Chem* 27:576, 1962
29. DeGraw JI, Marsh JP Jr, Acton EM, Crews OP, Mosher CW, Fujiwara AN, Goodman L: The synthesis of homofolic acid. *J Org Chem* 30:3404, 1965
30. DeGraw JI, Kisliuk RL, Baugh CM, Nair MG: Synthesis and antifolate activity of 10-deaza aminopterin. *J Med Chem* 17:552, 1974
31. DeGraw JI, Kisliuk RL, Gaumont Y, Baugh CM: Antimicrobial activity of 8-deazafolic acid. *J Med Chem* 17:470, 1974
32. DeGraw JI, Brown VH, Kisliuk RL, Sirotnak FM: Synthesis and antifolate activity of 10-deaza-minopterin. In: *Chemistry and Biology of Pteridines*, edited by Kisliuk RL, Brown GM, p. 225. Elsevier, North Holland, New York, 1979
33. DeGraw JI, Brown VH, Tagawa H, Kisliuk RL, Gaumont Y, Sirotnak FM: Synthesis and antitumor activity of 10-alkyl-10-deazaminopterins. A convenient synthesis of 10-deaza-minopterin. *J Med Chem* 25:1227, 1982
34. Djerassi I, Kim SJ, Nayak N, Ohanissian H, Alder S, Hseich S: *Cancer Treat Reports* 61:749, 1977
35. Djerassi I, Rominger CJ, Kim JS et al.: Phase I study of high dose methotrexate with citrovorum factor in patients with lung cancer. *Cancer* 30:22, 1972
36. Djerassi I, Royer AE et al.: Long term remission in childhood acute leukemia. Use of infrequent infusions of methotrexate; supportive role of platelet transfusions and citrovorum factor. *Clin Pediatr* 5:502, 1966
37. Djerassi I, Royer G, Treat C et al.: Management of childhood lymphosarcoma and reticulum cell sarcoma with high dose intermittent methotrexate and citrovorum factor. *Proc Am Assoc Cancer Res* 9:18, 1968
38. Dolnick BJ, Berenson RJ, Bertino JR, Kaufman RJ, Nunberg JH, Shimke RT, Correlation of dihydrofolate reductase elevation with gene amplification in a homogeneously staining chromosomal region in L5178 Y cells. *J Cell Biol* 83:394, 1979
39. Domin BA, Cheng YC, Nair MG: Effect of 11-oxahomofolate and its reduced derivatives on human dihydrofolate reductase and human cells having different amounts of dihydrofolate reductase. *Biochem Pharmacol* 31:255, 1982
40. Domin BA, Cheng YC, Hakala MT: Properties of dihydrofolate reductase from a methotrexate resistant subline of human KB cells, and it's interaction with polyglutamates. In: *Chemistry and Biology of Pteridines*, edited by Kisliuk RL, Brown GM, p. 395. Elsevier, North Holland, Inc., New York, 1979
41. Eisenstadt J, Lengyel P: Formylmethionyl-tRNA dependence of amino acid incorporation in extracts of trimethoprim treated *E. coli. Science* 154:524, 1966
42. El-Dareer SM, Tillery KF, Hill DL: Disposition of 5-methyl tetrahydrohomofolate in mice, dogs and monkeys. *Cancer Treat Reports* 63:201, 1979
43. Ervin TJ, Weichselbaum R, Miller D, Meshad M, Posner M, Fabian R: Treatment of advanced squamous cell carcinoma of the head and neck with cisplatin bleomycin and methotrexate. *Cancer Treat Reports* 65:787, 1981
44. Fontecilla-Camps JC, Bugg CE, Tample C, Rose JD, Montgomery JA, Kisliuk RL: In: *Chemistry and Biology of Pteridines*, edited by Kisliuk RL, Brown GM, p. 235. Elsevier, North Holland, New York, 1979
45. Freeman MV: The fluorometric measurement of the absorption, distribution, and excretion of single doses 4-amino-10-methyl-pteroyl glutamic acid (Amethopterin) in man. *J Pharmacol Exp Ther* 122:154, 1958
46. Friedkin M, Crawford EJ, Plante LT: Empirical vs rational approaches to cancer chemotherapy. *Annals NY Acad Sci* 186:209, 1971
47. Friedkin M, Crawford EJ, Humphreys SR, Goldin A: The association of increased dihydrofolate reductase with amethopterin resistance in mouse leukemia. *Cancer Res* 22:600, 1962
48. Fry DW, Anderson LA, Borst M, Goldman ID: Analysis of the role of membrane transport and polyglutamation of methotrexate in gut and Ehrlich tumor *in vivo* as factors in drug sensitivity and selectivity. *Cancer Res* 43:1087, 1983
49. Galivan J: Evidence for the cytotoxic activity of polyglutamate derivatives of methotrexate. *Mol Pharmacol* 17:105, 1980
50. Gaumont Y, Kisliuk RL: Action of diastereoisomers of tetrahydrohomofolate on the growth of *Lactobacillus casei. Annals NY Acad Sci* 186:438, 1971
51. Gewirtz AD, White JC, Randolph JK, Goldman ID: Formation of methotrexate polyglutamates in rat hepatocytes. *Cancer Res* 39:2914, 1979
52. Goldin A, Mantel D, Greenhouse S: Effect of delayed administration of citrovorum factor on the antileukemic effectiveness of aminopterin in mice. *Cancer Res* 14:43, 1954
53. Goldin A, Venditti J, Kline: Eradication of leukemia cells (L1210) by methotrexate plus citrovorum factor. *Nature* 212:1548, 1966
54. Goldman ID: The characteristics of the membrane transport of amethopterin and naturally occurring folates. *Annals NY Acad Sci* 186:400, 1971
55. Goldman ID: Analysis of the cytotoxic determinants for methotrexate (NSC 740). A role for intracellular drug. *Cancer Chemother Rep* 6:51, 1975
56. Goodman L, DeGraw J, Kisliuk RL, Friedkin M, Pastore EJ, Crawford EJ, Plante LT, Al-Nahas A, Morningstar JF, Kwok G, Wilson L, Donovan EF, Ratzan J: Tetrahydrohomofolate, a specific inhibitor of thymidylate synthetase. *J Amer Chem Soc* 86:308, 1964
57. Hakala MT: On the role of drug penetration in amethopterin resistance of sarcoma-180 cells *in vitro. Biochim Biophys Acta* 102:198, 1965
58. Harrap KR, Hill BT, Furness ME, Hart LI: Sites of action of amethopterin: Intrinsic and acquired drug resistance. *Annals NY Acad Sci* 186:312, 1971
59. Henderson ES, Adamson RH, Denham C, Olivero VT: The metabolic fate of tritiated methotrexate. 1. Absorption, excretion, and distribution in mice, rats, dogs and monkeys. *Cancer Res* 25:1008, 1965
60. Hertz R, Lewis J, Lipsett MB: Five years experience with the chemotherapy of metastatic choriocarcinoma and related trophoblastic tumors in women. *Am J Obstet Gynec* 82:631, 1961
61. Hertz R, Ross GT, Lipsett MB: Primary chemotherapy of non-metastatic trophoblastic disease in women. *Am J Obstet Gynec* 86:808, 1965
62. Hornbeak HR, Nair MG: Antifolate Activity of Isoaminopterin in HeLa Cells. *Antimicrobial Agents and Chemotherapy* 15:503, 1979
63. Hornbeak HR, Nair MG: Transport and inhibitory activity of new folate analogues in HeLa Cells. *Molecular Pharmacol* 14:299, 1978
64. Howell SB, Ensminger WD, Krishan A, Frie E: Thymidine rescue of high dose methotrexate in humans. *Cancer Res* 38:325, 1978

65. Huennekens FM, Henderson GB: Transport of folate compounds into mammalian and bacterial cells. In: *Chemistry and Biology of Pteridines*, edited by Pfleiderer W, p. 179. Walter de Gruyter, Berlin, New York, 1975

66. Hughes LR, Marsham PR, Oldfield J, Jones TR, O'Connor BM, Bishop JAM, Calvert AH, Jackman AL: Thymidylate synthase (TS) inhibitory and cytotoxic activity of a series of C^2 substituted-5,8-dideazafolates. *Proc Am Assoc Cancer Res* 29:286, 1988

67. Jackman AL, Taylor GA, Moran R, Bishop JAM, Bisset G, Pawelczak K, Balmanno K, Hughes LR, Calvert AH: Biological properties of 2-desamino-2-substituted-5,8-dideazafolates that inhibit thymidylate synthase. *Proc Am Assoc Cancer Res* 29:287, 1988

68. Jacobs SA, Derr CJ, Johns DG: Accumulation of methotrexate diglutamate in human liver during methotrexate therapy. *Biochem Pharmacol* 26:2310, 1977

69. Jacobs SA, Stoller RG, Chabner BA, Johns DG: 7-hydroxymethotrexate as a urinary metabolite in human subjects and Rhesus monkeys receiving high dose methotrexate. *J Clin Invest* 57:534, 1976

70. Jacobs SA, Adamson RH, Chabner BA, Derr CI, Johns DG: Stoichiometric inhibition of mammalian dihydrofolate reductase by the γ-glutamyl metabolite of methotrexate, 4-amino-4-deoxy-N[10]-methylpteroyl-glutamyl-γ-glutamate. *Biochem Biophys Res Commun* 63:692, 1975

71. Jaffe N, Paed D: Recent advances in the chemotherapy of metastatic osteogenic sarcoma. *Cancer* 30:1627, 1972

72. Johns DG, Valerino DM: Metabolism of folate antagonists. *Annals NY Acad Sci* 186:378, 1971

73. Johnson TB, Nair MG, Galivan J: Role of folylpolyglutamate synthetase in the regulation of methotrexate polyglutamate formation in H35 hepatoma cells. *Cancer Res* 48:2426, 1988

74. Jolivet J, Schilsky RL, Bailey BD, Drake JC, Chabner BC: Synthesis, retention, and biological activity of methotrexate polyglutamates in cultured human breast cancer cells. *Clin Invest* 70:351, 1982

75. Jones TR, Calvert AH, Jackman AL, Brown SJ, Jones M, Harrap KR: A potent antitumor quinazoline inhibitor of thymidylate synthase: synthesis, biological properties and therapeutic results in mice. *Europ J Cancer* 17:11, 1981

76. Kim YH, Gaumont Y, Kisliuk RL, Mautner HG: Synthesis and biological activity of 10-Thia-10-deaza analogues of folic acid, pteroic acid and related compounds. *J Med Chem* 18:776, 1975

77. Kisliuk RL: Homofolates and other 2-amino-4-oxy antifolates. In: *New Approaches to the Design of Antineoplastic Agents*, edited by Bardos, Kalman, p. 201. Elsevier Science Publishing Company, Inc., 1982

78. Kisliuk RL, Gaumont Y, Baugh CM, Galivan JH, Maley GF, Maley F: Inhibition of thymidylate synthase by poly-γ-glutamyl derivatives of folate and methotrexate. In: *Chemistry and Biology of Pteridines*, edited by Kisliuk RL, Brown GM, p. 431. Elsevier North Holland, Inc., New York, 1979

79. Kisliuk RL, Gaumont Y: Action of diastereomers of tetrahydrohomofolate on the growth of *L. casei*. *Annals NY Acad Sci* 186:438, 1971

80. Kisliuk RL, Gaumont Y: Tetrahydrohomofolate: an inhibitor of folate transport in *S. faecium*. In: *Chemistry and Biology of Pteridines*, edited by Iwai K, Akino M, Goto M, Iwanami Y, p. 357. International Academic Printing Co., Tokyo, 1970

81. Kisliuk RL, Tattersall MHN, Gaumont Y, Pastore EJ, Brown B: Aspects of reversal of methotrexate toxicity in rodents. *Cancer Treat Reports* 61:647, 1977

82. Lin RL, Narasimhachari N: Tetrahydrofolic acid: An inhibitor of the methyl tetrahydrofolic acid-mediated methylation of indol ethyl amines. *Biochemica et Biophysica Acta* 385:268, 1975

83. Livingston D, Crawford EJ, Friedkin M: Studies with tetrahydrohomofolate and thymidylate synthase from

84. Loo TL, Adamson RH: The metabolite of 3',5'-dichloro-4-amino-4-deoxy-N[10]-methyltroyl glutamic acid (dichloromethotrexate). *J Med Chem* 8:513, 1965

85. McCuen RW, Sirotnak FM: Thymidylate synthetase from *D. pneumoniae*. Properties and inhibition by folate analogues. *Biochim Biophys Acta* 384:369, 1975

86. Mastropaolo D, Camerman A: Folic acid: crystal structure and implications for enzyme binding. *Science* 210:334, 1980

87. Mead JAR, Goldin A, Kisliuk RL, Friedkin M, Plante L, Crawford EJ, Kwok G: Pharmacologic aspects of homofolate derivatives in relation to amethopterin-resistant murine leukemia. *Cancer Res* 26:2374, 1966

88. Mead JAR: Biochemical pharmacology and drug design. *Coll Pap Ann Symp Fundam Cancer Res* 27:197, 1975

89. Mead JAR: Rational design of folic acid antagonists. In: *Handbuch fuer Experimentelle Pharmakologie: Antineoplastic and Immuno Suppressive Agents*, p. 52. Springer-Verlag, New York, 1974

90. Mishra LC, Parmer AS, Mead JAR: The antileukemic activity of dihydrohomofolate (H_2HF) and its reduction to tetrahydrohomofolate (H_4HF) in mice. *Proc Am Assoc Cancer Res* 11:57, 1970

91. Montgomery JA, Rose JD, Temple C Jr, Piper JR: A convenient synthesis of methotrexate and related compounds. In: *Chemistry and Biology of Pteridines*, edited by Pfleiderer W, p. 485. Walter De Gruyter, Berlin, 1975

92. Nahas A, Nixon PF, Bertino JR: Uptake and metabolism of N[5]-formyl tetrahydrofolate by L1210 leukemia cells. *Cancer Res* 32:1416, 1972

93. Nair MG, Salter DC, Kisliuk RL, Gaumont Y, Sirotnak FM: Unpublished work, 1983

94. Nair MG, Salter DC, Kisliuk RL, Gaumont Y, North G, Sirotnak FM: Folate analogues, 21: synthesis and antifolate and antitumor activities of N[10]-(cyanomethyl)-5,8-dideaza folic acid. *J Med Chem* 26:605, 1983

95. Nair MG, Baugh CM: Synthesis and biological evaluation of poly-γ-glutamyl derivatives of methotrexate. *Biochem* 12:3923, 1973

96. Nair MG, Chen SY, Kisliuk RL, Gaumont Y, Strumpf D: Folate analogues altered in the C^9,N^{10}-bridge region 11-thiohomofolic acid. *J Med Chem* 22:850, 1979

97. Nair MG, Bridges TW, Henkel TJ, Kisliuk RL, Gaumont Y, Sirotnak FM: Folate analogues altered in the C^9,N^{10}-bridge region. 18. Synthesis and antitumor evaluation of 11-oxahomo aminopterin. *J Med Chem* 24:1058, 1981

98. Nair MG, Sanders C, Chen SY, Kisliuk RL, Gaumont Y: Folate analogues altered in the C^9,N^{10}-bridge region. 14. 11-oxahomofolic acid, a potential antitumor agent. *J Med Chem* 23:59, 1980

99. Nair MG, Campbell PT: Folate analogues altered in the C^9,N^{10}-bridge region: 10-oxafolic acid and 10-oxa aminopterin. *J Med Chem* 19:825, 1976

100. Nair MG, Campbell PT, Baugh CM: The synthesis of 10-thiofolic acid, a potential antitumor agent. *J Org Chem* 40:1745, 1975

101. Nair MG, Baugh CM: The synthesis and biological evaluation of isofolic acid. *J Med Chem* 17:223, 1974

102. Nair MG, Mehtha AP, Dair IG: The metabolism of 10-Propargyl-5,8-dideazafolate in mice. *Fed Proc* 45:821, 1986

103. Nair AG, Nanavati NT, Nair IG, Kisliuk RL, Gaumont Y, Hsiao MC, Kalman TI: Folate Analogues. 26. Synthesis and antifolate activity of 10-substituted derivatives of 5,8-dideazafolic acid and the polyglutamyl metabolites of N[10]-propargyl-5,8-dideazafolic acid (PDDF). *J Med Chem* 29:1754, 1986

104. Nair MG, Murthy BR, Patil SD, Kisliuk RL, Thorndike J, Gaumont Y, Ferone R, Duch DS, Edelstein MP: Folate Analogs. 31. Synthesis of the reduced derivatives of 11-deazahomofolic acid, 10-methyl-11-deazahomofolic acid and their evaluation as inhibitors of glycinamide ribonucleotide

formyltransferase. *J Med Chem* 32:1277, 1989

105. Niethammer D, Jackson RC: Transport of folate compounds through the membrane of human lymphoblastoid cells. In: *Chemistry and Biology of Pteridines*, edited by Pfleiderer W, p. 197. Walter de Gruyter, Berlin, 1975

106. Nunberg JH, Kaufman RJ, Schimke RT, Uerlab G, Chasin LA: Amplified dihydrofolate reductase genes are localized to a homogeneously staining region of a single chromosome in a methotrexate-resistant Chinese hamster ovary cell line. *Proc Natl Acad Sci USA* 75:5553, 1978

107. Oliverio VT, Zaharko DS: Tissue distribution of folate antagonists. *Annals NY Acad Sci* 186:387, 1971

108. Oliverio VT, Loo TL: Separation and isolation of metabolites of folic acid antagonists. *Proc Amer Assoc Cancer Res* 3:140, 1960

109. Patil SD, Jones C, Nair MG, Galivan J, Maley F, Kisliuk RL, Gaumont Y, Thorndike J, Duch D, Ferone R: Folate Analogues 32: Synthesis and biological evaluation of 2-desamino-2-methyl-N^{10}-propargyl-5,8-dideazafolic acid (DMPD DF) and related compounds. *J Med Chem* 32:1284, 1989

110. Peters TJ: Intestinal peptidases. *Gut* 11:720, 1970

111. Piper JR, McCaleb GS, Montgomery JA, Kisliuk RL, Gaumont Y, Sirotnak FM: 10-Propargylaminopterin and alkyl homologues of methotrexate as inhibitors of folate metabolism. *J Med Chem* 25:877, 1982

112. Piper WN, van Lier RBL, Hardwicke DM: Pteridine regulation of uroporphyrinogen I synthetase activity. In: *Chemistry and Biology of Pteridines*, edited by Kisliuk RL, Brown GM, p. 329. Elsevier, North Holland, New York, 1979

113. Poser RG, Sirotnak FM, Chello PL: Extracellular recovery of methotrexate polyglutamates following efflux from L1210 leukemia cells. *Biochem Pharmacol* 29:2701, 1980

114. Poser RG, Sirotnak FM, Chello PL: Differential synthesis of MTX polyglutamates in normal proliferative and neoplastic mouse tissues *in vivo*. *Cancer Res* 41:4441, 1981

115. Rosen G, Nirenberg: Chemotherapy of osteogenic sarcoma: An investigative method, not a recipe. *Cancer Treat Rep* 66:1687, 1982

116. Rosenblatt DS, Whitehead VM, Vera N, Pottier A, Dupont M, Vuchich MJ: Prolonged inhibition of DNA synthesis associated with the accumulation of methotrexate polyglutamates by cultured human cells. *Mol Pharmacol* 14:1143, 1978

117. Rueckert RR, Mueller GC: Studies on unbalanced growth in tissue culture. I. Induction and consequences of thymidine deficiency. *Cancer Res* 20:1584, 1960

118. Ryser HJP, Shen WC: Conjugation of methotrexate to poly (L-lysine) increases drug transport and overcomes drug resistance in cultured cells. *Proc Natl Acad Sci USA* 75:3867, 1978

119. Sartorelli AC, LePage GA: Effects of amethopterin on the purine biosynthesis of susceptible and resistant TA3 ascites cells. *Cancer Res* 18:1336, 1958

120. Sartorelli AC, Upchurch HF, Bolte BA: Effects of folinic acid on amethopterin induced inhibition of Ehrlich ascites carcinoma. *Cancer Res* 22:102, 1962

121. Scanlon KJ, Moroson BA, Bertino JR, Hynes JB: Quinazoline analogues of folic acid as inhibitors of thymidylate synthetase from bacterial and mammalian sources. *Molec Pharmacol* 16:261, 1979

122. Schimke RT: Gene amplification and drug resistance. *Sci Amer* 243:60, 1980

123. Seeger DR, Smith JM, Hultquist ME: Antagonist for pteroylglutamic acid. *J Amer Chem Soc* 69:2567, 1947

124. Seeger DR, Cosulich DB, Smith JM, Hultquist ME: Analogs of pteroyl glutamic acid. III. 4-amino derivatives. *J Amer Chem Soc* 71:1753, 1949

125. Shapiro WR: High-dose methotrexate in malignant gliomas. *Cancer Treat Reports* 61:753, 1977

126. Sirotnak FM, Donsbach RC, Dorick DM, Moccio DM: High dose methotrexate therapy with citrovorum factor: A pharmacologic perspective in murine tumor models. *Cancer Treat Reports* 61:565, 1977

127. Sirotnak FM, Kurita S, Hutchison DJ: On the nature of a transport alteration determining resistance to amethopterin in L1210 leukemia. *Cancer Res* 28:75, 1968

128. Sirotnak FM, Chello PL, Piper JR, Montgomery JA, DeGraw JI: Structural specificity of folate analog transport and binding to dihydrofolate reductase in murine tumor and normal cells: Relevance to therapeutic efficacy. *Chemistry and Biology of Pteridines*, edited by Kisliuk RL, Brown GM, p. 597. Elsevier North Holland, New York, 1979

129. Sirotnak FM: Correlates of folate analog transport, pharmacokinetics, and selective antitumor action. *Pharmacol Ther* 8:71, 1980

130. Sirotnak FM, DeGraw JI, Moccio DM, Dorick DM: Antitumor properties of a new folate analog, 10-deaza aminopterin in mice. *Cancer Treat Rep* 62:1047, 1978

131. Sirotnak FM: Private communication, 1983

132. Skipper HE, Mitchell JH, Bennett LL: Inhibition of nucleic acid synthesis by folic acid antagonists. *Cancer Res* 10:510, 1950

133. Skipper HE, Bennett LL, Law LW: Effects of amethopterin on formate incorporation into the nucleic acids of susceptible and resistant leukemic cells. *Cancer Res* 12:677, 1952

134. Smith GK, Benkovic PA, Benkovic SJ: L(−)-10-formyl tetrahydrofolate is the cofactor for glycinamide ribonucleotide transformylase from chicken liver. *Biochem* 20:4034, 1981

135. Steel GG: Cytokinetics in neoplasia. In: *Cancer Medicine*, edited by Holland JF, Frei III E, p. 125. Philadelphia: Lea and Febiger, 1973

136. Struck RF, Shealy YF, Montgomery JA: Potential folic acid antagonists. 5. Synthesis and biologic evaluation of N^{10}-deazapteroic acid and N^{10}-deazafolic acid and their 9,10-dihydro derivatives. *J Med Chem* 14:693, 1971

137. Taylor EC, Wong GSK, Fletcher SR, Harrington PJ, Beardsley PG, Shih CJ: Synthesis of 5,10-dideaza-5,6,7,8-tetrahydrofolic acid (DDATHF) and analogs. In: *Chemistry and Biology of Pteridines*, edited by Cooper BA and Whitehead VM, p 61, Walter de Gruyter, Berlin 1986

138. Totter JR, Best AN: The metabolism of formate ^{14}C by rabbit bone marrow *in vitro*. *Arch Biochem Biophys* 54:318, 1955

139. Thorndike J, Gaumont Y, Kisliuk RL et al.: Infiltration of glycinamide ribonucleotide formal transferase a.o. folic enzymes by homofolate folice glutamate in human lymphoma and murine leukemia cell extracts. *Cancer Res* 29, 1988 (in press)

140. Von Hoff DD, Penta JS, Helman LJ, Slavik M: Incidence of drug related deaths secondary to high dose methotrexate and citrovorum factor administration. *Cancer Treat Reports* 61:745, 1977

141. Waxman S: Studies on the origin of serum folate binding protein. In: *Chemistry and Biology of Pteridines*, edited by Kisliuk RL, Brown GM, p. 619. Elsevier North Holland, New York, 1979

142. Weiss HD, Walker MD, Niernik PH: Neurotoxicity of commonly used antineoplastic agents. *New Engl J Med* 291:75, 1974

143. Whitehead MV: Synthesis of methotrexate polyglutamates in L1210 murine leukemia cells. *Cancer Res* 37:408, 1977

144. Whitehead MV, Rosenblatt DS: Decreased synthesis of methotrexate polyglutamates in mutant hamster cells and in folinic acid-treated human fibroblasts. In: *Chemistry and Biology of Pteridines*, edited by Kisliuk RL, Brown GM, p. 689. Elsevier, North Holland, Inc., N.Y., 1979

145. Williams AD, Staler GG, Winzler RJ: The effect of amethopterin on formate-C^{14} incorporation of mouse leukemias *in vitro*. *Cancer Res* 15:532, 1955

For postscript see end of Volume, p. 243.

5

PURINE ANTIMETABOLITES

WOLFGANG SADÉE and BINH NGUYEN

The ever increasing number of purine analogs with potent biological properties, either isolated from various microorganisms or obtained by chemical synthesis, can elicit an unusual fascination with this subject. What are the unique features of purine metabolism in different species and cell types that allow one organism to accumulate high concentrations of cytotoxic purines, presumably as a defense mechanism without harm to itself? And more relevant to the present review, can these natural antipurines or their synthetic counterparts be utilized to preferentially kill cancer cells without affecting normal tissues? The answer to the latter question must be a qualified because with the exception of the 6-thiopurines there are no purine antimetabolites in general clinical use in the treatment of neoplasms. However, among the new anticancer drugs undergoing clinical evaluation, the purine antimetabolites indeed play a very prominent role. Of 37 experimental anticancer drugs for which INDA's were filed by the NCI during the period 1977–1983, no less than seven are purine antimetabolites (64). These experimental antipurines are:

> L-alanosine (NSC 51143)
> tiazofurin (NSC 286193)
> fludarabine phosphate; 5-fluoro-ara-AMP (NSC 312887)
> acivicin (NSC 163501)
> DON; 6-diazo-5-oxo-L-norleucine (NSC 7365)
> pentostatin; deoxycoformycin (NSC 218321) (potentiates araA activity)
> 9-arabinosyl adenine; araA (NSC 404241) (in combination with pentoatatin).

In this review we will briefly describe the purine metabolic network in order to provide a basic understanding of the current rationale underlying the use of purine antimetabolites against neoplasms. Furthermore, we will provide a summary of the currently available major antipurines and their mechanisms of action. Detailed discussion will be limited to the 6-thiopurines, and tiazofurin as an example of one of the experimental drugs.

Several antimetabolites are excluded since they do not act specifically on purine metabolism alone, e.g., the antifols and ribonucleotide reductase inhibitors. The listed glutamine analog acivicin acts on pyrimidine metabolism (e.g., CTP synthetase), but it also blocks two purine pathways (amidophosphoribosyl transferase and GMP synthetase) and therefore represents to a substantial degree a purine antimetabolite.

THE PURINE METABOLIC NETWORK

Cells can synthesize purine nucleotides either by the *de novo* pathway or by the salvage pathways that utilize preformed purine bases and nucleosides (Figure 1). (For review see: 20, 65-75). The first *de novo* enzyme committed to purine biosynthesis, amido phosphoribosyl transferase or PRPP amidotransferase, utilizes PRPP and glutamine to form phosphoribosylamine. It represents the rate limiting step for overall *de novo* purine biosynthesis and is the target of inhibition by purine nucleotide products. From phosphoribosylamine the purine ring system is constructed in a series of metabolic steps (Figure 1) with IMP as the first complete purine nucleotide, which represents the branching point for the biosynthesis of adenine and guanine nucleotides. IMP-Dehydrogenase is probably the enzyme of lowest capacity among the enzymes catalyzing purine ribonucleotide metabolism. Control at the IMP branching point is provided by both positive and negative feedback mechanisms: ATP is required for GTP synthesis, and GTP for ATP synthesis, while GMP and AMP inhibit their own production (20).

The rate limiting enzyme for the utilization of guanine and adenine for DNA synthesis is thought to be the ribonucleotide reductase which is capable of reducing all four (T, C, G, A) ribonucleotide diphosphates to the corresponding deoxyribonucleotides, which are subsequently phosphorylated to triphosphates and incorporated into DNA by DNA polymerase. It is possible that this sequence of events is mediated by a multienzyme complex, forming a metabolic channel that guides distant DNA precursors (e.g., GDP or ADP) directly into DNA without mixing with the general cellular pools of the intermediate products (e.g., (59)). While such channeling could be of biological importance in the control of cell replication, it has predominantly been studied for the pyrimidine nucleotides, while its significance remains largely unknown for the purine nucleotides. The control of ribonucleotide reductase is extremely complex, with ATP serving as an allosteric effector of CDP and UDP reduction, dGTP as an effector of ADP reduction and an inhibitor of UDP and CDP reduction, and dATP as a general feedback inhibitor (59, 62).

Because of the vital importance of purine nucleotides, it is not surprising that the cells can rely on an alternative purine supply system, namely the salvage pathways that largely consist of two phosphoribosyl transferases (APRTase and HGPRTase) and several nucleoside kinases. The salvage

P.V. Woolley (ed.), Cancer management in Man: Biological Response Modifiers, Chemotherapy, Antibiotics, Hyperthermia, Supporting Measures
© 1989. Kluwer Academic Publishers, Dordrecht.

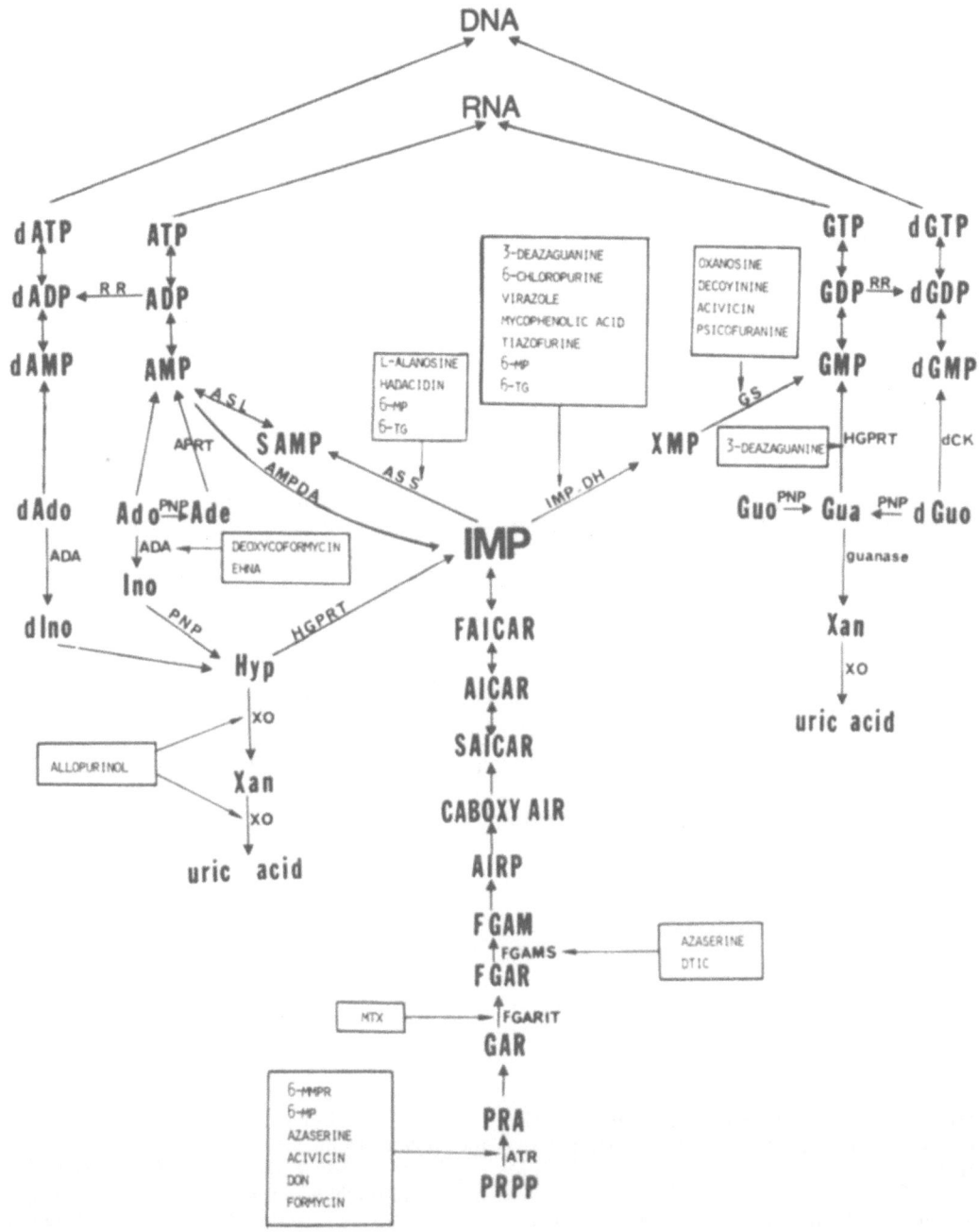

Figure 1. Purine metabolic network. Only major metabolic pathways are included; moreover, pathways leading to specialized products (SAM, NAD, GDP-mannose, etc.) are also omitted. The following abbreviations are used: Purine and their metabolic precursors: IMP, inosinate; XMP, xanthylate; SAMP, adenylosuccinate, FAICAR, formylaminoimidazolecarboximide ribonucleotide, AICRP aminoimidazole carboxamide ribosephosphate, AICAR, aminoimidazolecarboximide ribonucleotide, AIR, aminoimidazoleribonucleotide, AIRP, aminoimidazoleribonucleotide phosphate, FGAM, formylglycinamidine ribonucleotide, FGAR, formylglycine, amidoribonucleotide, GAR, glycine amidoribonucleotide, PRA, phosphoribosylamine; PRPP, phosphoribosylpyrophosphate. Selected enzymes: RR, ribonucleotide diphosphate reductase; ASS, adenylosuccinate synthetase; ASL, adenylosuccinate lyase; AMPDA, AMP deaminase; IMPDH, IMP dehydrogenase, GS, guanylate synthetase; FGAMS, FGAM synthetase; ATR, amidophosphoribosyl transferase; XO, xanthine oxidase. Salvage enzymes: APRT, adenine phosphoribosyl transferase, ADA, adenosine deaminase; HGPRT, hypoxanthine-guanine phosphoribosyltransferase; PNP, purine nucleotide phosphorylase. Purine anti metabolites: 6-MP; 6-mercaptopurine; 6-TG, 6-thioguanine; 6-MMPR, 6-methylmercaptopurine ribonucleoside; MA, mycophenolic acid, MTX, methotrexate; DON, 6-diazo-5-oxo-L-norleucine, DTIC, dimethyltriazenoimidazole carboxamide; EHNA, erythro-9-(2-hydroxynon-3-yl)-adenine.

enzymes in most tissues possess a greater biosynthetic capacity than the *de novo* enzymes (66, 67) and allow the cells to reuse circulating purine bases and nucleosides. Their biological importance is illustrated by the severe or lethal consequences of inborn deficiencies of HGPRTase (Lesh–Nyhan syndrome) and of PNPase and ADAase (immuno deficiencies). Moreover, most purine antimetabolites require activation by salvage enzymes to cytotoxic nucleotide analogs. This places added significance on the salvage pathways in the clinical use of antipurines against cancer. While adenine and guanine nucleotides serve many cellular functions, a generalization as to their predominant roles can be made (59, 62). The adenylates carry the major burden as energy donors and thus play an important role in metabolic processes, while the guanylates are more prominent as regulators of enzymatic processes than as energy donors and appear to exert a critical control over cell replication. Much more adenylates are required than guanylates which is reflected in the relative abundance of both (ATP 2–3 mM, GTP ~ 0.3 mM in mammalian liver). Moreover, inhibition of guanylate synthesis results in an immediate cessation of DNA synthesis, while inhibition of adenylate synthesis results in cell toxicity before any reduction in DNA synthesis is apparent (9). Other functions of GTP include: substrate for RNA, 5'-'cap' formation in messenger RNA, production of small nRNA species, polymerization of microtubules, lipid biosynthesis (GDP-mannose), cyclic GMP formation, protein synthesis, activator of CTP synthetase and adenylosuccinate synthetase, inhibitor of AMP deaminase. Therefore, depletion of guanine or the formation of toxic guanine nucleotide analogs may interfere with any of these diverse functions to a varying extent.

Finally, it should be noted that the pyrimidine nucleotide metabolism cannot be viewed independent of purine metabolism, since both networks may compete for the same substrate (PRPP, glutamine) or serve as mutual regulators. Examples of purines as regulators of the pyrimidine network are already mentioned above (GTP function for CTP synthetase (26) and the ribonucleotide reductase regulation) and further include GMP as an inhibitor of dCMP deaminase (36) and ATP as a primary donor in phosphorylation reactions.

CORRELATION BETWEEN CELLULAR TRANSFORMATION AND TUMOR PROGRESSION AND THE CONCURRENT CHANGE IN PURINE METABOLISM

Let us now consider the question how purine antimetabolites can selectively interfere with the metabolism of transformed cells. Weber (66, 67) has proposed the 'molecular correlation concept' as a biochemical strategy to develop anticancer drugs. This concept is based on key enzymes and metabolic pathways that are stringently linked with neoplastic transformation. Apparently, a reprogramming of gene expression occurs that is rather specific to the process of transformation, with quantitative and qualitative (isozyme shift) metabolic imbalance that is consistently found within several metabolic networks, e.g., the purine and pyrimidine pathways. Further changes during the progression stage of neoplasm may lead to additional progression-linked enzyme changes.

Weber and colleagues (66, 67) have identified a series of key enzymes among the purine pathways that lead to an enhanced synthesis and utilization of purines in neoplastic over that in normal cells. These studies were primarily conducted in hepatoma cell lines, but the same changes were found to occur in other cells as well. The following key enzymes of the synthetic pathways were elevated and can serve as enzyme markers of transformation: (see Figure 1)

amido-phosphoribosyl transferase
formylglycineamidine ribonucleotide synthetase
adenylosuccinate synthetase
adenylosuccinate lyase
AMP deaminase
IMP dehydrogenase
GMP synthetase

Among the degradative enzymes, the following were decreased, thereby providing a greater purine salvage supply:

5'-nucleotidases
inosine phosphorylase
xanthine oxidase

The synthetic enzymes are elevated 2–10-fold in tumor tissues, while the catabolic enzymes are drastically reduced. Because of their rate limiting capacity, their key location in the metabolic pathways, their sensitivity to feedback inhibition, and their stringent linking to transformation and progression, amidophosphoribosyl transferase, adenylosuccinate synthetase and IMP dehydrogenase have emerged as the primary targets of purine antimetabolites of potential promise as anticancer drugs.

A BRIEF SURVEY OF THE MAJOR PURINE ANTIMETABOLITES

Because of the varied functions of the purine nucleotides, it is not surprising that most antimetabolites display more than one type of cellular toxicity. The major challenge then is to elucidate the mechanism or mechanisms that are responsible for the antitumor effects, a question that remains elusive to a large extent. In principle, the purine metabolites can block certain enzymatic pathways or they can mimic the reactivity of the natural purines as substrates to be metabolized to their corresponding ribonucleotide and deoxyribonucleotide triphosphates and subsequently incorporated into DNA and RNA. Interference with nucleic acid synthesis and function causes multiple types of toxicities and will be discussed separately. Frequently, both inhibition of mononucleotide metabolism and nucleic acid incorporation occur (example: 6-thiopurines). The effects of purine analogs are either cytotoxic, a characteristic apparently inherent with any antitumor efficacy, or regulatory in particular with respect to external message/signal transduction through the cell membrane and intracellular processing of the message. These events involve GTP regulated membraneous coupling proteins, cyclic AMP and cyclic GMP, and protein kinases that are largely dependent on ATP. Purine analogs that interfere with these regulatory functions can produce muscle relaxation, hypothermia, antiallergic activity, inotropic effects on the heart, etc. (e.g., (2)). It is unknown whether such effects play any role in the antitumor effects of purine antimetabolites.

Most of the purine antimetabolites are applied in the form of bases or nucleosides which must rely on activation by the purine salvage enzymes for activation. Alterations or deletions of nonessential tumor salvage enzymes therefore represent a major mechanism of drug resistance (*vide infra*, 6-thiopurines). Robins (44) recently pointed out the advantages that could arise from the use of nucleotide analogs that do not need to be further activated and that do not enter RNA or DNA. He also reviewed the mechanisms by which the polar nucleotide analogs can enter the cells (44).

Antimetabolites that interfere with adenine metabolism. Adenine analogs of potential clinical utility include L-alanosine, fludarabine phosphate, pentostatin and 9-arabinosyl adenine (64). Further, adenine antimetabolites include tubercidine (7-deazaadenosine), 2-fluoroadenine, 8-azaadenine, formycin, toyocamycin, sangivamycin, cordycepin (3'-deoxyadenosine), psicofuranine, hadacidin, 2-chloro- and 2-bromo-2'-deoxyadenosine (19, 40, 41, 52, 69).

Of considerable interest are deoxyadenosine analogs or compounds that interfere with (deoxy)adenosine deaminase, (e.g., (19, 24)). The latter compounds include formycin, pentostatin (deoxycoformycin), EHNA. Deoxyadenosine is

formycin

highly toxic to the cells because of its potent feedback inhibition of ribonucleotide reductase after phosphorylation to dATP (e.g. (62)), although other mechanisms of cellular toxicity have also been proposed, e.g., deoxyadenosine incorporation into polyadenylated RNA and the accumulation of S-adenosylhomocysteine (e.g., (24)). The observation that an inborn deficiency of adenosine deaminase (ADA) leads to immunodeficiency because of T and B cell toxicity prompted the use of 2'-deoxyadenosine in combination with 2'-deoxycoformycin (to prevent dAdo deamination) in T lymphoblastic leukemia (12, 24). Another use of the ADA inhibitors is to block the deactivation of adenosine analogs, such as 9-arabinosyl adenine (64).

The inhibition of *de novo* adenylate formation represents another important target with two key enzymes, adenylosuccinate synthetase and adenylosuccinate lyase (Fig. 1). The amino acid analogs L-alanosine and hadacidin are either competitive with or replace aspartate in the formation of adenylosuccinate (21, 52). In particular, L-alanosine isolated from a Streptomyces (41), was found to be effective against certain viruses and transplanted fibrosarcoma induced by SV-40 virus in newborn hamsters. It undergoes

condensation with inosinate (IMP) (21) and also forms the alanosine analog of N-succinyl-carboxamide–amino imidazole riboside (28) which may represent the active conjugate that inhibits adenylsuccinate synthetase. Although the biological consequences of adenine nucleotide depletion remain unknown, cell toxicity by adenine starvation is apparently unrelated to RNA and DNA synthesis which continues at a normal rate at moderately toxic concentrations of L-alanosine (9). L-Alanosine is currently undergoing clinical testing (14).

Antimetabolites that interfere with guanine metabolism. In contrast to adenine starvation, guanine nucleotide starvation leads to a drastic reduction in DNA synthesis and to a lesser extent RNA synthesis, which occurs before the cellular pools of GTP and dGTP are fully exhausted (9). More recent studies with partially synchronized cell populations argue against the existence of separate cellular compartments of guanine nucleotides for nucleic acid synthesis. Again, our understanding of the biological consequences of guanine starvation is limited; nevertheless, with the rate limiting IMP dehydrogenase stringently linked to transformation and progression, inhibitors of this enzyme are potent antiviral drugs or antitumor agents in rodent tumor models: the 6-thiopurines, 3-deazaguanine, tiazofurin (see below), mycophenolic acid (see below), 6-chloropurine, virazol (1, 25, 43, 49, 50, 53, 56, 57). Mycophenolic acid is thought to represent a rather selective IMP dehydrogenase inhibitor with antiviral and antitumor activity, and limited antibacterial and antifungal activity. It was apparently isolated in 1896 by Gozio from the broth of penicillin glaucum and only much later proposed as a new lead compound in

mycophenolic acid

anticancer chemotherapy (57). Its major limitation for clinical use was thought to be its rapid *in vivo* inactivation by glucuronidation at the carboxyl function (56). Other IMP dehydrogenase inhibitors followed with tiazofurin representing one of the promising drugs. It will therefore be discussed separately.

Although guanylate synthetase usually displays a greater capacity than IMP dehydrogenase, there are several interesting antimetabolites that interfere at that point of guanylate formation *de novo*: acivicine, oxanosine, decoyinine, psicofuranine (66, 67, 72). In oxanosine, the N-1 is replaced by an oxygen which conveys its inhibitory properties against GMP synthetase (72).

Cadeguomycin represent just one more example of a guanosine analog isolated from microorganisms (58, 71). One can thus expect more guanine analogs of potential value in chemotherapy in the near future.

oxanosine

cadeguomycin

ANTIMETABOLITES THAT INTERFERE WITH EARLY *DE NOVO* PURINE BIOSYNTHESIS

The very first committed and rate limiting step of *de novo* purine biosynthesis is the target of several important antimetabolites that either afford allosteric inhibition of amidophosphoribosyl transferase (6-thiopurines, formycin) or compete with or mimick glutamine as the source of the amino group (azaserine, acivicin, DON). The glutamine antimetabolite acivicin interferes with several glutamine requiring reactions that appear to be transformation linked: amidophosphoribosyl transferase, GMP synthetase, carbamylphosphate synthetase and CTP synthetase, and it is therefore of considerable theoretical and possibly clinical interest (66). Azaserine also interferes with FGAM formation (Figure 1); however, it additionally acts as a potent mutagen-carcinogen by causing extensive DNA damage (34). The reaction thought to be responsible for the DNA toxicity is the α,β-elimination of diazoacetic acid which gives rise to carboxymethylated bases in DNA (75).

Antimetabolites that interfere with nucleic acids. The first example to be discovered of purine antimetabolite incorporation into nucleic acids was 8-azaguanine (40). Its toxicity is primarily a result of incorporation into RNA, which inhibits maturation of rRNA and thus protein synthesis (43, 69). Puromycin also inhibits protein synthesis at the ribosomal level. In contrast, 3-deazaguanine's toxicity is primarily directed against DNA after incorporation, although RNA related effects cannot be ruled out (43). A similar case can be made for 6-thioguanine. Other antimetabolites that are incorporated into nucleic acids or inhibit their functions or formation include tubercidine (7-deazaadenosine) and 2-fluoroadenosine (40). The mode of action of these agents is extremely diverse and often largely unaccounted for.

6-THIOPURINES

The thiopurines, 6-mercaptopurine and 6-thioguanine, represent the only purine antimetabolites that are currently in general clinical use as anticancer drugs. The 6-thiopurine derivative azathioprine is primarily used as an immunosuppressive agent and will not be discussed here. 6-Methylmercaptopurine ribonucleoside (6-MMPR), a metabolite of 6-mercaptopurine, is of interest since its toxicity is rather selectively a result of feedback inhibition of amidophosphoribosyl transferase by the nucleotide monophosphate of 6-MMPR (18). The 6-thiopurines are clinically used primarily in combination chemotherapy against various

leukemias (8); dose limiting toxicities of thioguanine include nausea and vomiting and myelosuppression (6, 8, 27). 6-Mercaptopurine is extensively metabolized along a number of pathways that include its conversion to 6-thioguanine 5'-monophosphate. The metabolism of both 6-mercaptopurine and 6-thioguanine is given in Figure 2. Degradative pathways primarily include liver microsomal cytochrome P450 enzymes and xanthine oxidase. Inhibition of the latter by concomitant administration of allopurinol can lead to a significant decrease of thiopurine catabolism following oral doses (73) during the first-pass metabolism in the liver. Salvage enzymes (HGPRTase) activate 6-mercaptopurine and 6-thioguanine to their corresponding nucleotides. 6-Mercaptopurine ribosyl 5'-phosphate (6-MPRP) is then either methylated to the active 6-MMPRP nucleotide or to 6-TGRP (Figure 2), which is subsequently elevated to the ribo- and deoxyribonucleotide triphosphates and incorporated into DNA and RNA (4, 15, 42, 60, 61, 68).

The mechanisms of action of the 6-thiopurines include the following (15, 42):

1. Inhibition of *de novo* purine biosynthesis by feedback inhibition of amidophosphoribosyltransferase by 6-MMPRP, 6-MPRP and 6-TGRP.
2. Sequential blockade of guanine nucleotide biosynthesis mostly by 6-TGMP.
3. Incorporation of 6-thioguanine into DNA.
4. Incorporation of 6-thioguanine into RNA with subsequent effects on rRNA maturation or translation.
5. 6-MPRP inhibits 3' to 5' exonuclease activity of DNA polymerase, thereby mimicking IMP effects (30).

Both purine biosynthesis inhibition and incorporation into nucleic acids were discovered rather early (4, 32, 33). However, the question as to which mechanism is the more important with regard to cytotoxicity (in particular of 6-mercaptopurine) remained controversial. An early study had revealed a greater degree of 6-thioguanine incorporation into DNA of 6-mercaptopurine resistant mouse tumor cells (4). However, Tidd and Paterson (60) showed that exposures of cells to equitoxic doses of 6-mercaptopurine and 6-thioguanine led to equal extents of 6-thioguanine incorporation into DNA at the time when toxicity became apparent. The same authors subsequently distinguished between the inhibition of purine nucleotide biosynthesis with immediate onset of cellular toxicity and the delayed toxicity associated with DNA incorporation (61).

The delayed DNA related toxicity of 6-thioguanine became the subject of intensive investigations. Weigent and Nelson (68) showed that one 6-thioguanine per 100 000 base units disrupts the transforming ability of *B. subtilis* DNA, and they concluded that 6-TG-DNA cannot serve as a template *in vitro* for transformation. With the use of a technique called premature chromatin condensation, Maybaum and Mandel (38, 39) were able to demonstrate severely disrupted chromatin in G2 cells that apparently occurred in only one of the sister chromatids with the delay of one cell cycle. They argued that 6-thioguanine readily incorporates into DNA, but that 6-TG-DNA fails to serve as an adequate template for DNA replication, which explains the delayed cytotoxicity.

The complexity of the mechanism of the thiopurine cytotoxicity is further demonstrated by the paradoxical behav-

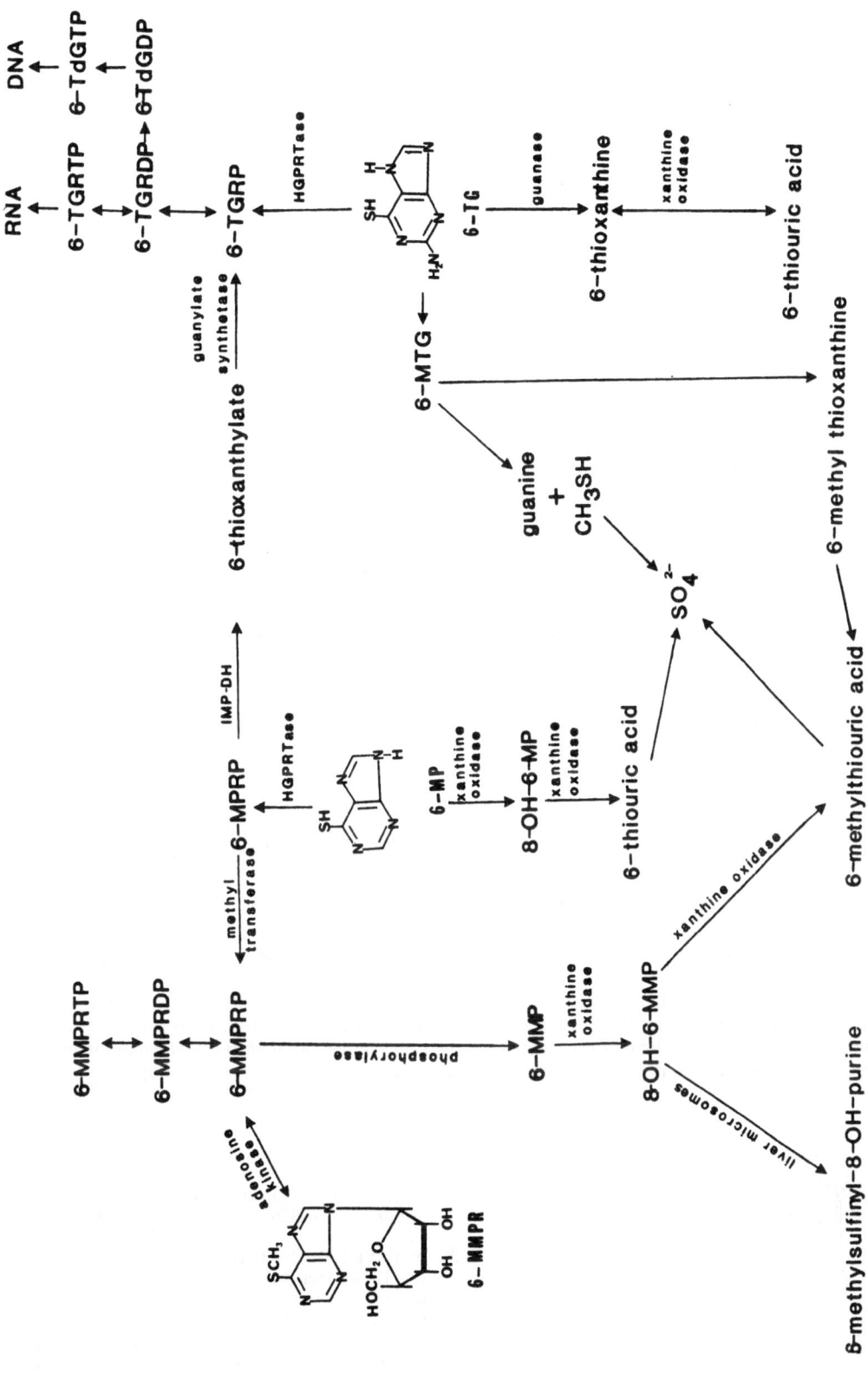

Figure 2. Metabolism of 6-mercaptopurine (6-MP), 6-thioguanine (6-TG), and 6-methylmercaptopurine ribonucleoside (6-MMPR). RP added to these abbreviations indicates the ribonucleoside 5′-monophosphate, and DP/TP stand for the 5′-di- and 5′-triphosphates.

ior of 6-mercaptopurine. With increasing doses, cytotoxicity reaches a plateau and subsequently decreases. Matsumura *et al.* (37) have attributed this behavior to a drug induced block of cell progression in G1, which prevents the cells from suffering lethal damage in G2.

Acquired resistance to the thiopurines presents a major problem with their clinical use (as well as that of other purine antimetabolites) and has, therefore, been extensively studied (3, 7, 18, 31, 47, 48, 63, 70). Alterations or deficiencies of HGPRTase were expected since this enzyme is required for thiopurine activation (e.g. (7)). Indeed, van Diggelen *et al.* (63) found 6-thioguanine resistance in cell cultures *in vitro* to be almost exclusively associated with HGPRTase deficiency, and Bennett *et al.* (3) suggested the ribonucleotide 6-MMPR as an alternative agent. Other mechanisms of resistance were also observed, including altered feedback inhibition of amidophosphoribosyl transferase (18) and increased nucleotide phosphohydrolyse activity to deactivate the thiopurine nucleotides (70). Furthermore, the frequency of the various biochemical modes of thiopurine resistance in cancer patients did not reveal a prevalence of HGPRTase deficiency (47, 48). Severe to moderate HGPRTase deficiency (determined by the APRTase/HGPRTase ratio) was only observed in 12% and 23%, respectively, of resistant tumors with acute nonlymphocytic leukemia. Altered HGPRTase (determined by the 6-MP/hypoxanthine specific activity ratio) was detected in 6 out of 18 resistant patients with acute leukemia. Finally, increased phosphohydrolase activity was present in 6 out of 7 resistant tumors with acute lymphatic leukemia (48) and in 5 out of 11 patients with lymphocytic leukemia (70). It may be of interest to search for drugs that show collateral sensitivity subsequent to these genetic enzyme changes.

TIAZOFURIN

The triazole derivative virazol (ribavirin) ranks among the first broad spectrum antiviral agents (53). It is promoted by adenosine kinase to the monophosphate and subsequently the triphosphate which interferes with nucleic acid functions. However, ribavirin also functions as a potent IMP dehydrogenase inhibitors, although its antitumor effects are rather limited (54). A systematic search for analogs with altered ring structure led to the thiazol derivative, tiazofurin (54). This agent was found to be among the most potent drugs against the Lewis lung tumor, which is used by the NCI screening program to identify compound of promise in

the treatment of lung tumors. With certain dosages, tiazofurin afforded complete protection and 10/10 long-term survivors in this model (45). It was subsequently found that tiazofurin is activated to its monophosphate by an as yet unidentified phosphotransferase activity (51) and that it inhibits GMP *de novo* biosynthesis (23). Further work revealed the formation of thiazol-4-carboxamide adenine dinucleotide (TAD), which functions as an NAD$^+$ analog and blocks IMP dehydrogenase in a highly selective fashion (10, 29). The molecular basis of the selective blockade of only IMP dehydrogenase, and no other NAD$^+$ utilizing

TAD

enzyme tested, remains unknown, but it is thought that guanine starvation is to a large part responsible for the antitumor effect of tiazofurin (16). Thus, polyADP ribosylation was also unaffected by TAD *in vitro* (11). Jayaram *et al.* (22) observed that cellular resistance to tiazofurin is associated with a lack of its anabolism to TAD while the monophosphate is formed in normal amounts.

It is currently unknown whether tiazofurin exhibits mechanisms of cellular toxicity other than IMP dehydrogenase inhibition. With the use of an *in vivo* labeling technique, Streeter and Miller (55) suggested the possibility that tiazofurin is also a potent inhibitor of GDP kinase, a finding that may be of importance *in vivo*, since such a block would not be bypassed by the guanine salvage pathways.

Current clinical testing will reveal the value of tiazofurin and other purine antimetabolites as anticancer agents. Whatever the clinical results, however, it is already clear that we have learned a great deal from these drugs about biochemical changes related to transformation and tumor progression.

tiazofurin   ribavirin

REFERENCES

1. Anderson JH, Sartorelli AC: Inhibition of inosinic acid dehydrogenase by 6-chloropurine nucleotide. *Biochem Pharmacol* 18:2737, 1969
2. Bartlett RT, Cook AF, Holman MJ, McComas WW, Nowoswait EF, Poonian MS: Synthesis and pharmacological evaluation of a series of analogues of 1-methylisoguanosine. *J Med Chem* 24:947, 1981
3. Bennett LL Jr *et al.*: Activity and mechanism of action of 6-methylthiopurine ribonucleoside in cancer cells resistant to 6-mercaptopurine. *Nature* 205:1275, 1965
4. Bieber S, Dietrich LS, Elion GB, Hitchings GH, Martin DS:

The incorporation of 6-mercaptopurine-S³⁵ into the nucleic acids of sensitive and nonsensitive transplantable mouse tumors. *Cancer Res* 21:228, 1961

5. Breter M-J, Zahn RK: The quantitative determination of metabolites of 6-mercaptopurine in biological materials. II. Advantages of a variable-wavelength detector for the determination of 6-thiopurines. *J Chromatogr* 137:61, 1977

6. Britell JC, Moertel CG, Kvols LK, O'Connell MJ, Rubin J, Schutt AJ: Phase II trial of i.v. 6-thioguanine in advanced colorectal carcinoma. *Cancer Treat Rep* 65:909, 1981

7. Brockman RW: Biochemical aspects of mercaptopurine inhibition and resistance. *Cancer Res* 23:1191, 1963

8. Brox LW, Birkett L, Belch A: Clinical pharmacology of oral thioguanine in acute myelogenous leukemia. *Cancer Chemother Pharmacol* 6:35, 1981

9. Cohen MB, Sadée W: The contributions of the depletion of guanine and adenine nucleotides to the toxicity of purine starvation. *Cancer Res* 43:158, 1983

10. Cooney DA, Jayaram HN, Gebeyehu G, Betts CR, Kelley JA, Marquez VE, Johns DG: The conversion of 2-β-D-ribofuranosylthiazole-4-carboxamide to an analogue of NAD with potent IMP dehydrogenase inhibitory properties. *Biochem Pharmacol* 31:2133, 1982

11. Cooney DA, Jayaram HN, Glazer RI, Kelley JA, Marquez VE, Gebeyehu G, Van Cott AC, Zwelling LA, Johns DA: Studies on the mechanism of action of tiazofurin. Metabolism to an analog of NAD with potent IMP dehydrogenase-inhibitory activity. *Adv Enz Reg* 21:271, 1983

12. Cowan MJ, Cashman D, Ammann AJ: Effects of formycin B on human lymphocyte deoxyribonucleic acid synthesis. Optimization of cell culture conditions. *Biochem Pharmacol* 30:2651, 1981

13. Day JL, Tterlikkis L, Niemann R, Mobley A, Spikes C: Assay of mercaptopurine in plasma using paired-ion high-performance liquid chromatography. *J Pharm Sci* 67:1027, 1978

14. Dosik GM, Stewart D, Valdivieso M, Burgess MA, Bodey GP: Phase I Study of L-alanosine using a daily × 3 schedule. *Cancer Treat Rep* 66:73, 1982

15. Drake S, Carpenter P, Nelson JA: Use of vaccinia, a DNA virus, to study the role of DNA incorporation in the mechanism of action of 6-thioguanine. *Biochem Pharmacol* 32:1448, 1983

16. Earle MF, Glaser RI: Activity and metabolism of 2-D-ribofuranosylthiazole-4-carboxamide in human lymphoid tumor cells in culture. *Cancer Res* 43:133, 1983

17. Elion GB, Callahan S, Rundles RW, Hitchings GH: Relationship between metabolic fates and antitumor activities of thiopurines. *Cancer Res* 23:1207, 1963

18. Henderson JF, Caldwell IC, Paterson ARP: Decreased feedback inhibition in a 6-methylmercaptopurine ribonucleoside-resistant tumor. *Cancer Res* 27:1773, 1967

19. Huang M-C, Hatfield K, Roether AW, Montgomery JA, Blakley RL: Analogs of 2'-deoxyadenosine: Facile enzymatic preparation and growth inhibitory effects on human cell lines. *Biochem Pharmacol* 30:2663, 1981

20. Jackson RC, Weber G, Morris HP: IMP Dehydrogenase, an enzyme linked with proliferation and malignancy. *Nature* 256:331, 1975

21. Jayaram HN, Tyagi AK, Anandaraj S, Montgomery JA, Kelley JA, Kelley J, Adamson RH, Cooney DA: Metabolites of alanosine, an antitumor antibiotic. *Biochem Pharmacol* 28:3551, 1979

22. Jayaram HN, Cooney DA, Glazer RI, Dion RL, Johns DG: Mechanism of resistance to the oncolytic C-nucleoside 2-β-D-ribofuranosylthiazol-4-carboxamide (NSC-286193). *Biochem Pharmacol* 31:2557, 1982

23. Jayaram HN, Dion RL, Glazer RI, Johns DG, Robins RK, Srivastava PC, Cooney DA: Initial studies on the mechanism of action of a new oncolytic thiazole nucleoside, 2-β-D-ribofuranosylthiazole-4-carboxamide (NSC 286193). *Biochem Pharmacol* 31:2371, 1982

24. Kefford RF, Taylor IW, Fox RM: Flow cytometric analysis of adenosine analogue lymphocytotoxicity. *Cancer Res* 43:5112, 1983

25. Khwaja TA: 3-Deazaguanine, a candidate drug for the chemotherapy of breast carcinomas? *Cancer Treat Rep* 66:1853, 1982

26. Kizaki H, Ohsaka F, Sakurada T: Role of GTP in CTP synthetase from Ehrlich Ascites tumor cells. *Biochem Biophys Res Commun* 108:286, 1982

27. Konits PH, Egorin MJ, Van Echo DA, Aisner J, Andrews PA, May ME, Bachur NR, Wiesnik PH: Phase II evaluation and plasma pharmacokinetics of high-dose intravenous 6-thioguanine in patients with colorectal carcinoma. *Cancer Chemother Pharmacol* 8:199, 1982

28. Kovach JS: L-Alanosine (NSC 153353). In: *Pharmacokinetics of Anticancer Agents in Humans*, edited by Ames MM, Powis G, Kovach JS, chapter 15, pp. 455–456. Elsevier, Amsterdam-New York–Oxford, 1983

29. Kuttan R, Robins RK, Saunders PP: Inhibition of inosinate dehydrogenase by metabolites of 2-β-D-ribofuranosylthiazole-4-carboxamide. *Biochem Biophys Res Commun* 107:862, 1982

30. Lee MYWT, Byrnes JJ, Downey KM, So AG: Mechanism of inhibition of deoxyribonucleic acid synthesis of 1-β-D-arabinofuranosyladenosine triphosphate and its potentiation by 6-mercaptopurine ribonucleoside 5'-monophosphate. *Biochem* 19:215, 1980

31. Lee SH, Sartorelli AC: Biochemical mechanism of resistance of cultured sarcoma 180 cells to 6-thioguanine. *Biochem Pharmacol* 30:3109, 1981

32. LePage GA: Basic biochemical effects and mechanism of action of 6-thioguanine. *Cancer Res* 23:1202, 1963

33. LePage GA, Jones M: Purinethiols as feedback inhibitors of purine synthesis in ascites tumor cells. *Cancer Res* 21:642, 1961

34. Lilja HS, Hyde E, Longnecker DS, Yager JD Jr: DNA damage and repair in rat tissues following administration of azaserine. *Cancer Res* 37:3925, 1977

35. Loo TL, Lu K, Benvenuto JA, Rosenblum MG: Disposition and metabolism of thiopurines III. 2'-Deoxythioguanosine and 6-thioguanine in the dog. *Cancer Chemother Pharmacol* 6:131, 1981

36. Mancini WR, Cheng YC: Human deoxycytidylate deaminase substrate and regulator specificities and their chemotherapeutic implications. *Molec Pharmacol* 23:159, 1983

37. Matsumura S, Hoshino T, Weizsaecker M, Deen DF: Paradoxical behavior of 6-mercaptopurine as a cytotoxic agent: Decreasing cell kill with increasing dose. *Cancer Treat Rep* 67:475, 1983

38. Maybaum J, Mandel HG: Differential chromatid damage induced by 6-thioguanine in CHO cells. *Exp Cell Res* 135:465, 1981

39. Maybaum J, Mandel HG: Unilateral chromatid damage: A new basis for 6-thioguanine cytotoxicity. *Cancer Res* 43:3852, 1983

40. Montgomery JA: The biochemical basis for the drug actions of purines. *Progr Med Chem* 7:69, 1970

41. Murthy YKS, Thiemann JE, Coronelli C, Sensi P: Alanosine, a new antiviral and antitumor agent isolated from a Streptomyces. *Nature* 211:1198, 1966

42. Nelson JA, Carpenter JW, Rose LM, Adamson DJ: Mechanism of action of 6-thioguanine, 6-mercaptopurine and 8-azaguanine, *Cancer Res* 35:2872, 1975

43. Rivest RS, Irwin D, Mandel HG: Purine analogs revisited: Interference in protein formation. *Adv Enzym Reg* 20:351, 1982

44. Robins RK: The potential of nucleotide analogs as inhibitors of retroviruses and tumors. *Pharm Res* 1:11, 1984

45. Robins RK, Srivastava PC, Narayanan VL, Plowman J, Paull KD: 2-D-Ribofuranosylthiazole-4-carboxamide, a novel potential antitumor agent for lung tumors and metastases. *J Med Chem* 25:107, 1982

46. Rosenfeld JM, Taguchi VY, Hillcoat BL, Kawal M: Determination of 6-mercaptopurine in plasma by mass spectrometry. *Anal Chem* 49:725, 1980

47. Rosman M, Williams HE: Leukocytic purine phosphoribosyl transferase in human leukemias sensitive and resistant to 6-thiopurines. *Cancer Res* 33:1202, 1973

48. Rosman M, Lee MH, Creasey WA, Sartorelli AC: Mechanism of resistance to 6-thiopurines in human leukemias. *Cancer Res* 34:1952, 1974

49. Saunders PP, Chao LY, Robins RK, Loo TL: Action of 3-deazaguanine in *Escherichia coli*. *Molec Pharmacol* 15:691, 1979

50. Saunders PP, Chao LY, Loo TL, Robins RK: Actions of 3-deazaguanine and 3-deazaguanosine on variant cell lines of Chinese hamster ovary cells. *Biochem Pharmacol* 30:2374, 1981

51. Saunders PP, Kuttan R, Lai MM, Robins RK: Action of 2-D-ribofuranosylthiazole-carboxamide (Tiazofurin) in Chinese hamster ovary and variant cell lines. *Molec Pharmacol* 23:534, 1983

52. Shigeura HT, Gordon CN: The mechanism of action of hadacidin. *J Biol Chem* 237:1937, 1962

53. Sidwell RW, Huffman JH, Khare GP, Allen LB, Witkowski JT, Robins RK: Broad spectrum antiviral activity of virazol: 1-D-Ribofuranosyl-1,2,4-triazol-3-carboxamide. *Science* 177:705, 1972

54. Srivastava PC, Pickering MV, Allen LB, Streeter DG, Campbell MT, Witkowski JT, Sidwell RW, Robins RK: Synthesis and antiviral activity of certain thiazole C-nucleosides. *J Med Chem* 20:256, 1977

55. Streeter DG, Miller JP: The *in vitro* inhibition of purine nucleotide biosynthesis of 2-D-ribofuranosylthiazole-4-carboxamide. *Biochem Biophys Res Commun* 103:1409, 1981

56. Sweeney MJ, Hoffman DH, Esterman MA: Metabolism and biochemistry of mycophenolic acid. *Cancer Res* 32:1803, 1972

57. Sweeney MJ, Gerzon K, Harris PN, Holmes RE, Poore GA, Williams RH: Experimental antitumor activity and preclinical toxicology of mycophenolic acid. *Cancer Res* 32:1795, 1972

58. Tanaka N, Wu RT, Okabe T, Yamashita H, Shimazu A, Nishimura T: Cadeguomycin, a novel nucleoside analog antibiotic. I. The producing organism, production and isolation of cadeguomycin. *J Antibiot* 35:272, 1982

59. Thelander L, Reichard P: Reduction of ribonucleotides. *Ann Rev Biochem* 48:133, 1979

60. Tidd DM, Paterson ARP: A biochemical mechanism for the delayed cytotoxic reactions of 6-mercaptopurine. *Cancer Res* 34:738, 1974

61. Tidd DM, Paterson ARP: Distinction between inhibition of purine nucleotide synthesis and the delayed cytotoxic reaction of 6-mercaptopurine. *Cancer Res* 34:733, 1974

62. Ullman B, Cliff SM, Gudas LJ, Levinson BB, Wormsted MA, Martin DW Jr: Alterations in deoxyribonucleotide metabolism is cultured cells with ribonucleotide reductase activities refractory to feedback inhibition by 2'-deoxyadenosine triphosphate. *J Biol Chem* 255:8308, 1980

63. Van Diggelen OP, Donahue TF, Shin SI: Basis of differential cellular sensitivity to 8-azaguanine and 6-thioguanine. *J Cell Physiol* 98:59, 1979

64. Venditti JM: The National Cancer Institute Antitumor Drug Discovery Program. Current and future perspectives: A commentary. *Cancer Treat Rep* 67:767, 1983

65. Watts RWE: Purine enzymes and immune function. *Clin Biochem* 16:48, 1983

66. Weber G: Biochemical strategy of cancer cells and the design of chemotherapy: G.H.A. Clowes Memorial Lecture. *Cancer Res* 43:3466, 1983

67. Weber G: Enzymes of purine metabolism in cancer. *Clin Biochem* 16:57, 1983

68. Weigent DA, Nelson JA: Reduction of DNA transforming activity in culture by 6-mercaptopurine. *Cancer Res* 40:4381, 1980

69. Weiss JW, Pitot HC: Inhibition of ribosomal RNA maturation in Novikoff hepatoma cells by toyocamycin, tubercidin, and 6-thioguanosine. *Cancer Res* 34:581, 1974

70. Wolpert MK, Damle SP, Brown JE, Sznycer E, Agrawal KC, Sartorelli AC: The role of phosphohydrolases in the mechanism of resistance of neoplastic cells to 6-thiopurines. *Cancer Res* 31:1620, 1971

71. Wu RT, Okabe T, Namikoshi M, Okuda S, Nishimura T, Tanaka N: Cadeguomycin, a novel nucleoside analog antibiotic II. Improved purification, physicochemical properties and structure assignment. *J Antibiotics* 35:279, 1982

72. Yagisawa N, Shimada N, Takita T, Ishizuka M, Takeuchi T, Umezawa M: Mode of action of oxanosine, a novel nucleoside antibiotic. *J Antibiot* 35:755, 1982

73. Zimm S, Collins JM, O'Neill D, Chabner BA, Poplack DG: Inhibition of first-pass metabolism in cancer chemotherapy: Interaction of 6-mercaptopurine and allopurinol. *Clin Pharmacol Ther* 34:810, 1983

74. Zimmerman TP, Chu L-C, Bugge CJL, Nelson DJ, Lyon GM, Elion GB: Identification of 6-methylmercaptopurine ribonucleoside 5'-diphosphate and 5'-triphosphate as metabolites of 6-mercaptopurine in man. *Cancer Res* 34:221, 1974

75. Zurlo J, Curphey TJ, Hiley R, Longnecker DS: Identification of 7-carboxymethylguanine in DNA from pancreatic acinar cells exposed to azaserine. *Cancer Res* 42:1286, 1982

For postscript see end of Volume, p. 244.

6

ALKYLATING AGENTS

D.E.V. WILMAN and P.B. FARMER

INTRODUCTION

Alkylating agents hold an important place in the array of drugs available for clinical cancer chemotherapy. Chemically alkylating agents are compounds (RX) which react with nucleophilic (electron-donating) centres (Y) to form covalently bound products (RY) containing the alkyl group (R). The binding of alkylating agents to cellular macromolecules is thought to be largely responsible for the *in vivo* cytotoxic action of these compounds. Unfortunately the chemical processes are not tumour-selective and the *in vivo* effects of alkylating agents are seen in all dividing cells to which these drugs have access. Frequently the side effects that occur with alkylating agent treatment limit the dose of the compound that can be used for tumour control. There has consequently been a great deal of interest in the development of alkylating agents which contain a structural molecular feature which might guide it more selectively towards a tumour cell rather than towards a normal cell. Selectivity of alkylating agent attack towards tumour cells may also be increased by clinical protection measures on normal tissues (e.g., by autologous bone marrow transplantation). The development of alkylating agent use has thus been an equal challenge to the drug-designers and to the clinical chemotherapists.

The clinically used alkylating agents described in this chapter, with the exception of the triazenes, all possess the chemical property of bifunctionality, i.e., they contain two centres capable of alkylating nucleophiles, and are thus able to cross-link two of these nucleophiles. DNA cross-linking has been demonstrated to be a general phenomenon for bifunctional alkylating agents *in vitro*, and there is a substantial amount of evidence now (e.g., (183)) to support the hypothesis of Brookes and Lawley in 1961 (32) that the formation of DNA strand cross-links is a major factor governing the cytotoxicity of bifunctional alkylating agents. Thus for example the *in vitro* cytotoxicity of several chloroethylnitrosoureas to human embryo cells appears to be related (though not quantitatively) to the extent of DNA cross-linking; the more resistant cells showed little or no DNA interstrand cross-linking, implying either the failure to form these linkages or their rapid repair (83). Similarly in three Burkitt's lymphoma cell lines the cytotoxicity of melphalan was correlated with interstrand cross-linking of DNA (76).

Although DNA cross-linking could satisfactorily explain the observed inhibition of the DNA template caused by alkylating agents, it is not an all-inclusive mechanism of alkylating action. Monofunctional agents such as DTIC (5-(3,3-dimethyl-1-triazeno)imidazole-4-carboxamide) and procarbazine do not appear to be chemically capable of producing cross-links, but show antitumour properties. Bifunctional alkylating agents also give rise to monofunctional DNA alkylations, and DNA-protein cross-links although the relevance of these to their antitumour effects is not yet understood.

Although alkylating agents have been studied as anticancer agents for about 40 years, and several thousand of these compounds have been synthesised and tested in that time, the number of alkylating agents in clinical practice is surprisingly small. For the reasons described above bi- or poly-functional compounds have been the most popular to investigate. Initially the pioneering work was carried out by Ross (200) who synthesised a variety of nitrogen mustards, including chlorambucil, which is still clinically used. Variations in the nature of the leaving group (X) in the alkylating agent could be used to increase or decrease the reactivity of the molecule, and other pharmacological and physicochemical parameters (e.g. lipid solubility, pK) could be altered by making modifications to the alkyl group (R) (Table 1). Melphalan for example contains an amino acid as the alkyl group, and was synthesised by Bergel and Stock (21) in the hope of interfering with malignant cell protein or DNA metabolism.

The concept of using prodrugs has also been attempted with nitrogen mustards. A prodrug is an agent whose activity is increased following some enzymic or chemical action that is specific to the target site for the drug's action. One of the earlier examples in the alkylating agent field was the azo-mustard CB1414 (4-[di-(2-chloroethyl)amino]-2-methylazobenzene-2'-carboxylic acid), which was designed by Ross and Warwick (204) for use against tumours which are high in levels of the enzyme azoreductase. The action of this enzyme on the azomustard is to release a *p*-phenylenediamine mustard which is of very much greater alkylating activity than the initial drug, and which will therefore cause toxicity specifically in the areas where the azoreductase enzyme is present. This concept has subsequently been applied with the compound CB10-252 (see below) which is currently undergoing development. The very widely used alkylating agent cyclophosphamide was also designed as a prodrug of a more active agent, although in this case the rationale was later shown to be unsatisfactory.

In parallel with the development of nitrogen mustards as anticancer agents came that of the other major classes of alkylating agents, methane sulphonates, aziridines, epoxides

63

P.V. Woolley (ed.), Cancer management in Man: Biological Response Modifiers, Chemotherapy, Antibiotics, Hyperthermia, Supporting Measures
© 1989. Kluwer Academic Publishers, Dordrecht.

Table 1. Nitrogen mustards R–N(CH$_2$CH$_2$Cl)$_2$.

Name	R group	Hypothesis for original synthesis
Melphalan		Imitation of endogenous compound
Chlorambucil		Altered lipophilicity and ionic charge
Prednimustine		Transport to areas high in glucocorticoid receptors
Sulphadiazene mustard		Concentration in tumours because of pH differences
p-Hydroxyaniline mustard glucuronide		Activated in areas containing β-glucuronidase
Cyclophosphamide		Activated by enzymatic hydrolysis[a]
Azo-mustard CB 10-252		Activated in areas containing azoreductase[b]
Spiromustine		High lipid solubility for concentration in CNS

[a] This hypotheses was later shown to be invalid. See text.
[b] The alkylating group in the azo-mustard CB 10-252 is N–(CH$_2$CH(CH$_3$)Br)$_2$.

and more recently triazenes and nitrosoureas (Table 2). Examples of drugs from each of these sections which have been in, or are approaching, clinical use, will be covered in some detail in subsequent sections of this chapter.

The most recent attempts to improve the selectivity of alkylating agents to tumour cells have concentrated on ways of delivering the agent more specifically to these cells. For example the linkage of the alkylating function to an antibody or to a hormone for which the tumour cell has receptors may result in a useful localisation of the alkylating

Table 2. L-Phenylalanine.

Class	Example	Structure
Alkanesulphonate	Busulphan	$CH_3SO_2OCH_2CH_2CH_2CH_2OSO_2CH_3$
Aziridine	Thio-TEPA	
Epoxide	Dianhydrogalactitol	
Triazene	DTIC	
Nitrosourea	BCNU	

agent's attack. Although these possibilities have been understood and exploited for many years there is as yet no dramatic improvement in the clinic of the new drugs' activity over that of the best established drugs such as cyclophosphamide.

Cancer chemotherapy does, however, continue to improve its effectiveness, both through the use of alkylating agents and the other drugs described elsewhere in this volume.

One of the drawbacks associated with the resulting increasing life span of cancer sufferers that is now being achieved is the development of long-term side effects following successful anticancer therapy. In particular many clinically used alkylating agents are carcinogenic (213) and mutagenic, and it is important that ways of minimising these genotoxic risks should be studied in parallel with the development of more powerful drugs. Protection against this carcinogenicity may in some cases be possible, a recent example being the use of mercaptoethanesulphonic acid (Mesna (29)) which decreases the incidence of bladder tumours in rats caused by cyclophosphamide therapy, in addition to its immediate protective effect against haemorrhagic cystitis. Attention should also be paid to the health of the nurses administering alkylating agents to patients. There have been recent reports of the increased mutagenicity of such nurses' urine (89), of increased sister chromatid exchange frequencies in nurses' lymphocytes (191), and even of the urinary excretion of cyclophosphamide by nurses handling this drug (128). At this stage, however, the number of cases studied has been extremely small and the results have been strongly criticised (77, 78). Furthermore rigorous studies of this problem are clearly necessary.

ANILINE MUSTARD

Aniline mustard (bis-(2-chloroethyl)aniline, I) was the first aromatic nitrogen mustard to be synthesised (197), although it was not until later (199) that it was prepared as an anticancer agent. To date the clinical potential of this drug has not been fully exploited. The particular interest in aniline mustard stems from the observation by Connors and Whisson (60) of its ability to eradicate the ADJ/PC5 mouse plasma cell tumour, it being the only compound capable of doing this. 4-Hydroxyaniline mustard is twelve times more toxic than aniline mustard in this system but both toxicity and antitumour activity of other parasubstituted derivatives are greatly reduced. These same authors later demonstrated a correlation between inhibitory action and β-glucuronidase activity in a variety of tumours (253). The sarcoma 180 and NK lymphoma with β-glucuronidase levels similar to liver were unaffected by aniline mustard whereas the ADJ/PC5 and ADJ/PC6A plasmacytomas, which have elevated levels of the enzyme, underwent total regression. Other tumours which are extremely sensitive to aniline mustard have also been shown to have high levels of β-glucuronidase (19, 73).

The hypothesis put forward for this activity by Connors and Whisson (60) was that aniline mustard is metabolised in the liver to 4-hydroxyaniline mustard (II), which although extremely reactive due to the electron donating character of the hydroxyl group, is rapidly conjugated to form the O-glucuronide (III). Subsequently, in tissue of high β-glucuronidase activity, the conjugate is cleaved back to the cytotoxic 4-hydroxyaniline mustard. Synthesis of various glucuronic acid derivatives and testing in the ADJ/PC6A tumour system gave added support to this theory (38).

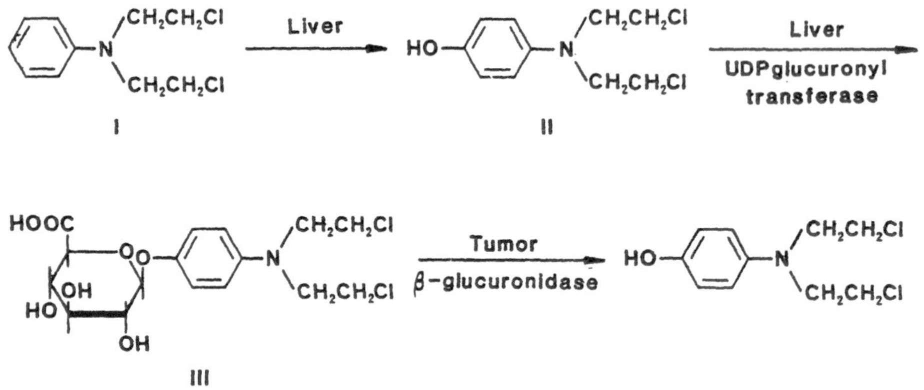

Figure 1. Aniline mustard metabolism.

Microsomal metabolism of aniline mustard *in vitro* yields the glucuronide which can also be identified in the serum and bile of treated rats (45, 56).

The most significant clinical report relating to aniline mustard was that of Young and his colleagues (261). The importance of this trial was that the tumour β-glucuronidase was measured in biopsy specimens from a number of patients. Although the number of significant responses was poor, 6 of 78 patients with advanced cancer treated, 5 of which were cancer of the prostate and one a renal tumour, some correlation was observed between β-glucuronidase level and tumour regression. Of particular interest was the observation that two of the tumours with a high β-glucuronidase level were sensitive to aniline mustard therapy initially, but upon relapse were both insensitive to the drug and lacking in the enzyme. To date no trial solely limited to β-glucuronidase positive tumours has been undertaken and until such happens the usefulness of this drug will remain unknown.

CHLORAMBUCIL

Chlorambucil (4-(bis-(2-chloroethyl)amino)phenylbutyric acid, Table 1) was the product of an investigation by Ross into the effect of changes in charge and lipophilicity on the activity of aniline mustard (86). It is water soluble as a salt, but has surface active properties due to the high lipophilicity of the remainder of the molecule. The drug was soon introduced into the clinic (98) and has since become established as of major importance in the treatment of malignant disease. It is routinely used in the treatment of chronic lymphoid leukaemia (209) and carcinoma of the ovary (172). Other clinical situations in which chlorambucil is of value are Hodgkin's disease and other lymphomas (87, 148) and a number of solid tumours (180). Chlorambucil has also been used in numerous combination regimes. Of particular note has been its incorporation into the MVPP (mustine, vinblastine, procarbazine and prednisone) combination for the treatment of advanced Hodgkin's disease (146, 175). Replacement of mustine by chlorambucil (ChlVPP) results in a combination which produces a similar remission rate to MVPP without the associated toxicity. It is only more re-

cently that details of the metabolism and mechanism of action of the drug have been elucidated.

Interest in this aspect was aroused by the suggestion that chlorambucil is metabolised into a more effective derivative. This metabolic activation is enhanced by phenobarbitone pretreatment (15, 124). Although chlorambucil is an active alkylating agent in its own right, and therefore unlike cyclophosphamide does not require metabolic activation, this does not preclude the possibility of metabolism resulting in a more active species. Subsequently Mitoma *et al.* (178) identified 10 urinary metabolites from rats treated with ^{14}C-labelled chlorambucil. The majority of these involved oxidative degradation of the butyric acid side chain to give phenylacetic and benzoic acid derivatives. Godeneche and co-workers (107) had also shown that β-oxidation of the side chain occurred.

An elegant chemical synthesis of 3,4-dehydro-chlorambucil, a postulated intermediate in the metabolism of chlorambucil, to phenylacetic acid mustard (2-(4-N,N-bis(2-chloroethyl)aminophenyl)acetic acid) enabled this pathway to be confirmed (176). Phenylacetic acid mustard was detected in the blood of rats injected with 3,4-dehydrochlorambucil, from which it would be formed by β-oxidation. These same workers showed that the major urinary metabolite was 2-(4-N-(2-chloroethyl)aminophenyl)acetic acid formed by dechloroethylation. As phenylacetic acid mustard has similar antitumor activity to chlorambucil but is more than twice as toxic (176) the metabolism of the parent drug must be regarded as disadvantageous from a therapeutic point of view. Attempts to improve the therapeutic efficiency of chlorambucil by inhibiting this metabolism have been investigated.

Farmer and co-workers (90) synthesised dideuterated analogues of chlorambucil with both deuterium atoms either α or β to the carboxylic acid group. In either case the first steps of metabolism, dehydrogenation to 3,4-dehydrochlorambucil followed by rehydration to the β-hydroxy derivative further dehydrogenation of which liberates the β-keto analogue, could be expected to show a deuterium isotope effect. Such an effect would be expected to reduce the rate at which chlorambucil is metabolised to phenylacetic acid mustard. The results obtained with these compounds, however, demonstrated a deuterium isotope effect only in the β-position but this was insufficient to alter the therapeutic response. Deuterium was lost rapidly from the α-position by an uncertain mechanism. The study of chlorambucil analogues in which the β-oxidation step is completely blocked by substitution at the β-position is in progress. Difluorination at this position removed the CNS toxicity observed with chlorambucil but caused severe haemorrhage in rats. Monomethylation or trifluoromethylation caused extreme toxicity (40). To date pharmacokinetic investigations have not been undertaken on these new analogues.

Chlorambucil has recently been reported as a radiosensitiser in experimental systems (122).

In experimental tumour systems the activity of chlorambucil is enhanced by prednisolone. Prednimustine, the prednisolone ester of chlorambucil (Table 1) is equally active as the combination (119). Prednimustine was originally synthesised to use the steroid as a carrier through the cell membrane for the cytotoxic drug (158). There is currently some discussion as to the utility of prednimustine in relation to a mixture of its components (185).

Pharmacokinetic studies have shown that prednimustine is not detectable in the plasma of patients whilst chlorambucil is (80). In fact the bioavailability of chlorambucil is some five times lower in prednimustine treated patients than in those receiving the parent alkylating drug. This confirmation in man of earlier studies in rodents (187) has led to the conclusion that the use of prednimustine in routine combination therapy cannot be recommended (186).

One of the ways under development of attacking tumour cells selectively is by attaching the cytotoxic entity to a tissue specific protein or more particularly a tumour specific antibody. Initially chlorambucil was used in this fashion either physically bound (102) or chemically bound (201, 202).

However, the number of cytotoxic molecules which can be attached to an antibody without denaturation is often insufficient for cell death. Despite this such chlorambucil–antibody complexes have shown activity in murine systems (70). Interest has therefore been focused on toxins such as ricin, abrin and diphtheria toxin, where a single A-chain is sufficient to kill the cell. Interest in chlorambucil has been maintained, however, as it is now used to provide selective attachment of the toxin to the antibody (234).

Chlorambucil has also recently been linked to an anti-CEA antibody (22), and the conjugate will be investigated for anticolon cancer properties.

MELPHALAN

L-Phenylalanine mustard (Table 2) variously known as melphalan and L-PAM is one of the optical isomers of the alanine derivatives of aniline mustard, and was first synthesised by Bergel and Stock (20, 21). The D-isomer (medphalan) was also synthesised at this time by Bergel and Stock, whilst the racemate (sarcolysin) was prepared by Larionov *et al.* (165) and shown to be half as potent as melphalan.

Despite the principle of its design melphalan has not shown clinical utility against melanoma, however, it has enjoyed widespread clinical use in the treatment of other tumours. Initially this was in the treatment of myeloma (26) and its effectiveness has been increased by combination with

prednisone (99). Other successfully treated malignancies include carcinoma of the ovary (193), testicular cancer (246), advanced breast cancer (133) and other solid tumours and leukaemias (102). It has also been suggested that it may have activity against disseminated carcinoma of the prostate (96). The response rate to melphalan as a single agent in breast cancer therapy varies between 16 and 30% (168), and it has shown some promise as an adjuvant to surgery in the treatment of this disease. However, whilst early results, particularly in menopausal women, were remarkably good (94), these have not always been born out in later trials. For instance, Glucksberg and co-workers (106) have shown that the CMFVP combination (cyclophosphamide, methotrexate, 5-fluorouracil, vincristine and prednisone) is superior to melphalan in terms of survival and recurrence in both pre- and post-menopausal women with breast cancer. However, Carpenter and Maddox (42) have recently pointed out that because of the variable absorption of oral melphalan (4) detailed patient comparisons are required before a definitive assessment of the benefit or otherwise of this drug in the adjuvant therapy of breast cancer can be made.

In normal clinical use the dosage of melphalan is limited to 20–25 mg/m^2 to avoid severe myelosuppression. A number of methods have been established over the past few years to enable larger doses to be given without causing unduly severe side effects.

The first of these, marrow rescue, was introduced by McElwain and his colleagues (173) as a treatment for malignant melanoma. Investigation of the *in vivo* plasma and urinary half-lives of melphalan by mass spectrometry showed that after six hours plasma levels of the drug following a 140 mg/m^2 dose would be insufficient to have a significantly toxic effect on bone marrow cells. In a Phase I study of 8 patients, marrow was removed, the drug administered and the marrow reinfused eight hours later after storage at 4°C. The tumours of 7 patients showed a response and there was 1 remission. The granulocyte count of these patients recovered more quickly than that of 4 patients receiving 60–125 mg/m^2 of melphalan without the marrow graft.

The other site of melphalan toxicity is gut epithelium. This can be ameliorated by administration of a 'priming' dose of cyclophosphamide a week prior to melphalan (63). The use of a priming dose of cyclophosphamide had previously been shown to be of value in overcoming the marrow toxicity of melphalan (120).

Such high dose therapy has also been used in the treatment of plasma cell leukemia and myeloma (174).

Prednisolone has been shown to enhance the antitumor activity of melphalan in mice but at the expense of some increase in toxicity (216). The nitroimidazole radiosensitisers are also capable of enhancing the toxicity of alkylating agents to hypoxic cells (49, 198). In the case of the sensitiser misonidazole the activity is observed when it is given shortly before or together with the alkylating agent. A recently reported Phase I trial of melphalan infusion 2 hours after oral misonidazole produced response or disease stabilisation in 50% of the patients (52) without apparent effect on the plasma pharmacokinetics of melphalan. Phase II trials in non-oat cell lung cancer and malignant melanoma are planned.

Pharmacokinetic and metabolism studies with melphalan have shown that it has a rapid terminal phase plasma half-life (3) and *in vitro* undergoes hydrolysis which is similar quantitively and qualitatively to degradation seen *in vivo*, there being no detectable metabolism (85). The hydrolysis is related to the intracellular concentration of glutathione (232).

Interestingly the entrapment of melphalan in liposomes reduces the drug's rate of clearance in mice and gives rise to higher activity against the PC6 plasma cell tumour (164).

A peptide analogue of phenylalanine mustard, peptichemio, has recently been developed. It has activity in breast cancer which is refractory to cyclophosphamide (112, 133). *In vitro* peptichemio is active against cyclophosphamide resistant L1210 cells but no better than L-PAM or medphalan (214), and it is cross resistant with these latter two drugs (215).

The clinical activity of peptichemio has led to further synthetic interest in peptide analogues of aniline mustard and melphalan. One of these, a tripeptide (PTT.119), has activity against a number of *in vitro* cell lines including human AML and ALL (260). Furthermore leukaemia cell lines resistant to melphalan were susceptible to PTT.119 (259).

AZOMUSTARDS

Another group of nitrogen mustards requiring bioactivation is the azomustards. First investigated by Ross and Warwick (203, 204) this class of nitrogen mustards is relatively unreactive chemically, due to the powerful electron withdrawing nature of the azo linkage. However, reduction of the azo group leads to an extremely reactive phenylenediamine mustard. The necessary enzyme azoreductase is present at high levels in normal liver (57) and is well retained in hepatoma (12). CB 10-252 (4-(N,N-bis(2-bromo-n-propyl)-amino-2'-carboxy-2-methylazobenzene, IV) was therefore designed to exploit these facts (37). In addition the cytotoxic metabolite (V) has a short half-life of 41 seconds so that little of it is likely to reach sensitive tissues such as bone marrow or gut epithelium. That the design of the prodrug works in principle was confirmed by Connors *et al.* (58). The Walker 256 tumour when implanted into the flank is sensitive to cyclophosphamide but not to CB 10-252. However, when

implanted in the liver the tumour is unaffected by cyclophosphamide and cured by azomustard.

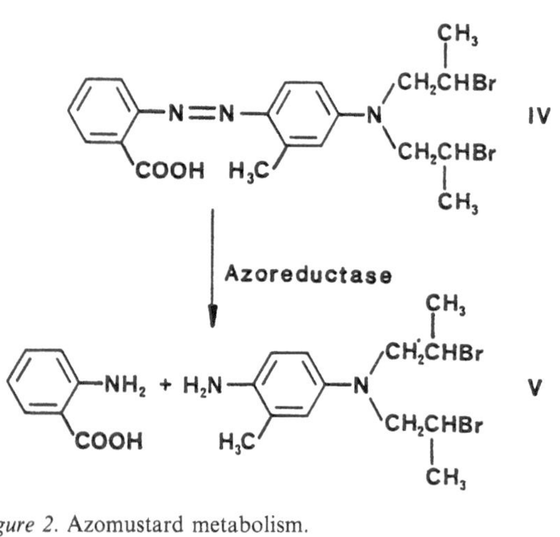

Although a trial in London (184) showed no clinical activity for this drug, the tumours used were not the rapidly proliferating primary hepatocellular carcinoma seen in Africa, for which CB 10-252 was designed. Attempts to undertake trials in Africa have proved inconclusive due to the problems associated with the lack of continued clinical observation of the patients. A recent study (152) has shown that the azo group can also be reduced by aldehyde oxidase. This means there is another enzyme for which elevated tumour levels could be exploited for the activation of CB 10-252. Also it may help to explain the myelosuppression observed in the European trial (184).

CYCLOPHOSPHAMIDE

Cyclophosphamide, VI (7) is one of most valuable alkylating agents in clinical practice, and is used alone or in combination against a wide range of tumours (e.g., acute and chronic lymphoblastic leukemia, Burkitt's lymphoma, Hodgkin's disease, lymphosarcoma and solid tumours of the breast, cervix, lung and ovary). The discovery of its anticancer activity was somewhat serendipidous, as the hypothesis for which it was originally designed was subsequently found to be invalid. The intention was that it would act as a prodrug being activated by, for example, a phosphamidase, to liberate an active alkylating agent (e.g., nornitrogen mustard) at the sites where this enzyme was abundant (believed then to include tumour cells). In fact cyclophosphamide is not a substrate for the enzyme, but it does become activated in a different way. The current understanding of the metabolism of cyclophosphamide is illustrated in Fig. 3. The initial site of metabolic attack is the 4-position of the oxazaphosphorine ring (adjacent to the nitrogen), which is hydroxylated to yield 4-hydroxycyclophosphamide, VII. This metabolism is carried out by the hepatic mixed function oxidase system; only a minor proportion of this metabolite is thought to be formed extrahepatically. 4-Hydroxycyclophosphamide is in equilibrium with its open-ring tautomer aldophosphamide, VIII, which is an unstable species and breaks down at pH 7 to give acrolein, IX and phosphoramide mustard, X. (This equilibrium and decomposition have been observed by proton magnetic resonance (242). The half-life for this non-enzymatic decomposition of 4-hydroxycyclophosphamide has been reported to be 100 min at pH 7 in 0.07 M phosphate buffer (30). However, Low, Borch and Sladek (170) have shown that the reaction is catalysed by the phosphate and thus the rate of generation of phosphoramide mustard from 4-hydroxycyclophosphamide *in vivo* will depend on the local concentration of phosphate and other bifunctional catalysts. The breakdown occurs via a chemical β-elimination process, which requires the existence of a hydrogen atom at the C-5 position. Cyclophosphamide analogues disubstituted at C-5 (e.g. 5,5-dimethylcyclophosphamide) are inactive as antitumour agents (8), which indicates that the breakdown to aldophosphamide and phosphoramide mustard is of importance for anti-cancer activity. (Although on the basis of this metabolic pathway it would be expected that analogues disubstituted at C-4 would also be inactive as

Figure 2. Azomustard metabolism.

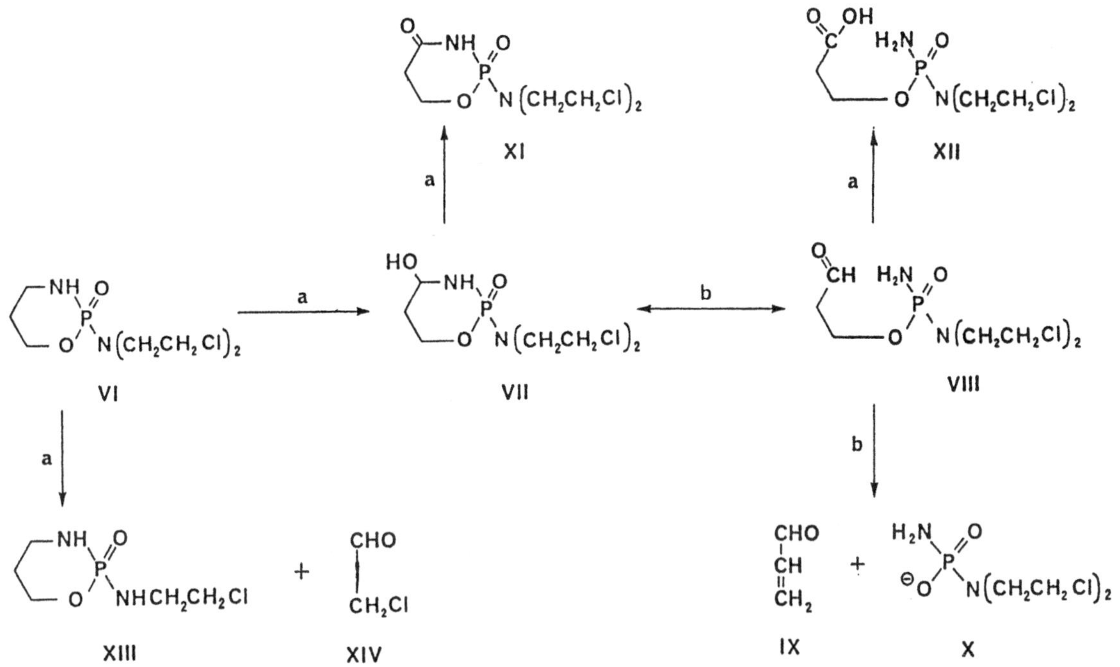

Figure 3. Metabolism of cyclophosphamide. (a) Pathways mediated by enzymes; (b) Pathways which proceed spontaneously.

anti-tumour agents, Sosnovksy and Paul (227) have reported on the activity of 4,4-dimethylcyclophosphamide against the P388 lymphocytic leukaemia in mice. Metabolism studies of this compound are clearly warranted.

In addition to the breakdown pathway for 4-hydroxycyclophosphamide and aldophosphamide, these compounds are oxidized by soluble enzymes to yield 4-ketocyclophosphamide, XI, and carboxyphosphamide, XII, respectively (231). 4-Hydroxycyclophosphamide may also form conjugates with, for example, glucuronic acid (16). Other minor metabolites include alcophosphamide, formed from the reduction of aldophosphamide (72), and the monochloroethyl analogue of cyclophosphamide, XIII, (55) which is produced following a hydroxylation at the carbon atom adjacent to the mustard nitrogen. The side product in this dechloroethylation is chloroacetaldehyde, XIV, which has also recently been detected as a urinary metabolite in animal experiments (219).

In vitro toxicity tests for cyclophosphamide and its metabolites have indicated that the parent drug is itself not very active, but that both phosphoramide mustard and acrolein are highly toxic. For example, the concentrations required to kill 50% of Walker tumour cells in culture are 23 mM, 1.9 μM, and 17.9 μM for cyclophosphamide, phosphoramide mustard and acrolein, respectively (68). Phosphoramide mustard is capable of cross-linking DNA (84) and is believed to be the ultimate alkylating agent responsible for the anti-tumour activity of cyclophosphamide. Acrolein, on the other hand is believed to be responsible for one of the major side-effects associated with cyclophosphamide therapy, haemorrhagic cystitis (31). This was elegantly demonstrated by Cox (63) who showed that bladder toxicity in rats was caused by the analogue of cyclophosphamide, in which the chloroethyl groups were replaced by ethyl groups,

in the same way as by cyclophosphamide. (This analogue was shown to be metabolised similarly to cyclophosphamide in that it produced acrolein, but it cannot give any other alkylating metabolites.) Much attention has recently been paid to ways of minimising the bladder toxicity caused by acrolein without affecting the anti-tumour activity. It appears that acrolein may be removed from the bladder by the use of N-acetylcysteine (25, 28, 63) or of sodium mercaptoethanesulphonic acid (mesna) (147, 210) and the use of the latter compound as a uroprotectant has now become well established.

Mesna administration prevents the induction of bladder cancer in rats treated with cyclophosphamide (212) and it is to be hoped that a similar reduction in the incidence of human cyclophosphamide-related bladder cancer (88) will also result from the use of mesna. No reduction of anti-tumour activity of cyclophosphamide in animal test systems is seen when mesna is concomitantly administered (114).

Various proposals have been made, based on a knowledge of the metabolic scheme for cyclophosphamide, to explain why the drug shows some oncostatic selectivity. It seems likely that 4-hydroxycyclophosphamide may be responsible for this selectivity, which is lost on liberation of the active agent phosphoramide mustard, i.e., that 4-hydroxycyclophosphamide is a carrier for the active metabolite. The possibility that normal and tumour tissues differ in their ability to carry out the detoxification pathways to 4-ketocyclophosphamide and to carboxyphosphamide received some support from the work of Cox, Phillips and Thomas (67), which showed that in rats the liver was 16 times more efficient at deactivating the primary cyclophosphamide metabolites than the Walker tumour. This hypothesis has not been supported by more studies in mice (127). 4-Hydroxycyclophosphamide also may be deactivated by the reaction of its 4-position with thiol compounds, and Brock and Hohorst (30) believe that this is of greater importance in governing the specificity of this metabolite. Thus for example 4-hydroxycyclophosphamide could be transported as a bound complex with a thiol-containing enzyme or with glutathione. Deconjugation could reliberate the active agent, although the reasons for any site specificity for this are as yet not understood.

Although 4-hydroxycyclophosphamide could not readily be used for human cancer treatment in view of its high chemical instability, 4-hydroperoxycyclophosphamide is a more stable analogue which decomposes *in vivo* to 4-hydroxycyclophosphamide. Against xenografted human breast tumours in mice (160), 4-hydroperoxycyclophosphamide shows activity greater than cyclophosphamide.

Compounds containing thioethers at the 4-position of cyclophosphamide have been synthesised and some show promising anticancer activity. Compounds of this type could have the clinical advantage over cyclophosphamide in that no metabolism is required to produce the active metabolite, and thus the pharmacokinetics could be better predicted. An interesting example of one of these compounds is ASTA Z7557 [4-(2-sulphonatoethylthio)-cyclophosphamide, i.e., a mesna complex with cyclophosphamide], which is stable at pH 4 but hydrolyses to an active alkylating agent at pH 7. Consequently good anti-tumour activity results and the compound does not give rise to significant bladder toxicity. Clinical trials are currently in progress on this compound, whose properties have recently been reviewed (*Investigational New Drugs*, 1984, Volume 2).

Studies of the clinical pharmacokinetics of cyclophosphamide are complicated because of the number and, in some cases, instability of the metabolites. Gas chromatography (GC) (143) or gas chromatography-mass spectrometry (GC-MS) (135) has been used for quantification of cyclophosphamide, phosphoramide mustard and nornitrogen mustard. 4-Hydroxycyclophosphamide is too unstable for GC or GC-MS but has been measured in the plasma of patients by converting it to a thioether derivative with benzyl mercaptan (244). Similarly aldophosphamide has been identified *in vivo* as a stable cyanohydrin derivative (92). A more recently developed method for detecting 4-hydroxycyclophosphamide and aldophosphamide, based on measurements of fluorescence of acrolein released from these compounds, has been used to study the pharmacokinetics of these metabolites in treated patients (243). 4-Ketocyclophosphamide and carboxyphosphamide have been measured using stable isotope labelled internal standards and direct insertion mass spectrometry (64, 111).

Cyclophosphamide may be administered orally or intravenously, although there is some divergence of opinion on the bioavailability of the drug (97%, (71); 34–90%, (142)). Intravenous administration shows dose-dependence of plasma levels of cyclophosphamide (see review by Colvin (53)), and maximum alkylating ability (which indicates the extent to which the active metabolite has been produced) is found after 2–3 hours (13). However, the plasma levels of phosphoramide mustard and of nornitrogen mustard have been shown to peak at a shorter time (< 1 hour) after *iv* injections of cyclophosphamide (143). Following single *iv* doses of cyclophosphamide the terminal phase plasma half-life ($t_{1/2}\beta$) of unchanged drug has been reported to be in the range 3–11 hours (e.g., 51, 135, 136, 137). That of phosphoramide mustard is 8.7 hours and nornitrogen mustard 3.3 hours (14).

The main urinary metabolites in animals and in man are carboxyphosphamide, nornitrogen mustard (which may be a breakdown product of carboxyphosphamide (135)) and 4-ketocyclophosphamide, although phosphoramide mustard and 4-hydroxycyclophosphamide have both also been reported to be in human urine (135, 244).

The use of high dose cyclophosphamide has been shown in animal experiments to cause damage to the hepatic cytochrome P450 mixed function oxidase system (24, 113). Thus repeated use of cyclophosphamide may partially destroy some of the enzymes responsible for the activation of the drug. Evidence exists (25) to suggest that this toxicity is caused by acrolein and thus that the concurrent use of a protector such as mesna may enhance the activity of cyclophosphamide on subsequent use. Another parameter of importance with regard to the repeated uses of cyclophosphamide is the 'priming effect'; the use of a small priming dose of the drug allows the subsequent successful administration, 4 days later, of a dose which could normally be in the toxic range (177). Although the mechanism for this phenomenon is as yet unknown it has been shown in experiments with mice (1) that the priming dose causes an increase after 5 days in the levels of glutathione and glutathione S-transferase in the bone marrow, which would thus be protected against the toxic effects of the second dose of the drug. Studies of this effect in treated patients would be of value in the assessment of the value of the priming technique in clinical practice.

The chemical structure of cyclophosphamide contains an asymmetric centre (phosphorus) and thus optical isomers exist. In 1975 the optical isomers were synthesised (151) and evaluated separately in comparison with the racemate in both animals and humans. Antitumour tests in mice (PC6 plasma cell tumour) indicated that one of the enantiomers (S-) was more active than the clinically used racemate (65) and metabolism studies in three animal species showed that there was stereoselective metabolism of the enantiomers (66). However, in patients treated with each of the enantiomers there was no consistent stereoselectivity in plasma half-life of cyclophosphamide or in carboxyphosphamide excretion (136). Although small differences in 4-ketocyclophosphamide excretion were seen there is currently no further interest in clinical studies of these isomers.

Of more relevance, however, is the report that samples of cyclophosphamide from different suppliers differ in their biological properties, e.g., toxic effects on the bladder (217). Structural differences between the two forms of the drug have been detected spectroscopically. Although one report suggests that the forms differ in their enantiomeric composition (218) this seems unlikely on the basis of their chemical preparation. A stereochemical variation in the confirmation of the six-membered ring in the structure seems a more likely possibility, and warrants further study.

ISOPHOSPHAMIDE

Isophosphamide, XV, is a structural isomer of cyclophosphamide and undergoes a similar metabolic transformation

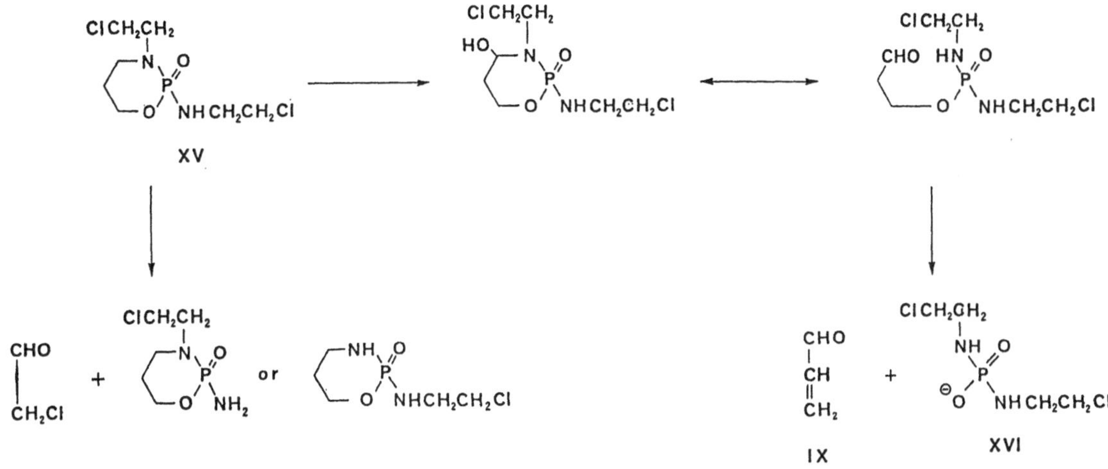

Figure 4. The metabolism of isophosphamide to the dechloroethylated derivatives and to isophosphoramide mustard.

to it (Fig. 4). The presumed active metabolite is isophosphoramide mustard, XVI, which has been determined in the plasma of patients receiving the drug by the use of a gas liquid chromatographic method (34). Peak plasma levels were seen 2–4 hours after *iv* administration of the parent drug. It is interesting to note that the cross-linking effects in macromolecules caused by isophosphoramide mustard may be different from those of the cyclophosphamide metabolite, phosphoramide mustard, X, as the two active centres of the former bifunctional molecule are separated by a greater chain length, and thus will give rise to longer DNA cross-links. Concurrent with the production of the active alkylating agent is that of acrolein, IX, which again has irritant properties against the bladder epithelium (31). Mesna has been successfully used to diminish this toxicity without affecting the metabolism of isophosphamide or the production of isophosphoramide mustard (35).

The N-dechloroethylation pathways, shown in Figure 4, which involve the loss of chloroacetaldehyde from the parent drug, appear to be more prevalent with isophosphamide than with cyclophosphamide (190), and the products from these pathways are abundant urinary metabolites.

Plasma pharmacokinetics of isophosphamide have been studied in detail by Allen, Creaven and Nelson (5), who administered the [^{14}C]-labelled drug to patients. The terminal plasma half-life is 15.2 hours following high single doses $(3.8–5\,g/m^2)$, which is around twice that reported for cyclophosphamide. The difference was reduced at lower doses. Less of the administered drug (49%) was metabolised compared with cyclophosphamide and thus, in view of the metabolic pattern (see above), it seems that less of the biologically active metabolite is produced *in vivo*.

Although isophosphamide has a wide range of antitumour activities and has been claimed to show lower toxicity to bone marrow than cyclophosphamide its use so far has been on a minor scale in comparison with that of cyclophosphamide.

ALKANESULPHONATES

The mode of alkylation by alkanesulphonates follows S_N2

kinetics, which means that the rate-determining step involves both the alkylating agent and the nucleophile being attacked. Consequently the rate of reaction will depend to an extent on the nature of the nucleophile being alkylated. Sulphur nucleophiles (e.g., cysteine, glutathione) are most reactive towards S_N2 alkylating agents, followed by nitrogen and oxygen nucleophiles.

Busulphan (myleran, 1,4-dimethylsulphonyloxybutane) (Table 2) is the only alkanesulphonate in widespread clinical use. Its preference for sulphur nucleophiles is illustrated by the fact that more than half of the urinary excreted metabolites in rat, rabbit and mouse derived from [^{14}C]-labelled busulphan is accounted for by 3-hydroxytetrahydrothiophene-1,1-dioxide (196), formed following the reaction of busulphan with a thiol group. Cross-linking of DNA does however occur, as illustrated by the work of Tong and Ludlum (237) who showed, in an *in vitro* experiment, the production of 1,4-di(7-guanyl)butane following incubation with busulphan.

DNA–DNA interstrand cross-linking has also been observed by Bedford and Fox (18) in Yoshida lymphosarcoma cells treated with busulphan. Also tested in this work were the analogs of busulphan with more (5–9) or less (1–3) methylene units in the chain linking the methanesulphonate residues. In most cases, interstrand cross-linking was correlated with *in vitro* cytotoxicity, six CH_2 groups showing the greatest effects. However, with this tumour *in vivo* the activity of the compounds was not closely correlated to interstrand cross-linking. The length of the cross-link produced by a bifunctional compound may be of particular importance in determining the therapeutic ratio of the compound.

Pharmacologically busulphan differs from the nitrogen mustards in that it has a more selective effect on myeloid cells (see review by Fox (95)). It is consequently used most extensively in the treatment of chronic myelogenous leukaemia. The reason for the drug's effectiveness against these cells is unknown. Busulphan was introduced to the clinic in the late 1950s, and as is often the case with the earlier alkylating agents, little satisfactory pharmacokinetic data is available for the compound. However, Ehrsson *et al.* (81) have recently quoted elimination half-lives of about $2\frac{1}{2}$ hours for patients with chronic myelocytic leukaemia receiving oral busulphan (2–6 mg). The drug was determined by gas chromatography–mass spectrometry after its conversion to 1,4-diiodobutane (79).

Treosulphan is a novel analogue of busulphan whose structure (L-threitol 1,4-bis-methanesulphonate) differs from busulphan only by the addition of two hydroxy groups. These groups are believed to play a part in the drug's metabolism which is thought to involve the intramolecular displacement of the methyl sulphonate groups by the hydroxylic groups, to yield the active metabolite L-diepoxybutane (see Epoxides). Unlike busulphan the pharmacokinetics of treosulphan have been well studied, using a GC quantitative method (250). The clinical application of treosulphan has been mainly in the treatment of ovarian cancer.

EPOXIDES

Epoxides are directly acting alkylating agents which react by a bimolecular process (see Alkanesulphonates). The leading epoxide in clinical practice is dianhydrogalactitol (Table 2) (82), but it should also be pointed out that dibromomannitol and dibromodulcitol, which are also under clinical evaluation, are believed to be active because of the conversion *in vivo* to mono- or diepoxides (131). The clinical trials that have been carried out on these three compounds have been surveyed by Chiuten *et al.* (46). Both dibromodulcitol and dianhydrogalactitol have the property of crossing the blood-brain barrier and much attention has been paid to the study of patients with intracranial tumours. Dibromomannitol has been used in the treatment of chronic myelogenous leukaemia but did not show any dramatic therapeutic advantages over the use of busulphan.

The human pharmacokinetics of dianhydrogalactitol have been studied in detail by Eagan *et al.* (76), using a high pressure liquid chromatographic method for quantitating the drug, following its conversion to a bis(dithiocarbamoyl)ester. The drug is rapidly removed from the plasma (initial half-life $t_{1/2}\alpha$ 3.9 min, terminal half-life $t_{1/2}\beta$ 31.3 min) following 1-hour infusions, and further studies on methods of administration that would result in maintained plasma concentration were recommended by these authors. Although there was only a low rate of tumour response in this Phase II/III study the observed regression of three tumours (large cell lung carcinoma, carcinoid of the thymus and a mixed adenocarcinoma/squamous cell carcinoma of the lung) suggests that further studies of the drug are necessary.

Further epoxides which are in an earlier stage of clinical development are di-acetyldianhydrogalactitol, di-succinyl dianhydrogalactitol and the triepoxide 1,3,4-triglycidylurazole.

AZIRIDINES

The mechanism of action of some nitrogen mustards is regarded as involving a cyclic aziridinium ion intermediate (200). This led to an interest in compounds containing the three-membered aziridine ring. Indeed it has subsequently been shown that 2-bromoethylaminonaphthoquinone is metabolised by rat hepatocytes to 2-aziridinylnaphthoqui-

none (247). They also found that the 4-chlorobutyl analogue cyclised under similar conditions to form a 5-membered pyrrolidine ring; which is similar to the intermediate postulated by Tisdale, Elson and Ross (235) to account for the activity of a series of halogenobutylethers.

The aziridine ring is chemically reactive, due to the strain imposed by its configuration. Ring opening which is promoted by acid results in the formation of an alkylating carbonium ion.

A number of aziridine derivatives have found clinical use, the two of most significance being thio-TEPA (Table 2) in the treatment of ovarian carcinoma, disseminated carcinoma of the breast and Hodgkin's disease, and in combination with an androgen for breast carcinoma (117, 241) and triethylenemelamine (TEM). Investigation of the mechanism of action of TEM and an attempt to prepare an inactive analogue led to the synthesis of hexamethylmelamine (36, 121) and its subsequent introduction into clinical use (166).

In addition to these multifunctional alkylating agents based on the active aziridine group a number of apparently monofunctional agents have been of interest, however, they all have the potential for metabolism of another part of the molecule to a reactive species. Tetramin (4-aziridinyl-3-hydroxybut-1-ene), which has shown activity against a number of tumours (254), has the possibility for *in vivo* epoxidation of its double bond to form a reactive difunctional derivative.

Of more general interest, though clinical application has yet to be achieved, are the dinitrophenylaziridines. 1-Aziridinyl-2,4-dinitrobenzene (XVII, R = H) was discovered over 30 years ago (6) and, with a therapeutic index of 10 against the Walker 256 carcinosarcoma, is comparable with clinically useful alkylating agents. A subsequent detailed structure-activity study (149, 150) established the structural requirements of this class of compounds and, more particularly, 5-(1-aziridinyl)-2,4-dinitrobenzamide (CB 1954, XVII, R = $CONH_2$) as the most active of the series. It has proved to be extremely selective for the Walker 256 carcinosarcoma with a therapeutic index of 70, the highest recorded in this system, and little or no activity against other tumours. Small variations in structure were sufficient to destroy the activity. This unusual selectivity has been the subject of considerable investigation but to date has failed to identify the mechanism of action. Metabolic studies have shown that, although CB 1954 is superficially a monofunctional alkylating agent, other reactive groups are introduced into the molecule by reduction *in vivo* (138). It has also been suggested that CB 1954 may be an inhibitor of ribonucleotide reductase (236).

CB 1954 has been shown to have other properties. It is a potent radiosensitiser and chemosensitiser. As a radiosensitiser it gives an enhancement ratio (the ratio of cell kill by a standard dose of X-rays with and without the drug) of 2.2 compared with 1.5 for misonidazole at the same molar concentration, in hypoxic Chinese hamster cells *in vitro*. This activity is reduced by 2-phenyl-5-aminoimidazo-4-carboxamide (2-phenylAIC) to the same level as misonidazole (230). As 2-phenylAIC inhibits the cytotoxicity of CB 1954 to the Walker tumour *in vitro* and *in vivo* the increase in the radiosensitising effect over the nitroimidazoles may result from the inherent cytotoxicity of the compound. In a similar fashion CB 1954 has been found to be a promoter of alkylating agent activity. It is as effective an enhancer of the antitumor activity of cyclophosphamide as misonidazole but less good in conjunction with melphalan (50). It is to be hoped that this reviewed interest in CB 1954 with provide a useful contribution for this drug in cancer treatment.

XVII   XVIII

Another series of aziridine derivatives has been developed over the past ten years. These are the aziridinylbenzoquinones. Based on the known ability of compounds of this type to inhibit intracerebrally implanted tumours in rodent test systems (74) molecules were designed which would retain the ability to penetrate the central nervous system and yet have sufficient aqueous solubility to facilitate administration and equal or improve antitumour activity (47, 144). This work has resulted in two compounds going forward for clinical evaluation.

The first of these AZQ (3,6-diaziridinyl-2,5-bis(carboethoxyamino)-1,4-benzoquinone, XVIII, R = NHCOO C_2H_5) has been under investigation in the clinic for some years. In its Phase I trial the major toxicity was myelosuppression at doses in excess of $10 \, mg/m^2$. Nausea, alopecia and anaemia were also observed. Although no significant responses were observed in 40 previously treated patients with advanced disease, minor objective responses were observed in three patients. AZQ was found in the CSF of the three patients investigated, in one case with a CSF to plasma ratio of 1:1 (211). A number of other Phase I trials have suggested that AZQ may be useful against CNS tumours (110, 171) and responses have been seen in grade III and IV astrocytomas (9, 69). Paediatric patients with CNS involvement in refractory acute leukaemia have shown response to AZQ (14). Most Phase II trials not involving CNS tumours have so far reported little or no response to this drug.

Although the aziridinyl groups of AZQ are chemically reactive, alone they are insufficient for antitumour activity (144). The reasons for this are still not clear nor is the importance or otherwise of metabolism. However, AZQ has been shown to form a semiquinone free radical on biochemical reduction (115), and to cause selective destruction to mitochondria in human glioma cell lines (192).

The poor aqueous solubility of AZQ ($200 \, \mu g/ml$) means that mixed solvent systems are necessary for clinical administration (194). A second generation analogue is therefore currently being developed with 10-fold greater aqueous solubility and similar antitumour activity. This is BZQ (3,6-diaziridinyl-2,5-bis(hydroxyethylamino)-1,4-benzoquinone, XVIII, R = NHCH$_2$CH$_2$OH) (47). In addition to being more soluble it is also active at considerably lower doses such that the aqueous solubility will be sufficient for

clinical administration although its partition coefficient is lower (118) and therefore its penetration of the blood brain barrier may be less efficient (167).

Two antitumour antibiotics contain an aziridine group which is responsible at least in part for their activity. These are mitomycin C and carzinophilin A. Reductive metabolism of the quinone portion of mitomycin C allows release of the indole nitrogen lone pair followed by loss of methanol resulting in activation of the aziridine and carbamate groups as potential alkylating functions (134). Mitomycin C is used clinically for the treatment of malignanices of the breast, lung, colon and stomach (43). Carzinophilin A, which has been used clinically to treat cancer of the skin and jejunum, reticulosarcoma and chronic leukaemia (161), requires no metabolic activation.

Other more recently developed antitumour agents containing the aziridine group include selenothiotepa (156) and nitroxyl spin-labelled thiotepa (157). For the latter compound electron spin resonance (esr) may be used to follow the intracellular fate of the drug.

NITROSOUREAS

The nitrosourea antitumor agents have been extensively studied since the early 1960's. *In vivo* these compounds decompose and liberate transiently an active alkylating agent, together with an isocyanate. The mechanism of this process is shown in Fig. 5. Many variants of the nitrosourea structure, containing different R and R' groups have been synthesised (see, e.g., (140, 141)) and tested for antitumour activity. The screening data indicated that the most active compounds were those with R = 2-chloroethyl, 2-fluoroethyl or a cycloalipathic group and R' = 2-chloroethyl or 2-fluoroethyl. Thus the first nitrosourea to be used extensively in the clinic was carmustine (BCNU, XIX, 1,3-bis(2-chloroethyl)-1-nitrosourea) where R and R' are 2-chloroethyl groups. There was also enthusiasm about the possible clinical use of lomustine (CCNU, 1-(2-chlorethyl)-3-cyclohexyl-1-nitrosourea), XX, and semustine (MeCCNU, 1-(2-chloroethyl)-3-(4-methylcyclohexyl)-1-nitrosourea), XXI, which like BCNU had high activity in the animal tumour screen and were lipid soluble, allowing their use for the treatment of brain tumours. The chloroethylnitrosoureas have been reviewed by Weiss and Issell (249) and by Weinkam and Lin (248).

BCNU, CCNU and MeCCNU are all believed to alkylate intracellular nucleophiles following the formation of a $ClCH_2CH_2^+$ ion. Cross-linking between DNA chains *in vivo* (153, 238) and cross-linking between two nucleophilic sites within the same DNA base molecule (108) have both been observed.

Indeed cross-linking of DNA by MeCCNU in sensitive and resistant murine colon tumours was correlated with the sensitivity to the drug (251), even though total DNA binding was the same in both tumours.

The fate and biological function of the isocyanate that is concomitantly produced (2-chloroethyl, cyclohexyl and 4-methylcyclohexyl isocyanates from BCNU, CCNU and MeCCNU respectively) is less certain. Nitrosourea-derived isocyanates react readily with amine groups, such as those in lysine residues in proteins (252) and this may be of impor-

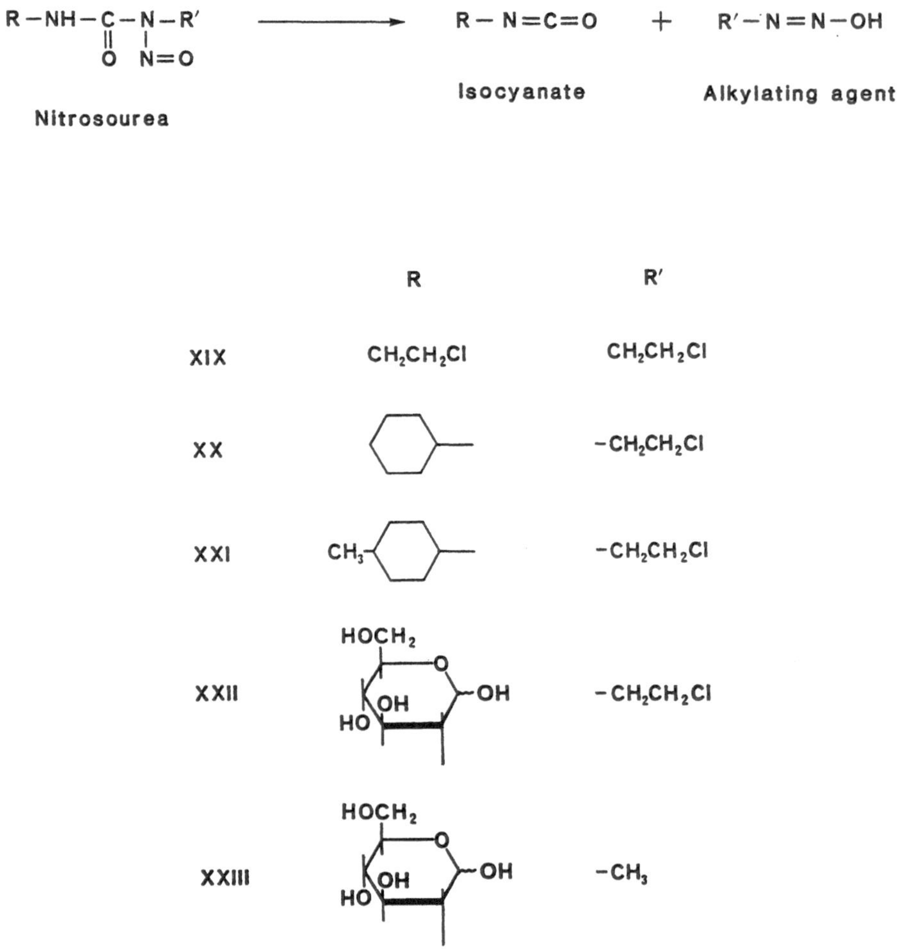

R — NH — C — N — R' ⟶ R — N=C=O + R' — N = N — OH
         ‖ |
         O N=O

Isocyanate   Alkylating agent

Nitrosourea

	R	R'
XIX	CH₂CH₂Cl	CH₂CH₂Cl
XX	(cyclohexyl)	-CH₂CH₂Cl
XXI	CH₃-(cyclohexyl)	-CH₂CH₂Cl
XXII	(sugar, HOCH₂, OH, HO, OH)	-CH₂CH₂Cl
XXIII	(sugar, HOCH₂, OH, HO, OH)	-CH₃

Figure 5. The decomposition of nitrosoureas.

tance with regard to the observed inhibition of DNA strand-break repair, DNA replication and RNA strand scission (see review by Kohn (154)) that is seen after nitrosourea treatment. Although the isocyanate has generally been thought to be more associated with unfavourable side effects than antitumour effects, Gibson and Hickman (103) have challenged this hypothesis with their studies on nitrosourea sensitive and resistant TLX5 lymphoma cell lines. The resistant line was cross-resistant to isocyanates, but not to alkylating agents, suggesting that the isocyanates were of considerable importance with regard to the cytotoxicity of nitrosoureas in this particular system. In general, however, nitrosoureas with low carbamoylating activity retain their antitumour properties. For example chlorozotocin, XXII, produces the alkylating species and the isocyanate in the normal way, but the latter compound inactivates itself by intramolecular cyclisation (carbamoylation of the sugar residue (116)). Chlorozotocin is an analog of the naturally occurring methyl nitrosourea streptozotocin, XXIII, and both of these compounds, which are currently undergoing clinical trial, cause lower myelosuppression than BCNU or CCNU.

Tsujihara *et al.* (239, 240) and Morikawa *et al.* (181) have synthesised a series of nitrosoureas disubstituted on the nitrogen bearing the R group, and with a β-hydroxy group on one of these substituents. Some of these compounds cannot form isocyanates but can form alkylating intermediates, and these were more active in animal tests than CCNU. Further work by this research group led to the synthesis of wide series of sugar containing nitrosoureas (e.g., (182)), some of which (e.g., 1-(2-chloroethyl)-3-isobutyl-3-(β-maltosyl)-1-nitrosourea) have promising antitumour activity (2).

Other nitrosoureas whose animal antitumour activity warrants their further investigation include the fluoroethyl nitrosoureas (139) and steroid linked nitrosoureas (212, 262).

Although the breakdown pathway illustrated in Fig. 5 is a major metabolic route other forms of metabolism have been identified, such as denitrosation (BCNU, (125)) and R-group hydroxylation (CCNU cyclohexyl ring, (126, 195)). In the latter case metabolism is extremely rapid and carbamoylation *in vivo* is likely to be by hydroxycyclohexyl isocyanates in addition to cyclohexyl isocyanate.

Despite the intense study of structure-activity relationships, metabolism and mechanism of action of the nitrosoureas over the past 20 years, the impact of these compounds on cancer chemotherapy has been greatly limited by

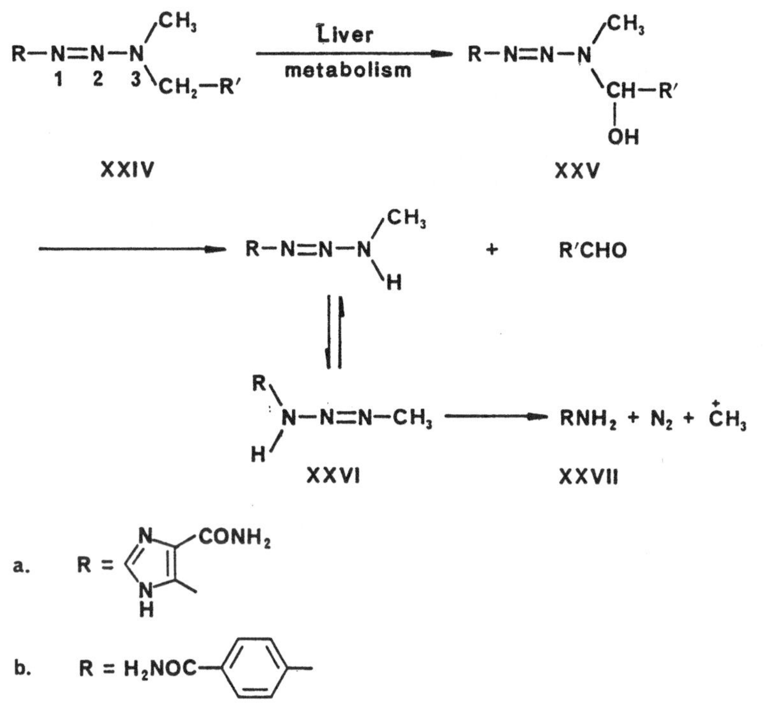

Figure 6. Triazene metabolism.

the severe and cumulative myelosuppression that they produce. The future of BCNU and CCNU is therefore uncertain, and attention is currently being focused on the more recently developed analogs such as chlorozotocin and streptozotocin. Another agent where clinical evaluation has started is PCNU (1-(2-chloroethyl)-3-(2,6-dioxo-3-piperidyl)-1-nitrosourea (258)). This has a higher alkylating activity than CCNU and is also lipid soluble making it suitable for brain penetration (97). Again, however, the dose-limiting toxicity was myelosuppression.

Regardless of the future of nitrosoureas in cancer chemotherapy they are extremely useful experimental tools for laboratory mechanistic studies. One of the major intracellular targets for nitrosoureas is transcriptionally active chromatin. An understanding of the molecular nature of these interactions (see review by Tew *et al.* (233)) may allow the development of nitrosoureas of greater selectivity against tumour cells, in addition to leading to a greater understanding of chromatin structure and function.

TRIAZENES

The rationale for including triazenes in a chapter on alkylating agents is perhaps questionable, however, their major route of metabolism results in the formation of an alkylating carbonium ion. Whether or not this carbonium ion or some other established metabolite is responsible for the antitumour activity observed with these compounds is still uncertain. Albeit the mechanism of action of the triazenes remains to be established, DTIC (5-(3,3-dimethyl-1-triazene-4-carboxamide, DIC, dacarbazine, XXIVa, R' = H) has found some clinical utility and second-generation agents are currently being investigated clinically.

The first synthesis of a triazene or diazoamino compound was by Wallach (245). Biological interest in such compounds did not occur until 70 years later, when it was shown that aryldialkyltriazenes had activity against the sarcoma 180 and leukaemia 82 (39, 48). However, these findings were largely ignored until well after the discovery of DTIC.

Shealy and his colleagues (222, 223, 224) designed DTIC to be a prodrug form of 5-diazoimidazo-4-carboxamide, a chemically unstable inhibitor of the Walker 256 carcinosarcoma. DTIC has since proved to have a different mechanism of action to that predicted and its photochemical decomposition to the diazo compound has been suggested as a contributory factor in its toxicity. The photodecomposition products of the clinically formulated material are different from those of pure DTIC (129, 130). However, means of administration which exclude light are now available such that this should no longer be such a critical problem (14, 159). Phototoxic effects have been reported (17) in patients exposed to sunlight within 24 hours of DTIC therapy, which might be attributable to photodecomposition of the drug.

DTIC has been studied clinically in a variety of tumour types (44). Its most significant activity as a single agent is to produce an overall 25% response rate in the treatment of metatastic malignant melanoma (54). This is the highest response rate of any single agent and a substantial improvement on other alkylating agents. Similar response rates are observed with high dose DTIC in combination with either actinomycin D or BCNU and hydroxyurea (61). Although it does not have the single agent activity of doxorubicin in the therapy of adult soft tissue sarcomas, DTIC in combination with doxorubicin shows a cumulative response which is further improved by the addition of cyclophosphamide and vincristine to the combination (CYVADIC) (109). These results are, however, not necessarily reproducible (105).

There are two combination chemotherapy regimes for the treatment of Hodgkin's disease, of which MOPP (mechlorethamine, vincristine, prednisone and procarbazine) is regarded as the standard therapy. However ABVD (doxorubicin, bleomycin, vinblastine and DTIC) has been shown not to be cross-resistant with MOPP (207, 208) and capable of producing 100% response and 100% 2-year survival if the two combinations are alternated (27).

DTIC also exhibits single agent activity in neuroblastoma and rhabdomyosarcoma (93) which although not as good in itself as established combinations warrants investigation of its possible inclusion.

Like all alkylating agents DTIC causes immune suppression clinically (33). However, in experimental systems a BCNU resistant EL4 leukaemia line showed altered immunogenicity and was curable by BCNU following DTIC treatment (189).

The metabolism and mechanism of action of DTIC has been studied in some detail although as yet its precise mechanism of action has not been determined. The work in this area related to DTIC must be considered in conjunction with that derived from the dialkylaryltriazenes. Originally DTIC was regarded as an antimetabolite of 5-aminoimidazole-4-carboxamide (AIC, XXVIIa) (223). The present evidence, although originating preponderantly from the aryl series, is that dialkyltriazenes require metabolic activation by the host in order to produce an antitumour effect (11, 59, 101).

The major urinary metabolite of DTIC in man is AIC (132, 225, 226) and it is also formed by mouse liver microsomes and human and animal tumour tissue (100, 179). Such evidence indicates a metabolic route via the monomethyl derivative, MIC (5-(3-methyl-1-triazeno)-imidazole-4-carboxamide, XXVIa, following oxidative metabolism and loss of formaldehyde. The detection of HMIC (5-(3-hydroxymethyl-3-methyl-1-triazeno)imidazole-4-carboxamide, XXVa, R' = H) and MIC in the plasma of DTIC treated patients (207) and of the primary oxidative metabolite HMIC as a urinary metabolite in rats (155) would seem to be final metabolic proof of this metabolic pathway. The surprisingly high stability of HMIC in polar solvents as compared with MIC led these authors to suggest that it may be the transport form of the activated drug.

Although the metabolites, HMIC and MIC, are observable in the plasma of DTIC treated patients there is a considerable species difference in metabolism between mouse, rat and man. Plasma clearance of DTIC is some 9 times more rapid in mice than man and is reflected in the higher levels of the metabolite seen in the mouse. Comparison of these data with *in vitro* cytotoxicity testing leads to the conclusion that in mice cytotoxic levels of HMIC and MIC may result from DTIC metabolism, a situation which is not achieved in rats and most patients even after high doses, suggesting that the relatively low clinical activity of DTIC, in relation to its effect in murine tumour systems is due to man's poor ability to metabolise the drug (206).

The toxicity observed with DTIC, in particular the severe nausea and vomiting, has led to interest in analogues in which this problem may be overcome. A number of studies have shown that the imidazole group may be replaced by various other ring systems without any major change in activity. Ring types investigated have included phenyl, pyrazole and γ-triazole (169). A detailed structure activity study

of dialkylaryltriazenes (59) demonstrated the structural requirements for activity against a murine plasmacytoma. These are an aryl or heteroaryl carrying group at N^1, a methyl group at N^3 and a readily metabolised group also at N^3 (XXIV).

The metabolism of the dialkylaryltriazenes is similar to that of the imidazotriazenes (59, 257) hence similar problems in relation to metabolic activation in man might be predicted. This is indeed the case, but in the rat levels of metabolites of 1-(4-carbamoylphenyl)-3,3-dimethyltriazene (XXIVb, R' = H) following phenobarbitone pretreatment are almost identical to those seen in the mouse, giving the hope that clinically this problem may be overcome (205).

The original intention behind the development of a second-generation triazene was to overcome the clinical side effects of DTIC and to produce a far more effective antimelanoma drug. Other properties of these compounds and the dialkylaryltriazenes in particular have evoked interest in the treatment of other tumour types. Farquhar (91) demonstrated the difference in CSF to plasma ratio of an aryltriazene (1-(4-carbamoylphenyl)-3,3-dimethyltriazene) and DTIC, in dogs. He found that this ratio was 1:1 for the aryltriazene but 1:10 for DTIC. The life span of mice carrying the intraperitoneally implanted L1210 was increased 40–50% by both drugs following i.p. administration but only the aryltriazene produced a similar response when the tumour was implanted intracerebrally. The most likely explanation of this difference in ability of the metabolites of these drugs to cross the blood-brain barrier (BBB) is the greater lipid solubility of the aryltriazene which meets Levin's criteria for drugs to cross the BBB (167). The findings are also in agreement with the differences in optimal partition coefficient of active drugs being dependent on the site of implant of the L1210 tumour (41).

More recent work in this direction has involved the use of human grade III and IV astrocytoma xenografts growing in immune deprived mice. When implanted subcutaneously in the flank these tumours are sensitive to drugs such as BCNU, procarbazine, DTIC and CB 10-350 (1-(4-carbamoylphenyl)-3-methyl-3-pentyltriazene, XXIV, R' = $CH_2CH_2CH_2CH_3$). Cyclophosphamide, vincristine, 5-FU and hexamethylmelamine have little or no activity. A somewhat different pattern emerges when the tumour is implanted intracerebrally, in this case only BCNU and CB 10-350 inhibit tumour growth (256). This data allows certain conclusions to be drawn, firstly because DTIC is not active on the intracerebral implant whereas CB 10-350 is, the BBB has remained intact and the tumour is located in this privileged site. Secondly, that CB 10-350 has the predicted criteria, high lipophilicity and molecular weight below 400 (167), for penetration of the BBB. Thirdly, a more generalised investigation of the aryltriazenes in this tumour system is warranted to establish a drug of choice for clinical study.

Although DTIC became the initial triazene of choice for clinical use BTIC (5-(3,3-bis(2-chloroethyl)-1-triazeno)imidazole-4-carboxamide, XXVIII) has better activity in murine tumours (221). The metabolism of BTIC parallels that of DTIC in leading to a monoalkyl, in this case a 2-chloroethyltriazene (MCTIC, (220)). A second series of compounds designed as chemically activated prodrug forms of these two cytotoxic imidazole derivatives has been pursued by Stevens and his colleagues (229) at the University of

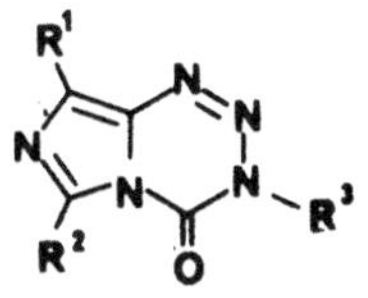

Figure 7. Structural requirements of imidazotetrazinones.

Aston. The first of these compounds 8-carbamoyl-3-(2-chloroethyl)imidazo[5,1-*d*]-1,2,3,5-tetrazin-4(3*H*)-one (mitozolamide, XXIX, R = CH_2CH_2Cl) cures many experimental tumours (123). It has been shown to decompose chemically, under mildly alkaline conditions, by opening of the tetrazine ring, to yield MCTIC (229). Biological evaluation of mitozolamide also points to the drug acting as a prodrug form of MCTIC (228).

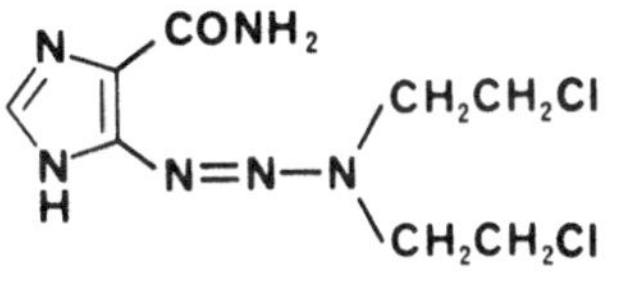

XXVIII 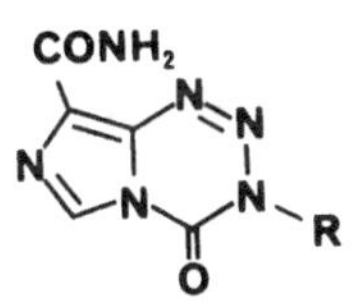   **XXIX**

The Phase I clinical study of mitozolamide (188) covered doses from 8 to 153 mg/m^2 and demonstrated dose-related but not severe vomiting, with thrombocytopenia as the dose-limiting toxic effect at doses greater than 115 mg/m^2. The plasma half-life of the drug was 1 to 1.3 hours and independent of the route of administration (i.v. or oral). Partial responses were seen in two patients with adenocarcinoma of the ovary who had received previous cisplatin therapy. Phase II studies with this drug are planned against melanoma and lung and ovarian tumours.

A detailed structure activity study (163, 228) has indicated the structural requirements for antitumour activity in this class of compounds (Fig. 7). The substituent at R^1 may be an amide, sulphonamide, sulphone or sulphoxide, that at R^2 a hydrogen or small alkyl group and R^3 must be either a methyl or 2-chloroethyl group. Antitumour evaluation of these compounds have indicated the most active to be CCRG 81045 (8-carbamoyl-3-methylimidazo[5,1-*d*]-1,2,3, 5-tetrazin-4(3*H*)-one, XXIX, R = CH$_3$). This compound decomposes chemically in a similar fashion to mitozolamide, in this case producing MTIC as the active metabolite, the presumed active metabolite of DTIC, without the need for biological activation. Extensive testing of CCRG 81045 in experimental tumour systems has shown it to be superior to DTIC and to have a different spectrum of activity to mitozolamide (162). Consequently it has been selected for toxicological evaluation prior to Phase 1 clinical trial (228).

CONCLUSION

New alkylating agents are constantly being synthesised and tested for anticancer activity. They are selected for toxicological and ultimately clinical trial on the basis of animal screening tests. Many of these novel compounds that have 'passed' these tests (e.g., PCNU, spiromustine, aziridinylbenzoquinone (AZQ), etc.) have promising activity, which clearly warrants their further clinical testing. It should be pointed out, however that there is a danger that the animal test systems may not be the best predictor for human drug activity. Most of the compounds going successfully through the preclinical development fall into the same general chemical classes as the earliest alkylating agents developed twenty or more years ago. Maybe our initial test systems are particularly sensitive to these classes of compounds and maybe our perspective should be extended towards broader based test systems, which might show up novel classes of compounds. The current use of human tumour xenografts in the drug development programmes of the NCI and other groups may well prove to give rise to the selection of drugs having more diverse structural properties and activity against the currently refractory types of human tumour.

REFERENCES

1. Adams DJ, Carmichael J, Smyth JF, Wolf CR: Relationship between bone marrow glutathione and glutathione S-transferase levels and drug priming. *Brit J Cancer* 50:268, 1984

2. Akaike Y, Arai Y, Taguchi H, Satoh H: Effect of 1-(2-chloroethyl)-3-isobutyl-3-(β-maltosyl)-1-nitrosourea on experimental tumours. *Gann* 73:480, 1982

3. Alberts D, Chang S, Melnick L, Himmelstein K, Walson P, Gross J, Salmon S: Melphalan (M) disposition in man. *Proc Am Assoc Cancer Res* 18:128, 1977

4. Alberts DS, Chang SY, Chen GH-S, Evans TL, Moon TE: Oral melphalan pharmacokinetics. *Clin Pharmacol Ther* 26:737, 1979

5. Allen CM, Creaven PJ, Nelson RL: Studies on the human pharmacokinetics of isophosphamide (NSC-109724). *Cancer Treat Rep* 60:451, 1976

6. Anonymous: Nucleotoxic and mutagenic nitrogen mustards, epoxides, ethyleneimines and related substances. *Ann Rept Brit Empire Cancer Campgn* 28:56, 1950

7. Arnold H, Bourseaux F: Synthese und Abbau cytostatisch wirksamer zyklischer N-Phosphamidester des Bis(β-chloroathyl)amins. *Angew Chem* 70:539, 1958

8. Arnold H, Bourseaux F, Brock N: Über Beziehung zwischen chemischer Konstitution und cancerotoxischer Wirkung in der Reihe der Phosphamidester des Bis(β-chloroathyl)amins. *Arzneimittelforschung* 11:143, 1961

9. Aroney RS, Kaplan RS, Saleman M, Montgomery E, Wiernik PH: A Phase II trial of AZQ (NSC-182986) in patients with recurrent primary or metastatic brain tumours. *Proc Am Soc Clin Oncol* 1:24, 1982

10. Astaldi G: Peptichemio: A multifaceted antiblastic drug. *Wadley Medical Bull* 5:303, 1975

11. Audette RCS, Connors TA, Mandel HG, Merai K, Ross WCJ: Studies on the mechanism of action of the tumour inhibitory triazenes. *Biochem Pharmac* 22:1855, 1973

12. Autrup H, Thurlow BJ, Warwick GP: Activation by reductive cleavage of potentially cytotoxic azo compounds by human hepatocellular carcinoma. *Biochem Pharmac* 23:2341, 1974

13. Bagley CM, Bostick FW, DeVita VT: Clinical pharmacology of cyclophosphamide. *Cancer Res* 33:226, 1973

14. Baird GM, Willoughby ML: Photodegradation of dacarbazine. *Lancet* ii:681, 1978

15. Basu TK, Bishun NP, Williams DC: Accentuation of the cell-killing effects of chlorambucil by phenobarbital, caffeine and vitamin A in culture. *Cytobios* 9:115, 1974

16. Bates DJ, Foster AB, Jarman M: The metabolism of cy-

clophosphamide by isolated rat hepatocytes. *Biochem Pharmac* 30:3055, 1981

17. Beck TH, Hart NE, Smith CE: Photosensitivity reaction following DTIC administration: Report of two cases. *Cancer Treat Rep* 64:725, 1980

18. Bedford P, Fox BW: DNA–DNA interstrand crosslinking by dimethanesulphonic acid esters. *Biochem Pharmac* 32:2297, 1983

19. Benckhuysen C, Ter Hart HGJ, Van Dijk PJ: Enhanced cytostatic effectiveness of aniline mustard against 7,12-dimethylbenz[a]anthracene induced rat mammary tumours during regression in response to ovariectomy. *Cancer Treat Rep* 65:567, 1981

20. Bergel F, Stock JA: Cytotoxic alpha amino acids and peptides. *Ann Rep Brit Empire Cancer Campgn* 31:6, 1953

21. Bergel F, Stock JA: Cytoactive amino acid and peptide derivatives. Part 1. Substituted phenylalanines. *J Chem Soc* 2409, 1954

22. Berger MR, Floride J, Schreiber J, Schmahl D, Eisenbrand G: Evaluation of new estrogen-linked 2-chloroethylnitrosoureas. I. Short term anticancer efficacy in methylnitrosourea-induced rat mammary carcinoma and hormonal activity in mice. *J Cancer Res Clin Oncol* 108:148, 1984

23. Bernier LG, Page M, Gaudreault RC, Joly LP: A chlorambucil-anti-CEA conjugate cytotoxic for human colon adenocarcinoma cells *in vitro*. *Br J Cancer* 49:245, 1984

24. Berrigan MJ, Gurtoo HL, Sharma SD, Struck RF, Marinello AJ: Protection by N-acetylcysteine of cyclophosphamide metabolism-related *in vivo* depression of mixed function oxygenase activity and *in vitro* denaturation of cytochrome P-450. *Biochem Biophys Res Commun* 93:797, 1980

25. Berrigan MJ, Marinello AJ, Pavelic Z, Williams CJ, Struck RF, Gurtoo HL: Protective role of thiols in cyclophosphamide-induced urotoxicity and depression of hepatic drug metabolism. *Cancer Res* 42:3688, 1982

26. Blokhin N, Larionov L, Perevodchikova N, Chebotareva L, Merkulova N: Clinical experiences with sarcolysin in neoplastic diseases. *Ann NY Acad Sci* 68:1128, 1958

27. Bonadonna G, Fossati V, De Lena M: MOPP vs MOPP plus ABVD in stage IV Hodgkin's disease. *Proc Am Soc Clin Oncol* 19:363, 1977

28. Botta JA, Nelson CW, Weikel JH: Acetylcysteine in the prevention of cyclophosphamide-induced cystitis in rats. *J Natl Cancer Inst* 51:1051, 1973

29. Brock N, Habs M, Pohl J, Schmahl D, Steckar J: Mesna (natrium-2-mercaptoethansulfonat). *Therapiewoche* 32:4977, 1982

30. Brock N, Hohorst H-J: The problem of specificity and selectivity of alkylating cytostatics: studies on N-2-chloroethylamido-oxazaphosphorines. *Z Krebsforsch* 88:185, 1977

31. Brock N, Steckar J, Pohl J, Niemeyer U, Scheffler G: Acrolein, the causative factor of urotoxic side-effects of cyclophosphamide, iphosphamide, trophosphamide and suphosphamide. *Arzneimittelforschung* 29:659, 1979

32. Brookes P, Lawley PD: The reaction of mono- and difunctional alkylating agents with nucleic acids. *Biochem J* 80:496, 1961

33. Bruckner HW, Mokyr MB, Mitchell MS: Effect of imidazole-4-carboxamide,5-(3,3-dimethyl-1-triazeno) on immunity in patients with malignant melanoma. *Cancer Res* 34:181, 1974

34. Bryant BM, Jarman M, Baker MH, Smith IE, Smyth JF: Quantification by gas chromatography of N,N-di-(2-chloroethyl)-phosphorodiamidic acid in the plasma of patients receiving isophosphamide. *Cancer Res* 40:4734, 1980

35. Bryant BM, Jarman M, Ford HT, Smith IE: Prevention of isophosphamide-induced urothelial toxicity with 2-mercaptoethanesulphonate sodium (mesnum) in patients with advanced carcinoma. *Lancet* ii:657, 1980

36. Buckley SM, Stock CC, Crossley ML, Rhoads CP: Inhibition of the Crocker mouse sarcoma 180 by certain ethyleneimine derivatives and related compounds. *Cancer Res* 10:207, 1950

37. Bukhari A, Connors TA, Gilsenan AM, Ross WCJ, Tisdale MJ, Warwick GP, Wilman DEV: Cytotoxic agents designed to be selective for liver tumours. *J Natl Cancer Inst* 50:243, 1973

38. Bukhari MA, Everett JL, Ross WCJ: Aryl-2-halogenoalkylamines. XXVI. Glucuronic, sulphuric and phosphoric esters of p-Di-2-chloroethylaminophenol. *Biochem Pharmac* 21:963, 1972

39. Burchenal JH, Dagg MK, Beger M, Stock CC: Chemotherapy of Leukaemia VII. Effect of substituted triazenes on transplanted mouse leukaemia. *Proc Soc Expt Biol Med* 91:398, 1956

40. Buss CW, Coe PL, Markou M, Foster AB: Unpublished data, 1984

41. Cain BF: The role of structure-activity studies in the design of antitumour agents. *Cancer Chemother Rep* 59:679, 1975

42. Carpenter JT, Maddox WA: Melphalan adjuvant therapy in breast cancer. *Lancet* ii:450, 1983

43. Carter SK, Crook ST: *Mitomycin C – Current Status and New Developments*. Academic Press, New York, 1979

44. Carter SK, Friedman MA: 5-(3,3-Dimethyl-1-triazeno)imidazole-4-carboxamide (DTIC, DIC, NSC-45388) – A new antitumour agent with activity against malignant melanoma. *Eur J Cancer* 8:85, 1972

45. Chipman JK, Hirom PC, Millburn P: Biliary excretion and enterohepatic circulation of aniline mustard metabolites in the rat and rabbit. *Biochem Pharmac* 29:1299, 1980

46. Chiuten DF, Rozencweig M, Von Hoff DD, Muggia FM: Clinical trials with the hexitol derivatives in the U.S. *Cancer* 47:442, 1981

47. Chou F, Khan AH, Driscoll JS: Potential central nervous system antitumour agents. Aziridinylbenzoquinones 2. *J Med Chem* 19:1302, 1976

48. Clarke DA, Barclay RK, Stock CC, Rondestvedt CS: Triazenes as inhibitors of mouse sarcoma 180. *Proc Soc Exptl Biol Med* 90:484, 1955

49. Clement JJ, Gorman MS, Wodinsky I, Catane R, Johnson RK: Enhancement of antitumour activity of alkylating agents by the radiation sensitiser misonidazole. *Cancer Res* 40:4165, 1980

50. Clement JJ, Johnson RK: Evaluation of radiosensitisers in combination with chemotherapeutic agents in solid tumours. *Int J Radiat Oncol Biol Phys* 8:631, 1982

51. Cohen JL, Jao JY, Jusko WJ: Pharmacokinetics of cyclophosphamide in man. *Brit J Pharmac* 43:677, 1971

52. Coleman CN, Friedman MK, Jacobs C, Halsey J, Ignoffo R, Leibel S, Hirst VK, Gribble M, Carter SK, Phillips TL: Phase I trial of intravenous 1-phenylalanine mustard plus the sensitiser misonidazole. *Cancer Res* 43:5022, 1983

53. Colvin M: In: *Pharmacological Principles of Cancer Treatment*, Chapter 13, pp. 276–308. Edited by B Chabner. W.B. Saunders Company, Philadelphia, 1982

54. Comis RL, Carter SK: Integration of chemotherapy into combined modality therapy of solid tumours. IV. Malignant melanoma. *Cancer Treat Rev* 1:285, 1974

55. Connors TA, Cox PJ, Farmer PB, Foster AB, Jarman M: Some studies of the active intermediates formed in the microsomal metabolism of cyclophosphamide and isophosphamide. *Biochem Pharmac* 23:115, 1974

56. Connors TA, Farmer PB, Foster AB, Gilsenan AM, Jarman M, Tisdale MJ: Metabolism of aniline mustard (N,N-di-(2-chloroethyl)-aniline). *Biochem Pharmac* 22:1971, 1973

57. Connors TA, Foster AB, Gilsenan AM, Jarman M, Tisdale MJ: Chemical trapping of a reactive metabolite. The metabolism of the azomustard 2'-carboxy-4-di-(2-chloroethyl)amino-2-methylazobenzene. *Biochem Pharmac* 21:1309, 1972

58. Connors TA, Gilsenan AM, Ross WCJ, Bukhari A, Tisdale MJ, Warwick GP: Agents designed specifically for the treatment of liver cancer. In: *Chemotherapy of Cancer Dissemination and Metastasis*, pp. 367–376. Edited by S Garattini, G Franchi. Raven Press, New York, 1973

59. Connors TA, Goddard PM, Merai K, Ross WCJ, Wilman DEV: Tumour inhibiting triazenes: structural requirements for an active metabolite. *Biochem Pharmac* 25:241, 1976

60. Connors TA, Whisson ME: Cure of mice bearing advanced plasma cell tumours with aniline mustard. *Nature, Lond* 206:689, 1965

61. Constanzi JJ, Fletcher WS, Balcerzak SP, Taylor S, Eyre HJ, O'Bryan RM, Al-Sarraf M, Frank J: Combination chemotherapy plus levamisole in the treatment of disseminated malignant melanoma. *Cancer* 53:833, 1984

62. Cornbleet MA, McElwain TJ, Kumar PJ, Filshie J, Selby P, Carter RL, Hedley DW, Clark ML, Millar JL: Treatment of advanced malignant melanoma with high-dose melphalan and autologous bone marrow transplantation. *Br J Cancer* 48:319, 1983

63. Cox PJ: Cyclophosphamide cystitis-identification of acrolein as causative agent. *Biochem Pharmac* 28:2045, 1979

64. Cox PJ, Farmer PB, Foster AB, Gilby ED, Jarman M: The use of deuterated analogues in qualitative and quantitative investigations of the metabolism of cyclophosphamide. (NSC-26271). *Cancer Treat Rep* 60:483, 1976

65. Cox PJ, Farmer PB, Jarman M, Jones M, Kinas R, Stec WJ: Observation on the differential metabolism and biological activity of the optical isomers of cyclophosphamide. *Biochem Pharmac* 25:993, 1976

66. Cox PJ, Farmer PB, Jarman M, Kinas RW, Stec WJ: Stereoselectivity in the metabolism of the enantiomers of cyclophosphamide in mice, rats and rabbits. *Drug Metab Dispos* 6:617, 1978

67. Cox PJ, Phillips BJ, Thomas P: The enzymatic basis of the selective action of cyclophosphamide. *Cancer Res* 35:3755, 1975

68. Cox PJ, Phillips BJ, Thomas P: Studies on the selective action of cyclophosphamide (NSC-26271) inactivation of the hydroxylated metabolite by tissue-soluble enzymes. *Cancer Treat Rep* 60:321, 1976

69. Curt GA, Schilsky R, Kelly J, Kufta C, Smith B, Thomas C, Young RC: Phase II study of aziridinylbenzoquinone (AZQ) in high grade gliomas. *Proc Am Soc Clin Oncol* 1:13, 1982

70. De Weger RA, Dullens HFJ, Den Otter W: Eradication of murine lymphoma and melanoma cells by chlorambucil-antibody complexes. *Immunological Rev* 62:29, 1982

71. D'Incalci M, Bolis G, Facchinetti T, Mangioni C, Morasca L, Morazzoni P, Salmona M: Decreased half-life of cyclophosphamide in patients under continual treatment. *Eur J Cancer* 15:7, 1979

72. Domeyer BE, Sladek NE: Metabolism of 4-hydroxycyclophosphamide/aldophosphamide *in vitro*. *Biochem Pharmac* 29:2903, 1980

73. Double JA, Workman P: A new high-glucuronidase mouse tumour curable by aniline mustard therapy. *Cancer Treat Rep* 61:909, 1977

74. Driscoll JS, Hazard GF, Wood HB, Goldin A: Structure – antitumour activity relationships among quinone derivatives. *Cancer Chemother Rep* Part 2, 4(2):1, 1974

75. Ducore JM, Erickson LC, Zwelling LA, Laurent G, Kohn KW: Comparative studies of cross-linking and cytotoxicity in Burkitt's lymphoma cell lines treated with *cis*-diamminedichloroplatinum (II) and L-phenylalanine mustard. *Cancer Res* 42:897, 1982

76. Eagan RT, Ames MM, Powis G, Kovach JS: Clinical and pharmacological evaluation of split-dose intermittent therapy with dianhydrogalactitol. *Cancer Treat Rep* 66:283, 1982

77. Editorial: Hazards of cancer chemotherapy. *Lancet* ii:1317, 1982

78. Editorial: How real is the hazard? *Lancet* i:203, 1984

79. Ehrsson H, Hassan M: Determination of busulfan in plasma by GC-MS with selected-ion monitoring. *J Pharm Sci* 72:1203, 1983

80. Ehrsson H, Hassan M, Ehrnebo M, Beran M: Busulfan kinetics. *Clin Pharmacol Ther* 34:86, 1983

81. Ehrsson H, Wallin I, Nilsson S-O, Johansson B: Pharmacokinetics of chlorambucil in man after administration of the free drug and its prednisolone ester (prednimustine, Leo 1031). *Eur J Clin Pharmac* 24:251, 1983

82. Elson LA, Jarman M, Ross WCJ: Toxicity, haematological effects and anti-tumour activity of epoxides derived from disubstituted hexitols. Mode of action of mannitol myleran and dibromomannitol. *Eur J Cancer* 4:617, 1968

83. Erickson LC, Bradley MO, Ducore JM, Ewig RAG, Kohn KW: DNA crosslinking and cytotoxicity in normal and transformed human cells treated with antitumour nitrosoureas. *Proc Natl Acad Sci USA* 77:467, 1980

84. Erickson LC, Ramonas LM, Zaharko MD, Kohn KW: Cytotoxicity and DNA cross-linking activity of 4-sulfidocyclophosphamides in mouse leukaemia cells *in vitro*. *Cancer Res* 40:4216, 1980

85. Evans TL, Chang SY, Alberts DS, Sipes IG, Brendil K: *In vitro* degradation of L-phenylalanine mustard (L-PAM). *Cancer Chemother Pharmac* 8:175, 1982

86. Everett JL, Roberts JJ, Ross WCJ: Aryl-2-halogenoalkylamines. XII. Some carboxylic derivatives of N,N-di-2-chloroethylaniline. *J Chem Soc* 2386, 1953

87. Ezdinli EZ, Stutzman L: Chlorambucil therapy for lymphomas and chronic lymphocytic leukaemia. *J Am Med Ass* 191:444, 1965

88. Fairchild WV, Spence R, Solomon HD, Gangai MP: The incidence of bladder cancer after cyclophosphamide therapy. *J Urol* 122:163, 1979

89. Falck K, Grohn P, Sorsa M, Vainio H, Heinonen E, Holsti LR: Mutagenicity in urine of nurses handling cytostatic drugs. *Lancet* i:1250, 1979

90. Farmer PB, Foster AB, Jarman M, Newell DR, Oddy MR, Kiburis JH: The metabolism of deuterated analogues of chlorambucil by the rat. *Chem–Biol Interactions* 28:211, 1979

91. Farquhar D: p-(3,3-Dimethyl-1-triazeno)benzamide (DTB): a potential central nervous system (CNS)-active analogue of dacarbazine (DTIC). *Proc Am Ass Cancer Res* 17:176, 1976

92. Fenselau C, Kan M-NN, Rao SS, Myles A, Friedman OM, Colvin M: Identification of aldophosphamide as a metabolite of cyclophosphamide *in vitro* and *in vivo* in humans. *Cancer Res* 37:2538, 1977

93. Finklestein JZ, Albo V, Ertel I, Hammond D: 5-(3,3-Dimethyl-1-triazeno)imidazole-4-carboxamide (NSC-45388) in the treatment of solid tumours in children. *Cancer Chemother Rep* 59:351, 1975

94. Fisher B, Carbone PP, Economow SG, Frelick R, Glass A, Lerner H, Redmond C, Zelen M, Katrych DL, Wolmark N, Band P, Fisher ER: 1-Phenylalanine mustard (L-PAM) in the management of primary breast cancer. *New England J Med* 292:117, 1975

95. Fox BW: Mechanism of action of methanesulphonates. In: *Handbook of Experimental Pharmacology*, Vol. 38, Part II, *Antineoplastic and Immunosuppressive Agents*, pp. 35–46. Edited by AC Sartorelli, DG Johns. Springer-Verlag, Berlin, 1975

96. Franks CR: Melphalan in metastatic cancer of the prostate. *Cancer Treat Rev* 6(Suppl):121, 1979

97. Friedman MA: PCNU Phase I study in the Northern California Oncology. *Group Rec Res Cancer Res* 76:125, 1981

98. Galton DAG, Israels LG, Nabarro JDN, Till M: Clinical trials of p-(di-2-chloroethylamino)phenylbutyric acid (CB

1348) in malignant lymphoma. *Brit Med J* ii:1172, 1955

99.   George RP, Poth JL, Gordon D, Schrier SL: Multiple myeloma – intermittent combination chemotherapy compared to continuous therapy. *Cancer* 29:1665, 1972

100. Gerulath AH, Loo TL: Mechanism of action of 5-(3,3-dimethyl-1-triazeno)imidazole-4-carboxamide in mammalian cells in culture. *Biochem Pharmac* 21:2335, 1972

101. Gescher A, Hickman JA, Simmonds RJ, Stevens MFG, Vaughan K: Studies of the mode of action of antitumour triazenes and triazines – II. Investigation of the selective toxicity of 1-aryl-3,3-dimethyltriazenes. *Biochem Pharmac* 30:89, 1981

102. Ghose T, Norvell ST, Guclu A, Cameron D, Bodurka A, McDonald AS: Immunochemotherapy of cancer with chlorambucil-carrying antibody. *Br Med J* 3:495, 1972

103. Gibson NW, Hickman JA: The role of isocyanates in the toxicity of antitumour haloalkylnitrosoureas. *Biochem Pharmac* 31:2795, 1982

104. Gingold N, Pitterman E, Stacker A: Peptichemio in the therapy of malignancies (Phase I study). *Int J Clin Pharmac Biopharm* 10:190, 1974

105. Giuliano AE, Larkin KL, Eilber FR, Morton DL: Failure of combination chemotherapy (CYVADIC) in metastatic soft tissue sarcomas: implications for adjuvant studies. *Proc Am Soc Clin Oncol* 19:359, 1977

106. Glucksberg H, Rivkin SE, Rasmussen S, Tranum B, Gad-el-Mawla N, Constanzi J, Hoogstraten B, Athens J, Maloney T, McCracken J, Vaughn C: Combination chemotherapy (CMFVP) versus L-phenylalanine mustard (L-PAM) for operable breast cancer with positive axillary nodes. *Cancer* 50:423, 1982

107. Godeneche D, Madelmont JC, Sauvezie B, Billaud A: Etude de la cinétique d'absorption de distribution et d'élimination de l'acide *N,N*-dichloro-2,ethyl,*p*-aminophenyl-4,butyrique (chloraminophène) marqué au ^{14}C chez le rat. *Biochem Pharmac* 24:1303, 1975

108. Gombar CT, Tong WP, Ludlum DB: Mechanisms of actions of the nitrosoureas – IV. Reactions of bis-chloroethyl nitrosourea and chloroethyl cyclohexyl nitrosourea with deoxyribonucleic acid. *Biochem Pharmac* 29:2639, 1981

109. Gottlieb JA, Baker LH, O'Bryan RM, Sinkovics JG, Hoogstraten B, Quagliana JM, Rivkin SE, Bodey GP, Rodriguez VT, Blumenschein GR, Saiki JH, Coltman C, Burgess MA, Sullivan P, Thigpen P, Bottomley R, Balcerzak S, Moon TE: Adriamycin (NSC-123127) used alone and in combination for soft tissue and bony sarcomas. *Cancer Chemotherap Rep Part 3*, 6:271, 1975

110. Griffin JP, Newman RA, McCormack JJ, Krakoff IH: Clinical and clinical pharmacological studies of aziridinylbenzoquinone. *Cancer Treat Rep* 66:1321, 1982

111. Griggs LJ, Jarman M: Synthesis of deuterium-labeled analogs of cyclophosphamide and its metabolites. *J Med Chem* 18:1102, 1975

112. Grose WE, Burgess MD, Bodey GP: Clinical evaluation of peptichemio. *Cancer Treat Rep* 63:385, 1979

113. Gurtoo HL, Gessner T, Culliton P: Studies of the effects of cyclophosphamide, vincristine and prednisone on some hepatic oxidations and conjugations. *Cancer Treat Rep* 60:1285, 1976

114. Gurtoo HL, Marinello AJ, Berrigan MJ, Bansal SK, Paul B, Pavelic ZP, Struck RF: Effect of thiols on toxicity and carcinostatic activity of cyclophosphamide. *Sem Oncol* 10 Suppl 1:35, 1983

115. Gutierrez PL, Friedman RD, Bachur NR: Biochemical activation of AZQ (3,6-diaziridinyl-2,5-bis(carboethoxyamino)-4-benzoquinone) to its free radical species. *Cancer Treat Rep* 66:339, 1982

116. Hammer CF, Loranger RA, Schein PS: Structures of the decomposition products of chlorozotocin: new intramolecular carbamates of 2-amino-2-deoxyhexoses. *J Org Chem* 46:1521, 1981

117. Hancock K, Peet BG, Price JJ, Watson GW, Stone J, Turner RL: Ten-year survival rates in breast cancer using combination chemotherapy. *Br J Surg* 64:134, 1977

118. Hansch C, Leo AJ: *Substituent Constants for Correlation Analysis in Chemistry and Biology.* John Wiley & Sons Inc, New York, 1979

119. Harrap KR, Riches PG, Gilby ED, Smallwood SM, Wilkinson R, Konyres I: Studies on the toxicity and antitumour activity of prednimustine, a prednisolone ester of chlorambucil. *Europ J Cancer* 13:873, 1977

120. Hedley DW, Millar JL, McElwain TJ, Gordon MY: Acceleration of bone-marrow recovery by pretreatment with cyclophosphamide in patients receiving high-dose melphalan. *Lancet* ii:966, 1978

121. Hendry JA, Homer RF, Rose FL, Walpole AL: Cytotoxic agents: III, derivatives of ethyleneimine. *Br J Pharmac* 6:357, 1951

122. Hetzel FW, Kaufman N: Chemotherapeutic drugs as indirect oxygen radiosensitisers. *Int J Radi Oncol Biol Phys* 9:751, 1983

123. Hickman JA, Stevens MFG, Gibson NW, Langdon SP, Fizames C, Lavelle F, Atassi G, Lunt E, Tilson RM: Experimental antitumor activity against murine tumor model systems of 8-carbamoyl-3-(2-chloroethyl)imidazo(5,1-d)-1,2,3,5-tetrazin-4(3H)-one (Mitozolomide), a novel broadspectrum agent. *Cancer Res* 45:3008, 1985

124. Hill BT, Douglas DC, Grover PL: Increased antitumour activity of chlorambucil following pretreatment with inducers of drug-metabolising enzymes. *Biochem Pharmac* 22:1083, 1973

125. Hill DL, Kirk MC, Struck RF: Microsomal metabolism of nitrosoureas. *Cancer Res* 35:296, 1975

126. Hilton J, Walker MD: Enzymic hydroxylation of CCNU. *Proc Amer Assoc Cancer Res* 16:103, 1975

127. Hipkins JH, Struck RF, Gurtoo HL: Role of aldehyde dehydrogenase in the metabolism-dependent biological activity of cyclophosphamide. *Cancer Res* 41:3571, 1981

128. Hirst M, Tse S, Mills DG, Levin L, White DF: Occupational exposure to cyclophosphamide. *Lancet* i:186, 1984

129. Horton JK, Stevens MFG: Triazines and related products, Part 23. New photoproducts from 5-diazoimidazole-4-carboxamide (Diazo-IC). *JCS Perkin Trans* 1:1433, 1981a

130. Horton JK, Stevens MFG: A new light on the photodecomposition of the antitumour drug DTIC. *J Pharm Pharmac* 33:808, 1981

131. Horvath IP, Csetenyi J, Kerpel-Fronius S, Hindy I, Eckhardt S: Metabolism and pharmacokinetics of dibromodulcitol (DBD, NSC-104800) in man. I. Metabolites of DBD. *Eur J Cancer* 15:337, 1979

132. Householder GE, Loo TL: Elevated urinary excretion of 4-aminoimidazole-5-carboxamide in patients after intravenous injection of 4-(3,3-dimethyl-1-triazeno)imidazole-5-carboxamide. *Life Sciences* 8:533, 1969

133. Hug V, Hortobaghi GN, Buzdar AU, Blumenschein GR, Grose W, Burgess MA, Bodey GP: A Phase II study of peptichemio in advanced breast cancer. *Cancer* 45:2524, 1980

134. Iyer VM, Szybalski W: A molecular mechanism of mitomycin action: linking of complementary DNA strands. *Proc Natl Ac Sci* 50:355, 1963

135. Jardine I, Fenselau C, Appler M, Kan M-N, Brundreth RB, Colvin M: Quantitation by gas chromatography-chemical ionisation mass spectrometry of cyclophosphamide, phosphoramide mustard and nornitrogen mustard, in the plasma and urine of patients receiving cyclophosphamide therapy. *Cancer Res* 38:408, 1978

136. Jarman M, Cox PJ, Farmer PB, Foster AB, Milsted RAV, Kinas RW, Stec WJ: The use of deuterium-labelled analogs

in a study of the metabolism of the enantiomers of cyclophosphamide. In: *Stable Isotopes, Proceedings of the Third International Conference*, pp. 363–370. Edited by ER Klein, PD Klein, Academic Press, New York, 1979

137. Jarman M, Gilby ED, Foster AB, Bondy PK: The quantitation of cyclophosphamide in human blood and urine by mass spectrometry-stable isotope dilution. *Clin Chim Acta* 58:61, 1975

138. Jarman M, Melzack DH, Ross WCJ: The metabolism of the antitumour agent 5-(1-aziridinyl)-2,4-dinitrobenzamide (CB 1954). *Biochem Pharmac* 25:2475, 1976

139. Johnson TP, Kussner CL, Carter RL, Frye JL, Lomax NR, Plowman J, Narayanan VL: Studies on synthesis and anticancer activity of selected N-(2-fluoroethyl)-N-nitrosoureas. *J Med Chem* 27:1422, 1984

140. Johnston TP, McCaleb GS, Montgomery JA: The synthesis of antineoplastic agents. XXXII. N-Nitrosoureas. I. *J Med Chem* 6:669, 1963

141. Johnston TP, McCaleb GS, Opliger PS, Montgomery JA: The synthesis of potential anti-cancer agents. XXXVI. N-Nitrosoureas. II. Haloalkylderivatives. *J Med Chem* 9:892, 1966

142. Juma FD, Rogers HJ, Trounce JR: Pharmacokinetics of cyclophosphamide and alkylating activity in man after intravenous and oral administration. *Br J Clin Pharmac* 8:209, 1979

143. Juma FD, Rogers HJ Trounce JR: The pharmacokinetics of cyclophosphamide, phosphoramide mustard and nornitrogen mustard studied by gas chromatography in patients receiving cyclophosphamide therapy. *Br J Clin Pharmac* 10:327, 1980

144. Kamen BA, Holcenberg JS, Siegel SE: Aziridinylbenzoquinone (AZQ) treatment of central nervous system leukemia. *Cancer Treat Rep* 66:2105, 1982

145. Kaung DT, Wittington RM, Spencer H, Patno ME: Comparison of chlorambucil and streptonigrin (NSC-45383) in the treatment of malignant lymphomas. *Cancer* 23:1280, 1969

146. Kaye SB, Juttner CA, Smith IE, Barrett A, Austin DE, Peckham MJ, McElwain TJ: Three years' experience with ChlVPP (a combination of drugs with low toxicity) for the treatment of Hodgkin's disease. *Brit J Cancer* 39:168, 1979

147. Kedar A, Simpson CL, Williams P, Moore R, Tritsch G, Murphy GP: The prevention of cyclophosphamide-induced bladder swelling in the rat by i.v. administration of sodium-2-mercaptethane sulfonate. *Res Commun Chem Pathol Pharmac* 29:339, 1980

148. Khan AH, Driscoll JS: Potential central nervous system antitumour agents. Aziridinylbenzoquinones. 1. *J Med Chem* 19:313, 1976

149. Khan AH, Ross WCJ: Tumour-growth inhibitory nitrophenylaziridines and related compounds: structure-activity relationships. II. *Chem-Biol Interact* 4:11, 1971/72

150. Khan AH, Ross WCJ: Tumour-growth inhibitory nitrophenylaziridines and related compounds: structure-activity relationships. II. *Chem-Biol Interact* 4:11, 1971/72

151. Kinas R, Pankiewicz K, Stec WJ: The synthesis of enantiomeric cyclophosphamides. *Bull Acad Pol Sci Ser Chim* 23:981, 1975

152. Kitamura S, Tatsumi K: Azoreductase activity of liver aldehyde oxidase. *Chem Pharm Bull* 31:3334, 1983

153. Kohn KW: Interstrand cross-linking of DNA by 1,3-bis(2-chloroethyl)-1-nitrosourea and other 1-(2-haloethyl)-1-nitrosoureas. *Cancer Res* 37:1450, 1977

154. Kohn KW: Mechanistic approaches to new nitrosourea development. *Rec Res Cancer Res* 76:141: 1981

155. Kolar GF, Maurer M, Wildsrhutte M: 5-(3-Hydroxymethyl-3-methyl-1-triazeno)imidazole-4-carboxamide is a metabolite of 5-(3,3-dimethyl-1-triazeno)imidazole-4-carboxamide (DIC, DTIC, NSC-45388). *Cancer Lett* 10:235, 1980

156. Konieczny M, Guiterrez PL, Sosnovsky G: In the search for new anticancer drugs. IV: Antitumor activity of seleno-TEPA. *Z Naturforsch, Teil B* 38:1138, 1983

157. Konieczny M. Gutierrez PL, Sosnovsky G: In the search for new anticancer drugs. V: Study of the binding of spin-labelled thio-TEPA to cells. *Z Naturforsch, Teil B* 38:1142, 1983

158. Könyves I, Fex H, Högberg B: Novel corticosteroid esters with alkylating properties. In: *Antineoplastic Chemotherapy*, pp. 791–795. Edited by GK Daikon. Proc 8th Int Congress of Chemoterapy, 1973

159. Koriech OM, Shükla VS: Dacarbazine (DTIC) in malignant melanoma: Reduced toxicity with protection from light. *Clin Radiol* 32:53, 1981

160. Kubota T, Hanatani Y, Tsuyuki K, Nakada M, Ishibiki K, Abe O, Kamabaki T, Kato R: Antitumor effect and metabolic activation of cyclophosphamide and 4-hydroperoxycyclophosphamide in the human breast carcinoma (MX-1) nude mouse system. *Gann* 74:437, 1983

161. Kuroyanagi S, Miyajima S, Hirota M, Yamana T: Effect of carzinophilin on malignant tumours. *Gann* 47:359, 1965

162. Langdon SP, Stevens MFG, Stone R, Gibson NW, Baig GU, Hickman JA, Newton CG, Lunt E: *Brit J Cancer* 52:439, 1985

163. Langdon SP, Chubb D, Vickers L, Stone R, Stevens MFG, Baig GU, Gibson NW, Hickman JA, Lunt E, Newton CG, Warren PJ, Smith CJ: *Brit J Cancer* 52:437, 1985

164. Large P, Gregoriadis G: Phospholipid composition of small unilamellar liposomes containing melphalan influences drug action in mice bearing PC6 tumours. *Biochem Pharmac* 32:1315, 1983

165. Larionov LF, Shkodinskaja EN, Troosheikina VI, Kholzhlov AS, Vasina OS, Novikova MA: Studies on antitumour activity of *p*-di(2-chloroethyl)aminophenylalanine (Sarcolysin). *Lancet* ii:169, 1955

166. Legha SS, Slavik M, Carter SK: Hexamethylmelamine. An evaluation of its role in the therapy of cancer. *Cancer* 38:27, 1976

167. Levin VA: Relationship of octanol/water partition coefficient and molecular weight to rat brain capillary permeability. *J Med Chem* 23:682, 1980

168. Livingstone RB, Carter SK: *Single Agents in Cancer Chemotherapy*, pp. 99–111. Plenum, New York, 1970

169. Loo TL: *Triazenoimidazole Derivatives* in '*Antineoplastic and Immunosuppressive Agents II*', pp. 544–553. Edited by AC Sartorelli, DG Johns. Springer-Verlag, Berlin, 1975

170. Low JE, Borch RF, Sladek NE: Conversion of 4-hydroperoxycyclophosphamide and 4-hydroxycyclophosphamide to phosphoramide mustard and acrolein mediated by bifunctional catalysts. *Cancer Res* 42:830, 1982

171. Lu K, Savaraj N, Yap BS, Bedikian AY, Feun L, Benjamin RS, Loo TL: Clinical pharmacology of 2,5-diaziridinyl-3,6-biscarboethoxyamino-1,4-benzoquinone (AZQ). *Eur J Cancer Clin Oncol* 19:603, 1983

172. Masterson JG, Calame RJ, Nelson J: A clinical study on the use of chlorambucil in the treatment of cancer of the ovary. *Am J Obstet Gynecol* 79:1002, 1960

173. McElwain TJ, Hedley DW, Burton G, Clink HM, Gordon MY, Jarman M, Juttner CA, Millar JL, Milsted RAV, Prentice G, Smith IE, Spence D, Woods M: Marrow autotransplantation accelerates haematological recovery in patients with malignant melanoma treated with high-dose melphalan. *Brit J Cancer* 40:72, 1979

174. McElwain TJ, Powles RL: High-dose intravenous melphalan for plasma-cell leukaemia and myeloma. *Lancet* ii:822, 1983

175. McElwain TJ, Toy J, Smith E, Peckham MJ, Austin DE: A combination of chlorambucil, vinblastine, procarbazine and prednisolone for treatment of Hodgkin's disease. *Brit J Cancer* 36:276, 1977

176. McLean A, Newell D, Baker G, Connors T: The metabolism of chlorambucil. *Biochem Pharmac* 29:2039, 1980

177. Millar JL, McElwain TJ: Combinations of cytotoxic agents that have less than expected toxicity on normal tissues in mice. *Antibiot Chemother* 23:271, 1978

178. Mitoma C, Onodera T, Takegoshi T, Thomas DW: Metabolic disposition of chlorambucil in rats. *Xenobiotica* 7:205, 1977

179. Mizuno NS, Humphrey EW: Metabolism of 5-(3,3-dimethyl-1-triazeno)imidazole-4-carboxamide (NSC-45388) in human and animal tumour tissue. *Cancer Chemother Rep* 56:465, 1972

180. Moore GE, Bross IDJ, Auman R, Nadler S, Jones R, Slack N, Rimm AA: Effects of chlorambucil (NSC-3088) in 374 patients with advanced cancer. *Cancer Chemother Rep* 52:661, 1968

181. Morikawa T, Ozeki M, Umino N, Karamori M, Arai Y, Tsujihara K: A new class of nitrosoureas. III. Synthesis and antitumour activity of 3,3-disubstituted-1-(2-chloroethyl)-1-nitrosoureas having an arabinopyranosyl, xylopyranosyl or ribopyranosyl moiety. *Chem Pharm Bull* 30:534, 1982

182. Morikawa T, Tsujihara K, Takeda M, Arai Y: A new class of nitrosoureas. VII. Synthesis and antitumor activity of 3-substituted 1-(2-chloroethyl)-3-(methyl-D-glucopyranosid-3-yl)-1-nitrosoureas. *Chem Pharm Bull* 30:4365, 1982

183. Murnane JP, Byfield JE: Irrepairable DNA cross-links and mammalian cell lethality with bifunctional alkylating agents. *Chem-Biol Interact* 38:75, 1981

184. Murray-Lyon IM, Tattersall MHB, Thomas H, Sherlock S, Cockrane M, Williams R, Read AE: CB 10-252 in the treatment of primary hepatocellular carcinoma. *Med Chir Dig* 7:425, 1978

185. Newell DR, Calvert AH, Harrap KR, McElwain TJ: Studies on the pharmacokinetics of chlorambucil and prednimustine in man. *Br J Clin Pharmac* 15:253, 1983

186. Newell DR, Calvert AH, Harrap KR, McElwain TJ: The clinical pharmacology of chlorambucil and prednimustine. *Br J Clin Pharmac* 16;762, 1983

187. Newell DR, Shepherd CR, Harrap KR: The pharmacokinetics of prednimustine and chlorambucil in the rat. *Cancer Chemother Pharmac* 6:85, 1981

188. Newlands ES, Blackledge G, Slack JA, Goddard C, Brindley CJ, Holden L, Stevens MFG: Phase I clinical trial of mitozodamide. *Cancer Treat Repts* 69:801, 1985

189. Nicolin A, Cavalli M, Missiroli A, Goldin A: Immunogenicity induced *in vivo* by DIC in relatively non-immunogenic leukaemias. *Europ J Cancer* 13:235, 1977

190. Norpoth K: Studies on the metabolism of isophosphamide (NSC-109724) in man. *Cancer Treat Rep* 60:437, 1976

191. Norppa H, Sorsa M, Vainio H, Grohn P, Heinonen E, Holsti L, Nordman E: Increased sister chromatid exchange frequencies in lymphocytes of nurses handling cytostatic drugs. *Scand J Work Environ Health* 6:299, 1980

192. Oberc-Greenwood MA, Smith BH, Cooke C, Ellis JR, Kornblith PL, McKeever PE: Mitochrondrial toxicity of 2,5-diaziridinyl-3,6-bis(carbethoxyamino)-1,4-benzoquinone. *J Natl Cancer Inst* 71:723, 1983

193. Piver MS, Barlow JJ, Lee FT, Vongtama V: Sequential therapy for advanced ovarian adenocarcinoma: operation, chemotherapy, second-look laparotomy and radiation therapy. *Am J Obstet Gynecol* 122:355, 1975

194. Poochikian GK, Cradock JC: 2,5-Diaziridinyl-3,6-bis(carboethoxyamino)-1,4-benzoquinone I: Kinetics in aqueous solutions by high performance liquid chromatography. *J Pharm Sci* 70:159, 1981

195. Reed DJ, May HE: Alkylation and carbamoylation intermediates from the carcinostatic 1-(2-chloroethyl)-3-cyclohexyl-1-nitrosourea (CCNU). *Life Sci* 16:1263, 1975

196. Roberts JJ, Warwick GP: The mode of action of alkylating agents. III. The formation of 3-hydroxytetrahydrothiophene-1:1-dioxide from 1:4-dimethanesulphonyloxybutane (myleran), S-β-L-alanyltetrahydrothiophenium mesylate, tetrahydrothiophene and tetrahydrothiophene-1:1-dioxide in rat, rabbit and mouse. *Biochem Pharmac* 6:217, 1961

197. Robinson R, Watt JS: Some derivatives of 3-ethylpyridine and 2:3-furano(2′:3′)pyridine. *J Chem Soc* 1536, 1934

198. Rose CM, Millar JL, Peacock JH, Phelps TA, Stevens TC: Differential enhancement of melphalan cytotoxicity in tumor and normal tissue by misonidazole. In: *Radiation Sensitisers. Their Use in the Clinical Management of Cancer*, pp. 250–257. Edited by LW Brady. Masson, New York, 1980

199. Ross WCJ: Aryl-2-halogenoalkylamines. Part I. *J Chem Soc* 183, 1949

200. Ross WCJ: *Biological Alkylating Agents.* Butterworth Press, London, 1962

201. Ross WCJ: The conjugation of chlorambucil with human γ-globulin. *Chem Biol Interact* 10:169, 1975

202. Ross WCJ: The conjugation of chlorambucil with human γ-globulin: confirmation that the drug is bound in an active form. *Chem-Biol Interact* 11:139, 1975

203. Ross WCJ, Warwick GP: Reduction of cytotoxic azo compounds by hydrazine and by the xanthine oxidase-xanthine system. *Nature* 176:298, 1955

204. Ross WCJ, Warwick GP: Aryl-2-halogeneoalkylamines. Part XVI. The preparation of derivatives of 4-(di(2-chloroalkyl)amino)azobenzenes. *J Chem Soc* 1364, 1956

205. Rutty CJ, Abel G, Vincent RB, Goddard PM, Harrap KR: Preliminary studies on the metabolism and pharmacokinetics of the dialkylphenyltriazenes. *Proceedings of the 10th International Symposium on the Biological Characterisation of Human Tumours*, 548, 1984

206. Rutty CJ, Newell DR, Vincent RB, Abel G, Goddard PM, Harland SJ, Calvert AH: The species dependent pharmacokinetics of DTIC. *Brit J Cancer* 48:140, 1983

207. Santoro A, Bonadonna G: Prolonged disease-free survival in MOPP-resistant Hodgkin's disease after treatment with adriamycin, bleomycin, vinblastine and dacarbazine (ABVD). *Cancer Chemother Pharmac* 2:101, 1979

208. Santoro A, Monfardini S, Bonadonna G: Treatment of MOPP-resistant Hodgkin's disease (HD) with adriamycin, bleomycin, vinblastine and dacarbazine (ABVD). *Proc Am Soc Clin Oncol* 19:363, 1978

209. Sawitsky A, Rai KR, Glidewell O, Silver RT: Comparison of daily versus intermittent chlorambucil and prednisone therapy in the treatment of patients with chronic lymphocytic leukaemia. *Blood* 50:1049, 1977

210. Scheef W, Klein HO, Brock N, Burkert H, Gunther U, Hoefer-Janker H, Mitrenga D, Schnitker J, Voigtmann R: Controlled clinical studies with an antidote against the urotoxicity of oxazaphosphorines: preliminary results. *Cancer Treat Rep* 63:501, 1979

211. Schilsky RL, Kelley JA, Ihde DC, et al.: Phase I trial and pharmakinetics of aziridinylbenzoquinone (NSC 182986) in humans. *Cancer Res* 42:1582, 1982

212. Schmahl D, Habs MR: Prevention of cyclophosphamide induced carcinogenesis in the urinary bladder of rats by administration of mesna. *Cancer Treat Rev* 10 Suppl A:57, 1983

213. Schmähl D, Habs M, Lorenz M, Wagner I: Occurrence of second tumours in man after anticancer treatment. *Cancer Treat Rev* 9:167, 1982

214. Schmid FA, Banks SE, Stock CC: Comparative antitumour effects of peptichemio and other alkylating agents. *Cancer Treat Rep* 51:473, 1977

215. Schmid FA, Stock CC: Antitumour activity of peptichemio. *Proc Am Assoc Cancer Res* 17:49, 1976

216. Selby PJ, Millar JL, Phelps TA, Gordon MY, Wilkinson R, McElwain TJ: The combination of melphalan with prednisolone. *Cancer Chemother Pharmac* 6:169, 1981

217. Shaw IC, Earl LK, McLean AEM, Mruzek MN, Souhami RL: Differences in the activity of two commercially available

preparations of cyclophosphamide. *Human Toxicol* 2:557, 1983

218. Shaw IC, Earl LK, Mruzek MN, Harper PG, McLean AEM, Souhami RL: Difference in bioactivity between two preparations of cyclophosphamide. *Lancet* i:709, 1983

219. Shaw IC, Graham MI, McLean AEM: 2-Chloroacetaldehyde, a metabolite of cyclophosphamide in the rat. *Xenobiotica* 13:433, 1983

220. Shealy YF: *J Pharm Sci* 64:177, 1975

221. Shealy YF, Krauth CA: Complete inhibition of mouse leukaemia L1210 by 5(or 4)-(3,3-bis(2-chloroethyl)-1-triazeno)imidazole-4(or 5)-carboxamide (NSC-82196). *Nature* 210:208, 1966

222. Shealy YF, Krauth CA, Montgomery JA: Imidazoles. 1. Coupling reactions of 5-diazoimidazole-4-carboxamide. *J Org Chem* 27:2150, 1962

223. Shealy YF, Montgomery JA, Laster WR: Antitumour activity of triazenoimidazoles. *Biochem Pharmac* 11:674, 1962

224. Shealy YF, Struck RF, Holum LB, Montgomery JA: Synthesis of potential anticancer agents. XXIX. 5-Diazoimidazole-4-carboxamide and 5-diazo-γ-triazole-4-carboxamide. *J Org Chem* 26:2396, 1961

225. Skibba JL, Beal DD, Ramirez G, Bryan GT: N-Dimethylation of the antineoplastic agent 4(5)-(3,3-dimethyl-1-triazeno)imidazole-5(4)-carboxamide in rats and man. *Cancer Res* 30:147, 1970

226. Skibba JL, Ramirez G, Beal DD, Bryan GT: Metabolism of 4(5)-(3,3-dimethyl-1-triazeno)imidazole-5(4)-carboxamide to 4(5)-aminoimidazole-5(4)-carboxamide in man. *Biochem Pharmac* 19:2043, 1970

227. Sosnovsky G, Paul BD: In the search for new anticancer drugs. VI: Structural modifications of cyclophosphamide. *Z Naturforsch, Teil B* 38:1146, 1983

228. Stevens MFG: Second-generation Azolotetrazinones. In: *Proceedings of the 8th Annual Bristol-Meyers Symposium on Cancer Research.* Edited by KR Harrap, TA Connors. Academic Press, New York, 335, 1986

229. Stevens MFG, Hickman JA, Stone R, Gibson NW, Baig GU, Lunt E, Newton CG: Antitumor imidazotetrazines. 1. Synthesis and chemistry of 8-carbamoyl-3-(2-chloroethyl)imidazo(5,1-*d*)-1,2,3,5-tetrazine-4(3H)-one, a novel broad spectrum antitumor agent. *J Med Chem* 27:196, 1984

230. Stratford IJ, Williamson C, Hoe S, Adams GE: Radiosensitising and cytotoxicity studies with CB 1954 (2,4-dinitro-5-aziridinylbenzamide). *Radiat Res* 88:502, 1981

231. Struck RF, Kirk MC, Mellett LB, El Dareer S, Hill DL: Urinary metabolites of the antitumor agent cyclophosphamide. *Mol Pharmac* 7:519, 1971

232. Suzukabe K, Vistica BP, Vistica DT: Dechlorination of L-phenylalanine mustard by sensitive and resistant tumour cells and its relationship to intracellular glutathione content. *Biochem Pharmac* 32:165, 1983

233. Tew KD, Smulson ME, Schein PS: Molecular pharmacology of nitrosoureas. *Rec Res Cancer Res* 76:130, 1981

234. Thorpe PE, Ross WCJ: The preparation and cytotoxic properties of anitbody-toxin conjugates. *Immunol Rev* 62:119, 1982

235. Tisdale MJ, Elson LA, Ross WCJ: Antitumour and haematological effects of δ-oxygen substituted butyl ethers. *Europ J Cancer* 8:255, 1972

236. Tisdale MJ, Habberfield AD: Selective inhibition of ribonucleotide reductase by the monofunctional alkylating agent 5-(1-aziridinyl)-2,4-dinitribenzamide (CB 1954). *Biochem Pharmac* 29:2845, 1980

237. Tong WP, Ludlum DB: Cross-linking of DNA by busulfan. Formation of diguanyl derivatives. *Biochim Biophys Acta* 608:174, 1980

238. Tong WP, Ludlum DB: Formation of the cross-linked base diguanylethane, in DNA treated with N,N′-bis(2-chloro-

239. ethyl)-N-nitrosourea. *Cancer Res* 41:380, 1981

239. Tsujihara K, Ozeki M, Morikawa T, Arai T: A new class of nitrosoureas. I. Synthesis and antitumor activity of 1-(2-chloroethyl)-3,3-disubstituted-1-nitrosoureas having a hydroxyl group at the β-position of the substituents. *Chem Pharm Bull* 29:2509, 19811.

240. Tsujihara K, Ozeki M, Morikawa T, Taga N, Miyazaki M, Kawamori M, Arai Y: A new class of nitrosoureas. II. Synthesis and antitumor activity of 1-(2-chloroethyl)-3,3-disubstituted-1-nitrosoureas having a glucopyranosyl, mannopyranosyl or galactopyranosyl moiety. *Chem Pharm Bull* 29:3262, 1981

241. Turner R: The value of anabolic sterols for patients receiving chemotherapy. *Excerpta Medica* APCS No 9, pp. 121–128, 1982

242. Valente EJ, Chan KK, Servis KL: Proton magnetic resonance studies of the decomposition of 4-hydroxycyclophosphamide, a microsomal metabolite of cyclophosphamide. *Pharm Res* 2:89, 1984

243. Wagner T, Heydrich D, Jork T, Voelcker G, Hohorst HJ: Comparative study on human pharmacokinetics of activated ifosfamide and cyclophosphamide by a modified fluorometric test. *J Cancer Res Clin Oncol* 100:95, 1981

244. Wagner T, Peter G, Voelcker G, Hohorst HJ: Characterisation and quantitative estimation of activated cyclophosphamide in blood and urine. *Cancer Res* 37:2592, 1977

245. Wallach O: Über das Verhalten einiger Diazo – und Diazoaminoverbindungen. *Ann Chem* 235:233, 1886

246. Wasserman TH, Comis RL, Goldsmith M, Handelsman H, Penta JS, Slavik M, Soper WT, Carter SK: Tabular analysis of the clinical chemotherapy of solid tumours. *Cancer Chemother Rep* Part 3, 6:399, 1975

247. Watanabe M, Tonda K, Hirata M, Hata Y: Enzyme-induced aziridine formation by isolated hepatocytes. *Biochem Biophys Res Commun* 112:356, 1983

248. Weinkam RJ, Lin H-S: Chlorethylnitrosourea cancer chemotherapeutic agents. *Adv Pharmacol Chemother* 19:1, 1982

249. Weiss RB, Issell BF: The nitrosoureas: carmustine (BCNU) and lomustine (CCNU). *Cancer Treat Rev* 9:313, 1982

250. Welsh J, Stuart JFB, Soukop M. Cunningham D, Blackie R, Sangster G, Kaye SB, Calman KC: The pharmacokinetics of oral and iv treosulfan. *Brit J Cancer* 46:467, 1982

251. Wheeler GP, Bowdon BJ, Torbet JW, Webster J, Alexander JA: Biological and biochemical effects of N-(2-chloroethyl)-N^1-(trans-4-methylcyclohexyl)-N-nitrosourea on two transplantable murine colon tumours. *Cancer Res* 43:5837, 1983

252. Wheeler GP, Bowdon BJ, Struck RF: Carbamoylation of amino acids, peptides and proteins by nitrosourea. *Cancer Res* 35:2974, 1975

253. Whisson ME, Connors TA: Cure of mice bearing advanced plasma cell tumours with aniline mustard: the relationship between glucuronidase activity and tumour sensitivity. *Nature*, Lond 210:866, 1966

254. White FR: New agent data summary: Tetramin. *Cancer Chemother Rep* 4:52, 1959

255. Wilman DEV, Connors TA: Molecular structure and antitumour activity of alkylating agents. In: *Molecular Aspects of Anti-cancer Drug Action.* Edited by S Neidle, MJ Waring. Macmillan Press, London, 1983

256. Wilman DEV, Bradley NJ, Richardson SG: Astrocytoma zenografts in the choice of a second generation triazene. *Br J Cancer* 50:277, 1984

257. Wilman DEV, Cox PJ, Goddard PM, Hart LI, Merai K, Newell DR: Tumor inhibitory triazenes. 3. Dealkylation within an homologous series and its relation to antitumor activity. *J Med Chem* 27:870, 1984

258. Woolley PV, Luc PVT, Rahman A, Korsmeyer SJ, Smith FP, Schein PS: Phase I trial and clinical pharmacology of 1-(2-chloroethyl)-3-(2,6-dioxo-3-piperidyl)-1-nitrosoureas. *Can-*

cer Res 41:3896, 1981

259. Yagi MJ, Chin SE, Scanlon KJ, Holland JF, Bekesi JG: PTT.119, p-F-Phe-m-bis-(2-chloroethyl) amino-L-Phe-Met ethoxy HCl, a new chemotherapeutic agent active against drug-resistant tumor cell lines. *Biochem Pharmac* 34:2347, 1985

260. Yagi MJ, Bekesi JG, Daniel MD, Holland JF, Barbieri AD: Increased cancericidal activity of PTT.119, a new synthetic bis-(2-chloroethyl)amino-L-phenylalanine derivative with carrier amino acids. *Cancer Chemother Pharmac* 12:70, 1984

261. Young CW, Yagoda A, Bitter ES, Smith SW, Grabstald H, Whitmore W: Therapeutic trial of aniline mustard in patients with advanced cancer. *Cancer* 38:1887, 1976

262. Zeller WJ, Schreiber J, Ho AD, Schmähl D, Eisenbrand G: Cytostatic activity of steroid linked nitrosoureas. *J Cancer Res Clin Oncol* 108:164, 1984

POSTSCRIPT

The peculiar sensitivity of the Walker tumour to CB 1954 has recently been reinvestigated by Roberts and his colleagues. CB 1954 forms DNA interstrand crosslinks time dependently in Walker tumour cells, but not in V79 cells which are unaffected by the drug (5). The V79 cells are, however, rendered sensitive to CB 1954 by co-culturing with Walker cells and interstrand crosslinks are formed in their DNA. This is indicative of the formation of a diffusible toxic metabolite by the Walker cells (3). The active metabolite has been identified as 5-(aziridin-1-yl)-4-hydroxylamino-2-nitrobenzamide by comparison with synthetic material (3). The metabolizing enzyme has been shown to be a form of NAD(P)H dehydrogenase (quinone) (DT diaphorase, quinone reductase) (4). The authors have suggested that this selective bio-activation could lead to the development of new anti-cancer strategies (1). Antibodies to the enzyme might lead to a screening system for CB 1954-sensitive tumours or the enzyme could be targeted to particular tumours by coupling to a tumour 'specific' antibody after the manner suggested by Bagshaw (1).

A phase I clinical study of 1-(4-carboxyphenyl)-3,3-dimethyl-triazene (CB 10-277) has been initiated (2) and 1 minor and 2 partial responses have been observed out of 4 melanoma patients treated.

POSTSCRIPT REFERENCES

1. Bagshaw KD: Antibody directed enzymes revive anti-cancer prodrugs concept. *Br J Cancer* 56:531, 1987

2. Foster BJ, Newell DR, Carmichael J, Harris AL, Gumbrell LA, Wilman DEV, Calvert AH: Clinical and preclinical pharmacokinetic studies with 1-4-(carboxyphenyl)-3,3-dimethyltriazene (CB 10-277). *Brit J Cancer* 58:276, 1988

3. Knox RJ, Friedlos F, Jarman M, Roberts JJ: A new cytotoxic, DNA interstrand crosslinking agent, 5-(aziridin-1-yl)-4-hydroxylamino-2-nitrobenzamide, is formed from 5-(aziridin-1-yl)2-,4-dinitrobenzamide (CB 1954) by a nitroreductase enzyme in Walker carcinoma cells. *Biochem Pharmacol* 37:4661, 1988

4. Knox RJ, Boland MP, Friedlos F, Coles B, Southan C, Roberts JJ: The nitroreductase enzyme in Walker cells that activates 5-(aziridin-1-yl)-2,4-dinitrobenzamide (CB 1954) to 5-(aziridin-1-yl)-4-hydroxylamino-2-nitrobenzamide is a form of NAD(P)H dehydrogenase (quinone) (EC 1.6.99.2). *Biochem Pharmac* 37:4671, 1988

5. Roberts JJ, Friedlos F, Knox RJ: CB 1954 (2,4-dinitro-5-aziridinyl-benzamide) becomes a DNA interstrand crosslinking agent in Walker tumour cells. *Biochem Biophys Res Commun* 140:1073, 1986

PLATINUM COMPOUNDS

CHARLES L. LITTERST and EDDIE REED

INTRODUCTION

cis-Diamminedichloroplatinum-II (DDP) is a relatively new antineoplastic drug with demonstrated activity against mainly ovarian and testicular cancers. The biological activity of DDP was discovered by accident when bacterial growth was observed to cease in the vicinity of a platinum electrode (170). The antibacterial effects of platinum were characterized as being mainly bacteriostatic, with an elongation of bacterial cells rather than actual cell death (170). Several platinum salts were screened for their antibacterial effects, and one of the most cytotoxic, DDP, was then tested against an animal tumor model (171). When DDP was discovered to prolong the life of tumored animals, large scale screening for antineoplastic activity was begun. DDP was screened against a large number of predominantly murine tumor models and found to have significant, confirmed activity against B16 melanoma, L1210 and P388 leukemias, and human mammary and colon xenographs, among others (212). In addition, DDP was found to be active by several treatment schedules, against rat as well as mouse tumors, and to be active against tumors of both chemical and biological origins (169). Clinical trials of DDP first began in the early 1970's.

CHEMISTRY

The relatively simple chemical structure of DDP (Fig. 1) belies an extensive series of spontaneous aquation reactions wherein the chlorine atoms of DDP are replaced with aquo and hydroxo groups (Fig. 2). These reactions, when allowed to proceed *in vitro*, will ultimately produce an equilibrium mixture of parent drug and the numerous aquated and hydroxylated products. In addition, the presence of di- and tri-aquo complexes also has been suggested (168). *In vivo*, the equilibrium probably never occurs because of selective removal of some of the reactants from the reaction mixture. Thus, the parent drug is rapidly excreted in urine and after removal of the chlorines from the molecule, extensive nucleophilic binding to proteins and other substances occurs, further depleting the pool of reactants. Although DDP has been shown to interact with various enzymes *in vivo* and *in*

The authors greatfully acknowledge the helpful guidance provided by Dr Len Zwelling in the preparation of portions of this review and wish to thank Mrs Beth Singer, Mrs Beverly Sisco, and Ms Laura Alpert for their skillful typing of the manuscript.

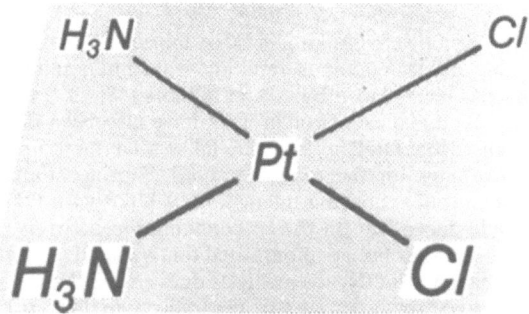

Figure 1. Chemical structure of *cis*-Diamminedichloroplatinum-II (DDP).

vitro (2, 3, 57, 121, 122, 132), no evidence for the catalysis of these aquation reactions by enzymatic means has appeared, nor has any enzyme-mediated metabolism of DDP been proposed. It has been inferred that biological activity resides with components other than the parent molecule but no identification of reactive products has been made. When DDP was incubated with plasma *in vitro* and ultrafilterable (nominal mw cutoff = 50000) as well as total platinum was analyzed, there was a gradual decrease in the concentration of filterable platinum (119), with a half time approximating that of the rate constant for the loss of the first chlorine atom (111). This suggested that DDP must undergo transformation to one or another of its byproducts prior to the appearance of the protein-bound platinum species. Additional work has shown that other effects on enzyme activity *in vitro* occur only after long incubation times (4, 57, 132). *In vitro* plasma binding curves are similar to those obtained in whole animals and in patients. Although the exact nature of the active species is unknown, the di- and tri-aquo polymers of DDP have been suggested to be extremely toxic (168).

ANTITUMOR MECHANISM

The mechanism by which DDP exerts its antitumor effect is thought to involve nucleophilic interaction with the DNA molecule and subsequent derangement of the structure and function of this nucleic acid. This thesis is based on the presence of platinum in cellular nuclei following DDP treatment (25, 101), its inhibition of DNA synthesis *in vitro* and *in vivo* (69, 84, 85, 136, 195), and the *in vitro* binding of DDP to DNA (48, 68, 93, 126, 150, 163, 220, 221). The mechanism of DNA binding and inactivation is thought to be denatura-

P.V. Woolley (ed.), Cancer management in Man: Biological Response Modifiers, Chemotherapy, Antibiotics, Hyperthermia, Supporting Measures
© 1989. Kluwer Academic Publishers, Dordrecht.

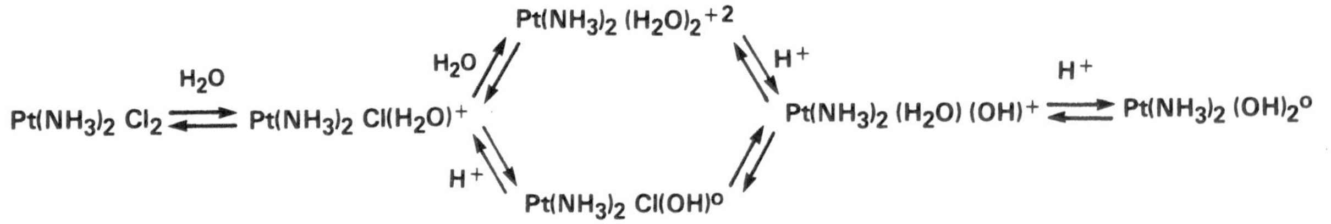

$$Pt(NH_3)_2 Cl_2 \underset{}{\overset{H_2O}{\rightleftharpoons}} Pt(NH_3)_2 Cl(H_2O)^+ \underset{H^+}{\overset{H_2O}{\rightleftharpoons}} Pt(NH_3)_2 (H_2O)_2^{+2} \underset{}{\overset{H^+}{\rightleftharpoons}} Pt(NH_3)_2 (H_2O)(OH)^+ \underset{}{\overset{H^+}{\rightleftharpoons}} Pt(NH_3)_2 (OH)_2^o$$

$$Pt(NH_3)_2 Cl(OH)^o$$

Figure 2. Chemical decomposition scheme of DDP in aqueous medium.

tion caused by crosslinking of DNA molecules. Thus, cross-linking of DNA strands resulting from interstrand cross links has been shown by several authors (48, 93, 150, 163, 220, 221) and DNA-protein links have also been demonstrated (220). DDP is bifunctional in that there are two reactive sites on the molecule (both chlorine atoms are leaving groups) and the interaction of DDP with DNA is strongly dependent on the *cis* configuration between these two sites. It has been demonstrated that *trans* DDP binds to mammalian cell DNA as avidly as does *cis* DDP and forms interstrand cross links even more rapidly than does *cis* DDP (48, 93, 150, 163, 220) but the *trans* configuration is much less cytotoxic. Hence, the difference in biological activity between the two isomers must not be in the initial binding to DNA or in the formation of interstrand cross links but in the intramolecular interactions between the second reactive site of *cis* DDP and various additional nucleophilic sites on the DNA molecule. Thus, it is thought that *cis* DDP initially interacts with nucleotides in DNA to form interstrand links but then subsequently interacts with other reactive sites on the same DNA strand to form intrastrand cross links that ultimately result in denaturation of the DNA molecules. In support of this theory, Eastman (48) concluded that the lack of denaturation of calf thymus DNA following *trans* DDP treatment was due to the inability of the *trans* molecule to form the same intrastrand cross links that were observed with *cis* DDP treatment. The binding of *cis* DDP to DNA is to the guanine bases and appears to mainly involve the N-7 positions (126). Support for guanine as the major binding site in DNA was obtained when intrastrand cross linking was shown to occur between adjacent guanine bases (164).

Although DDP-induced inhibition of DNA synthesis is widely recognized as being primarily responsible for the antitumor effects of DDP, the concentration of platinum found in tumors after administration of DDP to tumored animals is surprisingly low (80, 211). This had led to some speculation that a mechanism other than inhibition of DNA synthesis might also be operating to inhibit tumor growth. It has been postulated that DDP might interact with the host immune system to stimulate immune-mediated rejection of the tumor. Thus, Rosenberg first suggested that DDP may alter antigenic sites on tumor cell surfaces (167) and Sodhi and Aggarwal (189) showed an enhancement of cellular immunity in tumored animals treated with DDP. Subsequent work demonstrated that animals could be immunized against tumor cell challenge if previously treated with DDP-exposed tumor cells (178).

Although a good deal of animal work has been done with respect to DDP's effect on the immune system, work of only limited scope has been done in humans or with human tissues *in vitro*. Kleinerman *et al.* (104) reported that treating human monocytes with low concentrations of DDP (10^{-9} M) *in vitro* will cause enhancement of spontaneous monocyte-mediated cytotoxicity (SMMC). They cite literature suggesting that SMMC plays an important role in tumor cell kill in man. In a clinical study in ovarian cancer patients, all seven evaluable patients treated with a DDP-containing regimen showed at least a three-fold enhancement of cytotoxic function in the SMMC assay (105). This was thought to suggest that DDP may have some beneficial enhancement of immune function in treated patients. Howle *et al.* (85) reported that treating human monocytes *in vitro* with DDP in the 10^{-5} M range for up to 24 hr may actually suppress immune function. Kleinerman and Zwelling (103) studied the effects of *in vitro* DDP treatments in the 10^{-5} M range for one hour and reported no difference between treated cells and controls with respect to response to several mitogens and to ^{3}H-thymidine incorporation. These data, taken together with other animal data suggest that DDP may have an as yet incompletely understood but beneficial effect on the human immune system.

PHARMACOKINETICS AND DISTRIBUTION

Following a bolus intravenous administration of DDP to animals, platinum leaves the blood in a multi-compartmental fashion, with two major components. The initial distribution half time is 6–10 minutes in rats, dogs and rabbits (39, 42, 58, 119, 123, 156). The second major component is a very prolonged elimination half life reported to be 2–5 days in the same 3 species (39, 42, 58, 119, 123, 156). It is felt that these long half times reflect the biological half lives for various tissue proteins and thus the prolonged plasma platinum concentrations arise from platinum freed from tissue binding sites only by the normal endogenous catabolism of these proteins (RL Dedrick, personal communication). Plasma decay of platinum in humans following DDP administrations is similar to that in animals, with half times for the initial distribution phase of 23–24 min and for the elimination phase of 44–67 hr (21, 36, 63, 66, 89, 151). Variations in elimination half times may reflect variations in treatment regimens. The kinetic data reported above reflect determinations of total platinum in plasma. From earlier discussions (p. 1) it should be apparent that total platinum analysis reflects both protein-bound platinum and ultra-filterable platinum (i.e., either unbound platinum or platinum bound to low molecular weight components). Although the kinetic parameters for filterable platinum have not routinely been determined, many authors report that the plasma concentration of filterable platinum declines in a monoexponential fashion and is below the limits of detection by 1–2 hr after dosing in both animals and patients (21, 63, 66, 89, 119, 151).

Excretion of platinum is almost exclusively in the urine, with 30–50% of the administered dose appearing in urine within the first hour after dosing (8, 36, 39, 42, 119, 156) and 50–70% appearing by 24 hr (8, 39, 42, 58, 119, 123, 156). After that time only very small amounts of platinum are recovered in urine, although urinary platinum is still detectable 30 days after dosing (120). The large excretion of platinum during the first day after administration of DDP may be accounted for in part by the fact that DDP is a rather potent diuretic, with 2–3-fold increases in urine volume (8, 29, 61). This early diuretic effect has been shown to be due to an inhibition of release of vasopressin from the posterior pituitary (29). Total recoveries of platinum rarely exceed 70–80%, probably because of extensive binding in tissues of large mass, such as skin and liver. Consistent with the theory of platinum metabolism, 90% of the urinary platinum during the first hour is intact DDP (162). Fecal excretion has not been closely examined, probably due to esthetic considerations and to the obviously predominant role of renal excretory mechanisms. This seems justified because in one 48-hr stool collection no platinum was detected after adminstration of DDP to a patient (188). However, platinum has routinely been detected in bile in all studies where it has been examined (21, 119, 156, 187) and this has prompted examination of the biliary excretion of platinum following administration of DDP. In bile duct cannulated rats, only 1% of the administered dose was recovered in the bile in 24 hr (42, 187) and this is consistent with various studies that have extrapolated biliary excretion data to 2–3% of administered dose. Inconsistencies in plasma decay curves of platinum after DDP administration have been alleged to be due to enterohepatic recirculation of DDP in patients (201).

Following administration of DDP to animals, highest concentration of platinum is found in kidney (80, 118, 119, 156). Liver, skin, ovary and lung also have high concentrations of platinum (80, 118, 119, 156). The decay of platinum from these tissues is relatively slow, with substantial concentrations detected in kidney, liver and skin as long as 12 days after a single injection of DDP (119), and platinum was easily detectable in brain tumor and brain tissue 5 days after an injection of DDP (13, 78, 191). Tissue half lives of platinum in liver and kidney have been calculated to be 32 and 50 hr, respectively (25). Data on distribution of platinum in tissues of patients treated with DDP are uncommon but have appeared. Two days after DDP administration to a patient with Hodgkin's disease, platinum concentrations were highest in kidney, followed by liver, testes, lymph nodes and thymus, and in a lymphosarcoma patient 25 days after DDP extremely high concentrations of platinum were found in liver with high concentrations also found in testes and lung but only moderate concentrations in kidney (78).

The intracellular distribution of platinum in animals has been only recently investigated in much detail. As might be expected from DNA interactions of DDP, high concentrations of platinum have been found in nuclei, with microsomes also containing high concentrations (25, 101). Cytosol, however, contained 4–5 times more platinum than any other individual fraction (25). The presence of such high concentrations of platinum in cytosol may be attributable to high concentrations of glutathione and other thiol-containing chemicals in that fraction (121). Although there was some redistribution of platinum with time, both liver and kidney had similar subcellular distribution.

TOXICITY

DDP is a relatively toxic drug, with an intraperitoneal single dose mouse LD_{50} reported between 13.4–17.8 mg/kg (179, 183, 193). The single dose ip LD_{50} is 7.5 mg/kg for the rat (208) and is 9.7 mg/kg for the guinea pig (56). The dose-response curve is very steep. The spectrum of toxic effects observed clinically is similar to, but more extensive than that reported in animals. Potentially the most serious toxicity associated with DDP administration is to the kidney. An acute renal tubular necrosis characterized by azotemia, increased plasma creatinine, decreased creatinine clearance and proteinuria is widely reported. The lesion is best described as a renal proximal tubular degeneration and necrosis, mainly in the pars recta of the outer medulla or corticomedullary junction. Although some authors report regeneration (45), others claim no significant regeneration to occur (27). Single administration of nonlethal doses has been shown to produce a progressive chronic degeneration terminating in extensive cyst formation in renal tubules (27, 44) and reports of interstitial fibrosis (44). Chronic administration of very small doses twice weekly for 10 weeks also has been shown to produce interstitial fibrosis as well as a periglomerular fibrosis, both of which were concluded to represent irreversible damage (27). Glomerular damage has not been reported after acute doses in animals. Some clinical studies, however, report a decreased GFR in patients on combination regimens containing DDP (130). The mild proteinuria which is reported to occur is likely a reflection of the tubular lesion and is due to leakage of low molecular weight enzymes and microglobulins into the tubular fluid as a result of damage to epithelial and other cells lining the tubule (32, 107). Although not reported in animal studies, human studies have shown platinum blood concentrations to correlate with appearance of renal toxicity (19). However, toxicity was not correlated with the number of treatment cycles or with parameters of renal function (19). In patients dying of malignant disease after being treated with DDP a major distinction was the finding that lesions were mainly in the distal tubule, with the proximal tubule affected to a much lesser degree, particularly in low dose regimens (62). The explanation for this major discrepancy between animal models and human results is unexplained and should be addressed.

Related to the tubular lesions is a serious electrolyte wasting, which has resulted in occurrence of severe tetany in isolated patients (72). This presumed defect in tubular function affects mainly Mg^{2+} and Ca^{2+}, but K^+ is also affected. This defect has not been widely studied in animals and was not detected in early rodent studies (179, 208), possibly because these parameters are rarely studied in such investigations. However, both dogs and monkeys showed decreases in serum Ca^{2+} and K^+ (Mg^{2+} was not evaluated) in early preclinical toxicity studies (179). The demonstration that hypomagnesemia can persist for a number of years after treatment (181) supports this as a tubular malfunction and is consistent with the chronic effects on renal histology and tubular morphology cited above.

Of less life-threatening potential but greater practical significance to the patient is severe nausea and vomiting, beginning an hour after dosing and persisting for 24 hr. Dogs given high doses of DDP showed both emesis and severe hemorrhagic enterocolitis (179). No diarrhea was observed, however, even though this is a hallmark of DDP-induced gastrointestinal toxicity in rats (208) and has been reported in monkeys as well (179). The hemorrhagic enterocolitis has also been reported in rats (26). No mucosal necrosis or hemorrhage was reported in stomach or colon, but an increase in lesion severity occurred from the duodenum (35–40% decrease in crypt and villus cells) to the ileum (60–70% decrease in cells) of rats (26). Very high doses of DDP have been shown to affect the colon of the rat (208). Although of unknown significance a gastric distention has been reported in rodents (165) and may reflect the inability of the rat to vomit.

Clinically, bone marrow suppression by DDP has been minimal, possibly because severe renal impairment intervenes at doses below those required for significant marrow suppression. Mild marrow suppression, however, has been detected in numerous animal studies (70, 179, 208). At lethal doses in dogs only mild leukopenia and neutropenia were observed, but moderate anemia was present with no histologic evidence of hypocellularity (179). This is reminiscent of the hemolytic anemia observed in patients (60, 115). Hematologic effects of DDP in monkeys were restricted to anemia, reticulocytopenia, and neutropenia (179). All hematologic effects were mild and appeared to be reversible. Mice have been shown to manifest mainly a reticulocytopenia with no evidence of the anemia or leukopenia (70) observed in other species. The significance of the reticulocytopenia is unknown because this response is not commonly observed in patients.

Hearing loss following DDP treatment has been studied extensively in both monkeys and guinea pigs and reflects the effects observed in patients. High tone hearing loss measured in guinea pigs after either single or multiple doses of DDP occurred before lower tone loss and was dose related (56, 139). Furthermore, loss of hair cells in the lower turns of the organ of Corti correlated well with functional loss of hearing (56). Using different methods of evaluation, Naika *et al.* (139) came to essentially the same conclusions, and, in addition, detected a tendency toward recovery of hearing function in animals receiving very high doses of DDP. This is of interest because clinically, the decreased high-tone hearing loss has been shown to be irreversible (199). Hair cell degeneration observed following treatment has been elegantly described, but the mechanism of this effect is yet unknown.

Following the successful demonstration that renal toxicity could be dramatically lessened with the use of hydration and diuresis (37), numerous attempts were made to find other means of blocking or reversing toxicity. Thus, extensive work in this area has been reported using chemicals and drugs in animals (14, 64, 83, 87, 112, 117, 129, 172, 186, 207, 218). By-and-large, effects in animals have been equivocal or have not been suitable for clinical application. Two techniques, however, have been found to produce significant and reproducible decreases in clinical toxicity and deserve brief

mention. One of these is the use of sodium thiosulfate (TS) as an antidote and the other is the use of hyperosmotic NaCl as a vehicle for cisplatinum administration. Several authors have shown that TS could block cisplatinum-induced lethality and could decrease BUN elevations in a dose-dependent manner (83, 87). Recent work by Howell *et al.* (82) has shown a similar effect in patients. These authors administered DDP intraperitoneally for tumors confined to the peritoneal cavity and gave TS intravenously as an antidote. At doses up to 270 mg/m^2 there was no significant nephrotoxicity with minimal myelosuppression and no hearing loss or peripheral neuropathy. Previously, the maximum tolerated dose had been 100–120 mg/m^2. The elimination of nearly all toxic effects of DDP with this treatment suggests a dramatic change in overall biological activity of DDP and raises the question of the effect of TS on therapeutic efficacy. Results of Phase II and Phase III clinical trials of this regimen will have to be examined closely to determine if therapeutic effect also has been altered. The use of hyperosmotic saline to block lethality and renal accumulation of DDP was first shown to be effective in rodents (117) and has since undergone use in clinical trials of both testicular and ovarian cancer patients (145, 146). In both populations of patients, no consistent increases in BUN or creatinine were observed at doses exceeding 200 mg/m^2. Only one of 8 ovarian cancer patients had BUN elevations and when subsequently retreated there was no increase in this parameter. Responses have been observed in a population of ovarian cancer patients where no response had been previously observed. These 2 clinical uses of antidotes for systematic toxicity of DDP indicate that searches for new means of blocking potential dose limiting toxicities should not be abandoned because initial successes are modest in animal studies, or because there are difficulties in application of laboratory methods or chemicals to clinical use.

CLINICAL USE

Phase I clinical trials of DDP were started in 1971 (75, 76, 173, 192). These studies and others showed a good correlation between animal studies and human studies with respect to tumoricidal efficacy and toxicity. After reports of excellent clinical results using DDP, particularly in testicular cancer (51), the Food and Drug Administration approved this drug for human use in late 1978.

Spectrum of activity

Disseminated, non-seminomatous testicular cancer is one situation where DDP has become, without question, the mainstay of primary therapy. Higby *et al.* (75) showed in 1974 that DDP had significant activity when used as a single agent against refractory advanced testicular cancer. Prior to this time, single agent therapies and multiple drug combinations had been used with limited success (97, 125, 133, 176, 214). Single agents such as mithramycin and methotrexate, or combinations such as vinblastine-bleomycin gave long-term survival results ranging from 22% to 40% (97, 177, 214). In 1974, Indiana University started clinical trials with a platinum-vinblastine-bleomycin regimen (PVB) which was reported in detail in 1977 (51). Of the currently established chemotherapy regimens for testicular cancer, the PVB regimen appears to be the most efficacious. The "projected cure rate" for non-seminomatous stage III patients is now 70–80% using PVB regimen (152). It should be noted that all established first line regimens for testicular cancer now use DDP in combination with other drugs.

There are a number of malignancies for which DDP has been incorporated into combination chemotherapy regimens, but where it remains unclear if DDP containing regimens are truly superior to non-DDP containing regimens. Among these are neoplasms of the ovary, of the head and neck, and of the lung.

Single agent studies have shown that the response rate to DDP in ovarian cancer is in the 30% range (216). This is considerably less than with some alkylating agents such as thiotepa, cyclophosphamide, melphalan, or chlorambucil (216). Indeed, whereas protocols containing DDP show good response rates – CHAD* 90% (202), PAC-5* 65% (50), CHex-UP* 72% (217) – long-term survival data are not yet available. Further, these figures are in the same range as more established non-DDP containing regimens such as Hexa-CAF* 75% (215) and CHF* 83%* (40). A more certain role for DDP in the treatment of ovarian cancer may be as part of a second line regimen. Here, data from several centers show that DDP-containing regimens give superior results over non-DDP containing regimens (90, 202). There are data to suggest that "high dose" DDP may be superior to previous regimens in refractory cases (145, 146).

In head and neck malignancies, multiple studies have shown that methotrexate is probably the best single agent with response rates consistently reported in the 50–60% range (108, 109, 114, 149). DDP was initially reported to have response rates in the same range (116), however, subsequent studies have shown that even in DDP combinations, response rates in the 60–70% range are the best obtained to date (91, 159). There are multiple drug regimens containing no DDP which have response rates in the 60–70% range (81, 157). Once again, there is no clear advantage with the use of DDP. It should be noted, however, that published data are incomplete with respect to durability of response and to toxicity in most of the reports cited.

In non-small cell lung cancer (NSCLC), the response rate to DDP as a single agent has been reported to be 14–26% range (21, 148). This is similar to the response rates reported for other single agents such as vindesine (59), mitomycin C (175), adriamycin (10), and VP-16 (46). Although DDP-containing combinations have resulted in response rates of 40–50% (88, 153), there are several non-platinum containing regimens that have response rates in the same range (53, 138). Even though its popularity has increased in recent years in the treatment of NSCLC, DDP has yet to demonstrate clear advantage over other drugs used in this setting. In small cell lung cancer (SCLC), DDP has generally been felt to be of limited value. Minna *et al.* (135) classify DDP as being a drug "for which conflicting data exists" in the treatment of SCLC. More recent studies suggest that DDP may well be quite useful in SCLC when used in an intensive fashion in combination with VP-16 and/or other drugs, with

* See Table 3 for explanation.

Table 1. Rare tumors reported to have responded to DDP either as a single agent or in combination.

Type of cancer	Complete or partial response	Reference
Thymoma	CR	31, 20
Kidney	CR	196, 166
Adenoid Cystic Carcinoma	PR	185, 182
Hepatoblastoma	PR	3
Hepatocellular Carcinoma	PR	131
Vulvar Carcinoma	PR	86
Fallopian Tube	PR	43
Adrenal	PR	194
Thyroid	PR	190
Mesothelioma	PR	38
Suprasellar Germinoma		143

CR = complete response; PR = partial response

response rates in the 80–90% range even in extensive stage disease (71, 102, 141).

There are a number of malignancies in which DDP has begun to establish an important role in the treatment of inoperable, advanced disease; these include carcinomas of the endometrium (41, 184, 198), bladder (30, 140, 197), prostate (7, 28, 134), esophagus (94, 147, 203), melanoma (6, 142), cervix (1, 67, 204), brain (99, 106, 210), and osteogenic sarcoma (144). There are also a number of relatively rare malignancies where DDP has been used with good effect. Many of these are listed in Table 1. Even though there are not enough cases in any one disease listed to draw definite conclusions, literature reports such as these warrant consideration when the practitioner is posed with a similar problem requiring chemotherapeutic intervention.

Mode of administration

DDP is administered parenterally, usually in isotonic NaCl. NaCl is used because DDP may react with water at low chloride ion concentrations (47, 110, 160). The neutral DDP molecule can then become "aquated". The aquated DDP molecule may have different antineoplastic and toxic actions than the parent compound. DDP may form a precipitate when maintained in bicarbonate solutions (79), or when used with aluminum infusion needles (12, 155). For these reasons, stainless steel infusion needles should be used, and bicarbonate solutions should be avoided.

Many different treatment schedules have been used for administering DDP intravenously. These DDP schedules are usually part of the "larger" schedule of the particular multiple drug combination being used. It is difficult to determine what an "optimal" DDP schedule is for a given disease, as can be illustrated in the case of ovarian cancer. Table 3 lists several of the DDP treatment schedules that have been reported in "first-line" drug combinations used for ovarian cancer. There are no available data showing "true tissue exposure" to active DDP in patients treated with these regimens. From the schedules listed, one would guess that if "true tissue exposure" to active DDP were measured in a serum concentration × time fashion, these regimens would give significantly different results. However, response rates to these regimens are roughly comparable.

Table 2. Combination regimens used to treat cancer (all are administered on a 4 week cycle).

Acronym	Drugs	Dose and schedule
CHAD	Cyclophosphamide	600 mg/m^2 IV Day 1
	Hexamethylmelamine	200 mg/m^2 PO Days 8–22
	Adriamycin	25 mg/m^2 IV Day 1
	Cisplatinum	50 mg/m^2 IV Day 1
PAC-5	Cisplatinum	20 mg/m^2 IV Days 1–5
	Adriamycin	50 mg/m^2 IV Day 1
	Cyclophosphamide	750 mg/m^2 IV Day 1
CHEX-UP	Cyclophosphamide	150 mg/m^2 PO Days 2–16
	Hexamethylmelamine	150 mg/m^2 PO Days 2–16
	5-Fluorouracil	600 mg/m^2 IV Days 1 & 8
	Cisplatinum	30 mg/m^2 IV Days 1 & 8
HEXA-CAF	Hexamethylmelamine	150 mg/m^2 PO Days 1–14
	Cyclophosphamide	150 mg/m^2 PO Days 1–14
	Methotrexate	40 mg/m^2 IV Days 1 & 8
	5-Fluorouracil	600 mg/m^2 IV Days 1 & 8
CHF	Cyclophosphamide	100 mg/m^2 PO Days 1–14
	Hexamethylmelamine	150 mg/m^2 PO Days 1–14
	5-Fluorouracil	600 mg/m^2 IV Days 1 & 8

This leads one to assume that other drugs in these combinations play varying roles in tumor cell kill. This makes it extremely difficult to demonstrate an advantage of one DDP treatment schedule over another. Although some authors have suggested that scheduling may be used to minimize some of DDP toxicities (5), it has yet to be demonstrated that one can maintain tumoricidal efficacy and substantially reduce toxicity by scheduling alone.

Data on diseases discussed above resulted from intravenous administration of the drug. However, several centers have begun to use intraarterial and/or intracavitary administration in an effort to increase the amount of drug delivered to the tumor while minimizing systemic drug toxicity. Howell *et al.* (82) reported that using the intraperitoneal approach combined with systemic thiosulfate treatment per-

mitted administration of up to 270 mg/m^2 of DDP with peritoneal concentrations of drug reaching 21-fold higher than the concurrent plasma drug level. This resulted in disease regression in a number of cases of far-advanced previously treated ovarian carcinoma, mesothelioma, and malignant carcinoid. Blumenreich *et al.* (11) reported a 13% complete response rate for superficial bladder tumor using intravesicular administration. However, they concluded that this approach was ineffective in this setting. Compared to Howell's study (82), DDP doses used by Blumenreich were rather low ($50–150 \text{ mg/m}^2$) and systemic thiosulfate therapy was not given. Intraarterial drug administration has been used to treat osteogenic sarcoma, melanoma, and other regionally confined malignancies with response rates ranging from 45 to 75% (18, 128, 158). There are no studies reported to date comparing these "novel" treatment approaches to standard IV administration in a randomized controlled trial. Therefore, the true utility of these approaches has yet to be defined.

Toxicity

The major limiting toxicity in the clinical use of DDP is renal tubular dysfunction. Madias *et al.* reported that about 30% of patients receiving the drug may experience renal toxicity (127). Blachley *et al.* reported that this number may actually be as high as 75% (9). Associated with this may be electrolyte disturbances that may become quite profound including hypomagnesemia, hypocalcemia, and hypokalemia (9, 127, 180). Rossof *et al.* reported that renal dysfunction is cumulative in humans and is directly related to total dose (173). Whereas the renal toxicity of a single dose or course of treatment may be mild and reversible, after repeated courses and high doses, the toxicity may become severe and irreversible (219). Available data suggest that renal toxicity may be reduced by any of, or any combination of the following maneuvers: slow infusion rates (78); hydration before, during and after DDP administration (9); administration of mannitol; systemic administration of thiosulfate when the drug is given intraperitoneally (82); and possibly furosemide use (24). Concomitant aminoglycoside therapy should be avoided because of markedly increased risk of renal dysfunction (62).

The most pronounced immediate toxicity is nausea and vomiting. Multiple agents have been used with good control of this side effect including tetrahydrocannabinol (174), droperidol (65), metoclopramide, nabilone (74) and others. With some antiemetics, including droperidol and metoclopramide, some patients may experience severe extrapyramidal reactions which may necessitate intervention with cogentin or benadryl. The physician should be alert to this possibility and be prepared to switch to another antiemetic should this occur.

Although myelosuppression has been reported as being modest with DDP (205), some authors feel that this side effect assumes greater importance when DDP is used in combination with other myelosuppressive drugs (33, 209, 219). Table 2 lists other reported toxicities. These toxicities tend to occur rarely, or are mild when they occur. However, any of the side effects listed may be quite pronounced in a given patient.

Table 3. Side effects secondary to DDP administration.

Toxicity/side effect	Severity/frequency	Reference
Auditory dysfunction	Mild – Common	73, 154
Peripheral neuropathy	Mild – Common	92, 34
Hypomagnesemia	Moderate – Common	9, 180
Tetany*	Severe – Rare	72, 180
Seizures	Severe – Rare	155, 52
Anaphylaxis	Severe – Rare	98, 206
General allergic reactions	Mild – Not Common	98, 206, 100
Cerebral blindness	Severe – Rare	43
SIADH‡	Severe – Rare	113
Hemolytic anemia	Severe – Rare	60, 115
Mallory–Weiss syndrome	Severe – Rare	124
Toxic liver damage	Severe – Rare	23
Coronary artery disease	Severe – Rare	49
Platinum gum line	Mild – Rare	54

* Secondary to abnormally low serum magnesium.
‡ Syndrome of inappropriate anti-diuretic hormone secretion.

ANALOGS OF CISPLATINUM

Because of the severe nephrotoxicity, nausea and vomiting, and hearing loss associated with DDP administration, efforts have been underway to develop analogs of DDP which would retain the therapeutic efficacy but produce less toxicity. Hundreds of platinum containing analogs have been synthesized and subsequently screened for their antitumor effect in various animal systems (15, 213). Until recently only preliminary data in a very few patients were available regarding the efficacy of new analogs against human tumors and the associated human toxicity of these potential new drugs (77, 137, 161). Recently, however, large scale clinical testing of several of the DDP analogs was begun in both the US and in other countries, and efficacy and toxicity data are beginning to accumulate on the disease response and toxicity of these analogs. Several dozen abstracts have been presented at the recent meetings of the American Association of Clinical Oncology-American Association of Cancer Research, at the 4th International Symposium on Platinum Coordination complexes in Cancer Chemotherapy (1983) and elsewhere but the results to follow are from full length published manuscripts.

Cis-diammine-1,1-cyclobutane dicarboxylate platinum-II (Carboplatin; CBDCA) is an analog developed mainly in England but widely tested in other countries as well. At the present time at least 7 Phase I studies have been conducted and these are summarized by Calvert *et al.* (16). The most extensive work (17) reports carboplatin administration via 1 hr infusion to 60 patients (38 ovarian) in doses ranging from 100–520 mg/m^2. Dose limiting toxicity was thrombocytopenia, which was severe enough at 520 mg/m^2 to require platelet transfusions in 80% of the treated patients. Myelosuppression occurred at doses as low as 200 mg/m^2. Increases in urinary concentrations of leucine aminopeptidase, N-acetylglucosaminidase, and β_2-microglobulin (2–5 × greater than control) above a carboplatin dose of 320 mg/m^2 were the only evidence of renal toxicity. There appeared to be no significant dose-related increase in ^{51}Cr-EDTA clearance, even in patients with preexisting renal dysfunction. Nausea and vomiting were prominent but subjectively less severe than with DDP, and no hearing loss was noticed.

Table 4. Clinical results of Phase II trials with carboplatin in various human cancers.[1]

Disease	Evaluable patients	Number of responses[2]
Ovarian cancer[3]		
resistant	33	7
naive	34	19
Small cell lung cancer	36	12
Non small cell lung cancer	11	2
Testicular teratoma	9	0
Testicular seminoma	3	2
Mesothelioma	8	2
Thyroid carcinoma	5	1

[1] Summarized from Calvert *et al.* (190, 191).
[2] CR plus PR.
[3] Distinguished between having failed a DDP-containing regimen (resistant) or having not previously received DDP (naive).

Table 5. Clinical results of Phase II trials with DACCP in various human cancers.

Disease	Evaluable patients	Number of responses
Non-small cell lung cancer	29	1
Colon cancer	11	0
Ovarian cancer	8	1
Gastric cancer	9	1
Esophageal carcinoma	9	1
Testicular cancers	8	0
Bladder cancer	5	1

Eight percent of the patients showed signs of peripheral neurotoxicity. Response rate in the ovarian cancer patients was 39% (CR + PR) and another 39% had either no change in progression of disease. In 22 additional patients with various cancers there were 3 responses. No responses were seen in patients with testicular cancer. Results of Phase II evaluation of carboplatin against several cancers are summarized in Table 4. Of particular significance is the 21% response rate in ovarian patients previously failing DDP-containing regimens. Toxicity was mainly similar to that previously reported in the Phase I trials but with the previously unreported occurrence of leukopenia. In a Phase II trial against advanced ovarian carcinoma in 36 patients the overall response rate with carboplatin was 29% but more significant was a 25% response rate in heavily pretreated patients who had previously failed conventional cisplatinum therapy. At a dose of 300 mg/m^2 repeated monthly, hematologic toxicity (leukemia and thrombocytopenia) was severe and 14 patients required transfusions. Three patients with no prior chemotherapy showed no hematologic toxicity, however. Eighty-six percent of patients receiving 3 or more monthly courses showed no significant decrease in ^{151}Cr-EDTA clearance and the other 14% had a decrease of 20% or more. Emesis was common but not quantitated, either with respect to incidence or severity. There was no hearing loss but there appeared to be a progression of cisplatinum-induced peripheral neuropathy. The only Phase III trial involves ovarian carcinoma patients and although it is very early in the trial, response rates are equal in the carboplatin and DDP arms, although toxicity is less with carboplatin. Whether carboplatin will replace DDP as the first line platinum drug remains to be seen. The lack of renal toxicity observed at therapeutic doses is replaced by bone marrow toxicity, which is more reversible than renal toxicity but which may negate the advantage of DDP as a combination agent in regimens with marrow suppressive drugs.

A second drug whose Phase I and Phase II clinical trials have been reported (95, 96) is 4′-carboxyphthalato-(1,2-diaminocyclohexane)platinum-II (DACCP). Phase I studies were conducted in 45 patients using a rapid (15–20 min) iv infusion. As was true with carboplatin, the dose limiting toxicity seen with DACCP was thrombocytopenia. Leukopenia was observed only at the highest dose (800 mg/m^2). Significant renal toxicity was observed only at 640 and 800 mg/m^2 but nausea and vomiting were common, and fever with negative bacterial cultures occurred in 21% of the patients. Diarrhea was common (25%). Allergic reactions (other than fever) and peripheral neuropathy occurred in about 10% of patients. Four responses were recorded in 22 evaluable adult patients (all adenocarcinomas) and no responses were observed in 9 evaluable pediatric patients. The therapeutic response was considered encouraging (95) because responses were in tumors not highly responsive to DDP and in patients previously heavily pretreated with DDP. Phase II trials were conducted at 640-720 mg/m^2 in cancers shown in Table 5. In general, responses were less impressive than observed with carboplatin.

Results of Phase I studies have been reported (200) for 1,1-diamminomethylcyclohexane (sulphate) platinum-II (TNO-6), which is being developed and tested mainly in the Netherlands. Fifty-three patients were treated with a single iv injection at doses of 2.5-35 mg/m^2 or as a 3-6 hr infusion at 30-40 mg/m^2. Above 25 mg/m^2 there was a dose-dependent decrease in WBC with a nadir at day 14 and recovery by day 21-25. A similar nadir and recovery were observed with platelets. Patients receiving 30-40 mg/m^2 infusion occasionally required RBC transfusion to combat anemia. At 35-40 mg/m^2 renal toxicity was observed and was manifested by increased plasma creatinine and significant proteinuria. Infusion appeared to increase the risk of renal complication. Tubular damage also was evidenced by electrolyte abnormalities. Phlebitis, and nausea and vomiting were almost universal. Overall response rate was only 10%, but all responders had previously failed DDP-containing regimens.

Phase I trials also have been completed for *cis*-dichloro-*trans*-dihydroxy-bis-isopropylamine platinum-IV (CHIP) at doses of 40-350 mg/m^2 (35). Twenty-six patients were given a total of 40 courses as a 2 hr infusion repeated every four weeks. Dose limiting toxicity was myelosuppression with WBC nadir of 2500/mm^3 and a platelet nadir of 32,000/mm^3. The maximum tolerated dose (MTD) was 350 mg/m^2. Nausea and vomiting were universal, with 80% of the incidents classed as moderate (lasting 4 hours and easily controlled by antiemetics). No evidence of renal toxicity was observed, even in patients given the MTD with no hydration, or in patients receiving up to 5 treatment cycles. Hypersensitivity reactions were observed in two patients, but no evidence of hearing loss was found. No responses were obtained, but 5 patients had apparently stable disease. Starting dose for Phase II trials was recommended to be either 180 mg/m^2 or 270 mg/m^2 depending on bone marrow status.

Finally, malonato (1,2-diamminecyclohexane)platinum was studied in 49 patients at doses of 3-32 mg/kg (55). Gastrointestinal toxicity was nearly universal and at 24 mg/kg thrombocytopenia was moderate, with a nadir on day 15-21. There was no apparent renal, neurologic or ototoxicity, and hematologic effects did not appear to be cumulative. One of 36 evaluable patients had a partial response and 3 other patients had minor responses. Extensive Phase II trials apparently are not planned.

REFERENCES

1. Alberts DS, Martimbeau PW, Surwit EA, Oishi N: Mitomycin-C, bleomycin, vincristine, and *cis*-platinum in the treatment of advanced, recurrent squamous cell carcinoma of the cervix. *Cancer Clin Trials* 4:313, 1981
2. Allen R, Gale G, Oulla P, Gale A: Effects of certain antitumor platinum compounds on kidney esterases. *Bioinorg Chem* 8:83, 1978
3. Arshad RR, Woo SY, Abbassi V, Hoy GR, Sinks LF: Virilizing hepatoblastoma: precocious sexual development and partial response of pulmonary metastases to *cis*-platinum. *CA* 32:293, 1982
4. Aull JL, Allen RL, Bapat AR, Daron HH, Friedman ME, Wilson JF: Effects of platinum complexes on seven enzymes. *Biochim Biophys Acta* 571:352, 1979
5. Baker GH, Wiltshaw E: Use of high-dose *cis*-dichlorodiammine platinum (11) following failure of previous chemotherapy for advanced carcinoma of the ovary. *Brit J Ob and Gyn* 88:1192, 1981
6. Becher R, Seeber S, Schmidt CG: Combination chemotherapy with ifosfamide and *cis*-dichlorodiammineplatinum (II) in advanced malignant melanoma. *J Cancer Res Clin Oncol* 97:301, 1980
7. Berry J, MacDonald RN: Cisplatin, cyclophosphamide, and prednisone therapy for stage D prostatic cancer. *Cancer Treat Rep* 66:1403, 1982
8. Bertolero F, Litterst C: Changes in renal handling of platinum in *cis*platinum-treated rats following induction of metabolic acidosis or alkalosis. *Res Commun Chem Path Pharmacol* 36:273, 1982
9. Blachley JD, Hill JB: Renal and electrolyte disturbances associated with cisplatin. *Annals of Int Med* 95:628, 1981
10. Blum RH: An overview of studies with adriamycin in the United States. *Cancer Chemother Rep* 6:247, 1975
11. Blumenreich MS, Needles B, Yagoda A, Sogani P, Grabstald H, Whitmore WF Jr: Intravesical *cis*platin for superficial bladder tumors. *Cancer* 50:863, 1982
12. Bohart R, Ogawaq G: An observation on the stability of *cis*-dichlorodiammineplatinum(II): a caution regarding its administration. *Cancer Treat Rep* 63:2117, 1979
13. Bonnem EM, Litterst CL, Smith FP: Platinum concentrations in human glioblastoma multiforme following the use of cisplatinum. *Cancer Treat Rep* 66:1661, 1982
14. Borch RF, Pleasants ME: Inhibition of *cis*platinum nephrotoxicity by diethyldithiocarbamate rescue in a rat model. *Proc Natl Acad Sci (USA)* 76:6611, 1979
15. Bradner WT, Rose WC, Huftalen JB: Antitumor activity of platinum analogs. In: *Cisplatin*, edited by Prestayko AW, Crooke ST, Carter SK, pp. 171-182. New York Academic Press, 1980
16. Calvert AH, Harland SJ, Harrap KR, Wiltshaw E, Smith IE: JM-8 development and clinical projects: In: *Platinum Coordination Complexes in Cancer Chemotherapy*. Edited by Hacker M, Krakoff I, Douple E, Boston, Martinus Nijhoff 1984
17. Calvert AH, Harland SJ, Newell DR, Siddik ZH, Jones AC, McElwain TJ, Raju S, Wiltshaw E, Smith IE, Baker JM, Peckham MJ, Harrap KR: Early clinical studies with *cis*-diammine-1,1-cyclobutane dicarboxylate platinum. *Cancer Chemother Pharmacol* 9:140, 1982
18. Calvo DB, Patt YZ, Wallace S, Chuang VP, Benjamin RS, Pritchard JD, Hersh EM, Bodey GP Sr, Mavligit GM: Phase I–II trial of percutaneous intra-arterial *cis*-diamminedichloro platinum (II) for regionally confined malignancy. *Cancer* 45:1278, 1980
19. Campbell AB, Kalman SM, Jacobs C: Plasma platinum levels: relationship to cisplatin dose and nephrotoxicity. *Cancer Treat Reports* 67:169, 1983
20. Campbell MG, Pollard R, Al-Sarraf M: A complete response in metastatic malignant thymoma to cis-platinum, doxorubicin and cyclophosphamide: a case report. *Cancer* 48:1315, 1981
21. Casper ES, Goalla RJ, Kelsen DP, Cvitkovic E, Golbey RB: Phase II study of high-dose *cis*-dichlorodiammineplatinum(II) in the treatment of non-small cell lung cancer. *Cancer Treat Rep* 65:2107, 1974

22. Casper ES, Kelsen DP, Alcock NW, Young CW: Platinum concentrations in bile and plasma following rapid and 6 hr infusions of cisplatinum. *Cancer Treat Rep* 63:2023, 1979
23. Cavalli R, Tschopp L, Sonntag RW, Zimmerman A: A case of liver toxicity following *cis*-dichlorodiammineplatinum(II) treatment. *Cancer Treat Rep* 62:2125, 1978
24. Chary KK, Higby DJ, Henderson ES: A phase I study of high dose *cis*-diamminedichloroplatinum II (NSC 119875) with forced diuresis. *J Clin Hematol Oncol* 7:633, 1977
25. Choie D, del Campo A, Guarino A: Subcellular localization of *cis*-dichlorodiammineplatinum (II) in rat kidney and liver. *Toxicol Appl Pharmacol* 55:245, 1980
26. Choie DD, Longnecker DS, Copley MP: Cytotoxicity of cisplatin in rat intestine. *Tox Appl Pharmacol* 60:354, 1981
27. Choie DD, Longnecker DS, del Campo AA: Acute and chronic cisplatin nephropathy in rats. *Lab Invest* 44:397, 1981
28. Citrin DL, Hogan TF: A phase II evaluation of adriamycin and cis-platinum in hormone resistant prostate cancer. *Cancer* 50:201, 1982
29. Clifton GG, Pearce C, O'Neill WM, Wallin JD: Early polyuria in the rat following single-dose cisplatinum: effects on plasma vasopressin concentration and posterior pituitary function. *J Lab Clin Med* 100:659, 1982
30. Coates AS, Golovsky D, Freedman A: Prolonged remission in recurrent bladder carcinoma after chemotherapy with cisplatin. *Med J Aust* 16:533, 1981
31. Cocconi G, Boni C, Cuomo A: Long-lasting response to cis-platinum in recurrent malignant thymoma: case report. *Cancer* 49:1985, 1982
32. Cohen AI, Harberg J, Citrin DL: Measurement of urinary B₂-microglobulin in the detection of *cis*platin nephrotoxicity. *Cancer Treat Reports* 65:1083, 1981
33. Corder MP, Elliott TE, Bell SJ: Dose limiting myelotoxicity in absence of significant nephrotoxicity with a weekly outpatient schedule of cis-platinum(II) diamminedichloride. *J Clin Hematol Oncol* 7:645, 1977
34. Cowan JD, Klesms, Roth JL, Joyce R: Nerve conduction studies in patients treated with *cis*-diamminedichloroplatinum(II). A preliminary report. *Cancer Treat Rep* 64:1119, 1980
35. Creaven PJ, Madajewicz S, Pendayala L, Mittelman A, Pontes E, Spaulding M, Arbuch S, Solomon J: Phase I. Clinical trial of *cis*-dichloro *trans*-dihydroxy-bis-isopropylamine platinum (CHIP). *Cancer Treat Reports* 67(11):997, 1983
36. Crom WR, Evans WE, Pratt CB, Senzer N, Denison M, Green AA, Hayes FA, Yee GC: Cisplatin disposition in children and adolescents with cancer. *Cancer Chemother Pharmacol* 6:95, 1981
37. Cvitkovic E, Spaulding J, Bethune V, Martin J, Whitmore WF: Improvement of *cis*dichlorodiammineplatinum therapeutic index in an animal model. *Cancer* 39:1357, 1977
38. Dabouis G, Le Mevel B, Corroller J: Treatment of diffuse pleural malignant mesothelioma with *cis*dichlorodiammineplatinum (C.D.D.P.) in nine patients. *Cancer Chemother Pharmacol* 5:209, 1981
39. DeConti RC, Toftness BR, Lange RC, Creasey WA: Clinical and pharmacological studies with *cis*-diamminedichloroplatinum(II). *Cancer Res* 33:1310, 1973
40. Delgado G, Schein P, MacDonald J et al.: L-PAM vs cyclophosphamide, hexamethylmelamine, and 5-fluorouracil (CHF) for advanced ovarian cancer. *Proc Am Assoc Cancer Res* 20:434, 1979
41. Deppe G, Cohen CJ, Bruckner HW: Treatment of advanced endometrial adenocarcinoma with *cis*-dichlorodiammine platinum (II) after intensive prior therapy. *Gynecol Oncol* 10:51, 1980
42. DeSimone PA, Yancey RS, Coupal JJ, Butts J, Hoeschele J: Effect of a forced diuresis on the distribution and excretion (via urine and bile of ¹⁹⁵ᵐplatinum when given as ¹⁹⁵ᵐplati-

num *cis*dichlorodiammine-platinum(II). *Cancer Treat Rep* 63:951, 1979
43. Diamond SB, Rudolph SH, Lubicz SS, Deppe G, Cohen CJ: Cerebral blindness in association with cis-platinum chemotherapy for advanced carcinoma of the fallopian tube. *Obstet Gynecol* 59(Suppl):845, 1982
44. Dobyan DC, Hill D, Lewis T, Bulger RE: Cyst formation in rat kidney induced by cisplatinum administration. *Lab Invest* 45:260, 1981
45. Dobyan DC, Levi J, Jacobs C, Kosek J, Weiner MW: Mechanism of cisplatinum nephrotoxicity: II. Morphologic observations. *J Pharmacol Exp Therap* 213:551, 1980
46. Eagan RT, Ingle JN, Creagan ET, Frytak S, Kooks L, Rubin J, McMahon R: VP-16-213 chemotherapy for advanced squamous cell carcinoma and adenocarcinoma of the lung. *Cancer Treat Rep* 62:843, 1978
47. Earhart RH: Instability of *cis*-dichlorodiammineplatinum in dextrose solution. *Cancer Treat Rep* 62:1105, 1978
48. Eastman A: Comparison of the interaction of *cis* and *trans*-diamminedichloroplatinum(II) with DNA by a simple filter binding assay. *Biochem Biophys Res Commun* 105:869, 1982
49. Edwards GS, Lane M, Smith FE: Long-term treatment with *cis*-dichlorodiammineplatinum(II)-vinblastine-bleomycin: possible association with severe coronary artery disease. *Cancer Treat Rep* 63:551, 1979
50. Ehrlich CE, Einhorn L, Williams SD, Morgan J: Chemotherapy for Stage III-IV epithelial ovarian cancer with *cis*dichlorodiammineplatinum(II), adriamycin and cyclophosphamide: A preliminary report. *Cancer Treat Rep* 63:281, 1979
51. Einhorn LH, Donohue J: *Cis*-diamminedichloroplatinum, vinblastine, and bleomycin combination chemotherapy in disseminated testicular cancer. *Ann Intern Med* 87:293, 1977
52. Einhorn LH, Williams SD: The role of cis-platinum in solid-tumor therapy. *N Engl J Med* 300:289, 1979
53. Estape J, Milla A, Agusti A, Sanchez-Lloret J, Palacin A, Soriano E: VP16-213 (VP-16) and cyclophosphamide in the treatment of primitive lung cancer in phase M 1. *Cancer* 43:72, 1979
54. Ettinger LJ, Freeman AI: The gingival platinum line. A new finding following *cis*-dichlorodiammine platinum (II) treatment. *Cancer* 44:1882, 1979
55. Evans BD, Raju KS, Calvert AH, Harland SJ, Wiltshaw E: JM8 (*cis* diammine 1,1-cyclobutane dicarboxylate platinum II): a new platinum analog active in the treatment of advanced ovarian carcinoma. *Cancer Treat Reports* 67(9):795, 1983
56. Fleischman RW, Stadnicki SW, Etheir MF, Schaeppi U: Ototoxicity of *cis*dichlorodiammineplatinum(II) in the guinea pig. *Tox Appl Pharmacol* 33:320, 1975
57. Friedman ME, Melius P, Teggins JE, McAuliffe CA: Interactions of *cis* and *trans*-platinum(II) complexes with dehydrogenase enzymes in the presence of different mono- and polynucleotides: Evidence for a ternary complex. *Bioinorg Chem* 8:341, 1978
58. Friese J, Mueller WH, Magerstadt P, Schmoll HJ: Pharmacokinetics of liposome-encapsulated cisplatin in rats. *Arch Int Pharmacodyn et Therap* 258:180, 1982
59. Furnas BE, Williams SD, Einhorn LH, Cobleigh MA: Vindesine: An effective agent in the treatment of non-small cell lung cancer. *Cancer Treat Rep* 66:1709, 1982
60. Getaz EP, Beckley S, Fitzpatrick J, Dozier A: Cisplatin-induced hemolysis. *New Eng J Med* 302:334, 1980
61. Goldstein RS, Noordewier B, Bond JT, Hook JB, Mayor GH: Cis-dichlorodiammine platinum nephrotoxicity: time course and dose response of renal functional impairment. *Tox Appl Pharmacol* 60:163, 1981
62. Gonzalez-Vitale JC, Hayes DM, Cvitkovic E, Sternberg SS: Renal pathology in clinical trials of cisplatinum(II) diam-

minedichloride. *Cancer* 39:1362, 1977

63. Gormley PE, Bull JM, LeRoy AF, Cysyk R: Kinetics of cis-platinum. *Clin Pharmacol Therap* 25:351, 1979
64. Graziano J, Jones B, Pisciotto P: Effect of heavy metal chelators on the renal accumulation of platinum after *cis*dichlorodiammineplatinum-II administration to the rat. *Br J Pharmacol* 73:649, 1981
65. Grossman B, Lessin LS, Cohen P: Droperidol prevents nausea and vomiting from cis-platinum. *New Engl J Med* 301:47, 1979 (letter)
66. Gullo JJ, Litterst C, Maguire P, Sikic BL, Hoth DF, Woolley PV: Pharmacokinetics and protein binding of *cis*dichlorodiammineplatinum(II) administered as a one-hour or as a twenty-hour infusion. *Cancer Chem Pharmacol* 5:21, 1980
67. Hall DJ, Diasio R, Goplerud DR: Cis-platinum in gynecologic cancer. II. Squamous cell carcinoma of the cervix. *Am J Obstet Gynecol* 141:305, 1981
68. Harder HC: Renaturation effects of *cis-* and *trans-*platinum II and IV compounds on calf thymus deoxyribonucleic acid. *Chem Biol Interact* 10:27, 1975
69. Harder HC, Rosenberg B: Inhibitory effects of antitumor platinum compounds on DNA, RNA and protein synthesis in mammalian cells *in vitro. Int J Cancer* 6:207, 1970
70. Harrison SD: Toxicologic evaluation of *cis*-diamminedichloroplatinum-II in B6D2F$_1$ mice. *Fund Appl Tox* 1:382, 1981
71. Havemann K: Combination chemotherapy of small cell bronchogenic carcinoma with etoposide (VP-16) itosemide and vindesine (VPIV), and with adriamycin, cis-platinum and vincristine (APO). *Cancer Trat Rev* 9(A):95, 1982
72. Hayes FA, Green AA, Senzer N, Pratt CB: Tetany: a complication of *cis* dichlorodiammine platinum (II) therapy. *Cancer Treat Reports* 63:547, 1979
73. Helson L, Okonkwo E, Anton L, Cvitkovic E: Cis-platinum ototoxicity. *Clin Toxicol* 13:469, 1978
74. Herman TS, Einhorn LH, Jones SE, Nagy C, Charter A, Dean J, Furnas B, Williams S, Leigh S, Dunn R, Moon T: Superiority of nabilone over prochlorperazine as an antiemetic in patients receiving cancer chemotherapy. *N Engl J Med* 300:1295, 1979
75. Higby DJ, Wallace HJ Jr, Albert DJ, Holland JF: Diamminodichloroplatinum: a phase I study showing responses in testicular and other tumors. *Cancer* 33:1219, 1974
76. Higby DJ, Wallace HJ Jr, Holland JF: *Cis*-diamminedichloroplatinum (NSC-119875): a phase I study. *Cancer Chemother Rep* 57:459, 1973
77. Hill JM, Loeb E, Pardue A, Khan A, King JJ, Aleman C, Hill N: Platinum analogs of clinical interest. *Cancer Treat Reports* 63:1509, 1979
78. Hill JM, Loeb E, MacLellan A, Hill NO, Khan A, King JJ: Clinical studies of platinum coordination compounds in the treatment of various malignant diseases. *Cancer Chemother Rep* 59:647, 1975
79. Hincal AA, Long DF, Repta AJ: Cis-platin stability in aqueous parental vehicles. *J Parenteral Drug Assoc* 33:107, 1979
80. Hoeschele JD, Van Camp L: Whole body counting and the distribution of *cis* 195m Pt(NH$_3$)$_2$Cl$_2$) in the major organs of Swiss white mice. *Adv Antimicro & Antineoplastic Chemotherapy* II:241, 1972
81. Holoye PY, Byers RM, Gard DA, Goepfert H, Guillamondegui O, Jesse R: Combination chemotherapy of head and neck cancer. *Cancer* 42:1661, 1978
82. Howell SB, Pfeifle CL, Wung WE, Olshen RA, Lucas WE, Yon JL, Green M: Intraperitoneal cisplatin with systemic thiosulfate protection. *Ann Intern Med* 97:845, 1982
83. Howell S, Taetle R: Effect of sodium thiosulfate on *cis*dichlorodiammineplatinum(II) toxicity and antitumor activity in L1210 leukemia. *Cancer Treat Rep* 64:611, 1980
84. Howle J, Gale G: *Cis*dichlorodiammineplatinum(II). Persistent and selective inhibition of DNA synthesis *in vivo. Biochem Pharmacol* 19:2757, 1970

85. Howle JA, Thompson HS, Stone AE, Gale GR: *cis*-Dichlorodiammineplatinum(II): inhibition of nucleic acid synthesis in lymphocytes stimulated with phytohemagglutinin. *Proc Soc Exp Biol Med* 137:820, 1971
86. Hurley M, Stephens RL, Davidner ML, Magrina JF: Vulvar carcinoma. A case of DDP-induced neurotoxicity in chemotherapy. *J Kans Med Soc* 83:239, 1982
87. Ishizawa M, Taniguchi S, Baba T: Protection by sodium thiosulfate and thiourea against lethal toxicity of *cis*diamminedichloroplatinum(II) in bacteria and mice. *Jap J Pharmacol* 31:883, 1981
88. Issel BF, Valdivieso M, Bodey GP: Chemotherapy for adenocarcinoma and large cell anaplastic carcinoma of the lung with Ftorafur, adriamycin, and *cis*-dichlorodiammineplatinum (II). *Cancer Treat Rep* 62:1089, 1978
89. Jacobs C, Kalman SM, Tretton M, Weiner MW: Renal handling of cisplatinum. *Cancer Treat Rep* 64:1223, 1980
90. Kane R, Harvey H, Andrews T, Bernath A, Curry S, Dixon R, Gottlieb R, Kuhrika M, Lipton A, Maertel R, Ricci J, White D: Phase II trial of cyclophosphamide hexamethylmelamine, adriamycin, and *cis*-dichlorodiammineplatinum (II) combination chemotherapy in advanced ovarian carcinoma. *Cancer Treat Rep* 63:307, 1979
91. Kaplan BH, Vogl SE, Chiuten Det al.: Chemotherapy of advanced cancer of the head and neck (HNCa) with methotrexate (M), bleomycin (B), and *cis*-diamminedichloroplatinum (D) in combination. *Proc Am Assoc Cancer Res* 20:384, 1979
92. Kedar A, Cohen ME, Freeman AI: Peripheral neuropathy as a complication of *cis*-dichlorodiammineplatinum(II) treatment: a case report. *Cancer Treat Rep* 62:819, 1978
93. Kelman AD, Buchbinder M: Platinum-DNA crosslinking: platinum antitumor drug interactions with native γ-bacteriophage DNA studied using a restriction endonuclease. *Biochemie* 60:893, 1978
94. Kelsen DP, Bains M, Chapman R, Golbey R: Cisplatin, vindesine, and bleomycin (DVB) combination chemotherapy for esophageal carcinoma. *Cancer Treat Rep* 65:781, 1981
95. Kelsen DP, Scher H, Alcock N, Leyland-Jones B, Donner A, Williams L, Greene G, Burchenal JH, Tan C, Philips FS, Young CW: Phase I clinical trial and pharmacokinetics of 4'-carboxyphthalato-(1,2-diaminocyclohexane) platinum I (II). *Cancer Res* 42:4831, 1982
96. Kelsen DP, Scher H, Burchenal J: Phase I and early Phase II trials of 4' carboxyphthalato (1,2-diaminocyclohexane) platinum (II). In: *Platinum Coordination Complexes in Cancer Chemotherapy* (Edited by Hacker M, Douple E, Krakoff I) Boston, Martinus Nijhoff 1984
97. Kennedy BJ: Mithramycin therapy in advanced testicular neoplasms. *Cancer* 26:755, 1970
98. Khan A, Hill JM, Grater W, Loeb E, Maclellan A, Hill N: Atopic hypersensitivity to *cis*-dichlorodiammineplatinum(II) and other platinum complexes. *Cancer Res* 35:2766, 1975
99. Khan AG, D'Souza BJ, Wharam MD, Champion LA, Sinks LF, Woo SY, McCullough DC, Leventhal BG: Cisplatin therapy in recurrent childhood brain tumors. *Cancer Treat Rep* 66:2013, 1982
100. Khan A, Wakasugi K, Hill B, Richardson D, Disabato J, Hill J: Platinum complexes: immunology and allergy. *J Clin Hematol Oncol* 7:797, 1977
101. Khan MUA, Sadler PJ: Distribution of a platinum antitumor drug in HeLa cells by analytical electron microscopy. *Chem Biol Interact* 21:227, 1978
102. Klastersky J, Nicaise C, Longenal E, Strychmas P, EORTC Lung Cancer Working Party: Cisplatin, adriamycin and etoposide (CAV) for remission induction of small-cell bronchogenic carcinoma. *Cancer* 50:652, 1982
103. Kleinerman ES, Zwelling LA: The effect of *cis*-diamminedichloroplatinum(II) on immune function *in vitro* and *in vivo. Cancer Immunol Immunother* 12:191, 1982

104. Kleinerman ES, Zwelling LA, Muchmore AV: The enhancement of naturally occurring spontaneous monocyte-mediated cytotoxicity by *cis*-diamminedichloroplatinum(II). *Cancer Res* 40:3099, 1980

105. Kleinerman ES, Zwelling LA, Howser D, Barlock A, Young RC, Decker J, Bull JM, Muchmore AV: Defective monocyte killing in patients with malignancies and restoration of function during chemotherapy. *Lancet* 2:1102, 1980

106. Kolari'c K, Roth A, Jeli ci'c I, Matkovic A: Preliminary report on antitumorigenic activity of *cis*-dichlorodiammine platinum in metastatic brain tumors. *Tumori* 67:483, 1981

107. Kuhn JA, Argy WP, Rakowski TA, Moriarty JK, Schriener GE, Schein PS: Nephrotoxicity of *cis*diammine dichloroplatinum (II) as measured by urinary βglucuronidase. *Cancer Treat Reports* 64:1083, 1980

108. Lane M, Moore JE, Levin H et al.: Methotrexate therapy for squamous cell carcinoma of the head and neck. Intermittent intravenous dose program. *JAMA* 204:561, 1968

109. Leone LA, Albala MM, Rege VB: Treatment of carcinoma of the head and neck with intravenous methotrexate. *Cancer* 21:1729, 1973

110. LeRoy AF: Some quantitative data on *cis*-dichlorodiammineplatinum(II) species in solution. *Cancer Treat Rep* 63:231, 1979

111. LeRoy AF, Lutz RJ, Dedrick RL, Litterst CL, Guarino AM: Pharmacokinetic study of *cis*-dichlorodiammine platinum (II) (DDP) in the beagle dog. Thermodynamic and kinetic behavior of DDP in a biologic milieu. *Cancer Treat Rep* 63:59, 1979

112. Levi FA, Hrushesky WJ, Blomquist CH, Lakatua DJ, Haus E, Halberg F, Kennedy BJ: Reduction of *cis*diamminedichloroplatinum nephrotoxicity in rats by optimal circadian drug timing. *Cancer Res* 42:950, 1982

113. Levin L, Sealy R, Barron J: Syndrome of inappropriate antidiuretic hormone secretion following *cis*-dichlorodiammineplatinum II in a patient with malignant thymoma. *Cancer* 50:2279, 1982

114. Levitt M, Mosher MB, DeConti RC, Farher L, Skeel R, March J, Mitchell M, Papac R, Thomas E, Bertino J: Improved therapeutic index of methotrexate with "leucovorin rescue." *Cancer Res* 33:1729, 1973

115. Levy JA, Aroney RS, Dalley DM: Haemolytic anaemia after cisplatin treatment. *Brit Med J* 282:2003, 1981

116. Lippman AJ, Helson C, Helson L, Krakoff I: Clinical trials of *cis*-diamminedichloroplatinum (NSC-119875). *Cancer Chemother Rep* 57:191, 1973

117. Litterst CL: Alterations in the toxicity of *cis*-dichlorodiammineplatinum-II and in tissue localization of platinum as a function of NaCl concentration in the vehicle of administration. *Tox Appl Pharmacol* 61:99, 1981

118. Litterst CL: Plasma pharmacokinetics, urinary excretion and tissue distribution of platinum following IV administration of cyclobutane-dicarboxylate platinum (II) and cisplatinum to rabbits. In: *Platinum Coordination Complexes in Cancer Chemotherapy* (Edited by Hacker M, Douple E, Krakoff I), Nijhoff Publ, Boston, 1984

119. Litterst CL, Gram TE, Dedrick RL, LeRoy AF, Guarino AM: Distribution and disposition of platinum following IV administration of cisplatinum to dogs. *Cancer Res* 36:2340, 1976

120. Litterst CL, LeRoy AF, Guarino AM: Distribution and disposition of platinum following parenteral administration of *cis*-dichlorodiammineplatinum(II) to animals. *Cancer Treat Rep* 63:1485, 1979

121. Litterst CL, Tong S, Hirokata Y, Siddik Z: Stimulation of microsomal drug oxidation in liver and kidney of rats treated with the oncolytic agent *cis*-dichlordiammineplatinum-II. *Pharmacology* 26:46, 1983

122. Litterst CL, Tong S, Hirokata Y, Siddik Z: Alterations in

123. Litterst CL, Torres IJ, Guarino AM: Plasma levels and organ distribution of platinum in the rat, dog, and dog-fish shark following single intravenous administration of *cis*-dichlorodiammineplatinum(II). *j Clin Hematol Oncol* 7:169, 1976

124. Lubicz S, Shafir M, Diamond S, Monosan R, Cohen C: Mallory-Weiss syndrome secondary to cis-platinum chemotherapy: an unusual complication. *J Surg Oncol* 20:247, 1982

125. MacKenzie AR: Chemotherapy of metastatic testis cancer – results in 154 patients. *Cancer* 19:1369, 1966

126. Macquet JP, Butour JL: Modifications of the DNA secondary structure upon platinum binding: a proposed model. *Biochimie* 9:901, 1978

127. Madias NE, Harrington JT: Platinum nephrotoxicity. *Am J Med* 65:307, 1978

128. Mavligit GM, Benjamin R, Patt YZ, Jaffe N, Chuang V, Wallace S, Murray J, Ayala A, Johnston S, Hersh EM, Calvo DB 3d: Intraarterial cis-platinum for patients with inoperable skeletal tumors. *Cancer* 1:1, 1981

129. McGinnis JE, Proctor PH, Demopoulos HB, Hokanson JA, Kirkpatrick DS: Amelioration of cisplatinum nephrotoxicity by orgotein (Superoxide dismutase). *Physiol Chem Physics* 10:267, 1978

130. Meijer S, Mulder NH, Sleijfer DTh, deJong PD, Sluiter WJ, Koops HS, van der Hem GK: Nephrotoxicity of *cis*diamminedichloroplatinum (CDDP) during remission-induction and maintenance chemotherapy of testicular carcinoma. *Cancer Chemother Pharmacol* 8:27, 1982

131. Melia WM, Westaby D, Williams R: Diamminedichlorideplatinum (cis-platinum) in the treatment of hepatocellular carcinoma. *Clin Oncol* 7:275, 1981

132. Melius P, McAuliffe CA, Photake I, Sakarellou-Daitsiotou M: Interactions of platinum complexes, peptides, methionine, and dehydrogenases. *Bioinorg Chem* 7:203, 1977

133. Mendelson D, Serpic AA: Combination chemotherapy of testicular tumors. *J Urol* 103:619, 1970

134. Merrin CE: Treatment of previously untreated (by hormonal manipulation) stage D adenocarcinoma of prostate with combined archiectomy, estrogen, and cis-diamminedichloroplatinum. *Urology* 15:123, 1980

135. Minna JD, Higgins GA, Glatstein EJ: Cancer of the lung. In: *Cancer*. Edited by DeVita VT, Hellman S, Rosenberg SA, p. 452. Philadelphia, J.B. Lippincott Company, 1982

136. Muchausen L: The chemical and biological effects of *cis*-dichlorodiammine platinum (II), an antitumor agent, on DNA. *Proc Nat Acad Sci (USA)* 71:4519, 1974

137. Muggia FM, Wolpert-DeFillippes MK, Ribaud P, Mathe G: Clinical results with cisplatin analogs. In: *Cisplatin*. Edited by Prestayko AW, Crooke ST, Carter SK, pp. 517–527. New York Academic Press, 1980

138. Myers JW, Livingston RB, Coltman CA Jr: Combination chemotherapy of advanced adeno and large cell undifferentiated carcinoma of the lung with 5FU, vincristine and mitomycin-C (FOMi). *Proc AACR-ASCO* 21:453, 1980

139. Naika Y, Konishi K, Chang KC, Ohashi K, Morisaki N, Minowa Y, Morimoto A: Ototoxicity of the anticancer drug *cis*platin. An experimental study. *Acta Otolaryngol* 93:227, 1982

140. Narayana AS, Leoning SA, Culp DA: Chemotherapy for advanced carcinoma of the bladder. *J Urol* 126:594, 1981

141. Natale RB, Wittes RE: Combination cis-platinum and etoposide in small cell lung cancer. *Cancer Treat Res* 9(A):91, 1982

142. Nathanson L, Kaufman SD, Carey RW: Vinblastine, infusion, bleomycin, and cis-dichlorodiammine-platinum chemotherapy in metastatic melanoma. *Cancer* 48:1290, 1981

143. Neuwelt EA, Frankel EP, Smith RG: Suprasellar germinomas (etopic pinealomas): aspects of immunological characterization and successful chemotherapeutic responses in recurrent disease. *Neurosurgery* 7:352, 1980

144. Ochs JJ, Freeman AI, Douglass HO, Higby D, Mindall E, Sinks L: Cis-dichlorodiammineplatinum(II) in advanced osteogenic sarcoma. *Cancer Treat Rep* 62:239, 1978

145. Ozols RF: Renal effects and clinical pharmacokinetics of High dose cisplatin (40 mg/m² QD × 5) in hypertonic saline. In: *Platinum Coordination Complexes in Cancer Chemotherapy* (Edited by Hacker M, Douple E, Krakoff I), Boston Martinus Nijhoff 1984

146. Ozols RF, Deisseroth AB, Javadpour N, Barlock A, Messerschmidt G, Young RC: Treatment of poor prognosis nonseminomatous testicular cancer with a "high dose" platinum combination chemotherapy regimen. *Cancer* 51:1803, 1983

147. Panettiere FJ, Leichman L, O'Bryan R, Haas C, Fletcher W: Cis-diamminedichloride platinum(II), an effective agent in the treatment of epidermoid carcinoma of the esophagus. A preliminary report of an ongoing Southwest Oncology Group Study. *Cancer Clin Trials* 4:29, 1981

148. Panettiere FJ, Vonie RB, Stuckey WJ, Coltran CA, Costopzi JJ, Chen TT: Evaluation of Single-Agent Cisplatin in the Management of Non-Small Cell Carcinoma of the Lung: A Southwest Oncology Group Study. *Cancer Treat Rep* 67:399, 1983

149. Papac R, Lefkowitz E, Bertino JR: Methotrexate (NSC-740) in squamous cell carcinoma of the head and neck. II. Intermittent intravenous therapy. *Cancer Chemother Rep* 51:69, 1967

150. Pascoe JM, Roberts JJ: Interaction between mammalian cell DNA and inorganic platinum compounds. I. DNA interstrand crosslinking and cytotoxic properties of platinum (II) compounds. *Biochem. Pharmacol.* 23:1345, 1974

151. Patton TF, Repta AJ, Sternson LA, Belt RJ: Pharmacokinetics of intact cisplatin in plasma. Infusion versus bolus dosing. *Int J Pharmaceut* 10:77, 1982

152. Paulson DF, Einhorn L, Peckham M, Williams SD: Cancer of the testis. In: *Cancer* (Edited by DeVita VT, Hellman S, Rosenberg SA), p. 820. Philadelphia, JB Lippincott Company, 1982

153. Pearlman NW, Meyers TJ, Siebert PE, Wallner SF, Carson SD, Campbell DN, Johnson FB, Kennaugh R, Rempel P: Cyclophosphamide, Vincristine, Lomustine, Cisplatin, and Doxorubicin in the Treatment of Non-Small Cell Lung Cancer. *Cancer Treat Rep* 67:375, 1983

154. Piel IJ, Meyer D, Perlia C, Wolfe V: Effects of *cis*-diamminedichloroplatinum (NSC-119875) on hearing function in man. *Cancer Chemother Rep* 58:871, 1974

155. Prestayko AW, Cadiz M, Crooke ST: Incompatibility of aluminum-containing IV administration equipment with *cis*-dichlorodiammineplatinum(II) administration. *Cancer Treat Rep* 63:2218, 1979

156. Pretorius RG, Petrilli ES, Kean C, Ford LC, Hoeschele JD, Lagasse LD: Comparison of the IV and IP routes of administration of cisplatin in dogs. *Cancer Treat Rep* 65:1055, 1981

157. Price LA, Hill BT, Calvert AH, Dalley M, Levene A, Bushy E, Schachter M, Shaw H: Improved results in combination chemotherapy of head and neck cancer using a kinetically-based approach: A randomized study with and without adriamycin. *Oncology* 35:26, 1978

158. Pritchard J, Mauligit G, Benjamin R, Pratt Y, Calvo D, Hall S, Bodey G, Wallace S: Regression of regionally confined melanoma with intraarterial *cis*-dichlorodiammineplatinum(II). *Cancer Chemother Rep* 63:555, 1979

159. Randolph VL, Vallejo A, Spiro RH, Shah J, Strong E, Huvas A, Wittes R: Combination therapy of advanced head and neck cancer: Induction of remissions with diamminedichloroplatinum (II), bleomycin, and radiation therapy. *Cancer*

41:460, 1978

160. Repta AJ, Long DF, Hincal AA: *cis*-Dichlorodiammineplatinum(II) stability in aqueous vehicles: an alternative view. *Cancer Treat Rep* 63:229, 1979

161. Ribaud P, Gouveia J, Bonnay M, Mathe G: Clinical pharmacology and pharmacokinetics of cisplatinum and analogs. *Cancer Treat Reports* 65(suppl 3):97, 1981

162. Riley CM, Sternson LA, Repta AJ, Bannister SJ: Intact cisplatin in urine following IV infusion. *J Pharm Pharmacol* 34:826, 1982 (letter)

163. Roberts JJ, Pascoe JM: Cross-linking of complementary strands of DNA in mammalian cells by antitumor platinum compounds. *Nature* 235:282, 1973

164. Roos IA: Interaction of an antitumor platinum complex with DNA. *Chem-Biol Interact* 16:39, 1977

165. Roos IA, Fairlie DP, Whitehouse MW: A peculiar toxicity manifested by platinum(II)amines in rats: gastric distension after intraperitoneal administration. *Chem-Biol Interactions* 35:111, 1981

166. Roper M, Parmley RT, Crist WM, Kelly DR, Hyland CH, Salter M: Rhabdoid tumor of the kidney: complete remission induced by cis-platinum and adriamycin. *Med Pediatr Oncol* 9:175, 1981

167. Rosenberg B: Possible mechanisms for the antitumor activity of platinum coordination complexes. *Cancer Chemother Reports* 59(part i):589, 1975

168. Rosenberg B: Platinum complex-DNA interactions and anticancer activity. *Biochimie* 60:859, 1978

169. Rosenberg B: Cisplatin: Its history and possible mechanisms of action. In: *Cisplatin: Current Status and New Developments*. Edited by Prestayko AW, Crooke ST, Carter SK, pp. 9–20. Academic Press NY, 1980

170. Rosenberg B, Van Camp L, Krigas T: Inhibition of cell division in *Escherichia coli* by electrolysis products from a platinum electrode. *Nature* 205:698, 1965

171. Rosenberg B, Van Camp L, Trosko JR, Mansour V: Platinum compounds: a new class of potent antitumour agents. *Nature* 222:385, 1969

172. Ross DA, Gale GR: Reduction of the renal toxicity of *cis*-dichlorodiammineplatinum(II) by probenecid. *Cancer Treat Rep* 63:781, 1979

173. Rossof AH, Slayton RE, Perlia CP: Preliminary clinical experience with *cis*-diamminedichloroplatinum(II) (NSC-119875, CACP). *Cancer* 30:1451, 1972

174. Sallan SE, Zanberg NE, Frei E: Anti-emetic effects of delta-9-tetrahydrocannabinol in patients receiving cancer chemotherapy. *N Engl J Med* 293:795, 1975

175. Samson MK, Comis RL, Baker LH, Ginsberg S, Fraile R, Crooke S: Mitomycin C in advanced adenocarcinoma and large cell carcinoma of the lung. *Cancer Treat Rep* 62:163, 1978

176. Samuels ML, Howe CD: Vinblastine in the management of testicular cancer. *Cancer* 25:1009, 1970

177. Samuels ML, Johnson DE, Holoye PY: Continuous intravenous bleomycin (NSC-125066) therapy with vinblastine (NSC-49842) in stage III testicular neoplasia. *Cancer Chemother Rep* 59:563, 1975

178. Sarna S, Sodhi A: Chemo-immunotherapeutical studies on a fibrosarcoma with cisplatinum. *Indian J Exper Biol* 16:1236, 1978

179. Schaeppi U, Heyman IA, Fleischman RW, Rosenkrantz H, Illeivski V, Phelan R, Cooney DA, Davis RD: *cis*-dichlorodiammineplatinum(II): preclinical toxicologic evaluation of intravenous injection in dogs, monkeys and mice. *Tox Appl Pharmacol* 25:230, 1973

180. Schilsky RL, Anderson T: Hypomagnesemia and renal magnesium wasting in patients receiving *cis*platin. *Ann Intern Med* 90:929, 1979

181. Schilsky SRL, Barlock A, Ozols RF: Persistent hypomagnesemia following *cis*platin chemotherapy for testicular can-

cer. *Cancer Treat Rep* 66:1767, 1982

182. Schramm VL Jr, Srodes C, Myers EN: Cisplatin therapy for adenoid cystic carcinoma. *Arch Otolaryngol* 107:739, 1981

183. Schurig JE, Bradner WT, Huftalen GJ, Gylys JA: Toxic side effects of platinum analogs. In: *Cisplatin, Current Status and New Developments*. (Edited by Prestayko AW, Crooke ST, Carter SK), pp. 227–236. Academic Press, 1980

184. Seski JC, Edwards CL, Hérson J, Rutledge FN: Cisplatin chemotherapy for disseminated endometrial cancer. *Obstet Gynecol* 59:225, 1982

185. Sessions RB, Lehane DE, Smith RJ, Bryan RN, Suen JY: Intra-arterial cisplatin treatment of adenoid cystic carcinoma. *Arch Otolaryngol* 108:221, 1981

186. Shrieve DC, Harris JW: Protection against *cis*dichlorodiammine platinum (II) cytotoxicity *in vitro* by cysteamine. *Int J Radiation Oncology Biol Phys* 8:585, 1982

187. Siddik ZH, Newell DR, Boxall FE, Jones M, McGhee KG, Harrap KR: Biliary excretion, renal handling and red cell uptake of cisplatin and CBDCA in animals. In: *Platinum Coordination Complexes in Cancer Chemotherapy* (Edited by Hacker M, Douple E, Krakoff I), 1984

188. Smith PH, Taylor DM: Distribution and retention of the antitumor agent ^{195m}Pt-cisplatinum in man. *J Nuclear Med* 15:349, 19??

189. Sodhi A, Aggarwal SK: Effects of cisplatinum in the regression of sarcoma 180: A fine structural study. *J Natl Cancer Inst* 53:85, 1974

190. Spanos GA, Wolk D, Desner MR, Khan A, Platt N, Khafif RA, Cortes EP: Preoperative chemotherapy for giant cell carcinoma of the thyroid. *Cancer* 50:2252, 1982

191. Stewart DJ, Leavens M, Maor M, Feun L, Luna M, Bonura J, Caprioli R, Loo TL, Benjamin RS: Human central nervous system distribution of *cis*-diammine dichloroplatinum and use as a radiosensitizer in malignant brain tumors. *Cancer Res* 42:2474, 1982

192. Talley RW, O'Bryan RM, Gutterman JU, Brownlee RW, McCreedie KB: Clinical evaluation of toxic effects of *cis*-diamminedichloroplatinum (NSC-119875) – a phase I clinical study. *Cancer Chemother Rep* 57:465, 1973

193. Taniguchi S, Baba T: "Two route chemotherapy" using *cis*-diamminedichloroplatinum and its antidote, sodium thiosulfate, for peritoneally disseminated cancer in rats. *Gann* 73:475, 1982

194. Tattersall MH, Lander H, Bain B, Stocks AE, Woods RL, Fox RM, Byrne E, Trotten JR, Roos I: Cis-platinum treatment of metastatic adrenal carcinoma. *Med J Aust* 1:419, 1980

195. Taylor DM, Tews KD, Jones JD: Effects of *cis*-dichlorodiammineplatinum(II) in DNA synthesis in kidney and other tissues of normal and tumor-bearing rats. *Eur J Canc* 12:249, 1976

196. Trindade A, Samuels ML, Logothetis CJ: Chemotherapy of carcinoma of renal pelvis: preliminary report. *Urology* 18:54, 1981

197. Troner MB, Hemstreet GP 3d: Cyclophosphamide, doxorubicin, and cisplatin (CAP) in the treatment of urothelial malignancy: a pilot study of the Southeastern Cancer Study Group. *Cancer Treat Rep* 65:29, 1981

198. Trop'e C, Grundsell H, Johnsson JE, Cavallin-St'ahl E: A phase II study of cis-platinum for recurrent corpus cancer. *Eur J Cancer* 16:1025, 1980

199. Vermorken JB, Kapteijn TS, Hart AA, Pinedo HM: Ototoxicity of *cis*-diamminedichloroplatinum (II): Influence of dose, schedule and mode administration. *Eur J Cancer Clin Oncol* 19:53, 1983

200. Vermoken JB, Ten Bokkel Huinink WW, McVie JG, Van der Vijgh WJF, Pinedo HM: Clinical experience with 1,1-diaminomethylcyclohexane(sulphato)platinum(II) (TNO-6). In: *Proceedings of the 4th International Symposium on Platinum*

Coordination Complexes in Cancer Chemotherapy (Edited by Hacker M, Krakoff I, Douple E), 1983

201. Vermorken JB, Van der Vijgh WJ, Pinedo HM: Pharmacokinetic evidence for enterhepatic circulation in a patient treated with *cis*platinum. *Res Commun Chem Path Pharmacol* 28:319, 1980

202. Vogl SE, Berenzweig M, Kaplan BH, Moukhtar M, Bulkin W: The CHAD and HAD regimens in advanced ovarian cancer: Combination chemotherapy including hexamethylmelamine, adriamycin and *cis*dichlorodiammineplatinum (II). *Cancer Treat Rep* 63:311, 1979

203. Vogl SE, Greenwald E, Kaplan BH: Effective chemotherapy for esophageal cancer with methotrexate, bleomycin, and *cis*-diamminedichloroplatinum II. *Cancer* 48:2555, 1981

204. Vogl SE, Seltzer V, Camacho R, Calanog A: Dianhydrogalactitol and cisplatin in combination for advanced cancer of the uterine cervix. *Cancer Treat Rep* 66:1809, 1982

205. Von Hoff DD, Schilsky R, Reichert CM, Reddick R, Rozenzweig M, Young R, Muggie F: Toxic effects of *cis*-dichlorodiammineplatinum (II) in man. *Cancer Treat Rep* 63:1527, 1979

206. Von Hoff DD, Slavik M, Muggia FM: Allergic reactions to *cis*-platinum. *Lancet* 1:90, 1976 (letter)

207. Walker EM, Gale GR: Methods of reduction of cisplatin nephrotoxicity. *Ann Clin Lab Sci* 11:397, 1981

208. Ward JM, Fauvie KA: Nephrotoxic effects of *cis*-diamminedichloroplatinum(II) in male F344 rats. *Tox Appl Pharmacol* 38:535, 1976

209. Wiltshaw E: A review of clinical experience with cis-platinum diammine dichloride: 1972–1978. *Biochemie* 60:925, 1978

210. Witman G, Cadman E, Kapp D, Wagner F: The use of cisplatinum for treatment of malignant glioma. *Med Hypotheses* 8:335, 1982

211. Wolf W, Manaka R: Synthesis and distribution of ^{195m}Pt *cis*-dichlorodiammine platinum II. *J Clin Hematol Oncol* 7:79, 1977

212. Wolpert-DeFillipes MK: Antitumor activity of *cis*-dichlorodiammineplatinum (II). *Cancer Treat Rep* 63:1453, 1979

213. Wolpert-DeFillipes MK: Antitumor activity of cisplatinum analogs. In: Cisplatin. (Edited by Prestayko AW, Crooke ST, Carter SK), pp. 183–192. New York Academic Press, 1980

214. Wyatt JK, McAninch LH: A chemotherapeutic approach to advanced testicular carcinoma. *Can J Surg* 10:421, 1967

215. Young RC, Chabner BA, Hubbard SP: Prospective trial of melphalan (L-PAM) versus combination chemotherapy (Hexa-CAF) in ovarian adenocarcinoma. *N Engl J Med* 299:1261, 1978

216. Young RC, Hubbard SP, DeVita VT: The chemotherapy of ovarian carcinoma. *Cancer Treat Rev* 1:99, 1974

217. Young RC, Von Hoff DD, Gormley P, Makuch R, Cassidy J, Howser D, Bull JM: Cis-dichlorodiammineplatinum(II) for the treatment of advanced ovarian cancer. *Cancer Treat Rep* 63:1539, 1979

218. Yuhas JM, Culo R: Selective inhibition of the nephrotoxicity of *cis*dichlorodiammineplatinum(II) by WR-2721 without altering its antitumor properties. *Cancer Treat Rep* 64:57, 1980

219. Zwelling LA, Kohn KW: Platinum Complexes. In: *Cancer* (Edited by DeVita VT, Hellman S, Rosenberg SA), p. 329. Philadelphia, J.B. Lippincott Company, 1982

220. Zwelling LA, Andersen T, Kohn KW: DNA-protein and DNA interstrand cross linking by *cis* + *trans* platinum (II) diamminedichloride in: L1210 mouse leukemia cells and relative to cytotoxicity. *Cancer Res* 39:365, 1979

221. Zwelling LA, Kohn KW, Ross WE, Ewig R, Anderson T: Kinetics of formation and disappearance of a DNA cross-linking effect in mouse leukemia L1210 cells treated with *cis*- and *trans*-diamminedichloroplatinum(II). *Cancer Res* 38:1762, 1978

For postscript see end of Volume, p. 245.

8

NITROSOUREAS

GARTH POWIS

INTRODUCTION

The nitrosoureas represent a large and extensively studied family of antitumor agents. They exhibit a broader spectrum of activity against experimental tumors than any other class of agents and are one of the few groups of compounds to cross the so-called blood–brain barrier at therapeutically effective concentrations. Clinically the nitrosoureas are used against a variety of human solid tumors. There continues to be of interest in the development of new nitrosourea analogs with greater activity and reduced toxicity. The basic nitrosourea structure and analogs discussed in this chapter are shown in Fig. 1. Observations in the late 1950's that N-methyl-N'-nitro-N-nitrosoguanidine, a precursor of the methylating agent diazomethane, had activity against murine L1210 leukemia led to studies identifying the N-nitroso function as important for cytotoxicity. Nitrosoureas were the most active N-nitroso agents (81, 82 and references therein). Structure-activity studies led to the development of chloroethylnitrosoureas and observations that one analog, BCNU,* was curative against L1210 leukemia implanted intracranially or intraperitoneally (51, 105). Further structure-activity studies revealed that CCNU (2) and PCNU (5) were among the most active nitrosourea analogs against intraperitoneally and intracerebrally implanted L1210 leukemia and that MeCCNU (3) had high activity against implanted Lewis lung carcinoma (83, 84). BCNU (1), CCNU (2) and MeCCNU (3) are all lipid-soluble chloroethylnitrosoureas and were of great interest because of their ability to cross the blood–brain barrier and exhibit antitumor activity in experimental brain tumor models. MeCCNU exhibited a high level of antitumor activity but its low water solubility made it unsuitable for intravenous administration, although it could be given by mouth. Subsequently the water soluble carboxy analog CCNU (4) and acetic acid analog ACCNU (5) were synthesized and were

found to have activity against experimental tumors equal to, or greater than MeCCNU (48). Streptozocin (streptozotocin, **10**), a naturally occurring nitrosourea and a derivative of 2-amino-2-deoxyglucose, was isolated from a fermentation broth of *Streptomyces achromogenes*. Streptozocin was found to have only marginal activity against experimental leukemia but to be a potent toxin for the pancreatic islet beta cell and to exhibit clinical activity against pancreatic islet cell carcinomas (125). The 2-chloroethyl analog of streptozocin, chlorozotocin (**11**) has been synthesized (49) and like streptozocin shows less bone marrow toxicity than other nitrosoureas, but unlike streptozocin is not diabetogenic. Streptozocin and chlorozotocin do not cross the blood–brain barrier and are inactive against intracerebrally implanted L1210 leukemia. Some newer water soluble nitrosourea analogs currently undergoing clinical study are PCNU (**6**), MCNU (**7**), GANU (**8**), and ACNU (**9**).

MECHANISM OF ACTION

The antitumor activity of nitrosoureas appears to be related to their ability to bind irreversibly to cellular macromolecules. There are two chemical activities of the nitrosoureas, alkylation and carbamoylation (128). The chemical decomposition of chloroethylnitrosoureas in aqueous solutions leads to formation of chloroethyl carbonium ion (III) and a substituted isocyanate (I) as shown in Fig. 2. Evidence, summarized by Weinkam and Lin (123), suggests that at pHs greater than neutrality, including physiologic pH, there is formation of 2-chloroethylazohydroxide (II), which is kinetically indistinguishable from 2-chloroethyldiazonium ion, followed by nucleophilic attack on this species ($S_N 2$), or less likely, nucleophilic attack by the free carbonium ion. Evidence that the spontaneous decomposition of the chloroethylnitrosoureas is important to their antitumor activity is provided by studies where the proton on the non-nitroso nitrogen (i.e., –NHR in Fig. 2) is replaced with a methyl moiety producing a molecule which is much more stable in aqueous solution and which has a greatly reduced *in vitro* cytotoxicity (19). It should be noted that such non-nitroso nitrogen disubstituted derivatives retain *in vivo* antitumor activity since the alkyl group can be enzymatically removed. The cytotoxicity of BCNU, CCNU, and PCNU at the cellular level has been shown to correlate with the amount of 2-chloroethylazohydroxide formed by breakdown of chloroethylnitrosourea within the cell during the period of drug

---

* Chemical names and abbreviations of nitrosoureas discussed in this chapter are as follows: BCNU, N,N'-bis(2-chloroethyl)-N-nitrosourea; CCNU, N-(2-chloroethyl)-N'-cyclohexyl-N-nitrosourea; MeCCNU, N-(2-chloroethyl)-N'-(*trans*-4-methylcyclohexyl)-N-nitro-sourea; PCNU, N-(2-chloroethyl)-N'-2,6-dioxo-3-piperidyl)-N-nitrosourea; ACNU, N-(2-chloroethyl)-N'-[(4-amino-2-methyl-5-pyrimidinyl)methyl]-N-nitrosourea hydrochloride; GANU, N-(2-chloroethyl)-N'-(β-D-glucopyranosyl)-N-nitrosourea; MCNU, N-(2-chloroethyl)-N'-(methyl-α-D-glucopyranose-6-yl)-N-nitro-sourea; RFCNU, N-(2-chloroethyl)-N'-[1'-(5'-l-nitrobenzoyl-2',3'-isopropylidene)-α,β-D-ribofuranosyl]-N-nitrosourea.

P.V. Woolley (ed.), Cancer management in Man: Biological Response Modifiers, Chemotherapy, Antibiotics, Hyperthermia, Supporting Measures
© 1989. Kluwer Academic Publishers, Dordrecht

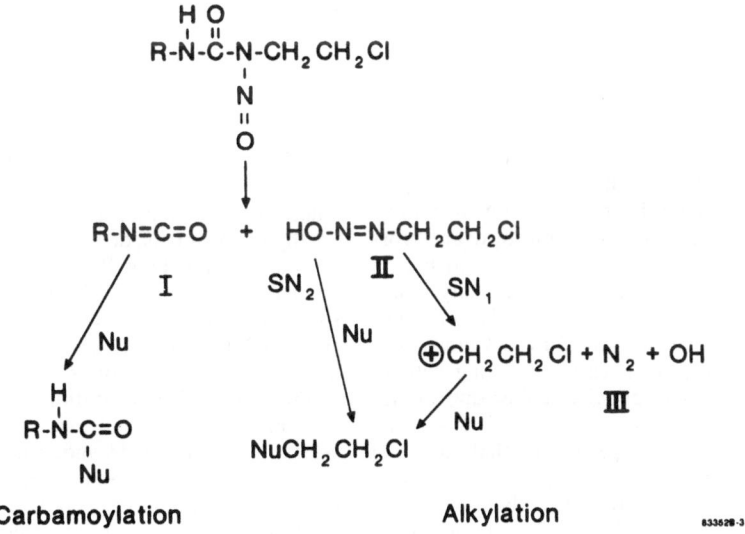

Figure 1. Structure of substituted chloroethylnitrosoureas, streptozocin and chlorozotocin.

Figure 2. Decomposition of chloroethylnitrosourea in aqueous solution to a substituted isocyanate (I) and 2-chloroethylazohydroxide (II). Alkylation of macromolecules by II proceeds either directly via an S_N2 reaction or via formation of the chloroethyl carbonium ion (III).

exposure rather than to the concentration of parent chloroethylnitrosourea (122, 123). There is no apparent effect due to the different carbamoylating species and different levels of carbamoylating activity of the agents. Chlorozotocin requires a two-fold higher concentration to produce the same toxic effect as the other chloroethylnitrosoureas probably because of the slow uptake of chlorozotocin by cells relative to its rate of conversion to the active species (122).

There are many studies focusing on the reaction of nitrosourea decomposition products with cellular macromolecules. In general, the chloroethyl (or methyl moiety) of nitrosoureas alkylate nucleic acids while the isocyanate portion of the molecule carbamoylates protein. For example, Cheng *et al.* (16) carried out *in vivo* and *in vitro* studies, and demonstrated that when the radiolabel of CCNU was in the chloroethyl moiety, radioactivity was preferentially associated with DNA. When the radiolabel was associated with the cyclohexyl moiety, radioactivity was bound to protein. Ludlum and Tong (71) have summarized studies, primarily from their laboratory, on the modification of DNA and RNA bases by the chloroethyl function of chloroethylnitrosoureas. Incubation of synthetic polynucleotides or DNA with BCNU followed by isolation and digestion of nucleotide reaction products resulted in identification of haloethyl, hydroxyethyl, and aminoethyl nucleoside or base products (71, 115, 116). Modification of nitrosourea substituents influenced the distribution of modified base products, and Tong *et al.* (114) noted that such changes in the base products might play a role in the biological activity of individual nitrosoureas. A number of investigators, most notably Kohn and colleagues, have shown that chloroethylnitrosoureas can crosslink either purified DNA or DNA in cells (24, 56, 57, 70). Crosslinking is due to the ethylene portion of the chloroethyl group. It is believed that the 2-chloroethylazohydroxide moiety or possibly the free chloroethyl carbonium ion first alkylates a heteroatom on a DNA base, such as the O–6 of guanine, and that the resulting guanine O-chloroethyl moiety undergoes rearrangement and reacts with its base sharing partner cytosine in the opposite DNA strand (113). DNA-protein crosslinks are also formed (24). DNA crosslinking by methylnitrosoureas is much reduced compared to chloroethylnitrosoureas, and methylnitrosoureas have less antitumor activity compared to chloroethylnitrosoureas (8).

Alkylation is thought to be the principal mechanism of nitrosourea antitumor activity. Nitrosoureas have a spectrum of antitumor activity similar to that of nitrogen mustard and tumors resistant to nitrogen mustard are cross resistant to nitrosoureas (105). Evidence for a contribution of carbamoylation to antitumor activity or toxicity is less decisive. Some results suggest that carbamoylation is not required for antitumor activity of nitrosoureas. Chlorozotocin, which has very little protein carbamoylating activity (128), has significant antitumor activity against several murine model systems (40). Reed (100) has pointed out that carbamoylation reactions can be specific and that the use of a single *in vitro* criterion for carbamoylating activity may lead to assumptions that are incorrect for carbamoylation *in vivo*. An example is ACNU which has virtually no carbamoylating activity with lysine *in vitro* but is a potent carbamoylating agent against gluthathione reductase (4). One can speculate, therefore, that even chlorozotocin may be capable

of some carbamoylation *in vivo*. Wheeler *et al.* (128) compared toxicity and antitumor activity for a number of nitrosoureas against intraperitoneally implanted L1210 in mice, to alkylation, carbamoylation and lipid solubility of these agents. They found that carbamoylation correlated with toxicity and alkylation correlated with cytotoxicity measured either by cell kill or 45-day survival. These data support the premise that carbamoylation is not required for antitumor activity, and suggest that toxicity may be reduced by reducing carbamoylation activity of nitrosoureas. However, while some nitrosoureas with low carbamoylating activity are less toxic than analogs with high carbamoylating activity, more recent structure-activity studies (39, 93, 94) suggest that carbamoylation may not be a primary factor in nitrosourea toxicity. The demonstration that carbamoylation inhibits radiation induced repair of DNA damage (52, 53) presents the intriguing possibility that inhibition of repair processes could enhance the therapeutic and toxic effects of alkylating agents, including the cytotoxic effects of the nitrosoureas themselves.

IN VITRO DECOMPOSITION

Chloroethylnitrosoureas decompose spontaneously by a base catalyzed reaction in pH 7.4 phosphate buffered saline with half-lives in the range of 25 to 53 min (60). The products formed by spontaneous breakdown of BCNU are shown in Fig. 3. The rate of decomposition of the lipophilic chloroethylnitrosoureas BCNU, CCNU and MeCCNU, although not of the more hydrophilic chloroethylnitrosoureas PCNU and ACNU, is enhanced in the presence of serum due to a nonspecific interaction between the lipophilic chloroethylnitrosoureas and serum proteins (124). The half-life of BCNU, for example, is 49 min in buffer but 14 min in serum (66). The products of the protein catalyzed decomposition are the same as the products of the base catalyzed reaction (124). The high reactivity of the decomposition products means that a large proportion probably react with and are covalently bound to albumin. This could explain the long half-lives of total radioactivity in plasma when radiolabeled chloroethylnitrosoureas are administered *in vivo* (21).

IN VITRO METABOLISM STUDIES

There are two major pathways for metabolism of chloroethylnitrosoureas, denitrosation and hydroxylation of the cyclohexyl ring. Thus BCNU which has no cyclohexyl ring is metabolized by denitrosation while CCNU and, at a slower rate MeCCNU, are hydroxylated on the cyclohexyl ring. CCNU and MeCCNU also undergo denitrosation but at a slower rate than BCNU.

Two types of denitrosation reactions have been reported for chloroethylnitrosoureas, reductive denitrosation with release of nitric oxide and, for BCNU only, glutathione conjugation with release of nitrite (Fig. 3). Denitrosation of chloroethylnitrosoureas was first reported for BCNU and N-methyl-N-nitrosourea by microsomes from mouse liver and lung (42). The product formed from BCNU was 1,3-bis-(2-chloroethyl)urea. Lin and Weinkam (69) have subsequently shown that 1,3-bis(2-chloroethyl)urea is subject to

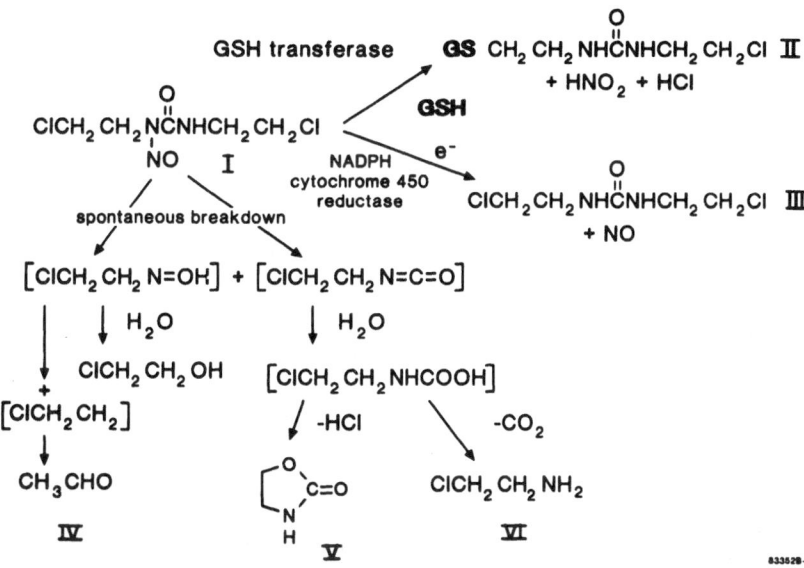

Figure 3. Chemical breakdown and metabolism of BCNU (I). Metabolism yields 2-chloroethyl-3-ethylglutathionylurea (II) and 1,3-bis(2-chloroethyl)urea (III). Chemical breakdown yields acetaldehyde (IV), 2-oxazolidone (V) and 2-chloroethylamine (VI).

further slow metabolism by microsomal preparations. Hill *et al.* (42) found very little denitrosation of BCNU in the absence of microsomes or NADPH and the reaction was only partly blocked by the inhibitors of cytochrome P-450, CO, 2-diethylaminoethyl 2,2-diphenylvalerate (SKF-525A) and by the absence of oxygen. Under similar incubation conditions Hill *et al.* (42) found that CCNU and MeCCNU formed only cyclohexyl ring hydroxylated metabolites and they concluded that if denitrosation of CCNU and MeCC-NU occurred it was at the rate less than 5% of that for hydroxylation. May *et al.* (77) subsequently showed that during hepatic microsomal metabolism of MeCCNU there was denitrosation of MeCCNU to the parent urea (MeCNU) by both rat and mouse liver microsomes. The rate of denitrosation by mouse liver microsomes was much slower than by rat liver microsomes. Only about half of the MeCCU formed required microsomes and NADPH, the remainder appeared to be formed as an artifact during the extraction procedure. When allowance was made for the nonenzymatic reaction, denitrosation of MeCCNU by phenobarbital induced rat liver microsomes appeared to be completely inhibited by CO. Potter and Reed (97) reported denitrosation of BCNU and CCNU by rat liver microsomes under anaerobic conditions with formation of the parent ureas and nitric oxide. Nitric oxide binds to hepatic microsomal cytochrome P-450 producing a characteristic Soret maximum at 444 nm which was used to measure denitrosation. Denitrosation of BCNU proceeded at about 3 times the rate of denitrosation of CCNU. Denitrosation required NADPH, was induced by phenobarbital but was only partly inhibited by SKF-525A, α-naphthoflavone, metyrapone and CO. Although the results suggested a possible role for cytochrome P-450 in denitrosation it was also shown that a reconstituted system of purified microsomal NADPH-cytochrome P-450 reductase, dilauroylphosphatidylcholine and NADPH was able to catalyze denitrosation of CCNU. The results were initially taken to indicate a dual catalytic

site on NADPH-cytochrome P-450 reductase and cytochrome P-450 for denitrosation of nitrosourea (97). Further work by the same authors (98) using NADPH-cytochrome P-450 reductase, dilauroylphosphatidylcholine and NADPH showed that denitrosation of CCNU was stimulated by addition of not only cytochrome P-450 but also by cytochrome c. Stimulation of denitrosation was maximal when the ratio of cytochrome to NADPH-cytochrome P-67450 reductase was 1:1 and decreased when the cytochrome was in excess. The results of these studies were taken to indicate that NADPH-cytochrome P-450 reductase rather than cytochrome P-450 was the microsomal enzyme responsible for denitrosation of CCNU. Although BCNU, CCNU and MeCCNU are the only nitrosoureas for which denitrosation has so far been reported, Potter and Reed (97) indicate that eight of nine other nitrosoureas studied by them were denitrosated.

BCNU has also been shown to undergo denitrosation when incubated with glutathione-supplemented mouse liver cytosol to form 1-chloroethyl-3-glutathionylurea (41) and nitrite (112) in a reaction catalyzed by glutathione-S-transferase. The reaction is increased by phenobarbital pretreatment (112). The apparent Km of the denitrosating enzyme for glutathione is 2 mM, a value that is below the normal glutathione concentration in mouse liver, indicating a possible role for the reaction under physiological conditions. Conjugation of BCNU with glutathione might explain the decrease in hepatic glutathione levels in mice treated with BCNU (78). However, BCNU is also an irreversible inhibitor of glutathione reductase in mouse and other species (3, 73) which result in a lowering of hepatic glutathione levels (3). Glutathione dependent denitrosation of BCNU has been reported not to occur in rat liver preparations (68). CCNU and MeCCNU are not substrates for glutathione dependent denitrosation by mouse liver cytosol (41).

Hydroxylation of the cyclohexyl ring is the major pathway of metabolism for CCNU and MeCCNU. Hydroxyla-

Table 1. Microsomal metabolism of CCNU in mouse and rat.

| Species | *Percent total hydroxylated metabolites* | | | | | |
| | 2-OH CCNU | | 3-OH CCNU | | 4-OH CCNU | |
	cis	*trans*	*cis*	*trans*	*cis*	*trans*
Rat (76)						
Control	–	–	30	39	21	9
PB	–	–	16	13	67	5
3-MC	–	–	25	40	30	5
Rat (43)						
Control	–	14	trace[a]	31	54	3
PB	–	3	3[a]	11	77	5
Rat (25)						
PB	trace	2	20	6	62	6
Mouse (129)						
Control	–	1	13	12	46	28

Data taken from Reed (100).
PB, phenobarbital induced; 3-MC, 3-methylcholanthrene induced.
[a] This value is probably an underestimate, see text for explanations.

tion occurs very rapidly when CCNU is incubated with hepatic microsomes, O_2 and NADPH (42, 43, 75) forming 5 of the 6 possible isomeric monohydroxylated metabolites (Table 1). Using rat hepatic microsomes the principal products found by May *et al.* (76) were *cis* and *trans*-3-hydroxy-CCNU while Hilton and Walker (43) found mostly *cis*-4-hydroxy-CCNU with some *trans*-3-hydroxy-CCNU. Reed (100) has pointed out that the analytical technique used by Hilton and Walker (43) would permit decomposition of the intrinsically unstable *cis*-3-hydroxy-CCNU, probably leading to its underestimation. Phenobarbital pretreatment leads to an increased stereochemical specificity for 4-axial hydroxylation of CCNU with *cis*-4-hydroxy-CCNU being the major metabolite. Pretreatment of rats with 3-methylcholanthrene does not change the pattern of hydroxylated CCNU metabolites. The principal hydroxylated metabolite of CCNU formed by uninduced mouse microsomes is *cis*-4-hydroxy-CCNU with some *trans*-4-hydroxy-CCNU (129). MeCCNU exhibits a slower rate of microsomal hydroxylation than CCNU but forms at least 7

metabolites including a metabolite resulting from α-hydroxylation of the ethylene side chain (Table 2). A different spectrum of metabolites is produced from MeCCNU by mouse microsomes compared to rat microsomes. *Trans*-4-hydroxy-methyl-CCNU predominates in the mouse but in the rat *trans*-4-hydroxymethyl-CCNU and a combination of methyl-CCU and *trans*-4-hydroxy-*cis*-methyl-CCNU are formed in equal amounts. Induction with phenobarbital leads to an increase in the rate of formation of *cis*-4-hydroxy-*trans*-4-methyl-CCNU in both rat and mouse, and although *trans*-4-hydroxymethyl-CCNU formation is increased in mouse, in rat its formation is decreased. Phenobarbital induction does not show as much stereospecificity for 4-axial hydroxylation with MeCCNU as with CCNU, possibly due to steric hindrance by the *trans*-4-methyl group. An unusual feature of metabolism of MeCCNU is inversion of the methyl group to the opposite side of the alicyclic ring during hydroxylation at the 4-position to yield *trans*-4-hydroxy-*cis*-4-methyl-CCNU (Table 2). Inversion has been shown to occur in the opposite direction during hydroxylation of *cis*-MeCCNU (96). A mechanism involving a transitory free radical intermediate has been proposed by Reed (100) which would permit a limited loss of stereospecificity during 4-hydroxylation.

IN VIVO METABOLISM STUDIES

Although chloroethylnitrosoureas break down spontaneously under physiological conditions comparison of the rates of chloroethylnitrosourea elimination *in vivo* with the rates of metabolism observed *in vitro* suggest that a considerable proportion of a dose of chloroethylnitrosourea might be metabolized before chemical breakdown can occur (42, 63, 75). Lee and Workman (59) reported metabolites of CCNU in plasma of mice after intraperitoneal administration of CCNU. CCNU disappeared rapidly from plasma in a biphasic manner with an initial half-life of 2 min and a terminal half-life of 53 min. Hydroxylated metabolites were detected in plasma as early as 1 min after CCNU administration. Five of the six possible isomeric mono-hydroxylated metabolites were detected in plasma although *trans*-2-hydroxy-CCNU was present in only trace amounts. *cis*-2-

Table 2. Microsomal metabolism of MeCCNU in mouse and rat.

| | *nmol/min/mg* | | | |
| | *Rat* | | *Mouse* | |
	Control	*Pb*	*Control*	*Pb*
*trans*3-OH-*trans*-4-MeCCNU	0.11	0.15	0.04	0.29
cis-3-OH-*trans*-4-MeCCNU	0.13	0.37	0.08	0.17
cis-4-OH-*trans*-4-MeCCNU	0.16	1.11	0.12	1.85
α-OH-*trans*-4-MeCCNU	0.07	0.48	0.04	0.40
trans-4-OH-MeCCNU	0.50	0.35	0.21	0.77
MeCCNU + *trans*-4-OH-*cis*-MeCCNU[a]	0.51	1.45	0.06	0.91

Data taken from May *et al.* (77).
Pb, phenobarbital induced.
[a] These two metabolites were not resolved by the analytical technique employed. Further evidence for formation of *trans*-4-OH-*cis*-4-MeCCNU was provided by Potter and Reed (96).

Table 3. Terminal half-life and $AUC_{0 \to \infty}$ for CCNU metabolites in mouse plasma.

Parameter	CCNU	3-OH CCNU		4-OH CCNU	
		cis	trans	cis	trans
t1/2β (min)	53.0	108.1	64.3	91.7	86.4
$AUC_{0 \to \infty}$ (μg·min/ml)	43.0	24	13	67	370

Data taken from Lee and Workman (59).
CCNU was administered to mice at a dose of 20 mg/kg.
$AUC_{0 \to \infty}$ is the area under the plasma concentration time curve from time = 0 to infinity.

hydroxy-CCNU was not detected. 4-Hydroxylated metabolites predominated in plasma similar to results *in vitro*, although in contrast to *in vivo* results *trans*-4-hydroxy-CCNU was present in excess of *cis*-4-hydroxy-CCNU. Maximum metabolite concentrations were reached within 10 to 20 min of administration of CCNU and their elimination was biphasic. Values for pharmacokinetic parameters of CCNU and the four major hydroxylated metabolites are shown in Table 3. It is interesting that the $AUC_{0 \to \infty}$ for total hydroxylated metabolites was 10-fold that for parent CCNU. Reed and May (102) and Reed (100) reported studies where [cyclohexyl-1-^{14}C] CCNU was administered intravenously to phenobarbital induced rats and the rats killed after 2 min. Brain and intestine contained mostly unchanged CCNU and monohydroxylated metabolites. Liver and blood contained a large proportion of unextractable radioactivity, presumably representing carbamoylated protein, as well as metabolites more polar than monohydroxylated CCNUs. In excess of 50% of the extractable radioactivity in liver was present as these unidentified polar metabolites, which it was suggested, might be N-hydroxy or N-amino derivatives formed by reduction of the nitroso group. [Ethylene-^{14}C] CCNU was not transformed into unextractable products, possibly indicating a high degree of protection by the ethyl moiety against alkylation of intracellular thiols such as glutathione. Reed and May (101) have shown that the 2-chloroethyl alkylating moiety of CCNU readily forms conjugates with glutathione or cysteine and 62% of a dose of [ethylene-^{14}C] CCNU administered intraperitoneally to uninduced rats is excreted in urine in 24 hr, mostly as thiodiacetic acid and S-carboxymethyl L-cysteine. Examination of urine of rats receiving [cyclohexyl-1-^{14}C] CCNU in the study of Reed (100) revealed that 44% of the dose of radioactivity was excreted in 24 hr, mostly as cyclohexylamine containing carbamoylated peptides, which on acid hydrolysis gave predominantly cysteine and serine residues. A small amount (12%) of radioactivity was excreted in urine as free cyclohexylamines with approximately equal amounts of cyclohexylamine, *cis*-3- and *cis*-4-hydroxycyclohexylamine and lesser amounts of *trans*-3- and *trans*-4-hydroxycyclohexylamine. Phenobarbital pretreatment increased the relative proportion of *cis*-4- and *trans*-4-hydroxyisomers.

Streptozocin breaks down extensively *in vivo* and at least 5 components have been detected in plasma and urine of mice given radiolabeled streptozocin (7). Two of these components were thought to be the α- and β- anomers of streptozocin itself while the other 3 components, which comprised 50% of the radioactivity in plasma 30 min after giving the drug and 51% in the urine in 4 hr, were not identified. Six components have been detected in urine of rat after giving radiolabeled streptozocin (54).

Guarino (34) has reported preliminary work on the distribution of radiolabeled BCNU and CCNU in shark. Although parent drug and metabolites were not separated this is an interesting comparative study. Slow plasma elimination of radiolabel was observed with half-lives in the range of 20–30 hr, presumably due to binding of radiolabel to plasma proteins as reported in other species (21). There was localization of radiolabel in hepatic and renal compartments while radiolabel could be detected in brain after 24 hr.

Despite the extensive work in animals there has been little work on metabolism of nitrosoureas in man. It is not known whether BCNU is metabolized in man. Clemens *et al* (17) reported the presence of vinyl chloride in blood and exhaled air of patients receiving BCNU. Vinyl chloride has been reported to be a volatile decomposition product of BCNU in aqueous buffer (19). However, Clemens *et al.* (17) only found vinyl chloride formed *in vitro* when BCNU was incubated with erythrocytes, but not when incubated in saline or plasma. Lin and Weinkam (69) were unable to find 1,3-bis(2-chloroethyl)urea, the product of BCNU denitrosation, in urine of patients receiving BCNU therapy. Hilton and Walker (44) studied plasma of four patients receiving [ethylene-^{14}C] CCNU at therapeutic doses. At the end of intravenous infusion three quarters of the plasma radioactivity was hydroxylated products. Approximately one-third was *cis*-4-hydroxy-CCNU, two-thirds was *trans*-4-hydroxy-CCNU and there was a little *trans*-3-hydroxy-CCNU. These were preliminary results and few other details were given in the report. Since these compounds can only derive from metabolism and not breakdown this finding, if confirmed, would indicate significant metabolism of CCNU in human.

EFFECT OF METABOLISM ON ACTIVITY

Removal of the nitroso function from nitrosoureas results in compounds lacking antitumor activity (42, 81). Not surprisingly, therefore, metabolic denitrosation of BCNU leads to a decrease in antitumor activity of BCNU. This has been shown *in vitro* with isolated hepatocytes coincubated with cultured human tumor cells (2) and *in vivo*. Levin *et al.* (63) reported that in rats pretreated with phenobarbital the area under the plasma concentration time curve (AUC) for BCNU following intraperitoneal administration of drug was decreased by 90% and antitumor activity against intracerebrally implanted brain tumor was abolished. Phenobarbital pretreatment of rats also reduced the lethality of BCNU. The reduction in BNCNU lethality appeared to be less than the reduction in antitumor activity suggesting that phenobarbital pretreatment produces a decrease in the therapeutic index of BCNU. A surprising finding, in view of the presumed inactivation of BCNU by microsomal metabolism, was a report that incubation with an Aroclor 1254 induced rat liver microsomal preparation increased the mutagenicity of BCNU as well as CCNU, MeCCNU, streptozocin and chlorozotocin in the Ames *S. typhimurium* assay (26). Work by Suling *et al.* (111) suggests, however, that the major part of the enhanced mutagenicity of BCNU and CCNU is not due to metabolism but to nonspecific factors that are present in the liver enzyme preparation.

Hydroxylation of the cyclohexyl ring of chloroethylnitrosoureas leaving the chloroethylnitrosourea moiety intact gives compounds with antitumor activity similar to, or even greater than the parent compound (50, 81, 129). Phenobarbital pretreatment, which *in vitro* increases microsomal hydroxylation of CCNU, was found by Levin *et al.* (63) to produce a small although non-significant decrease in the antitumor activity of CCNU against brain tumor in rat. On the other hand, Muller *et al.* (86) found that in mouse phenobarbital pretreatment markedly reduced the toxicity and the antitumor activity of CCNU against brain tumor, as well as against tumor at a subcutaneous site. These results suggest that denitrosation, which is also increased by phenobarbital pretreatment, may be a more important pathway for elimination of CCNU in mouse than in rat. Phenobarbital pretreatment has been shown to significantly reduce the antitumor activity and toxicity of MeCCNU, CCNU and ACNU in rats and mice, although with no change in therapeutic index of the drugs (55, 87, 109).

Administration of the radiosensitizing drug misonidazole to mice increases the toxicity and to a greater extent the antitumor activity of CCNU with a consequent increase in the therapeutic index (45, 117). This appears to be due to a pharmacokinetic mechanism. Lee and Workman (59) have shown that administration of misonidazole to mice prolongs the initial phase of plasma elimination of CCNU and increases the concentration of hydroxylated CCNU metabolites in plasma. There was, however, no effect of misonidazole on the terminal phase of plasma elimination of CCNU or its hydroxylated metabolites. The authors suggested that this indicated that the terminal phase of elimination was not dependent on hepatic metabolism but on the redistribution of drug from depots such as adipose tissue back into plasma. They also suggested that misonidazole might inhibit subsequent metabolism of hydroxylated CCNU derivatives to unknown species. In contrast to results in mouse Urtasun *et al.* (118) have reported that misonidazole has no effect of the plasma kinetics of BCNU in man. Whether this represents a true species difference between mouse and man, or is due to other factors remains to be seen. SKF-525A, an inhibitor of microsomal mixed function oxidase, increases the toxicity and antitumor activity of both CCNU and MeCCNU in mice although, unlike misonidazole, SKF-525A produces no gain in therapeutic index of CCNU or MeCCNU (55, 109, 117).

PHARMACOKINETICS OF PARENT NITROSOUREAS

Many early studies on the disposition of nitrosoureas employed ^{14}C-labeled drug. The label was either incorporated uniformly or in the alkylating or carbamoylating portions of the molecule. Elimination of radiolabel from plasma was relatively slow with half-lives in the order of days. The long half-life is probably due to the covalent binding of nitrosourea breakdown products or metabolites to plasma proteins. In some of these studies radiolabeled drug and metabolites were separated by thin layer chromatography and pharmacokinetic parameters for unchanged drug obtained. Sensitive and specific mass spectrometric and hplc assays capable of measuring parent drug have recently become

available and have been used to obtain reliable pharmacokinetic parameters for unchanged nitrosoureas. Tables 4 and 5 summarize pharmacokinetic parameters for parent nitrosoureas in animals and in man. The biologic half-life for unchanged nitrosoureas in plasma is relatively short, on the order of 25 to 100 min, and does not vary much between animals and man. BCNU appears to have the largest steady state apparent volume of distribution. Steady state apparent volume of distribution decreases with increasing hydrophilicity and for ACNU and MCNU, two water soluble nitrosoureas, in man is about the same as total body water, that is, 0.55 to 0.65 l/kg. Total body plasma clearance of nitrosoureas is generally higher for more lipophilic nitrosoureas. The contribution of metabolism to the elimination of nitrosoureas in man is not known except for a preliminary study by Hilton and Walker (44) showing formation of hydroxylated metabolites from CCNU, already referred to. Levin *et al.* (66) suggested that serum factors might play a major role in the *in vivo* pharmacokinetics of BCNU in man because of the similarity of the apparent first order rate constant for elimination of BCNU, $0.0324 \, min^{-1}$, and the decomposition rate observed for BCNU in serum *in vitro* of $0.044 \, min^{-1}$. Similar arguments for a major role for serum factors in *in vivo* elimination could be advanced for PCNU where the apparent first order rate constant for elimination is $0.028 \, min^{-1}$ and the decomposition rate in plasma *in vitro* $0.027 \, min$ (60). In the absence of studies on metabolism of nitrosoureas in man it is difficult to arrive at a conclusion concerning the relative contribution of chemical breakdown and metabolism to elimination. Parent chloroethylnitrosoureas are not the biologically active species so that plasma concentrations of an unchanged drug are unlikely to relate directly to antitumor activity. Physical properties of the drug such as lipophilicity and size, as well as tumor vascularity, blood flow and capillary permeability will determine the amount of drug reaching the tumor for a given plasma concentration. Conversion to compounds with antitumor activity equal to, or greater than the parent drug will also obscure the relationship between concentrations of parent chloroethylnitrosourea and antitumor activity. Some chloroethylnitrosoureas retain antitumor activity when given by mouth. It is unlikely that after oral administration much unchanged drug will reach the systemic circulation because of chemical breakdown in the gastrointestinal tract and first-pass metabolism by the liver. Unfortunately there have been no studies using newer analytical techniques on the pharmacokinetics of orally administered nitrosoureas.

ANTITUMOR ACTIVITY

Animals

Studies in tumored mice have shown a correlation between antitumor activity of nitrosoureas and their alkylating activity (128). Lipid solubility, which is a critical determinant of the ease with which nitrosoureas cross cell membranes and the blood–brain barrier, also contributes to the antitumor activity of the nitrosoureas. Structure activity relationships by Montgomery *et al.* (83) have shown a parabolic relationship between antitumor activity against Lewis lung carcinoma in mice and log of the octanol–water partition coef-

Table 4. Pharmacokinetic parameters of parent nitrosoureas in animals.

Species	Parameter	BCNU	CCNU		PCNU	RFCNU	Streptozocin	Chlorotozocin
Mouse	t1/2α min		5[a]*	2.3[b]	–		10–15[d]	5[e]*
	t1/2β min		100	53	29[c]*			
	Vd l/kg		–	35.6	1.6			
	CĪ ml/min/kg		–	463.0	39			
Rat	t1/2α min	5[f]				< 5[g]*		
	t1/2β min	26						
	Vd l/kg	1.9						
	CĪ ml/min/kg	40						
Dog	t1/2α min	15[h]	5[a]*				5[d]	
	t1/2β min	–	> 120				15	

t1/2α, initial half-life; t1/2β, terminal half-life; Vd, apparent volume of distribution; CĪ, total body plasma clearance.
* Studies using radioactively labeled drug.
[a] Oliverio *et al.* (92); [b] Lee and Workman (59); [c] Rahman *et al.* (99); [d] Bhuyan *et al.* (7); [e] Mhatre *et al.* (80); [f] Levin *et al.* (63); [g] Godeneche *et al.* (30); [h] Hochberg *et al.* (46).

Table 5. Pharmacokinetic parameter of parent nitrosoureas in man.

Drug	Dose	Route	t1/2α min	t1/2β min	t1/2γ min	Vd$_{ss}$ l/kg	CĪ ml/min/kg	Reference
BCNU	30–175 mg/m^2	i.v.	3.5[a]	69.0[a]	–	3.25	56	Levin *et al.* (66)
	50 mg	i.v.	1.4	17.8	59	2.59	16.7	Russo *et al.* (103)
MeCCNU	100 mg	p.o.	–	96	–	–	–	Caddy *et al.* (12)
PCNU	90–100 mg/m^2	i.v.	4.7[a]	45.1[a]	–	1.9	33	Levin *et al.* (67)
	94 mg/m^2	i.v.	–	24.7	–	3.2[b]		Smith *et al.* (110)
ACNU	100–150 mg	i.v.	1.3	35	–	0.49	16	Mori *et al.* (85)
	100–150 mg	i.v.	6.5	49	–	0.55	NS	Harada *et al.* (37)
	70–140 mg	i.v.	3.4	50	–	0.57[b]	NS	Hara *et al.* (35)
MCNU	NS	i.v.	4.5	44	–	0.65	NS	Harada *et al.* (36)
GANU	120 mg/m^2	i.v.	4.6	–	–	0.14[b]	21	Nakajima *et al.* (88)
Streptozocin	1500–2460 mg	i.v.	5	35	–	NS	NS	Adolphe *et al.* (1)

t1/2α, initial half-life; t1/2β, terminal half-life; Vd$_{ss}$, steady state apparent volume of distribution, CĪ, total body plasma clearance.
[a] Calculated values.
[b] Calculated for a 70 kg, 1.8 m^2 individual.
– Means there is no appropriate value, NS means not stated or insufficient information given to be calculated.

ficient (log *P*) of the nitrosourea, with maximum antitumor activity obtained for values of log *P* between −0.20 and +1.34. Levin and Kabra (62) found that antitumor activity against rat brain tumor decreased with increasing log *P* between 0.37 and 3.3. In this study insufficient drugs with log *P* lower than 0.37 were tested to determine if the relationship was parabolic. Subsequent studies by Panasci *et al.* (93, 94) demonstrated a significant correlation between lethality and alkylating activity of nitrosoureas, although no correlation was found with carbamoylating activity and neither parameter showed any correlation with antitumor activity. If, as suggested by *in vitro* studies, the activity of lipid soluble chloroethylnitrosoureas at the cellular level is related to the amount of active species formed within the cell and is relatively independent of structural parameters of the parent drug (122), then diffferences in *in vivo* disposition of the drugs could be a major factor in determining differences in antitumor activity between the chloroethylnitrosoureas.

Chloroethylnitrosoureas exhibit a wide range of activity against transplantable tumors in mice. Table 6 shows the activity of BCNU, CCNU, MeCCNU, PCNU and chlorozotocin against the National Cancer Institute tumor screening panel of experimental tumors which includes murine tumors and human tumor xenografts growing in nude (immunodeficient) mice. Activity in the screening panel ranges from 69% of tumors tested for BCNU, to 83% for CCNU, which is similar to the activity seen for alkylating agents such as nitrogen mustard, melphalan, cyclophosphamide and cisplatin, and exceeds the activity of most other clinically active antitumor agents (31). The chloroethylnitrosoureas exhibit activity against nearly all the murine tumors but show less activity against human tumor xenografts. The clinically established chloroethylnitrosoureas, BCNU, CCNU, and MeCCNU show activity in 33% to 60% of human tumor xenograft systems tested. In this respect they differ from the alkylating agents which generally exhibit activity greater than 60% in human tumor xenograft test systems. PCNU, a new chloroethylnitrosourea, is active in 67% of human tumor xenograft test systems. Not only are the nitrosoureas active in a wide range of animal tumors but

Table 6. Activity of chloroethylnitrosoureas against transplantable tumors in mice.

	BCNU	CCNU	MeCCNU	PCNU	Chlorozotocin
Mouse tumors					
L1210 leukemia	+	+	+	+	+
P388 leukemia	+	+	+	−	+
B16 melanoma	+	+	+	+	+
Lewis lung	+	+	+	+	+
Colon 26	+	+	+	+	+
Colon 38	+	+	+	+	+
CD8F$_1$ mammary	+	+	+	+	+
Human tumor xenografts					
Mammary MX-1, sc	−	−	+	+	−
Mammary MX-1, src	+	+	NT	+	NT
Lung LX-1, sc	−	+	−	+	−
Lung LX-1, src	+	+	NT	+	NT
Colon CX-1, sc	−	−	−	−	−
Colon CX-1, src	−	NT	NT	−	NT
Number	9/13	10/12	8/10	10/13	7/10
Percent	69	83	80	77	70

Data taken from Goldin *et al.* (31).
Human tumor xenografts were grown in nude mice either at a subcutaneous site (sc), or at a subrenal capsule site (src).
Response criteria; survival times, P388 $\geqslant$ 120%; L1210, B16 $\geqslant$ 125%; Colon 26 $\geqslant$ 130%, Lewis lung $\geqslant$ 140%; tumor weight inhibition, Colon 38, MX-1 sc, LX-1 sc, and CX-1 sc $\leqslant$ 42%; MX-1 src, and CX-1 $\leqslant$ 20%.
+ Signifies activity, − signifies no activity, NT = not tested.

they can cure some animals of tumor with a single dose (83, 104).

An important feature of the chloroethylnitrosoureas is their activity against experimental brain tumor (6, 62, 79, 104). This appears to be related to their lipid solubility and the ease with which the parent drug and/or metabolites cross the blood–brain barrier. Studies in a number of animals have shown the presence of parent drug and metabolites in the brain after systemic administration of chloroethylnitrosourea (21, 34. 79, 99, 100).

Man

The spectrum of antitumor activity of the nitrosoureas in man is shown in Table 7. BCNU, CCNU and MeCCNU have received extensive clinical trials and their antitumor activity is discussed below. A major problem with the nitrosoureas is that relatively few comparative studies have been conducted in man and there is a lack of information to show whether any of the compounds are clearly superior to the other compounds for a given tumor type (13).

Observations that nitrosoureas were active against intracerebrally implanted tumors in animals and confirmation that some nitrosoureas penetrate the blood–brain barriers led to studies demonstrating significant activity of BCNU and CCNU against human glioma (61, 65, 119). The ability of unchanged nitrosoureas to penetrate into the brain in man is shown in Table 8. The promise of the early clinical studies has, however, not been borne out in subsequent trials. A large 4 arm study comparing radiation, BCNU, radiation plus BCNU, or the best conventional care but no radiation or chemotherapy, in the post-surgical treatment of primary malignant glioma demonstrated a modest but significant role for BCNU in prolonging survival when used alone (120). BCNU did not, however, further improve the increased survival offered by radiation, although the number of long-term survivors (alive at 18 months) was significantly greater in the group receiving BCNU plus radiation than radiation alone. It is important to note, however, that few patients survive more than one year and it is only in these patients that BCNU may be of additional benefit. MeCCNU plus radiation offered no advantage over BCNU plus radiation (121). Based on these and other clinical trials

Table 7. Antitumor activity of nitrosoureas in man.

Drug	Brain	Colon	Stomach	Hodgkin's disease	Lung	Melanoma	Islet cell
BCNU	+	+	±	+	±	+	?
CCNU	+	±	±	+	+	±	?
MeCCNU	±	+	+	+	±	+	?
Streptozocin	−	−	?	+	−	?	+
Chlorozotocin	?	?	?	?	?	?	?

Data taken from Carter (13).

Table 8. Brain or CSF concentrations of unchanged nitrosoureas in man.

Drug	Dose	Tissue	Concentration µg/g	Tissue/blood[a] ratio	Ref.
BCNU	30–200 mg/m^2	CSF	~1	1.0	Levin *et al.* (64)
ACNU	100–150 mg	CSF	0.6[b]	0.3	Mori *et al.* (85)
	100–150 mg	Glioma	>1[c]	1.6[d]	Harada *et al.* (37)
MCNU	NS	CSF	0.4[e]	0.3	Harada *et al.* (36)

[a] Concomitantly measured blood or plasma concentration. [b] Peak value at 30 min. [c] Mean value over 60 min. [d] Peak value at 50 min. [e] Value at 40 min. NS = not stated.

BCNU in conjunction with whole brain irradiation is now widely used for treatment of malignant glioma. Although not curable, meaningful survival prolongation and palliation of neurologic deficits can be achieved with this combined treatment. BCNU appears equivalent to CCNU in this respect (126). Combinations of nitrosoureas with agents such as 5-fluorouracil, procarbazine and vincristine may increase the response rate of recurrent brain tumors but have little impact on duration of response (119).

Nitrosourea-containing regimens have established a role in the treatment of Hodgkin's lymphoma. Schein (106) and Gottlieb *et al.* (33) have reviewed the extensive Cancer and Leukemia Group B experience with nitrosoureas in the treatment of Hodgkin's lymphoma. Single agent studies demonstrated that CCNU was more effective than either BCNU or MeCCNU in the treatment of relapsed Hodgkin's patients (74, 107). Subsequent studies included three and four drug regimens, and focused on comparisons with the "MOPP" (nitrogen mustard, vincristine, procarbazine and prednisone) regimen for Hodgkin's disease (23). Replacement of nitrogen mustard with BCNU (BOPP) or CCNU (COPP) gave comparable periods of remission to MOPP in the treatment of advanced Hodgkin's disease (20, 90). Addition of CCNU to several regimens such as CVPP (CCNU, vinblastine, procarbazine and prednisone) also resulted in effective therapies for treatment of advanced Hodgkin's disease (20). Toxicities of these therapies appear to be equal to or less than those encountered with MOPP (233). The Eastern Cooperative Oncology Group has recently published results of ten years experience in the treatment of advanced Hodgkin's disease (29). After studying several regimens, the group found that the five drug regimen of BCNU, cyclophosphamide, vinblastine, procarbazine and prednisone (BCVPP) provided significantly longer complete response durations than did MOPP, and reduced gastrointestinal toxicity and neurotoxicity. While MOPP continues to be widely used in the treatment of Hodgkin's disease (22), nitrosourea-containing regimens have become clearly established as important in the treatment of this disease. Nitrosourea-containing regimens are also employed in the treatment of non-Hodgkin's lymphomas (22).

Nitrosoureas, as part of combination regimens, play a role in the treatment of small-cell lung cancer. Chemotherapy is particularly important in this disease since surgery and radiotherapy have not proven to be satisfactory treatment. Single agent therapy (9) have given way to combination regimens, many of which include nitrosoureas, primarily CCNU. Common nitrosourea-containing regimens include cyclophosphamide, methotrexate and CCNU, and methotrexate, adriamycin, CCNU and cyclophosphamide (MACC). A summary of studies by Bunn and Ihde (11) do not indicate any clear superiority for nitrosourea-containing combinations over non-nitroso containing combinations. Nitrosoureas do not appear to reduce the incidence of CNS relapse (10). Similar nitrosourea-containing combinations have been studied in non-small cell lung cancer. Unfortunately, there appears to be little long-term patient benefit from such treatment (18).

The nitrosoureas have been widely used in the treatment of gastrointestinal cancers. The activity of BCNU and CCNU as single agents against upper gastrointestinal tract cancer is low although the combination of BCNU and 5-fluorouracil for gastric cancer offers superior response rates and survival compared to either drug alone (58). BCNU is now little used in therapy of gastric cancer having been replaced by MeCCNU (126). BCNU and MeCCNU as single agents have low activity against advanced colorectal cancer while combination of MeCCNU with 5-fluorouracil offers a response advantage over 5-fluorouracil alone, but no survival advantage (5). Other cancers where nitrosoureas may be of some benefit are previously untreated melanoma and myeloma where BCNU may be useful as a substitute for melphalan as initial treatment (126).

Streptozocin has a limited use in the treatment of pancreatic islet cell (beta and non-beta) carcinomas. It has some activity against carcinoid tumors but negligible activity against most other cancer types (126). Despite arguments based on physical and chemical properties of the drug and results in animal tumor models PCNU does not appear clinically to be a notably superior drug to other chloroethyl-nitrosoureas (28).

TOXICITY

Animals

The most dramatic and consistent toxicities of the chloroethylnitrosoureas in animals involve the bone marrow, lymphoid tissues, liver, kidney and gastrointestinal tract (14). Initially the drugs deplete several hematopoietic elements of the marrow and lymphoidal components of the spleen and nodes. Escalation of the dose leads to damage to the liver, first with congestion and later cirrhosis, and renal damage at comparable doses. Delayed hepatotoxicity is striking and severe. In general, toxicities reported in animals resemble those seen in man (Table 9). Pulmonary toxicity and encephalopathy reported with BCNU in man were not

Table 9. Comparison of toxicities of nitrosoureas in dog and man.

Drug	Gastrointestinal	Hepatic	Hematopoietic	Nervous	Renal	Pulmonary
BCNU	+(++)	+(+)	+(++)	(+)	+(+)	(+)
CCNU	+(++)	+	+(++)		+(+)	
Streptozocin	+(++)	(+)			+(++)	
Chlorozotocin	+(+)	+(+)	+(++)		+(+)	

+ Toxicity seen in dog, (++) Major toxicity seen in man, (+) Minor toxicity seen in man.
Data taken from Carter and Newman (14); Guarino (34); Weiss and Issell (126); MacDonald *et al.* (72); Hoth and Duque-Hammershaimb (47).

however, seen in preclinical toxicology studies. BCNU, CCNU and MeCCNU are almost equitoxic in mouse (128) while PCNU is less toxic (28).

Man

When the dose of nitrosourea is expressed in terms of body surface area (mg/m^2) rather than weight, thus permitting an interspecies comparison (27), man exhibits the same or slightly less sensitivity to the toxic effects of nitrosoureas than mouse, dog or monkey (Table 10). Administration of the chloroethylnitrosoureas BCNU, CCNU and MeCCNU to man is associated with a number of acute toxicities including nausea and vomiting, and myelosuppression (thrombocytopenia and leukopenia). Myelosuppression is the dose-limiting toxicity and is delayed with nadirs 4 to 6 weeks after treatment (72, 126). Leukopenia and thrombocytopenia may be protracted, particularly in patients who received extensive prior chemotherapy (15). The methyl nitrosourea streptozocin does not cause myelosuppression and its dose-limiting toxicity is renal tubular toxicity (125).

Nitrosourea therapy can lead to less frequent chronic toxicities in man which appear more related to the total dose of nitrosourea rather than to time of exposure. An example is pulmonary toxicity observed following chronic administration of BCNU (72, 108, 127). This toxicity is characterized by dyspnea, tachypnea, reduced pulmonary function and pulmonary fibrosis. The reported incidence of BCNU pulmonary toxicity varies but approximates between 20% and 30% of patients receiving high doses of drug. The cumulative dose of BCNU producing pulmonary toxicity is 1.2 to $1.5 \, g/m^2$ and time from initial therapy to toxicity can

be several months to 3 years. There have been a few reports of pulmonary toxicity in patients receiving MeCCNU and chlorozotocin, but no reports of pulmonary toxicity associated with CCNU or streptozocin. With the exception of the dose-limiting renal toxicity secondary to therapy with streptozocin (125) renal toxicity with clinically used nitrosoureas is unusual (72). In a series of 857 patients receiving MeCCNU reviewed by Nichols and Moertel (89) only 4 (0.5%) exhibited drug associated nephrotoxicity. Three of these 4 patients had received more than $1 \, g/m^2$ MeCCNU and duration of therapy was more than 15 months. Renal toxicity has been reported in 35% of pediatric brain tumor patients receiving doses of MeCCNU greater than $1.5 \, g/m^2$ (38). Renal toxicity has also been associated with administration of BCNU, CCNU and chlorozotocin, although at very low incidence. Two other unusual toxicities of nitrosoureas are encephalopathy and optic neuritis (72, 126). Encephalopathy has only been reported at extraordinarily high doses ($> 1.2 \, g/m^2$) of BCNU in preparation for bone marrow transplantation while optic neuritis has not been unequivocably demonstrated to be associated with nitrosourea therapy. Of growing concern are reports that nitrosoureas, particularly MeCCNU are leukemogenic in man. There are a number of reports in which patients have been diagnosed with acute non-lymphocytic leukemia at least two years after diagnosis of primary malignant disease. All patients received high cumulative doses of nitrosoureas or extensive combined dose modality therapy with radiation or other chemotherapy and nitrosoureas (72).

The major toxicities of PCNU are similar to those of the chloroethylnitrosoureas, although perhaps it is less emetogenic. In contrast to findings in animals PCNU is relatively more toxic than BCNU in man and only about one-half as

Table 10. Toxicity ratios for man compared to various animal species.

Drug	Schedule[d]	Route	Toxicity ratio		
			Man/mouse[c]	Man/dog[d]	Man/monkey[d]
BCNU	Single dose	i.v.	2.1	0.9	0.6
CCNU	Single dose	p.o.	0.7	3.2	5.4
MeCCNU	Single dose	p.o.	1.5	1.8	1.5
Streptozocin	Daily × 5	i.v.	–	7.8	–

Data taken from Goldsmith *et al.* (32).
[a] Dose schedules are shown for man; where equivalent animal dose schedules were not available appropriate toxic doses were calculated for the human dose schedule.
[b] I.P. in mouse is considered the same as i.v. in human. Dose comparisons are made in mg/m^2.
[c] Toxicity ratio = maximum tolerated dose in man/LD_{10} in mouse.
[d] Toxicity ratio = maximum tolerated dose in man/toxic dose low in dog or monkey.

much can be administered (28, 95). Chlorozotocin was originally developed because of evidence in mice of a lack of myelosuppression. This has not been confirmed by studies in man where chlorozotocin demonstrates all of the major toxicities of the other chloroethylnitrosoureas (47). The dose-limiting toxicity of the remaining chloroethylnitrosoureas that have been used clinically, namely ACNU, GANU and MCNU, is myelosuppression (91).

CONCLUSIONS

An attempt has been made in this chapter to compare and contrast the distribution and metabolism of different nitrosoureas, together with their toxicity and antitumor activity, in animals and man. Physical properties of the nitrosoureas play a large role in determining their biological activity. However, distribution and metabolism can also influence biological activity. Extensive metabolism of the nitrosoureas has been demonstrated *in vitro* and *in vivo* for animals, but their is much less evidence that nitrosoureas are extensively metabolized in man. Studies in animals have shown that concomitantly administered drugs can modify the metabolism of nitrosoureas and alter their antitumor activity. It is not known if these findings can be extrapolated to man but they are important because of the implications for drug interactions and modulation of therapeutic activity. There is not much difference, qualitatively or quantitatively in the toxicities observed with nitrosoureas in animals or man. Man may be somewhat less sensitive to nitrosourea toxicity but exhibits all the major toxicities seen in animals. Delayed myelosuppression is the principal dose-limiting toxicity of all nitrosoureas, except streptozocin. Despite the promising activity of nitrosoureas in animals against a wide range of tumors their impact on the treatment of human cancer has been relatively modest (126). The lipid solubility of nitrosoureas allows their entry into brain and BCNU and CCNU favorably affect the course of human brain tumors, but only in association with whole brain irradiation. As sole therapy for brain tumor the nitrosoureas so far evaluated provide no survival benefit. The nitrosoureas can be useful for treatment of other cancers, primarily as a reasonable substitute for other drugs in combination regimens when there are concerns about specific side effects or means of administration. It remains to be seen whether new nitrosourea derivatives will exhibit greater antitumor acitivity than those tested so far in man.

ACKNOWLEDGEMENTS

The excellent secretarial assistance of Ms Wanda Rhodes in preparing this manuscript is gratefully acknowledged.

REFERENCES

1. Adolphe AB, Glasofer EP, Troetel WM, Ziegenfuss J, Stambaugh JE, Weiss AJ, Manthei RW: Fate of streptozotocin (NSC-85988) in patients with advanced cancer. *Cancer Chemother Rep* 59: 547, 1975
2. Alley MC, Powis G, Appel PL, Kooistra KL, Lieber MM: Activation and inactivation of cancer chemotherapeutic agents by rat hepatocytes cocultured with human tumor cell lines. *Cancer Res* 44: 549, 1984
3. Babson JR, Abell NS, Reed DJ: Protective role of glutathione redox cycle against adriamycin-mediated toxicity in isolated hepatocytes. *Biochem Pharmacol* 30: 2299, 1981
4. Babson JR, Reed DJ: Inactivation of glutathione reductase by 2-chloroethylnitrosourea-derived isocyanates. *Biochem Biophys Res Commun* 83: 754, 1978
5. Baker LH, Vaitkevicius VK, Gehan E: Randomized prospective trial company 5-fluorouracil (NSC-19893) to 5-fluorouracil and methyl-CCNU (NSC-95441) in advanced gastrointestinal cancer. *Cancer Treat Rep* 60: 733, 1976
6. Barker M, Hoshino T, Gurcay O, Wilson CB, Nielsen SL, Downie R, Eliason J: Development of an animal brain tumor model and its response to therapy with 1,3-bis(2-chloroethyl)-1-nitrosourea. *Cancer Res* 33: 976, 1973
7. Bhuyan BK, Kuentzel SL, Gray LG, Fraser TJ, Wallach D, Neil GL: Tissue distribution of streptozocin (NSC-85998). *Cancer Chemother Rep* 58: 157, 1974
8. Bradley MO, Sharkey NA, Kohn KW: Mutagenicity and cytotoxicity of various nitrosoureas in V-79 Chinese hamster cells. *Cancer Res* 40: 2719, 1980
9. Broder LE, Cohen MH, Selawry OS: Treatment of bronchogenic carcinoma II small cell. *Cancer Treat Rev* 4: 219, 1977
10. Bunn PA: Nitrosourea-containing combinations in small cell lung cancer. In: *Nitrosoureas: Current Status and New Developments*, Chapter 18, pp. 233–244. Edited by AW Prestayko, ST Crooke, LH Baker, SK Carter, PS Schein. Academic Press, New York, 1981
11. Bunn PA, Ihde DC: In: *Lung Cancer: Advances in Research and Treatment*. Edited by WL McGuire. Martinus Nijhoff, Boston, 1981
12. Caddy B, Idowu OR, Stuart JF: A high pressure liquid chromatographic procedure for monitoring 1-(2-chloroethyl)-3-(4-*trans*-methylcyclohexyl)-1-nitrosourea levels in body fluids. *Therap Drug Mont* 4: 389, 1982
13. Carter SK: The clinical evaluation of analogues. IV. Nitrosoureas. *Recent Results in Cancer Res* 70: 119, 1980
14. Carter SK, Newman JW: Nitrosoureas: 1,3-bis(2-chloroethyl)-1-nitrosourea (NSC-409962, BCNU) and 1-(2-chloroethyl)-3-cyclohexyl-1-nitrosourea (NSC-79037, CCNU). *Clinical Brochure Cancer Chemother Rep* Part 3: 1, 115, 1968
15. Chabner BA, Myers CE: Clinical pharmacology of cancer chemotherapy. In: *Cancer Principles and Practice of Oncology*, Chapter 9, pp. 156–197. Edited by VT DeVita Jr, S Hellman, SA Rosenberg. Lippincott Co., Philadelphia, 1982
16. Cheng CJ, Fujimura S, Grunberger D, Weinstein IB: Interaction of 1-(2-chloroethyl)-3-cyclohexyl-1-nitrosourea (NSC-79037) with nucleic acids and proteins *in vivo* and *in vitro*. *Cancer Res* 32: 22, 1972
17. Clemens MR, Frank H, Remmer H, Waller HD: Vinylchloride: Decomposition product of BCNU *in vivo* and *in vitro*. *Cancer Chemother Pharm* 10: 70, 1982
18. Cohen MH: In: *Nitrosoureas: Current Status and New Developments*, Chapter 19, pp. 245–258. Edited by AW Prestayko, ST Crooke, LH Baker, SK Carter, PS Schein. Academic Press, New York, 1981
19. Colvin M, Brundett RB, Cowens JW, Jardine I, Ludlum DB: A chemical basis for the antitumor activity of chloroethylnitrosoureas. *Biochem Pharmacol* 25: 695, 1976
20. Cooper MR, Pajak TF, Nissen NI, Stutzman L, Brunner K, Cuttner J, Falkson G, Grunwald H, Bank A, Leone L, Seligman BR, Silver RT, Weiss RB, Haurani F, Blom J, Spurr CL, Glidewell OJ, Gottlieb AJ, Holland JF: A new effective four-drug combination of CCNU (1-[2-chloroethyl]-3-cyclohexyl-1-nitrosourea) (NSC-79038), vinblastine, prednisone and procarbazine for treatment of advanced Hodgkin's disease. *Cancer* 46: 654, 1980

21. DeVita VT, Denham C, Davidson JD, Oliverio VT: The physiologic disposition of the carcinostatic 1,3-bis(2-chloroethyl)-1-nitrosourea (BCNU) in man and animals. *Clin Pharm Ther* 8: 566, 1967

22. DeVita VT Jr, Hellman S: Hodgkin's disease and non-Hodgkin's lymphomas. In: *Cancer: Principles and Practice of Oncology*, Chapter 35, pp. 1331–1401. Edited by VT DeVita Jr, S Hellman, SA Rosenberg. Lippincott Co., Philadelphia, 1982

23. DeVita VT, Serpick AA, Carbonne PP: Combination chemotherapy in the treatment of advanced Hodgkin's disease. *Ann Intern Med* 73: 881, 1970

24. Ewig RAG, Kohn KW: DNA-protein cross-linking and DNA interstrand cross-linking by haloethylnitrosoureas in L1210 cells. *Cancer Res* 38: 3197, 1978

25. Farmer PB, Foster AB, Jarman M, Oddy MR, Reed DJ: Synthesis, metabolism and antitumor activity of ducterated analogues of 1-(2-chloroethyl)-3-cyclohexyl-1-nitrosourea. *J Med Chem* 21: 514, 1978

26. Franza BR, Oeschger NS, Oeschger MP, Schein PS: Mutagenic activity of nitrosourea agents. *J Natl Cancer Inst* 65: 149, 1980

27. Freireich EJ, Gehan EA, Rall DP, Schmidt LH, Skipper HE: Quantitative comparison of toxicity and anticancer agents in mouse, rat, hamster, dog, monkey and man. *Cancer Chemother Rep* 50: 219, 1966

28. Friedman MA: Phase I and Phase II studies of PCNU. In *Nitrosoureas: Current Status and New Developments*, Chapter 32, pp. 379–398. Edited by AW Prestayko, ST Crooke, LH Baker, SK Carter, PS Schein. Academic Press, New York, 1981

29. Glick JH, Barnes JM, Bakemeier RF, Prosnite LR, Bennett JM, Neiman RS, Costello W, Orlow EL: Treatment of advanced Hodgkin's disease: 10-year experience in the Eastern Cooperative Oncology Group. *Cancer Treat Rep* 66: 855, 1982

30. Godenéche D, Madelmont JC, Moreau MF, Montoloy D, Plagne R: Disposition of the carcinostatic agent 1-(2-chloroethyl)-3-[1'-(5'-*p*-nitrobenzyl 2',3'-isopropylidene)-α,β-D-ribofuranosyl]-1-nitrosourea in animals. *Cancer Res* 40: 3351, 1980

31. Goldin A, Venditti JM, MacDonald JS, Muggia FM, Henrey JE, DeVita VT; Current results of the screening program at the division of cancer treatment, National Cancer Institute. *Europ J Cancer* 7: 129, 1981

32. Goldsmith MA, Slavik M, Carter K: Quantitative prediction of drug toxicity in humans from toxicology in small and large animals. *Cancer Res* 35: 1354, 1975

33. Gottlieb AJ, Bloomfield CD, Glickman AS, Nissen NI, Cooper MR, Pajak TF, Holland JF: In: *Nitrosoureas: Current Status and New Developments*, Chapter 14, pp. 181–197. Edited by AW Prestayko, ST Crooke, LH Baker, SK Carter, PS Schein. Academic Press, New York, 1981

34. Guarino AM: Pharmacologic and toxicologic studies of anticancer drug: Of sharks, mice and men (and dogs and monekys). *Methods Cancer Res* 17: 91, 1979

35. Hara M, Takeuchi K: Pharmacokinetic analysis of ACNU in brain tumors. *No To Shinkei* 31: 1289, 1979

36. Harada K, Kiya K, Okamato H, Uozomi T: Pharmacokinetics of water soluble nitrosoureas, ACNU and MCNU, used in treatment of brain tumors in humans. *Proc 13th Int Cancer Congress*, p. 55. Seattle, Washington, 1982

37. Harada K, Kiya K, Uozumi T: Pharmacokinetics of a new water-soluble nitrosourea derivative (ACNU) in human gliomas. *Surg Neurol* 15: 410, 1981

38. Harmon WE, Cohen HS, Schneeberger EE, Grape WG: Chronic renal failure in children treated with methyl CCNU. *N Engl J Med* 300: 1200, 1979

39. Heal JM, Fox P, Schein PS: A structure-activity study of

40. Helman LJ, Louie A, Slavik M: Chlorozotocin (NSC-178248) Clinical Brochure, Investigational Drug Branch, Cancer Therapy Evaluation Program, Division of Cancer Treatment, National Cancer Institute, August, 1976

41. Hill DL: N,N'-bis(2-chloroethyl)-N-nitrosourea (BCNU), a substrate for glutathione (GSH) S-transferase. *Proc Amer Assoc Cancer Res* 17: 52, 1976

42. Hill DL, Kirk MC, Struck RF: Microsomal metabolism of nitrosoureas. *Cancer Res* 35: 296, 1975

43. Hilton J, Walker MD: Hydroxylation of 1-(2-chloroethyl)-3-cyclo-hexyl-1-nitrosourea. *Biochem Pharmacol* 24: 2153, 1975

44. Hilton MD, Walker J: Nitrosourea pharmacodynamics in relation to the central nervous system. *Cancer Treat Rep* 60: 725, 1976

45. Hirst DG, Brown JM, Hazelhurst JL: Enhancement of CCNU cytotoxicity by misonidazole. Possible therapeutic gain. *Br J Cancer* 46: 109, 1982

46. Hochberg FH, Poletti CE, Krull IS, Strauss J: Analysis and distribution of 1,3-bis(2-chloroethyl)-1-nitrosourea (BCNU) in biological specimens. *Neurosurg* 13: 230, 1983

47. Hoth DF, Duque-Hammershaimb L: Chlorozotocin: Clinical trials. In: *Nitrosoureas: Current Status and New Developments*, Chapter 33. Edited by AW Prestayko, ST Crooke, LH Baker, SK Carter, PS Schein. Academic Press, New York, 1981

48. Johnston TP, McCaleb GS, Clayton SD, Frye JL, Krauth CA, Montgomery JA: Synthesis of analogues of N-(2-chloroethyl)-N'-(*trans*-4-methylcyclohexyl)-N-nitrosourea for evaluation as anticancer agents. *J Med Chem* 20: 279, 1977

49. Johnston TP, McCaleb GS, Montgomery JA: Synthesis of chlorozotocin, the 2-chloroethyl analog of the anticancer antibiotic streptozotocin. *J Med Chem* 18: 104, 1975

50. Johnston TP, McCaleb GS, Montgomery JA: Synthesis and biologic evaluation of major metabolites of N-(2-chloroethyl)-N'-cyclohexyl-N-nitrosoures. *J Med Chem* 18: 634, 1975

51. Johnston TP, McCaleb GS, Opliger PS, Montgomery JA: The synthesis of potential anticancer agents XXXVI. N-nitrosoureas. II. Haloalkyl derivatives. *J Med Chem* 9, 892, 1966

52. Kann HE Jr: Carbamoylating activity of nitrosoureas in the body. In: *Nitrosoureas: Current Status and New Developments*, Chapter 8, pp. 95–105. Edited by AW Prestayko, ST Crooke, LH Baker, SK Carter, PS Schein. Academic Press, New York, 1981

53. Kann HE Jr, Schott MA, Petkas A: Effect of structure and chemical activity of nitrosoureas to inhibit DNA repair. *Cancer Res* 40: 50, 1980

54. Karuananayake EH, Hearse DJ, Mellows G: The metabolic fate and elimination of streptozotocin. *Biochem Soc Trans* 3: 410, 1975

55. Klubes P, Miller HG, Cerna I, Trevithick J: Alterations in the toxicity of antitumor activity of methyl-CCNU in mice following pretreatment with either phenobarbital or SKF525A. *Cancer Treat Rep* 63: 1901, 1979

56. Kohn KW: Interstrand cross-linking of DNA by 1,3-bis(2-chloroethyl)-1-nitrosourea and other 1-(2-haloethyl)-1-nitrosoureas. *Cancer Res* 37, 1450, 1977

57. Kohn KW, Erickson LC, Laurent G, Ducore J, Sharkey N, Ewig RA: DNA crosslinking and the origin of sensitivity to chloroethylnitrosoureas. In: *Nitrosoureas: Current Status and New Developments*, Chapter 6, pp. 69–83. Edited by AW Prestayko, ST Crooke, LH Baker, SK Carter, PS Schein. Academic Press, New York, 1981

58. Kovach JS, Moertel CG, Schutt AJ, Hahn RG, Reitemeier J: A controlled study of combined 1,3-bis(2-chloroethyl)-1-

nitrosourea and 5-fluorouracil therapy for advanced gastric and pancreatic cancer. *Cancer* 33: 563, 1974

59. Lee FYF, Workman P: Modification of CCNU pharmacokinetics by misondazole – A major mechanism of chemosensitization in mice. *Br J Cancer* 47: 659, 1983

60. Levin VA: Clinical pharmacology of nitrosoureas. In: *Nitrosoureas: Current Status and New Developments*, Chapter 30, pp. 171–180. Edited by AW Prestayko, ST Crooke, LH Baker, SK Carter, PS Schein. Academic Press, New York, 1981

61. Levin VA: Chemotherapy of recurrent brain tumors. In: *Nitrosoureas: Current Status and New Developments*, Chapter 20, pp. 259–268.Edited by AW Prestayko, ST Crooke, LH Baker, SK Carter, PS Schein. Academic Press, New York, 1981

62. Levin VA, Kabra P: Effectiveness of the nitrosoureas as a function of their lipid solubility in the chemotherapy of experimental rat brain tumors. *Cancer Chemother Rep* 58: 787, 1974

63. Levin VA, Stearns J, Byrd A, Finn A, Weinkam RJ: Effect of phenobarbital pretreatment on antitumor activity of 1,3-bis-(2-chloroethyl)-1-nitrosoureas (BCNU), 1-(2-chloroethyl)-3-cyclohexyl-1-nitrosourea (CCNU) and 1-(2-chloroethyl)-3-(2,6-dioxo-3-piperidyl)-1-nitrosourea (PCNU) and on the plasma pharmacokinetics and biotransformation of BCNU. *J Pharmacol Exp Ther* 208: 1, 1979

64. Levin VA, Weinkam RJ, Hoffman W, Wilson CB: Pharmacokinetics of BCNU in humans. *Proc Amer Assoc Cancer Res* 18: 76, 1977

65. Levin VA, Wilson GB: Chemotherapy: The agents in current use. *Semin Oncol* 2: 63, 1975

66. Levin VA, Hoffman W, Weinkam RJ: Pharmacokinetics of BCNU in man: A preliminary study of 20 patients. *Cancer Treat Rep* 62: 1305, 1978

67. Levin VA, Liu J, Weinkam RJ: Comparative pharmacokinetics of 1-(2-chloroethyl)-3-(2,6-dioxo-1-piperidyl)-1-nitrosourea in rats and patients and extrapolation to clinical trials. *Cancer Res* 41: 3475, 1981

68. Lin HS: Quoted in Weinkam RJ, Lin HS (1982) Chloroethylnitrosourea cancer chemotherapeutic agents. *Adv Pharmacol Chemother* 19: 1, 1980

69. Lin HS, Weinkam RJ: Metabolism of 1,3-bis(2-chloroethyl)-1-nitrosourea by rat hepatic microsomes. *J Med Chem* 24: 761, 1981

70. Lown JW, McLaughlin LW, Chang YM: Mechanism of action of 2-haloethylnitrosoureas on DNA and its relation to their antileukemic properties. *Bioorganic Chem* 7: 97, 1978

71. Ludlum DB, Tong WP: Modification of DNA and RNA bases. In: *Nitrosoureas: Current Status and New Developments*. Edited by AW Prestayko, ST Crooke, LH Baker, SK Carter, PS Schein. Academic Press, New York, 1981

72. MacDonald JS, Weiss RB, Poster D, Hammershaimb L: Subacute and chronic toxicities associated with nitrosourea therapy. In: *Nitrosoureas: Current Status and New Developments*, Chapter 11, pp. 145–154. Edited by AW Prestayko, ST Crooke, LH Baker, SK Carter, PS Schein. Academic Press, New York, 1981

73. Maker HS, Weiss C, Brannan TS: The effects of BCNU (1,3-bis-(2-chloroethyl)-1-nitrosourea) and CCNU (1-(2-chloroethyl)-3-cyclohexyl-1-nitrosourea) on glutathione reductase and other enzymes in mouse tissue. *Res Comm Chem Path Pharm* 40: 355, 1983

74. Maurice P, Glidewell G, Jacquillat C, Silver RT, Carey R, TenPas A, Cornell CJ, Burningham RA, Nissen NI, Holland JF: Comparison of methyl-CCNU and CCNU in patients with advanced forms of Hodgkin's disease, lymphosarcoma and reticulum cell sarcoma. *Cancer* 41: 1658, 1978

75. May HE, Boose R, Reed DJ: Hydroxylation of the carcinostatic 1-(2-chloroethyl)-3-cyclohexyl-1-nitrosourea (CCNU) by rat liver microsomes. *Biochem Biophys Res Commun* 57:

426, 1974

76. May HE, Boose R, Reed DJ: Microsomal monooxygenation of the carcinostatic (1-2-chloroethyl)-3-cyclohexyl-1-nitrosourea. Synthesis and identification of *cis* and *trans* monohydroxylated product. *Biochem* 14: 4723, 1975

77. May HE, Kohlhepp SJ, Boose RB, Reed DJ: Synthesis and identification of products derived from the metabolism of the carcinostatic 1-(2-chloroethyl)-3-(*trans*-4-methylcyclohexyl)-1-nitrosourea by rat liver microsomes. *Cancer Res* 39: 762, 1979

78. McConnell WR, Suling WJ, Rice LS, Shannon M, Hill DL: Reduction of glutathione levels in livers of mice treated with N,N′-bis(2-chloroethyl)-N-nitrosourea. *Cancer Chemother Pharmacol* 2: 221, 1979

79. Merker PC, Wodinsky I, Geran RI: Review of selected experimental brain tumor models used in chemotherapy experiments. *Cancer Chemother Rep* 59: 729, 1975

80. Mhatre RM, Green D, Panasci LC, Fox P, Woolley PV, Schein PS: Pharmacologic disposition of chlorozotocin in mice. *Cancer Treat Rep* 62: 1145, 1978

81. Montgomery JA: Chemistry and structure-activity studies of nitrosoureas. *Cancer Treat Rep* 60: 651, 1976

82. Montgomery JA: The development of the nitrosoureas: A study in congener synthesis. In: *Nitrosoureas: Current Status and New Developments*, Chapter 0, pp. 3–8. Edited by AW Prestayko, ST Crooke, LH Baker, SK Carter, PS Schein. Academic Press, New York, 1981

83. Montgomery JA, Mayo JG, Hansch C: Quantitative structure-activity relationships on anticancer agents. Activity of selected nitrosoureas against a solid tumor, the Lewis lung carcinoma. *J Med Chem* 17: 477, 1974

84. Montgomery JA, McCaleb GS, Johnston TP, Mayo JG, Laster WR: Inhibition of solid tumors by nitrosoureas. 1. Lewis lung carcinoma. *J Med Chem* 20: 291, 1977

85. Mori T, Katsuyoshi M, Katakura R: A consideration on pharmacokinetics of a new water-soluble antitumor nitrosourea, ACNU, in patients with malignant brain tumor. *No To Shinkei* 31: 601, 1979

86. Muller PJ, Tator CH, Bloom M: The effect of phenobarbital on the toxicity and tumoricidal activity of CCNU in a murine brain tumor model. *J Neurosurg* 52: 359, 1980

87. Nagashima T, Matsutani M, Kohono T: Effects of phenobarbital on the metabolism of ACNU *in vivo*. *No To Shinkei* 35: 677, 1983

88. Nakajima O, Yoshida Y, Kubota T, Takemasa Y, Koyama Y: Quantitative determination of 1-(2-chloroethyl)-3-(beta-D-glucopyranosyl)-1-nitrosourea in blood and urine of man. *J Chromatogr* 229: 481, 1982

89. Nichols WC, Moertel CG: Nephrotoxicity of methyl-CCNU. *N Engl J Med* 301: 1181, 1979

90. Nissen NI, Pajak TF, Glidewell O, Pedersen-Bjergaard J, Stutzman L, Falkson G, Cuttner J, Blom J, Leone L, Sawitsky A, Coleman M, Haurani F, Spurr CL, Harley JB, Seligman JB, Cornell C, Henry P, Senn H, Brunner K, Martz G, Maurice P, Bank A, Shapiro L, James GW, Holland JF: A comparative study of BCNU containing 4-drug program versus MOPP versus 3-drug combinations in advanced Hodgkin's disease. *Cancer* 43: 31, 1979

91. Ogawa M: Current status of nitrosoureas under development in Japan. In: *Nitrosoureas: Current Status and New Developments*, Chapter 34, pp. 399–499. Edited by AW Prestayko, ST Crooke, LH Baker, SK Carter, PS Schein. Academic Press, New York, 1981

92. Oliverio VT, Vietzke M, Williams MK, Adamson RH: The absorption, distribution, excretion and biotransformation of the carcinostatic 1-(2-chloroethyl)-3-cyclohexyl-1-nitrosourea in animals. *Cancer Res* 30: 1330, 1970

93. Panasci L, Fox PA, Schein PS: Structure-activity studies of methylnitrosourea antitumor agents with reduced bone marrow toxicity. *cancer Res* 37: 3321, 1977

94. Panasci LC, Green D, Nagourney R, Fox P, Schein PS: A structure-activity analysis of chemical and biological parameters of chloroethylnitrosourea in mice. *Cancer Res* 37: 2615, 1977
95. Poster DS, Penta JS, Bruno S: A new nitrosourea in clinical oncology. *Amer J Clin Oncol* 5: 9, 1982
96. Potter DW, Reed DJ: Loss of methylcyclohexyl stereospecificity during cytochrome P-450-dependent monooxygenation. In: *Microsomes and Drug Oxidations, and Chemical Carcinogenesis*, pp. 371–374. Edited by MJ Coon, AH Conney. Academic Press, New York, 1980
97. Potter DW, Reed DJ: Denitrosation of carcinostatic nitrosoureas by purified NADPH cytochrome P-450 reductase and rat liver microsomes to yield nitric oxide under anaerobic conditions. *Arch Biochem Biophys* 216: 158, 1982
98. Potter DW, Reed DJ: Involvement of FMN and phenobarbital cytochrome P-450 in stimulating a one-electron reductive denitrosation of 1-(2-chloroethyl)-3-(cyclohexyl)-1-nitrosourea catalyzed by NADPH-cytochrome P-450 reductase. *J Biol Chem* 258: 6096, 1983
99. Rahman A, Luc PVT, Schein PS, Woolley PV: Pharmacological disposition of 1-(2-chloroethyl)-3-(2,6-diozo-3-piperidyl)-1-nitrosourea in mice. *Cancer Res* 44: 149, 1984
100. Reed DJ: Metabolism of nitrosoureas. In: *Nitrosoureas: Current Status and New Developments*, Chapter 15, pp. 51–67. Edited by AW Prestayko, ST Crooke, LH Baker, SK Carter, PS Schein. Academic Press, New York, 1981
101. Reed DJ, May HE: Alkylation and carbamylation intermediates from the carcinostatic 1-(2-chloroethyl)-3-cyclohexyl-1-nitrosourea (CCNU). *Life Sci* 16: 1263, 1975
102. Reed DJ, May HE: Formation of alkylation and carbamoylation intermediates and cytochrome P-450 catalyzed monooxygenation of the 2-chloroethylnitrosourea CCNU and methyl-CCNU. In: *Microsomes and Drug Oxidations*, pp. 680–687. Edited by V Ulrich, I Roots, A Hildebrandt, RW Estabrook, AH Conney. Pergamon, Oxford, 1977
103. Russo R, Bartosek I, Piazza E, Santi AM, Libretti A, Garattini S: Differential pulse polarographic determinations of BCNU pharmacokinetics in patients with lung cancer. *Cancer Treat Rep* 65: 555, 1981
104. Schabel FM: Nitrosoureas: A review of experimental antitumor activity. *Cancer Treat Rep* 60: 665, 1976
105. Schabel FM, Johnston TP, McCaleb GS, Montgomery JA, Luster WR, Skipper HE: Experimental evaluation of potential anticancer agents. VIII. Effects of certain nitrosoureas and intracerebral L1210 leukemia. *Cancer Res* 23: 725, 1963
106. Schein PS: Nitrosoureas. In: *Cancer and Chemotherapy*, Vol. III, Chapter 3, pp. 37–48. Edited by ST Crooke, AW Prestayko. Academic Press, 1981
107. Selawry OS, Hansen HH: Superiority of CCNU (1-(2-chloroethyl)-3-cyclohexyl-1-nitrosourea) over BCNU (1,3-bis(2-chloroethyl)-1-nitrosourea) in treatment of advanced Hodgkin's disease. *Proc Am Assoc Cancer Res* 13: 46, 1972
108. Selker RG, Jacobs SA, Moore PB, Wald M, Fisher ER, Coehn M, Bellot P: BCNU (1-3-bis(2-chloroethyl)-1-nitrosourea) induced pulmonary fibrosis. *Neurosurgery* 7: 560, 1980
109. Siemann DW: The effect of pretreatment with phenobarbitone or SKF525A on the toxicity and antitumor activity of CCNU. *Cancer Treat Rep* 67: 259, 1983
110. Smith RG, Cheung LK, Feun LG, Loo TL: Determination of 1-(2-chloroethyl)-3-(2,6-dioxo-3-piperidyl)-1-nitrosourea in plasma by negative chemical ionization mass spectrometry. *Biomed Mass Spectrom* 10: 404, 1983
111. Suling WJ, Rice LS, Shannon WM: Increased mutagenicity of chloroethylnitrosoureas in the presence of a rat liver S9 microsome mixture. *J Natl Cancer Inst* 70: 767, 1983
112. Talcott RE, Levin VA: Glutathione-dependent denitrosation of N,N'-bis(2-chloroethyl)-N-nitrosourea (BCNU). Nitrite release catalyzed by mouse liver cytosol *in vitro*. *Drug Metab Disp* 11: 175, 1983
113. Tong WP, Kirk MC, Ludlum DB: Mechanism of action of the nitrosoureas – V. Formation of O^6-(2-fluoroethyl)-guanine and its probable role in the crosslinking of deoxyribonucleic acid. *Biochem Pharmacol* 32: 2011, 1983
114. Tong WP, Kohn KW, Ludlum DP: Modifications of DNA by different haloethylnitrosoureas. *Cancer Res* 42: 4460, 1982
115. Tong WP, Ludlum DP: Mechanisms of action of nitrosoureas – I. Role of fluoroethylcytidine in the reaction of bis-fluoroethyl nitrosourea with nucleic acid. *Biochem Pharmacol* 27: 77, 1978
116. Tong WP, Ludlum DP: Mechanism of action of nitrosoureas – III. Reaction of bis-chloroethylnitrosourea and bis-fluorethylnitrosourea with adenosine. *Biochem Pharmacol* 28: 1175, 1979
117. Twentyman P, Workman P: Effect of misonidazole or metronidazole pretreatment on the response of the RIF-1 mouse sarcoma to melphalan, cyclophosphamide, chlorambucil and CCNU. *Br J Cancer* 45: 447, 1982
118. Urtasun RC, Tanasichuk H, Fulton D, Raleigh J, Rabin HR, Turner R, Kozol D, Agboola O: Pharmacokinetic interaction of BCNU and misonidazole in humans. *Int J Rad Oncol Biol Phys* 8: 381, 1982
119. Walker MD: Nitrosoureas in central nervous system tumors. *Cancer Chemother Rep* Part 3, 4: 21, 1973
120. Walker MD, Alexander E, Hunt WE, MacCarty CS, Mahaley MS, Mealey J, Norrell HA, Owens G, Ransohoff J, Wilson CB, Gehan EA, Strike TA: Evaluation of BCNU and/or radiotherapy in the treatment of anaplastic gliomas. *J Neurosurg* 49: 333, 1978
121. Walker MD, Green SB, Byar DP, Alexander E, Batzdorf U, Brooks WH, Hunt WE, MacCarty CS, Mahley MS, Mealey J, Owens G, Ransohoft J, Robertson JT, Shapiro WR, Smith KR, Wilson CB, Strike TA: Randomized comparisons of radiotherapy and nitrosoureas for the treatment of malignant glioma after surgery. *N Engl J Med* 303: 1323, 1980
122. Weinkam RJ, Dolan ME: An analysis of 1-(2-chloroethyl)-1-nitrosourea activity at the cellular level. *J Med Chem* 26: 1656, 1983
123. Weinkam RJ, Lin HS: Chloroethylnitrosourea cancer chemotherapeutic agents. *Adv Pharmacol Chemother* 19: 1, 1982
124. Weinkam RJ, Liu TYJ, Lin HS: Protein mediated chemical reactions of chloroethylnitrosoureas. *Chem Biol Interact* 31: 167, 1980b
125. Weiss RB: Streptozocin: A review of its pharmacology, efficacy, and toxicity. *Cancer Treat Rep* 66: 427, 1982
126. Weiss RB, Issell BF: The nitrosoureas: carmustine (BCNU) and lomustine (CCNU). *Cancer Treat Rep* 9: 313, 1982
127. Weiss RB, Poster PS, Penta JS: The nitrosoureas and pulmonary toxicity. *Cancer Treat Rep* 8: 111, 1981
128. Wheeler GP, Bowdon BJ, Grimsley JA, Lloyd HH: Interrelationships of some chemical, physicochemical and biological activities of several 1-(2-haloethyl)-1-nitrosoureas. *Cancer Res* 34: 194, 1974
129. Wheeler GP, Johnston TP, Bowdon BJ, McCaleb GS, Hill DL, Montgomery JA: Comparison of the properties of metabolites of CCNU. *Biochem Pharmacol* 26: 2331, 1977
130. Woolley P, Luc V, Smyth A, Rahman A, Hoth D, Smith F, Schein PS: Phase I trial and pharmacology of 1-(2-chloroethyl)-3-(2,6-diozo-1-piperidyl)-1-nitrosourea (PCNU). *Proc Amer Soc Clin Oncol* 21: 336, 1980
131. Workman P, Twentyman PR: Enhancement by electron-affinic agents of the therapeutic effects of cytotoxic agents against the KHT tumor: structure-activity relationships. *Int J Radiat Oncol Biol Phys* 8: 623, 1982

9

TRIAZINE AND HYDRAZINE DERIVATIVES

GARTH POWIS

TRIAZINES

Background

Compounds containing the s-triazine moiety have long been of interest to cancer chemotherapists and, while hexamethylmelamine is currently the only triazine derivative in widespread clinical use, efforts continue to develop new s-triazine antitumor agents. The structures of some s-triazines with antitumor activity are shown in Fig. 1.

Triethylenemelamine (TEM) was the first s-triazine found to have antitumor activity against experimental tumors and leukemia in mice in 1950 (60). Clinical studies on triethylenemelamine were soon undertaken. The antitumor activity of triethylenemelamine was found to be similar to that of nitrogen mustard producing transitory responses in lymphomas, chronic lymphocytic leukemia and ovarian cancer (80, 91). Triethylenemelamine offered advantages over nitrogen mustard because it could be administered orally and had a lower incidence of acute side effects (73). Triethylenemelamine is not now used clinically. The synthesis of hexamethylmelamine (HMM) was first reported in 1951 (50) and it was introduced into clinical trial in 1965. Hexamethyl-

melamine has been found to be of use in combination with other drugs for the treatment of ovarian cancer, small cell carcinoma of the lung, breast cancer and lymphomas (47, 58). Due to its poor aqueous solubility hexamethylmelamine is administered orally. Attempts to develop a parenteral formulation of hexamethylmelamine as a complex with gentisic acid were unsuccessful (53). Recently, hexamethylmelamine hydrochloride has been reported to be well tolerated when given intravenously to dogs (49) although earlier studies using hexamethylmelamine formulated as the hydrochloride at pH 3 showed venous irritation and thrombophlebitis (57). A parenteral formulation of hexamethylmelamine in lipid used for parenteral nutrition has been described (3) and is currently in clinical trial. Pentamethylmelamine (PMM) was developed as a more water soluble analog of hexamethylmelamine and it can be given intravenously. Unfortunately pentamethylmelamine causes severe central nervous system and gastrointestinal toxicity which limits its clinical usefulness (67). Synthesis of a number of melamine analogs with antitumor activity have been reported (25) and one of them, N^2,N^4,N^6-trimethyl-N^2,N^4,N^6-trimethylolmelamine (TMTMM), is currently undergoing clinical trial. Melamine and all the methylmelamines exhibit

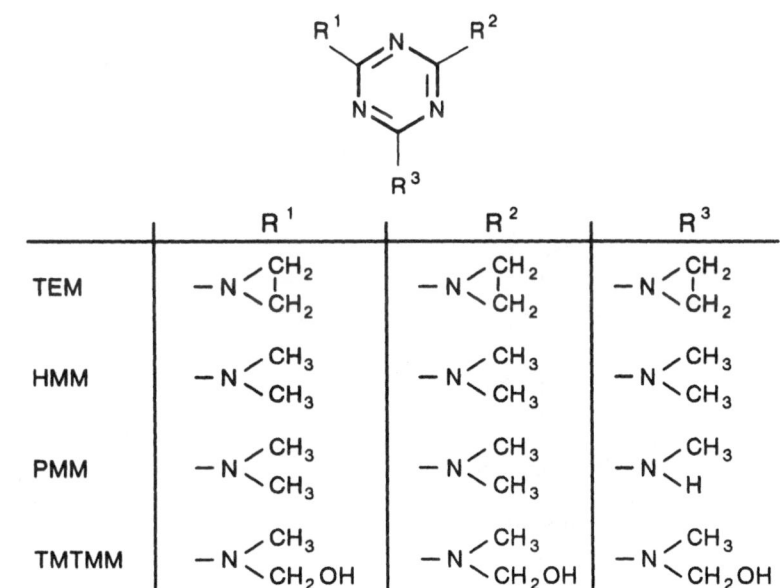

Figure 1. Structures of TEM, HMM, PMM and N^2,N^4,N^6-trimethyl-N^2,N^4,N^6-trimethylolmelamine (TMTMM).

113

P.V. Woolley (ed.), Cancer management in Man: Biological Response Modifiers, Chemotherapy, Antibiotics, Hyperthermia, Supporting Measures
© 1989. Kluwer Academic Publishers, Dordrecht.

chemosterilizing properties in houseflies and hexamethylmelamine in particular, received extensive study as a chemosterilant (13, 19).

Mechanism of action

Triethylenemelamine is a direct acting bifunctional alkylating agent and does not require metabolic activation (99). In this respect it differs from hexamethylmelamine and other methylmelamines which have little or no acute cytotoxic effect of their own on cells in culture. Acute cytotoxicity of the methylmelamines is greatly enhanced in the presence of a hepatic microsomal activating system (64, 82). The best available evidence suggests that hexamethylmelamine produces its antitumor activity by acting as an alkylating agent. Hexamethylmelamine is not, however, an alkylating agent itself and does not react with 4-(*p*-nitrobenzyl)pyridine (66, 99). Incubation of [^{14}C-ring]- or [^{14}C-methyl]-labeled hexamethylmelamine and pentamethylmelamine

with rat and mouse liver microsomes without NADPH results in no covalent binding, but when incubated with microsomes and NADPH there is covalent binding of radiolabel to microsomal macromolecules as well as to added DNA (6, 7). Administration of either [^{14}C-ring]- or [^{14}C-methyl]-moiety labeled hexamethylmelamine to mice results in binding of radiolabel to nucleic acids and/or proteins, in tumor and normal tissues (40, 83). Although it is tempting to speculate that the alkylating species formed during metabolism of hexamethylmelamine is also the species responsible for antitumor activity, other mechanisms might explain the antitumor activity. Hexamethylmelamine lacks cross-resistance with conventional alkylating agents (92) and is much less myelosuppressive than other alkylating agents (58). There are reports that prolonged exposure of tumor cells in culture to hexamethylmelamine results in cytotoxicity without the need for microsomal activation and without measurable metabolism of hexamethylmelamine (33, 81). The lack of cytotoxic activation of hexamethylmelamine by isolated hepatocytes co-cultured with tumor cells *in vitro*,

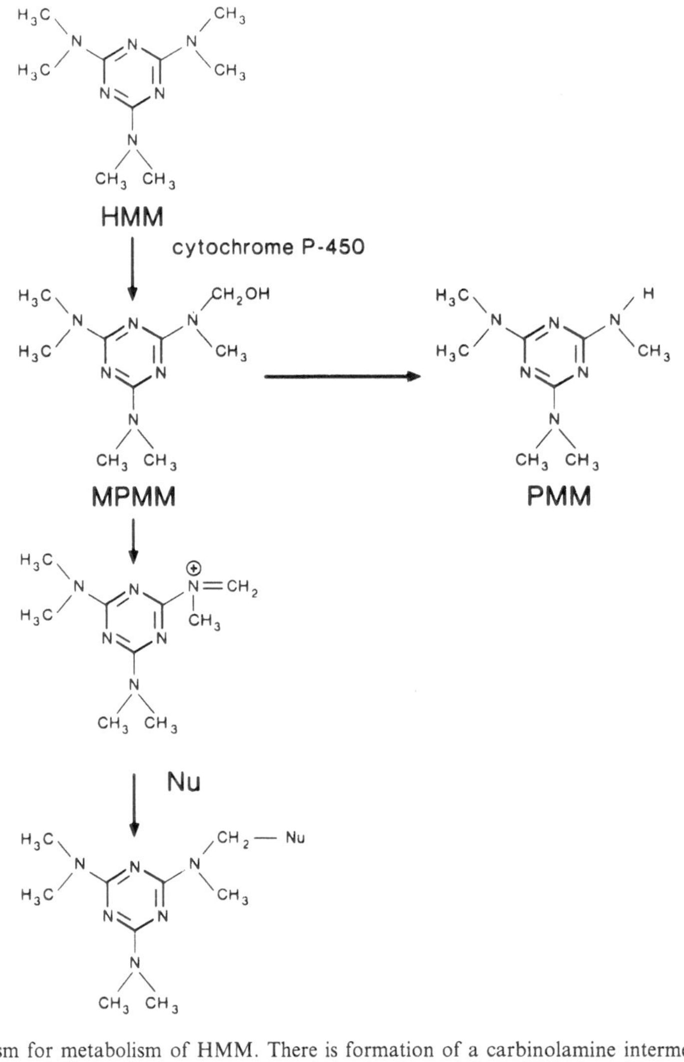

Figure 2. Suggested mechanism for metabolism of HMM. There is formation of a carbinolamine intermediate, N^2-monomethylolpentamethylmelamine, which preferentially breaks down to pentamethylmelamine and formaldehyde or forms a iminium ion which can react with cellular nucleophiles (from Ames *et al.* (7)).

where reactive metabolites have to diffuse out of the hepatocyte to reach the tumor cell as opposed to microsomal preparations where the reactive metabolite is formed in close contact with the tumor cell (21), also raise doubt that hepatic microsomal activation is essential for the antitumor activity of hexamethylmelamine. The possibility remains that the antitumor activity and alkylating properties of metabolically activated hexamethylmelamine are not related.

The identity of the alkylating species and the species responsible for antitumor activity, whether the same or different, are unknown. Formaldehyde, which is released during metabolism of hexamethylmelamine, is mildly cytotoxic but cannot be the species responsible for antitumor activity, since metabolism of trimethylmelamine which lacks antitumor activity produces plasma concentrations of formaldehyde similar to those produced by hexamethylmelamine (83). Furthermore, formaldehyde produces extensive DNA-protein cross-linking in L1210 cells at nontoxic concentrations and yet following treatment of L1210 cells with cytotoxic concentrations of microsomally activated hexamethylmelamine or pentamethylmelamine the frequency of DNA-protein cross-links is very low (79). N-methylolmelamines formed by metabolic C-hydroxylation of methylmelamines are the most likely candidates for the alkylating species. A pathway for alkylation by hexamethylmelamine via an N-methylol metabolite which could in turn form a reactive iminium ion is shown in Fig. 2 (7). The monomethylol metabolites of hexamethylmelamine, N^2-monomethylolpentamethylmelamine, is formed *in vitro* during metabolism of hexamethylmelamine (41) and methylol metabolites of methylmelamines have been detected *in vivo* (25, 84). N-methylolmelamines are more toxic than methylmelamines to tumor cells in culture (33, 81) and show antitumor activity *in vivo* (23, 42). Monomethylolmelamines can only act as a monofunctional alkylating agent and do not cross-link strands of DNA (79). The trimethylol derivative of hexamethylmelamine, N^2,N^4,N^6-trimethyl-N^2,N^4,N^6-trimethylolmelamine, has been shown to cross-link DNA of L1210 cells in culture (79). It would be expected that dimethylolmelamines could also function as bifunctional alkylating agents. However, dimethylol and trimethylol derivatives of methylmelamines do not appear to be formed under physiological conditions.

Metabolism

In vitro
Oxidative N-demethylation is the only known metabolic

pathway for the methylmelamines. Hexamethylmelamine is metabolized by the hepatic microsomal mixed funciton oxidase of rat and mouse in the presence of NADPH and O_2, to pentamethylmelamine and N^2,N^2,N^4,N^6-tetramethylmelamine (41, 82). A decreasing extent of methylation of the melamine leads to a decreased affinity for the hepatic microsomal mixed function oxygenase (Table 1) (4, 15). Further metabolism of N^2,N^2,N^4,N^6-tetramethylmelamine by rat hepatic microsomal fraction was not detected by Rutty and Connors (82). N^2-monomethylolpentamethylmelamine is the first product of metabolism of hexamethylmelamine and breaks down spontaneously to pentamethylmelamine and formaldehyde (41). Rat intestinal mitochondria have been shown to metabolize hexamethylmelamine in the presence of NADPH and O_2 to N^2-monomethylolpentamethylmelamine possibly by a cytochrome P-450 dependent mechanism, at the same rate as intestinal microsomal preparations (14). It is assumed that methylol intermediates are formed during N-demethylation of other methylmelamines, in addition to hexamethylmelamine, but individual N-methylolmelamines, apart from N^2-monomethylolpentamethylmelamine, have not been demonstrated. N-demethylation of hexamethylmelamine and other methylmelamines results in decreased toxicity and decreased antitumor activity in direct relation to the number of methyl groups removed (56, 81). Melamine, which has no N-methyl groups, lacks antitumor activity. Hexaethylmelamine lacks antitumor activity (82) and undergoes N-demethylation at a much slower rate than hexamethylmelamine (82).

In vivo
Triethylenemelamine is rapidly broken down *in vivo* and 78% of a dose of [^{14}C-ring]-labeled triethylenemelamine is excreted in the urine of mice in 24 hr, mostly in the first 2 hr after administration (68). The fact that the major urinary metabolite is 1,3-β-trihydroxy-s-triazine (cyanuric acid) and the virtual absence of radioactivity in exhaled carbon dioxide indicate that the s-triazine nucleus remains intact. Disposition of hexamethylmelamine *in vivo* has been studied in a number of species including housefly (19), dogfish (45), mouse (16), rat (21, 99, 100), rabbit (5), and man (31, 99). In rat, approximately 40% of a dose of hexamethylmelamine is excreted in the urine as metabolites in 48 hr, while biliary excretion accounts for only 5% of the dose (21, 99). Metabolism of hexamethylmelamine is qualitatively similar in all species studied (Table 2). N-demethylation of methylmelamines proceeds further *in vivo* than *in vitro* and can go as far as the completely demethylated melamine. The s-triazine ring is not, however, metabolically cleaved. The major urinary metabolites of hexamethylmelamine in most mammalian species are N^2,N^4-dimethylmelamine and monomethylmelamine, and in rat, for example, they account for more than 95% of the total metabolites in urine (21). In rabbit N^2,N^4,N^6-trimethylmelamine is also a major urinary metabolite (5). Conjugates of methylmelamines with glucuronic acid or sulfate are present in urine but only in minute quantities. Metabolism of pentamethylmelamine has been studied in rat (21), rabbit (5) and man (5, 10, 31) with similar results to hexamethylmelamine. The fact that methylmelamines containing completely N-demethylated

Table 1. In vitro metabolism of melamines by hepatic microsomes.

Substrate	Mouse[a]		Rat[b]	
	km mm	Vmax nmol/min/mg	km mm	Vmax nmol/min/mg
HMM	0.09	3.4	0.18	9.0
PMM	0.23	4.2	0.50	10.8
N^2,N^2,N^4,N^6-tetraMM	0.91	5.1	–	–
N^2,N^4,N^6-triMM	1.7	2.9	–	–

[a] Brindley *et al.* (15).
[b] Ames and Powis (4).

Table 2. Metabolism of hexamethylmelamine in different species.

Product	Housefly[a]	Rat[b]	Rat[c]	Rabbit[d]	Man[e]
HMM	−	−	−	−	−
PMM	+	+	+	+	++
N^2,N^2,N^4,N^6-tetraMM	+	+	+	++	+
N^2,N^2,N^4,N^4-tetraMM	−	−	−	−	−
N^2,N^4,N^6-triMM	+	++	++	+++	++
N^2,N^2,N^4-triMM	+	+	+	+	+
N^2,N^2-diMM	−	−	−	−	−
N^2,N^4-diMM	−	+++	+++	+++	+++
monoMM	−	+++	+++	++	+++
Melamine	−		+	+	++

+ + + Major metabolites; + + Present, but in smaller amounts; + Minor metabolites; − Not detected. All studies represent urinary metabolites except housefly where metabolites were isolated from treated flies and their excreta.
[a] Chang et al. (19); [b] Colombo et al. (21); [c] Worzalla et al. (99); [d] Ames et al. (3); [e] Worzalla et al. (100).

primary amine functions, that is N^2,N^2,N^4,N^4-tetramethyl-melamine and N^2,N^2-demethylmelamine, are not formed *in vivo* suggest that the mixed function oxidase exhibits greater affinity for dimethyl-substituted tertiary amines than for monomethyl-substituted secondary amines.

Pentamethylmelamine is eliminated more rapidly from plasma than hexamethylmelamine. The plasma half-life of pentamethylmelamine in mice is 8 min and the half-life of hexamethylmelamine 47 min (16). In rabbit half-lives are 22 min and 67 min, respectively (5). N-demethylated metabolites are found in plasma and tissues after administration of hexamethylmelamine and pentamethylmelamine (5, 16, 22, 31, 34, 40). The plasma half-lives of demethylated metabolites increases with decreasing number of methyl groups (10). Metabolites detected in plasma after administration of hexamethylmelamine to mice are pentamethylmelamine, N^2,N^2,N^4,N^6-tetramethylmelamine and N^2,N^4,N^6-trimethylmelamine (16). Demethylated metabolites are formed rapidly and the area under the plasma concentration time curve for N^2,N^2,N^4,N^6-tetramethylmelamine exceeds that of parent compound by seven- to ten-fold in mice. Metabolites detected in plasma of patients receiving pentamethylmelamine are N^2,N^2,N^4,N^6-tetramethylmelamine, N^2,N^2, N^4- and N^2,N^4,N^6-trimethylmelamine, dimethylmelamine and monomethylmelamine (5, 10, 31). In man, the area under the plasma concentration time curve for N^2,N^2,N^4, N^6-tetramethylmelamine and N^2,N^4,N^6-trimethylamine is less than that for parent compound (31). Rutty *et al.* (84) have reported a study directly comparing the metabolism of pentamethylmelamine in mouse, rat and man. The plasma half-life of pentamethylmelamine in mouse was less than 15 min, in rat 40 min and in man 102 min. In all species the major plasma metabolites of pentamethylmelamine were N^2, N^2,N^4,N^6-tetramethylmelamine and N^2,N^4,N^6-trimethylmelamine. Peak plasma concentration of total N-methylolmelamine was higher in mouse (6×10^{-4} M) than in rat (2×10^{-4} M) while in man N-methylolmelamine could not be detected ($< 5 \times 10^{-5}$ M). In tissues of mice administered hexamethylmelamine the major metabolite is N^2,N^4,N^6-trimethylmelamine and in brain the area under concentration time curve for N^2,N^4,N^6-trimethylmelamine exceeds that of parent drug by more than 20-fold (17, 40). Covalent binding of radiolabel from [^{14}C-methyl]-labeled hexamethylmelamine is highest in liver and intestine, and lowest in brain and heart. Except in the small intestine, where a decrease is observed between 2 and 10 hr, binding of radiolabel is complete by 2 hr and constant up to 40 hr (40, 83).

Hexamethylmelamine and its metabolites have been found in the cerebrospinal fluid of a patient after a single oral dose of hexamethylmelamine (34). The cerebrospinal fluid:plasma concentration ratio 230 min after giving the drug was, for hexamethylmelamine 0.06. for pentamethylmelamine 0.24, for N^2,N^2,N^4,N^6-tetramethylmelamine 0.47 and for N^2,N^4,N^6-trimethylmelamine 1.0. The difference in the ratios is probably due to differences in plasma protein binding which for hexamethylmelamine is 94% and which decreases with decreasing number of methyl groups.

Hexamethylmelamine administered orally has a low and variable bioavailability, probably because of a large first-pass metabolism (31, 32). First-pass metabolism of hexamethylmelamine after oral administration has been reported in both rat (52) and rabbit (5). The systemic bioavailability of oral hexamethylmelamine in rat is 8% and in rabbit 25%, despite complete absorption as judged from metabolite data. Both the intestine and liver contribute to first-pass metabolism in the rat with extraction ratios for intestine of 71% and for liver of 73% (52). Hexamethylmelamine is not appreciably metabolized by lung (52).

TOXICITY

Triethylenemelamine produces toxic effects in mice, rats, cats and dogs similar to those of nitrogen mustards, with myelosuppression, gastrointestinal lesions and parasympathetic stimulation. In addition there is delayed motor incoordination which may be central in origin (73). Toxic effects of triethylenemelamine in man are anorexia, nausea and vomiting, diarrhea and myelosuppression (80). The lowest dose of triethylenemelamine administered intravenously producing death in cat is 1 mg/kg, in dog 400 µg/kg and in monkey 100 µg/kg (86). A clinically effective dose of triethylenemelamine in man is 2 to 3 mg daily, for 2 to 3 days (80).

Toxic effects of hexamethylmelamine given orally to rodents are ulceration and hemorrhage of the gastrointestinal tract, inhibition of spermatogenesis and, at high doses, sedation and ataxia. Dogs and monkeys receiving intravenous hexamethylmelamine exhibit vomiting and, upon autopsy have evidence of pulmonary edema and hemorrhagic lesions of the lungs and gastrointestinal tract (57). Hexamethylmelamine is only mildly myelosuppressive in all species studied (57, 86). Hexamethylmelamine, unlike triethylenemelamine, is not teratogenic (9). Hexamethylmelamine appears to be equitoxic in most species studied, the LD_{50} for orally administered drug being in mouse 437 mg/kg, in rat 350 mg/kg, in guinea pig 255 mg/kg, and in chicken 341 mg/kg (93). A typical dosage schedule for hexamethylmelamine in man is 4 to 12 mg/kg by mouth daily for 21 to 90 days, depending on the daily dose. Dose-limiting toxicity of hexamethylmelamine in man is nausea and vomiting, and cumulative neurological toxicity, with myelosuppression occurring rarely (47, 58). The mechanism of nausea and vomiting, which occurs in 50 to 70% of patients, is unknown but may be a central effect rather than local irritation because it usually occurs some days after beginning treatment. Neurological toxicity occurs in about 20% of patients and paresthesias, hyperreflexias, muscle weakness, peripheral numbness, ataxia and Parkinson's disease-like symptoms have been reported. It has been suggested that neurological toxicity results from hexamethylmelamine reacting with pyridoxine to cause a pyridoxine deficiency, and concomitant pyridoxine has been recommended although its efficacy in ameliorating neurological toxicity has not been demonstrated (59). Moderate leukopenia and to a lesser degree thrombocytopenia occur in up to 40% patients receiving hexamethylmelamine.

Pentamethylmelamine administered to mice, dog, guinea pig, rabbit and rhesus monkey produces symptoms indicative of gastrointestinal disturbances and central neurologic toxicity, in addition to toxic lesions at the injection site and lesions to the lymphatic, renal and male reproductive systems (72). In man, pentamethylmelamine produces severe, dose-limiting nausea and vomiting, and central nervous system toxicities (47). Nausea and vomiting is evident a few hours after giving drug and can last several days. Central nervous system toxicity consists of somnolence, depression, headache, confusion, agitation and, at higher doses, visual hallucinations, electroencephalographic changes, including diffuse slowing of α- or β-waves and loss of consciousness. Myelosuppression, however, is mild and occurs only occasionally. Because of its toxicity pentamethylmelamine appears to offer no advantage over hexamethylmelamine and its further clinical development of pentamethylmelamine is unlikely.

Antitumor activity

Triethylenemelamine is a directly acting alkylating agent and has high activity against several animal tumors including rat Walker carcinosarcoma 256 (48, 60). Triethylenemelamine is not now used clinically but has been reported to have activity against Hodgkin's and non-Hodgkin's lymphoma, chronic lymphocytic leukemia and advanced ovarian carcinoma (80, 91). Hexamethylmelamine has only borderline activity against transplantable murine tumors such as sarcoma 180 and the murine tumors of the National Cancer Institute screening panel shown in Table 3 (42, 65). Hexamethylmelamine does, however, show significant activity against murine PC6 plasmacytoma (15, 81) and exhibits considerably greater antitumor activity against transplantable rat tumors including Walker carcinosarcoma 256, L5178Y lymphatic leukemia, Dunning's leukemia and Yoshida sarcoma (57, 71, 72). Hexamethylmelamine also has activity against human tumor xenografts, for example, lung carcinoma P246 growing in immune-deprived mice (65) and breast MX-1 xenograft growing in nude mice (42). Pentamethylmelamine shows more activity than hexamethylmelamine against human breast MX-2 xenograft and is equally active against human breast MX-1 xenograft (72). Pentamethylmelamine, N^2-monomethylolpentamethylmelamine and N^2,N^4,N^6-trimethyl-N^2,N^4,N^6-trimethylolmelamine exhibit antitumor activity against lung carcinoma P246 in immune-deprived mice (23). N^2,N^4,N^6-Trimethyl-N^2,N^4,N^6-trimethylolmelamine has activity against several murine tumors of the National Cancer Institute screening panel and against human tumor xenografts growing in nude mice (Table 3).

Hexamethylmelamine is potentially a valuable drug for treating cancer in man in combination with other anticancer agents because of its mild myelotoxicity. In ovarian cancer hexamethylmelamine appears to be at least as active as alkylating agents. Because there is no cross resistance between hexamethylmelamine and alkylating agents it appears logical to combine them together, or to use one therapy after the patient fails to respond to the other (58). Hexamethylmelamine is frequently used in combination with cyclophosphamide, cisplatin and adriamycin in the treatment of advanced ovarian cancer. Hexamethylmelamine containing regimens have produced moderate response rates with previously treated patients, although little or no change in median survival. Studies are now focusing on the use of hexamethylmelamine containing drug combinations in previously untreated patients with ovarian cancer (47). In lung cancer hexamethylmelamine continues to be a part of intensive and other regimens for the treatment of small cell and non-small cell carcinoma, but its value has yet to be determined. Hexamethylmelamine has been reported to have activity as a single agent against lymphomas, carcinoma of the cervix and breast carcinoma (58). Future trials have been recommended to determine the value of hexamethylmelamine in the treatment of endometrial and prostatic carcinomas (47).

HYDRAZINES

Background

Procarbazine (N-isopropyl-α-(2-methylhydrazino)-p-toluamide hydrochloride) is the only hydrazine antitumor agent in clinical use today. It was synthesized together with other methylhydrazines in the early 1960's as a potential inhibitor of monoamine oxidase (101). The finding that l-methyl-2-benzylhydrazine had significant antitumor activity against several transplantable tumors, although too hepatotoxic to be of clinical use, led to the search for antitumor activity among other methylhydrazine derivatives (11). The N-carbamoyl analog of l-methyl-2-benzylhydrazine and procarbazine were chosen for further screening and procarbazine hydrochloride, which was the less toxic of the two compounds, was introduced into clinical trial in 1963 (62). Procarbazine is now primarily used in combination with other chemotherapeutic agents in the treatment of Hodgkin's disease.

Mechanism of action

Procarbazine itself is not cytotoxic and has to undergo chemical or metabolic activation (39, 46). Chemical breakdown of procarbazine to potentially toxic substances complicates the study of the cytotoxicity of procarbazine *in vitro*. Procarbazine in solution at physiologic pH undergoes rapid chemical oxidation by molecular oxygen with a half-life of about 15 min, to yield azoprocarbazine (N-isopropyl α-[2-methyldiazeno)-p-toluamide) and hydrogen peroxide (1, 95). Azoprocarbazine slowly isomerizes, with a half-life of 50 min, to the conjugated hydrazone N-isopropyl-p-formyl-benzamide methylhydrazone which, in turn, hydrolyses to give the aldehyde N-isopropyl p-formyl-benzamide and, it is postulated, methylhydrazine which reacts with oxygen to form methane (94). Metabolism of procarbazine *in vivo* proceeds by a similar initial step forming azoprocarbazine and it is probable that both chemical oxidation and metabolism contribute to the formation of azoprocarbazine *in vivo*. Subsequent *in vivo* metabolism of azoprocarbazine is much more rapid than tautomerization to the hydrazone and little hydrazone is formed *in vivo*. It is unlikely that chemical breakdown products of procarbazine contribute significantly to the *in vivo* antitumor activity of procarbazine (1, 37). The antitumor activity of procarbazine *in vivo* is probably due to metabolic conversion to alkylating and/or free radical intermediates. Evidence supporting the view that procarbazine acts as an alkylating agent is the rapid incorporation of radiolabel from [N-methyl-^{14}C]-labeled

Table 3. Activity against transplantable tumors in mice.

	Hexamethylmelamine	Pentamethylmelamine	Trimethylol-TMM	Procarbazine
Mouse tumors				
L1210 leukemia	−	−	(+)	+
P388 leukemia	−	(+)	NT	+
B16 melanoma	−	−	(+)	+
Lewis lung	−	−	−	+
Colon 26	NT	NT	+	−
Colon 38	(+)	(+)	+	(+)
CD8F$_1$ mammary			+	−
Human tumor xenografts				
Mammary MX-1, sc	+	+	+	−
Mammary MX-1, src	+	+	+	NT
Lung LX-1, sc	−	−	(+)	+
Lung LX-1, src	−	−	−	+
Colon CX-1, sc		−	NT	−
Colon CX-1, src	+	−	+	NT

Data taken from Goldin et al. (42); Legha et al. (57); and Pentamethylmelamine Clinical Brochure (72).
+ Signifies activity; (+) signifies marginal activity; − signifies no activity; NT = not tested.
Human tumor xenografts were grown in nude mice either at a subcutaneous site (sc), or at a subrenal capsule site (src).
Response criteria; survival times, P388 $\geq$ 120%; L1210, B16 $\geq$ 125%; Colon 26 $\geq$ 130%; Lewis lung $\geq$ 140%; tumor weight inhibition, Colon 38, CD8F$_1$, MX-1 sc, LX-1 sc, and CX-1 sc $\leq$ 42%; MX-1 src, LX-1 src, and CX-1 $\leq$ 20%.

procarbazine into DNA, RNA, protein and phospholipids of P815 leukemic cells in tumored mice given the drug (57). Nucleic acid has been shown to be methylated on the [7]N-atom of guanine by transfer of an intact methyl group (63). The N-demethylated analogue of procarbazine lacks antitumor activity showing the importance of the N-methyl group for antitumor activity (11). Incubation of [^{14}C-ring]- or [N-methyl-^{14}C]-labeled azoprocarbazine with hepatic microsomes and NADPH under aerobic conditions results in covalent binding of radiolabel to microsomal protein (97).

More radiolabel is covalently bound using [N-methyl-^{14}C]-labeled azoprocarbazine than using [^{14}C-ring]-labeled azoprocarbazine further implicating the N-methyl group as forming a reactive species which might be responsible for the antitumor activity of procarbazine. A possible pathway leading to formation of a reactive methyldiazonium ion during the metabolism of procarbazine by hydroxylation of the benzyl carbon adjacent to an azoxy function to form a carbinolamine-like intermediate, as suggested by Weinkam and Shiba (96), is shown in Fig. 3. An alternative pathway for forming an alkylating species during metabolism of procarbazine is by hydroxylation of the methyl group adjacent to an azoxy function, which would also give a carbinolamine-like intermediate and an alkyldiazonium ion. Although Fig. 3 shows azoxyprocarbazine metabolites as intermediates in the formation of proposed alkylating species, Prough *et al.* (75) have reported that [methyl-^{14}C]-labeled methylazoxyprocarbazine and benzylazoxyprocarbazine, unlike [methyl-^{14}C]-labeled azoprocarbazine, do not bind covalently to liver microsomal protein suggesting that azoxyprocarbazines are not intermediates in the formation of alkylating species from procarbazine. An alternative mechanism for the antitumor activity of procarbazine involves the formation of reactive free radical intermediates (8, 95). Hydroxylation of azoprocarbazine in a manner analogous to that proposed for azoxy metabolites previously, would yield products that would rapidly hydrolyze to an aldehyde and diazene. Diazenes rapidly decompose in the presence of molecular oxygen to give molecular nitrogen and free radicals. Hydrogen abstraction by the free radical could ultimately lead to formation of methane and N-isopropyl-*p*-toluamide, both of which are detected as metabolites of procarbazine *in vivo* (61, 77, 96). Since metabolism of procarbazine is catalyzed by cytochrome P-450 and cytochrome P450 is not found in most tumors it must be assumed that one or more of the metabolites of procarbazine is the transport form of the drug in plasma and is taken up by tumor cells to produce a cytotoxic effect. At the present time the exact mechanism for the antitumor effect of procarbazine has not been established.

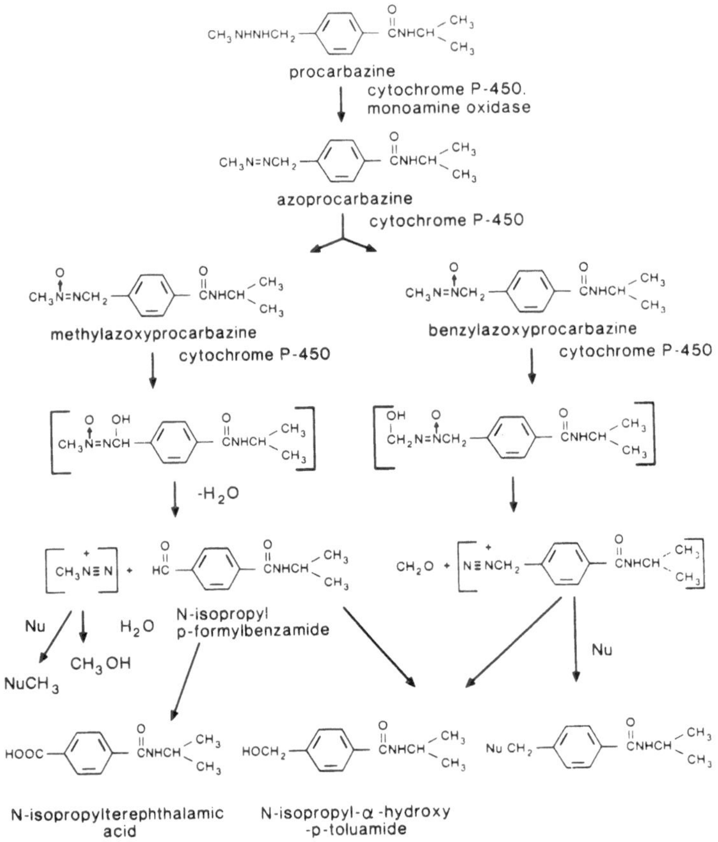

Figure 3. Metabolism of procarbazine to form of alkylating intermediates. Postulated metabolites are shown in parenthesis. Alkylating intermediates can react with water or cellular nucleophile (NU) (adapted from Shiba and Weinkam (88)).

Metabolism

In vitro

The metabolism of procarbazine has been extensively studied *in vitro* (8, 26, 30, 37, 76, 96, 97, 98) and *in vivo* (30, 36, 43, 55, 85, 88, 96). Pathways for the metabolism of procarbazine are shown in Fig. 3. Work, primarily by Prough and his colleagues (37, 76, 97), has shown that cytochrome P-450 catalyzes both the oxidation of procarbazine to azoprocarbazine and the subsequent oxidation of azoprocarbazine to the 2-isomeric azoxy derivatives, benzylazoxy- and methylazoxyprocarbazine. Azoprocarbazine has a greater affinity for cytochrome P-450 (Km 0.1 mm) than procarbazine (Km 0.6 mM) (97). Coomes and Prough (24) have shown that monoamine oxidase in rat liver mitochondria can also convert procarbazine to azoprocarbazine. Formation of the azoxy derivatives from azoprocarbazine is stereoselective and species dependent (Table 4). In rat two isozymes of cytochrome P-450 have been identified as being responsible for the major portion of microsomal metabolism of azoprocarbazine to azoxyprocarbazine (74). The formation of azoxyprocarbazine, methylazoxyprocarbazine, benzylazoxyprocarbazine, N-isopropyl-*p*-formylbenzamide, N-isopropyl-α-hydroxy-*p*-toluamide and N-isopropyl-terephthalamic acid from procarbazine by a rat liver 9000 × g supernatant in the presence of NADPH and oxygen has been reported by Shiba and Weinkam (88). Cummings *et al.* (26) have presented evidence that N-isopropyl-α-hydroxy-*p*-toluamide can be formed by two pathways, either by reduction of N-isopropyl-*p*-formylbenzamide by microsomal aldehyde reductase or by solvolysis of a benzyldiazonium ion formed by cytochrome P-450 dependent oxidation of azoprocarbazine. Cummings *et al.* (26) also presented evidence that the azoxyprocarbazine isomers are not intermediate in the formation of N-isopropyl-α-hydroxy-*p*-toluamide or perhaps even N-isopropyl-*p*-formylbenzamide.

In vivo

In vivo studies with radiolabeled procarbazine have shown that the major metabolites of procarbazine are carbon dioxide, which in rat accounts for up to 30% of a dose of [N-methyl-^{14}C]-labeled procarbazine (78, 85), and N-isopropyl-terephthalamic acid which is the only urinary metabolite of procarbazine so far identified in mouse, rat, dog and man (8, 69, 70, 77). The percent of a dose [CO-^{14}C]-labeled procarbazine excreted as radiolabel in the urine in 24 hr is, in rat 74%, in dog 81% and in man 73% (85).

Table 4. Metabolism of azoprocarbazine by hepatic microsomes.

Metabolites	nmol/min/mg			
	Rat		Rabbit	
	−	pB	−	Pb
Benzylazoxy	ND	0.39	0.09	0.32
Methylazoxy	0.35	1.50	0.35	0.96
p-Formyl-N-isopropylbenzamide	0.14	0.36	0.02	0.04

Pb – phenobarbital induced.
ND – not detectable.
Data taken from Wiebkin and Prough (97).

Kuttab *et al.* (55), using direct probe electron impact mass spectrometry and ether extraction of plasma, have reported that 15 min after intraperitoneal administration of procarbazine to rat azoprocarbazine is the principal metabolite in plasma. No parent drug of other metabolites were detected by these authors apart from a small amount of azoxyprocarbazine. Gorsen *et al.* (43), using gas chromatography-mass spectrometry and toluene extraction of plasma, found that 1 hr after an oral dose of procarbazine 70% of total drug and metabolites in plasma of rat was N-isopropyl-*p*-formylbenzamide with much smaller amounts (in decreasing order) of N-isopropyl-α-hydroxy-*p*-toluamide, azoxyprocarbazine, N-isopropyl-*p*-formylbenzamide methylhydrazone, N-isopropyl-*p*-toluamide, azoxyprocarbazine and procarbazine itself. N-isopropyl-terephthalamic acid could not be detected under the conditions used in the assay. Shiba and Weinkam (88), using high performance liquid chromatography and ether extraction of plasma, reported the time course of several metabolites in plasma of rats given procarbazine intraperitoneally. N-isopropyl-terephthalamic acid was present in the highest concentrations. Azoprocarbazine was less abundant than methylazoxyprocarbazine while benzylazoxyprocarbazine and N-isopropyl-*p*-formaldehyde were present in trace amounts. Shiba and Weinkam (88) also reported that in a patient receiving procarbazine the major circulating metabolite was methylazoxyprocarbazine with benzylazoxyprocarbazine and azoxyprocarbazine present at lower concentrations. It should be noted that azoxyprocarbazine and the isomeric azoxy compounds, methylazoxy- and benzylazoxyprocarbazine exhibit antitumor activity *in vivo* (87). Which of the metabolites of procarbazine in plasma represent the active form(s) of the drug is not clear.

Toxicity

Most methylhydrazines with antitumor activity depress hemopoiesis in animals, leucopoiesis and thrombopoiesis being most markedly inhibited and erythropoiesis much less affected (12). The extent of inhibition of leucopoiesis varies considerably with species. Procarbazine depresses lymphopoiesis in rats whereas in dogs it depresses predominantly granulopoiesis. Hemolysis with the appearance of Heinz-Ehrlich inclusion bodies in erythrocytes is a feature common to many hydrazine derivatives. Methylhydrazines cause marked depression of spermatogenesis and atrophy of the testis in mouse, rat and monkey (90). Some methylhydrazines are hepatotoxic, but one reason procarbazine was chosen for clinical trial was its lack of hepatotoxicity. Neurologic toxicity produced by procarbazine in monkeys includes loss of coordination, emesis, depression and marked anorexia before death (69, 70, 90). Procarbazine has been shown to be carcinogenic and to induce pulmonary tumors, leukemia and mammary carcinoma in rodents and myelogenous leukemia in monkeys (51, 90). Procarbazine can also suppress the immune system (38) and in animals is teratogenic (20).

Toxicity of procarbazine in man includes nausea and vomiting, myelosuppression resulting in thrombocytopenia and leukopenia, neurotoxicity and sterility (90). Male patients receiving procarbazine can develop persistent azoospermia and testicular biopsies show a microscopic picture of total germinal cell aplasia (89). There is some evidence that the germinal cell aplasia is reversible after treatment with procarbazine is stopped. The neurologic toxicity of procarbazine includes somnolence, confusion, hyperirritability, euphoria and cerebellar ataxia (27, 28). The neurologic toxicity of procarbazine has been suggested to be due to inhibition of monoamine oxidase (27) or to decreased levels of pyridoxal phosphate (18).

Antitumor activity

Procarbazine has activity against a wide range of transplantable tumors in mouse (see Table 3) (11, 42, 69, 70), rat (11, 69), and hamster (44). Procarbazine retains antitumor activity when administered orally and is active against intracerebrally implanted leukemia L1210 in mice (69, 70). Procarbazine is used clinically primarily in combination with other drugs for treatment of Hodgkin's disease as, for example, the MOPP regimen which consists of mechlorethamine, vincristine (Oncovine®), procarbazine and prednisone (29). Procarbazine is used less frequently in treatment of non-Hodgkin's lymphoma, malignant melanoma, multiple myeloma, bronchogenic carcinoma and, because of its good penetration into cerebrospinal fluid, brain tumor (35).

CONCLUSION

Methylmelamines and methylhydrazines are two distinct classes of compounds with antitumor activity and, yet, have several features in common., Both classes of compounds are represented by only one member that is used clinically. Both classes of compounds appear to act as alkylating agents and require metabolic activation to form alkylating species and, probably, to express antitumor activity. An N-methyl group appears to be important for the antitumor activity of both classes of compound. Drugs of both classes undergo extensive, rapid metabolism, primarily by the hepatic microsomal mixed function oxidase, *in vitro* and *in vivo*. Both classes of drugs are used in combination chemotherapy to treat specific human cancers and do not cross react with other alkylating agents. Nausea and vomiting and neurotoxicity are side effects common to both classes of compounds, but while methylmelamines are free of myelosuppression, methylhydrazines produce marked myelosuppression. Differences in antitumor activity exist between methylmelamines and methylhydrazines, with the former compounds exhibiting activity against a limited range of animal tumors while the latter group exhibit a wide range of activity against animal tumors.

ACKNOWLEDGEMENTS

The excellent secretarial assistance of Ms Wanda Rhodes in preparing this manuscript is gratefully acknowledged.

REFERENCES

1. Aebi H, DeWald B, Suter H: Autoxydation N²-substituierter Methylhydrazine Beeinflussung der cu und fe Katalyse durch Proteine. *Helv Chim Acta* 48: 656, 1965
2. Alley MC, Powis G, Appel PL, Kooistra KL, Lieber MM: Activation and inactivation of cancer chemotherapeutic agents by rat hepatocytes cocultured with human tumor cell lines. *Cancer Res* 44: 549, 1984
3. Ames MM, Kovach JS: Parenteral formulation of hexamethylmelamine potentially suitable for use in man. *Cancer Treat Rep* 66: 1579, 1982
4. Ames MM, Powis G: Metabolism of hexamethylmelamine and pentamethylmelamine by rat liver microsomes and isolated hepatocytes. *Proc Amer Assoc Cancer Res* 21: 257, 1980
5. Ames MM, Powis G, Kovach JS, Eagan RT: Disposition and metabolism of pentamethylmelamine and hexamethylmelamine in rabbits and humans. *Cancer Res* 39: 5016, 1979
6. Ames MM, Sanders ME, Tiede WS: Metabolic activation of hexamethylmelamine and pentamethylmelamine by liver microsomal preparations. *Life Sci* 29: 1591, 1981
7. Ames MM, Sanders ME, Tiede WS: Role of N-methylolpentamethylmelamine in the metabolic activation of hexamethylmelamine. *Cancer Res* 43: 500, 1983
8. Baggiolini M, DeWald B, Aebi H: Oxidation of *p*-(N¹-methylhydrazino methyl)-N-isopropyl benzamide (procarbazine) to the methylazo derivative and oxidative cleavage of the N²–C bond in the isolated perfused liver. *Biochem Pharmacol* 18: 2187, 1969
9. Barnes TC, Frances S: Toxicity of hexamethylmelamine in rats. *Arch Int Pharmacodyn* 160: 83, 1966
10. Benvenuto JA, Stewart DJ, Benjamin RS, Loo TL: Pharmacology of pentamethylmelamine in humans. *Cancer Res* 41: 566, 1981
11. Bollag W, Grunberg E: Tumor inhibitory effects of a new class of cytotoxic agents: methylhydrazine derivatives. *Experientia* 19: 130, 1963
12. Bollag W, Theiss E: Methylhydrazine derivatives. In: *International Symposium on Chemotherapy of Cancer*. Edited by PA Plattner Lugano, pp. 311–314. Elsevier, Amsterdam
13. Bořkovec AB, DeMilo AB: Insect chemosterilants. V. Derivatives of melamine. *J Med Chem* 10: 457, 1967
14. Borm P, Mingels MJ, Hulshoff A, Frankhuyen-Sierevogel A, Noordhoek J: Rapid formation of N-hydroxymethylpentamethylmelamine by mitochondria from rat small intestinal epithelium. *Life Sci* 33: 2113, 1983
15. Brindley C, Gescher A, Langdon SP, Broggini M, Colombo T, D'Incalci M: Studies of the mode of action of antitumor triazenes and triazines – III Metabolism studies on hexamethylmelamine. *Biochem Pharmacol* 31: 625, 1982
16. Broggini M, Colombo T, D'Incalci MD, Donelli MG, Gescher A, Garattini S: Pharmacokinetics of hexamethylmelamine and pentamethylmelamine in mice. *Cancer Treat Rep* 65: 669, 1981
17. Broggini M, Rossi C, Colombo T, D'Incalci M: Hexamethylmelamine and pentamethylmelamine tissue distribution in M5076/73A ovarian cancer-bearing mice. *Cancer Treat Rep* 66: 127, 1982
18. Chabner BA, DeVita V, Considine N, Oliverio VT: Plasma pyridoxal phosphate depletion by the carcinostatic procarbazine. *Proc Soc Exp Biol Med* 132: 1119, 1969
19. Chang SC, DeMilo AB, Woods CW, Bořkovec AB: Metabolism of C¹⁴-labeled hemel in male houseflies. *J Econ Entomol* 61: 1357, 1968
20. Chaube S, Murphy MC: Fetal malformations produced in rats by N-isopropyl-α-(2-methylhydrazine)-*p*-toluamide hydrochloride (procarbazine). *Teratology* 2: 23, 1969
21. Colombo T, Broggini M, Gescher A, D'Incalci M: Routes of elimination of hexamethylmelamine and pentamethylmelamine in the rat. *Xenobiotica* 12: 315, 1982
22. Colombo T, Torti L, D'Incalci MD: Dose-dependent pharmacokinetics of PMM in the rat. *Cancer Chemother Pharmacol* 5: 201, 1981

23. Connors TA, Cumber AJ, Ross WCJ, Clarke SA, Mitchley BCV: Regression of human lung tumor xenografts induced by water soluble analogs of hexamethylmelamine. *Cancer Treat Rep* 61: 927, 1977

24. Coomes MW, Prough RA: The mitochondrial metabolism of 1,2-disubstituted hydrazines procarbazine and 1,2-dimethylhydrazine. *Drug Metab Disp* 11: 550, 1983

25. Cumber AJ, Ross WCJ: Analogues of hexamethylmelamine: The antineoplastic activity of derivatives with enhanced water solubility. *Chem Biol Interact* 17: 349, 1977

26. Cummings SW, Guengerich FP, Prough RA: The characterization of N-isopropyl-*p*-hydroxymethylbenzamide formed during the oxidative metabolism of azo-procarbazine. *Drug Metab Disp* 10: 459, 1982

27. DeVita VT, Hahn MA, Oliverio VT: Monoamine oxide inhibition by a new carcinostatic agent N-isopropyl-α-(2-methylhydrazino)-*p*-toluamide. *Proc Soc Exp Biol Med* 120: 561, 1965

28. DeVita VT, Serpick A, Carbone PP: Preliminary clinical studies with ibenzmethyzin. *Clin Pharmacol Ther* 7: 542, 1966

29. DeVita VT, Serpick A, Carbone PP: Combination chemotherapy in the treatment of advanced Hodgkin's disease. *Ann Inter Med* 73: 881, 1970

30. DeWald B, Baggiolini M, Aebi H: N-Demethylation of *p*-N[1]-methyl-hydrazino methyl)-N-isopropyl benzamide (procarbazine), a cytostatically active methylhydrazine derivative, in the intact rat and in the isolated perfused rat liver. *Biochem Pharmacol* 18: 2179, 1969

31. D'Incalci M, Beggiolin G, Sessa C, Mangione C: Influence of ascites on pharmacokinetics of hexamethylmelamine and N-demethylated metabolites in ovarian cancer patients. *Eur J Cancer* 7: 1331, 1981

32. D'Incalci M, Bolis G, Mangioni C, Masca L, Garrattini S: Variable oral absorption of hexamethylmelamine in man. *Cancer Treat Rep* 62: 2117, 1978

33. D'Incalci M, Erba E, Balconi G, Morasca L, Garrattini S: Time dependence of the *in vitro* cytotoxicity of hexamethylmelamine and its metabolites. *Br J Cancer* 41: 630, 1980

34. D'Incalci M, Sessa C, Beggiolin G, Mangioni C: Cerebrospinal fluid levels of hexamethylmelamine and N-demethylated metabolites. *Cancer Treat Rep* 65: 350, 1981

35. Dorr RT, Fritz WL: Procarbazine. In: *Cancer Chemotherapy Handbook*, pp. 593–601. Elsevier, New York, 1980

36. Dost FN, Reed DJ: Methane formation *in vivo* from N-isopropyl-α-(2-methylhydrazino)-*p*-toluamide hydrochloride, a tumor inhibiting methylhydrazine derivative. *Biochem Pharmacol* 16: 1741, 1967

37. Dunn DL, Lubet RA, Prough RA: Oxidative metabolism of N-isopropyl-α-(2-methylhydrazino)-*p*-toluamide hydrochloride (procarbazine) by rat liver microsomes. *Cancer Res* 39: 4555, 1979

38. Floersheim GL: Verlängerte Überlebenszeit von Hauthomotransplantaten bei Mäusen durch ein Methylhydrazinderivat. *Experientia* 19: 546, 1963

39. Gale GR, Simpson JG, Smith AB: Studies of the mode of action of N-isopropyl-α-(2-methylhydrazine)-*p*-toluamide. *Cancer Res* 27: 1186, 1967

40. Garattini E, Colombo T, Donelli MG, Catalani P, Bianchi M, D'Incalci M, Pantorotto C: Distribution, metabolism and irreversible binding of hexamethylmelamine in mice bearing ovarian carcinoma. *Cancer Chemother Pharmacol* 11: 51, 1983

41. Gescher A, D'Incalci M, Fanelli R, Farina P: N-Hydroxymethylpentamethylmelamine, a major *in vitro* metabolite of hexamethylmelamine. *Life Sci* 26: 147, 1980

42. Goldin A, Venditti JM, MacDonald JS, Muggia FM, Henney JE, DeVita V: Current results of the screening program at the Division of Cancer Treatment, National Cancer Institute. *Eur J Cancer* 17: 129, 1981

43. Gorsen RM, Weiss AJ, Manthei RW: Analysis of procarbazine and metabolites by gas chromatography-mass spectrometry. *J Chromatogr* 221: 309, 1980

44. Grunberg E, Prince HN: The activity of ibenzmethyzin hydrochloride against the human transplantable tumors human epithelioma No. 3 and human adenocarcinoma No. 1. *Experientia* 22: 324, 1966

45. Guarino AM: Pharmacologic and toxicologic studies of anticancer drugs: of sharks, mice, and men (and dogs and monkeys) methods. *Cancer Res* 17: 91, 1979

46. Gutterman J, Huang A, Hochstein P: Studies on the mode of action of N-isopropyl-α-(2-methylhydrazine)-*p*-toluamide. *Proc Soc Exp Biol Med* 130: 797, 1979

47. Hahn DA: Hexamethylmelamine and pentamethylmelamine: An update. *Drug Intell Clin Pharm* 17: 418, 1983

48. Hendry JA, Homer RF, Rose FL, Walpole AL: Cytotoxic agents. III. Derivatives of ethyleneimine. *Brit J Pharmacol* 6: 357, 1951

49. Hulshoff A, Neyt JP, Smulders CFA, van Loenen AC: The intravenous injection of hexamethylmelamine (HMM) as its monohydrochloride. *Proc Amer Assoc Cancer Res* 21: 301, 1980

50. Kaiser DW, Thurston IT, Dudley JR, Schaeffer FC, Hechenbleikner I, Holm-Hansen D: Cyanuric chloride derivatives. II. Substituted melamines. *J Amer Chem Soc* 73: 2984, 1951

51. Kelly MG, O'Gara RW, Gadekan K, Yancey ST, Oliverio VT: Carcinogenic activity of new antitumor agent, N-isopropyl-α-(2-methylhydrazino)-*p*-toluamide hydrochloride (NSC 77213). *Cancer Chemother Rep* 39: 77, 1964

52. Klippert PJ, Hulshoff A, Mingels MJ, Hofman G, Noordhoek J: Low oral bioavailability of hexamethylmelamine in the rat due to simultaneous hepatic and intestinal metabolism. *Cancer Res* 43: 3160, 1983

53. Kreilgard B, Higuchi T, Repta AJ: Complexation in formulation of parenteral solutions. Solubilization of the cytotoxic agent hexamethylmelamine by complexation with gentisic and species. *J Pharmacol Sci* 64: 1850, 1975

54. Kries W, Yen Y: An antineoplastic C[14]-labeled methylhydrazine derivative in P815 mouse leukemia. A metabolic study. *Experientia* 21: 284, 1965

55. Kuttab SH, Vouros P, Tanglertpaibul S: Studies on the metabolism of procarbazine by mass spectrometry. *Biomed Mass Spec* 9: 78, 1982

56. Lake LM, Grunden EE, Johnson BM: Toxicity and antitumor activity of hexamethylmelamine and its N-demethylated metabolites in mice with transplantable tumors. *Cancer Res* 34: 2858, 1975

57. Legha SS, Slavik M, Livingston RB, Carter SK: Hexamethylmelamine (NSC 13875). Clinical Brochure, National Cancer Institute, Bethesda, Maryland, 1974

58. Legha SS, Slavik M, Carter SK: Hexamethylmelamine – an evaluation of its role in the therapy of cancer. *Cancer* 38: 27, 1976

59. Leite C: Hexamethylmelamine with or without pyridoxine in refractory breast cancer. *Proc Amer Assoc Cancer Res* 38: 27, 1978

60. Lewis MR, Crossley ML: Retardation of tumor growth in mice by oral administration of ethyleneimine derivatives. *Arch Biochem* 26: 319, 1950

61. Maloney SJ, Prough PA: Studies on the pathway of methane formation from procarbazine, a 2-methylbenzylhydrazine derivative, by rat liver microsomes. *Arch Biochem Biophys* 221: 577, 1983

62. Martz G: Clinical results with a methylhydrazine derivative. In: *Proc Int Symp Chemother Cancer*. Edited by PA Plattner. Lugano, Switzerland, p. 198, 2–63, Elsevier, New York, 1964

63. Matsumoto H, Higa HH: Studies on methylazoxymethanol, the aglycone of cycasin: methylation of nucleic acids *in vitro*.

Biochem J 98: 20c, 1966

64. Miller-Hatch KJ, Ames MM, Kovach JS, Ahmann DL: Cytotoxic activity of hexamethylmelamine in human tumor cell lines in the presence of rat hepatic preparations. *Proc Amer Assoc Cancer Res* 24: 247, 1983

65. Mitchley BCV, Clarke SA, Connors TA, Neville AM: Hexamethylmelamine-induced regression of human lung tumors growing in immune deprived mice. *Cancer Res* 35: 1099, 1975

66. Morimoto M, Green D, Rahman A, Goldin A, Schein PS: Comparative pharmacology of pentamethylmelamine and hexamethylmelamine in mice. *Cancer Res* 40: 2762, 1980

67. Muindi JR, Newell DR, Smith IE, Harrap KR: Pentamethylmelamine (PMM): Phase I clinical and pharmacokinetic studies. *Br J Cancer* 47: 27, 1983

68. Nadkarni MV, Goldenthal EI, Smith PK: The distribution of radioactivity following administration of triethyleneimino-s-triazine-C^{14} in tumor bearing and control mice. *Cancer Res* 14: 559, 1954

69. Oliverio VT, Kelly MG: Contributions to the biological and clinical effect of a methylhydrazine derivative. In: *Proc Int Symp Chemother Cancer*. Edited by PA Plattner. Lugano, Switzerland, pp. 221–226. Elsevier, New York, 1964

70. Oliverio VT, Kelly MG: Some pharmacological properties of a tumor inhibitory methylhydrazine derivative. *Proc Amer Assoc Cancer Res* 5: 49, 1964

71. Osswald H: The curative action of hexamethylmelamine on intramuscularly or intracerebrally implanted Yoshida sarcoma. *Cancer Lett* 21: 343, 1984

72. Pentamethylmelamine NSC 118742, Clinical Brochure: National Cancer Institute, Bethesda, Maryland, 1978

73. Philips FS, Thiersch JB: The nitrogen mustard-like actions 2,4,6-tris(ethyleneimino)-s-triazine and other bis(ethyleneimines). *J Pharmacol Exp Ther* 100: 398, 1950

74. Prough RA, Brown MI, Dannan GA, Guengerich FP: Major isoenzymes of rat liver microsomal cytochrome P-450 involved in the N-oxidation of N-isopropyl-alpha-(2-methylazo)-ρ-toluamide, the azo derivative of procarbazine. *Cancer Res* 44: 543, 1984

75. Prough RA, Coomes MW, Cummings SW, Wiebkin P: Metabolism of procarbazine [N-isopropyl-α-(2-methylhydrazine)-ρ-toluamide HCl]. *Adv Exp Med Biol* 136: 983, 1980

76. Prough RA, Coomes MW, Dunn DL: The microsomal metabolism of carcinogenic and/or therapeutic hydrazine. In: *Microsomes and Drug Oxidations, Volume 3*, pp. 600–607. Edited by V Ullrich, I Roots, AG Hildebrandt, RW Estabrook, AH Conney. Pergamon Press, New York, 1977

77. Raaflaub J, Schwartz DE: Über den Metabolismus eines cytostatisch wirksamen Methylhydrazin-derivates (Natulan). *Experientia* 21: 44, 1965

78. Reed D, Dost F: Methane and CO_2 formation by rats during metabolism of a methylhydrazine (Natulan). *Proc Am Assoc Cancer Res* 7: 57, 1965

79. Ross WE, McMillan DR, Ross CF: Comparative of DNA damage by methylmelamines and formaldehyde. *J Natl Cancer Inst* 67: 217, 1981

80. Rundles RW, Barton WB: Triethylenemelamine in the treatment of neoplastic disease. *Blood* 7: 483, 1952

81. Rutty CJ, Abel G: *In vitro* cytotoxicity of the methylmelamines. *Chem Biol Interact* 29: 235, 1980

82. Rutty CJ, Connors TA: *In vitro* studies with hexamethylmelamine. *Biochem Pharmacol* 26: 2385, 1977

83. Rutty CJ, Connors TA, Nguyen HN, Hoellinger H: *In vivo* studies with hexamethylmelamine. *Eur J Cancer* 14: 713, 1978

84. Rutty CJ, Newell DR, Muindi JRF, Harrap KR: The comparative pharmacokinetics of pentamethylmelamine in man, rat and mouse. *Cancer Chemother Pharm* 8: 105, 1982

85. Schwartz DE, Bollag W, Obrecht P: Distribution and excretion studies of procarbazine in animals and man. *Arzneim Forsch* 17: 1389, 1967

86. Sherman M, Herrick RB: Acute toxicity of five insect chemosterilants, hemel, hempa, TEPA, MeTEPA and methotrexate, for cockerels. *Tox Appl Pharm* 16: 100, 1970

87. Shiba DA, Weinkam RJ: Metabolic activation of procarbazine: activity of the intermediates and the effects of pretreatment. *Proc Am Assoc Cancer Res* 20: 139, 1979

88. Shiba DA, Weinkam RJ: Quantitative analysis of procarbazine, procarbazine metabolites and chemical degradation products with application to pharmacokinetic studies. *J Chromatogr* 229: 397, 1982

89. Sieber SM, Adamson RH: Toxicity of antineoplastic agents in man: Chromosomal aberrations, antifertility effects, congenital malformations and carcinogenic potential. *Adv Cancer Res* 22: 57, 1975

90. Sieber SM, Correa P, Dalgard DW, Adamson RH: Carcinogenesis and other adverse effects of procarbazine in nonhuman primates. *Cancer Res* 38: 2125, 1978

91. Sykes MR, Rundles RW, Pierce VK, Karnofsky PA: Triethylenemelamine in the management of far advanced ovarian cancer. *Surg Gynecol Obst* 101: 133, 1955

92. Takida H, Didolkar MS: Effect of hexamethylmelamine (NSC-13875) on small cell carcinoma of the lung (Phase II study). *Cancer Chemother Rep* 58: 371, 1974

93. Tatken RL, Lewis RJ: *Registry of Toxic Effects of Chemical Substances, 1981–1982 Edition*, Volume 2, p. 651. US Department of Health and Human Services, Cincinnati, OH 1983

94. Tsuji T, Kosower E: Diazenes. VI. Alkyldiazenes. *J Am Chem Soc* 93: 1992, 1971

95. Weinkam RJ, Shiba D: *Procarbazine in Pharmacologic Principles of Cancer Treatment*. Edited by B Chabner, pp. 340–362. Saunders, Philadelphia, 1982

96. Weinkam RJ, Shiba D: Metabolic activation of procarbazine. *Life Sci* 22: 937, 1978

97. Wiebkin P, Prough RA: Oxidative metabolism of N-isopropyl-α-(2-methylazo)-ρ-toluamide (Azoprocarbazine) by rodent liver microsomes. *Cancer Res* 40: 3524, 1980

98. Wittkop JA, Prough RA, Reed DJ: Oxidative demethylation of N-methylhydrazines by rat liver microsomes. *Arch Biochem Biophys* 134: 308, 1969

99. Worzalla JF, Johnson BM, Ramirez G, Bryan GT: N-demethylation of the antineoplastic agent hexamethylmelamine by rats and man. *Cancer Res* 33: 2810, 1973

100. Worzalla JF, Kaiman BD, Johnson BM, Ramirez G, Bryan GT: Metabolism of hexamethylmelamine-ring-^{14}C in rats and man. *Cancer Res* 34: 2669, 1974

101. Zeller P, Gutmann H, Hegedus B, Kaiser A, Langemann A, Muller M: Methylhydrazine derivatives, a new class of cytotoxic agents. *Experientia* 19: 129, 1963

10

ANTHRACYCLINE ANTIBIOTICS

N.R. BACHUR

MICROBIAL ORIGIN AND HISTORY

Although the anthracycline antibiotics were first discovered in 1939, as red substances derived from microorganisms, very little was understood of their chemical structure and composition until the 1950s when a series of anthracyclines from *Streptomyces* were systematically studied through definitive chemical analysis in Brockman's laboratory. These research studies which lasted more than a decade formed the groundwork for understanding the chemistry of this very important, interesting and useful family of antibiotics. Although the time of the 1950s and 1960s was an era when the discovery and utilization of antibiotics was a booming and even dazzling scientific developmental era, the anthracyclines resisted inclusion into the fold of useful antibiotics. Time after time, anthracycline antibiotics were isolated by research groups and showed very promising antibacterial activity only to prove to be much too toxic in animal toxicology studies. So it was with interest when in the early 1960s anthracycline isolates tested for antitumor bearing mice showed activity against these tumors. These findings heralded the entry of this important class of antibiotics into useful application against human disease.

Brockman's laboratory in the 50s established that separation of the anthracyclines could be accomplished into identifiable fractions. Their studies went on to show that anthracyclines consisted of an anthracyclinone portion and a varying number of sugars attached to this fundamental conjugated planar ring system, therefore they may be classified as glycosides. The sugars belong to one family, and are daunosamine, rhodosamine, 2-deoxy L-fucose and rhodi-

nose. The anthracyclinone was shown to be fused ring systems which contained conjugated systems and quinone groups with phenolic groups substituted at various ring positions. Subsequently many anthracyclinones have been discovered with varying substitution arrangements (Figure 1).

In the 1960s the anthracyclines discovered in Italy and France proved to excite the medical world with regard to their anticancer activity. From the *Streptomyces peucitius* daunomycin or what later came to be named daunorubicin was isolated at Farmitalia (Figure 2). Meanwhile the French investigators at Rhone-Poulec isolated an identical substance named rubidomycin from *Streptomyces coerubleo-rubidus*. Testing of this substance on animal tumors showed significant antitumor activities. These antibiotics were rapidly developed through animal toxicology and formulation to go into clinical testing against human malignancy where the remarkable activity of daunorubicin against adult acute leukemia had a stimulating effect on research into the anthracycline family. New analogs were produced by medicinal chemists whereas old molecules were reisolated from various strains of the *Streptomyces*. However, the single most important discovery to date among the anthracycline molecules was the discovery of adriamycin (doxorubicin) in 1967 at Farmitalia in Italy. Clinical testing of doxorubicin

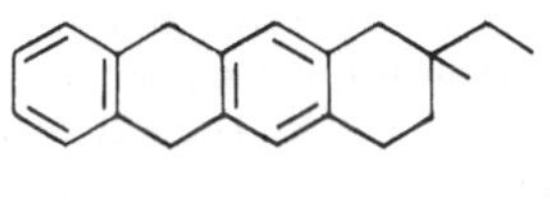

Anthracycline Aglycone	Phenolic groups		
Aklavinone	4, 6	OH	Sugars and other
Citromycinone	4, 11	OH	substituents at
Pyrromycinone	1, 4, 6	OH	other positions
Rhodomycinone	4, 6, 11	OH	
Isorhodomycinone	1, 4, 6, 11	OH	
Daunomycinone	6, 11, OH;	4 methoxy	

Figure 1. Anthracyclinones.

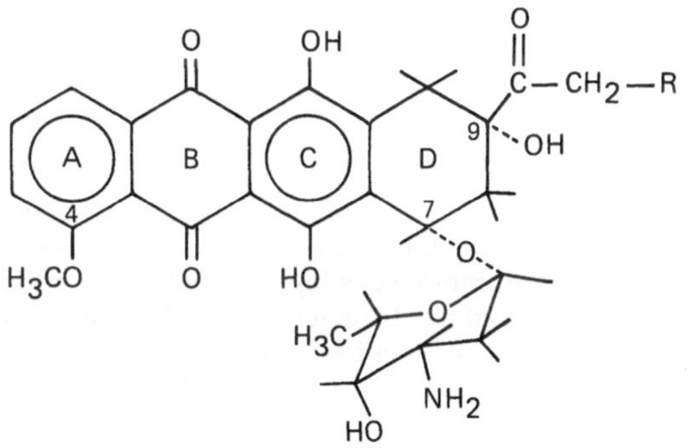

	R
DOXORUBICIN	OH
DAUNORUBICIN	H

Figure 2. Daunorubicin.

125

P.V. Woolley (ed.), Cancer management in Man: Biological Response Modifiers, Chemotherapy, Antibiotics, Hyperthermia, Supporting Measures
© 1989. Kluwer Academic Publishers, Dordrecht.

showed the antibiotic to have even more remarkable anti-cancer activities than daunorubicin since doxorubicin was quite effective against a rather wide spectrum of solid tumors as well as leukemias.

With the rash of excitement accompanying the discovery of the utility of daunorubicin and doxorubicin, other anthracyclines have been discovered and/or chemically modified to produce potentially useful compounds both for fundamental studies as well as for clinical usage. In the early 1970s, carminomycin an analog of daunorubicin was announced from the USSR. In the mid 1970s, aclacinomycin described by a Japanese group has shown to have antitumor activity and went into clinical testing. Since those important discoveries, thousands of anthracyclines have been isolated, characterized and tested for activity both as antibiotics and as antitumor agents. Today, a significant number of active and potentially active anthracycline analogs are available, although the major ones for clinical use at the present time remain as adriamycin (doxorubicin) and daunorubicin.

CHEMISTRY

Although the structures of many of anthracyclines have been determined, it is beyond the scope of this chapter to discuss each one. It is appropriate to focus on the clinically useful compounds that have been described since a great deal of corresponding comparative chemical and biological data are known for these compounds. However, despite this large amount of comparative data for both doxorubicin and daunorubicin, the correlation of chemical structure with specific biological actions lags. The red–orange doxorubicin and daunorubicin have the planar ring system of the anthraquinone with resonating electronic structure in the A and C rings and conjugated quinone structure in the B ring. Paired phenolic groups on the C ring supply hydrogen bonding, and a methoxy group at position 4 completes substituents on Rings A, B and C. The highly conjugated nature of the anthraquinone nucleus gives doxorubicin and daunorubicin their brilliant red–orange color. This distinctive color as well as the highly fluorescent nature of these compounds are very useful for chemical, biological and pharmacological studies.

The anthraquinone portion of doxorubicin or daunorubicin is by itself quite water insoluble and lipophilic. This gives the intact antibiotic molecules a highly lipophilic head which lends important binding characteristics to the molecules.

Although the D ring is not part of the conjugated electron system, its nonplanar characteristics are important for binding to macromolecules. Through the D ring at position 7 is linked the amino sugar, daunosamine, which is critical for water solubility of the molecules as well as their amphoteric properties. Under normal physiologic conditions at pH 7.4, the amino group of daunosamine is protonated and positively charged. The sugar linkage at position 7 as well as the side chain and hydroxy group at position 9 are optically active; and strict adherence to the proper stereochemical structure is essential for biological activity.

The only structural difference between doxorubicin and daunorubicin is the hydroxy group on carbon 14 of the methyl ketone side chain. It is an interesting and well established fact that this small chemical modification on so large and complex a molecule has such profound biological and pharmacological effects which will be discussed later. The differences in the chemistries of doxorubicin and daunorubicin are seen in increased instability for doxorubicin in solution and increased hydrophilicity.

Both doxorubicin and daunorubicin are sensitive to strong acid and alkali. Acids hydrolyze the glycosidic linkage to give the aglycones, doxorubicinone and daunorubicinone respectively and the aminosugar daunosamine. Alkaline treatment gives the fully anionic forms of the phenolic substituents at positions 6 and 11 which in time break down irreversibly.

Because of the quinone structure in the anthraquinone nucleus, doxorubicin and daunorubicin can undergo reversible oxidation reduction reactions. Under normal conditions, the quinones are in an oxidized state but can be reduced either chemically or biochemically. Reduction can occur either by single electron reduction or two electron reductions. A semiquinone free radical is the product of single electron reduction, whereas hydroquinone is the product of two electron reductions. The reactions appear to be important in the cytotoxic activity of the anthracycline antibiotics and will be discussed further.

A great deal of work has been done on the structure activity characteristics of anthracycline antibiotics, but no single conceptual picture of anthracycline model activity has evolved. This may be because no single site in eukaryotic cells is responsible for anthracycline cytotoxicity. Many modifications can be made to the doxorubicin and daunorubicin molecules to raise or lower activities. The sugar can be widely altered with no loss of activity – even with an increase in activity as seen in the cyanomorpholyno compounds. However, some groups of the anthraquinone are sensitive to change. These are the 6 and 11 phenolic hydroxyl groups and the 7 and 9 position groups. Loss or modification of the 6 and 11 phenolic hydroxyls reduces or destroys antitumor activity as does modification at the 7 and 9 position.

MOLECULAR INTERACTIONS

Probably the first predicted action of the anthracycline antibiotics was their binding to nuclear double stranded DNA. This was predictable since the anthracycline structural anthraquinone system is quite similar to other compounds which bind to helical DNA. The flat planar rings of the anthracycline quinone nucleus are an appropriate size and shape to slip into and between the base pair systems of stacked DNA bases in helically coiled DNA. This interaction has been studied extensively since the 1960s, and a substantial number of scientific papers describe the interactions. Despite all these studies it is still not clear what the exact molecular interaction is that accounts for anthracycline binding with DNA. Studies that utilize X-ray crystallography propose that the planar ring system slides between stacked bases and distorts the DNA helix. Projecting out from the intercalated anthracycline is the amino sugar which can be rotated and positioned so that the positively charged amino group can bind ionically with negatively charged phosphate groups of the DNA sugar phosphate backbone. Several variations of this type of binding have been published, and the intercalative mode is accepted as probably the most likely type of primary bonding. In addition, other types of non-intercalative DNA binding have been proposed for the anthracyclines.

The binding of doxorubicin and daunorubicin to DNA is easily demonstrated in tissue culture with live cells. The drugs readily concentrate in the nucleus of a cell or in chromosomal bands and will fluoresce strongly from these sites.

Several changes in the physical chemical properties of both the anthracycline antibiotics as well as the DNA occurs with binding of doxorubicin or daunorubicin to DNA. The drugs undergo spectral changes, with quenching of drug fluorescence as well and alterations of absorption spectra, and the quinone groups are limited in their ability to undergo redox changes. For the DNA, there is a decreasing buoyant density and sedimentation coefficient as well as an increase in melting temperature and viscosity. These are changes that would be expected of an intercalation reaction between drug and DNA.

Physical chemical measurement studies as well as studies utilizing X-ray crystallography and defraction, and NMR techniques have led to conflicting conclusions concerning the exact molecular interaction between anthracyclines and DNA. Most recently, an interesting question has arisen as to whether the different configurations of DNA show selective or specific binding to anthracyclines.

Another characteristic of DNA binding which has been investigated with the anthracyclines yet remains unresolved is the specificity of anthracyclines for base pair types. Although early studies describe a preferential binding to AT base pairs whereas more recent studies have leaned to preferential binding to GC bases, in fact, there are data which indicate that the binding to GC is an absolute requirement for DNA binding.

Recently interesting experiments have suggested a binding of DNA and anthracyclines through metal ion participation. This opens several possibilities concerning mechanism of action and may be useful for understanding DNA interactions. Because of the location of quinone and phenolic hydroxyl groups on the planar ring systems, the oxygens in these groups serve to share their abundant electron shells with positively charged divalent and trivalent cations such as Mg^{2+}, Cu^{2+}, Al^{3+}, Fe^{2+}, and Fe^{3+}. The chelation of metal cations by anthracyclines and the properties of these chelates have been studied extensively. The chelates with Cu^{2+} and Fe^{2+}, Fe^{3+} are most interesting also because of their possible involvement in free radical generation.

Although the binding of the anthracyclines to DNA has taken a paramount position with regard to molecular interactions in cells, these versatile molecules, because of charge characteristics and amphipathic nature, bind to numerous protein macromolecules as well as lipids and polysaccharides. In addition to extensive binding to cellular membrane and architectural structures such as the cell envelope, microsomal membranes, mitochondrial membranes and nuclear membranes, the anthracycline drugs also bind to soluble proteins. Examples of proteins that bind anthracyclines are spectrin, tubulin, histones, casin, fibrinogen, gammaglobulins, catalase, etc. Anthracycline binding can affect both the reactivity of a number of these proteins as well as protein interconversions. However, the binding affin-

ities to proteins are sufficiently weak that protein binding is not considered to be a primary site of action of the anthracyclines in the cell; but the protein–anthracycline interactions may mediate other actions and may lead to secondary affects which are important.

As part of the protein–membrane interactions, both the phospholipids as well as the polysaccharides play an important role in these functions. Cardiolipin has been shown to be a selective lipid component which binds to anthracyclines and is responsible for a significant portion of anthracycline membrane interactions. More recently, the doxorubicin effect on solid to fluid state transition in membranes of liposomes has been studied extensively with regard to lipid-anthracycline binding. It is possible that membrane located receptors may play an important role in anthracycline action and toxicity. Studies with anthracyclines bound to insoluble support show very high cytotoxicity for these drugs which do not penetrate the cell. This implies that the anthracyclines are acting at the membrane site.

Several respiratory enzymes are known to interact with the anthracycline antibiotics. First the flavoproteins NADPH Cytochrome P-450 Reductase and Xanthine Oxidase will reduce doxorubicin and daunorubicin to semiquinone products. In mitochondria coenzyme Q_{10} enzymes such as NADH-oxidase and succinoxidase are inhibited by the same anthracycline molecules. Of these reactions, no direct effect of the coenzyme Q_{10} enzymes has been observed. However, *in vivo* evidence of the reduction by flavoproteins is clear since the 7-deoxyaglycone products of this reaction are seen in tissues and metabolism products.

The anthracyclines belong to a group of natural products including mitomycin C, the vinca alkaloids, actinomycin D and antitumor substance which show a cross-resistance in some tumor cells. This cross-resistance is a characteristic which can be induced in the tumor cells and has been narrowed down to be caused by an increased ability of the resistant cell to excrete or eliminate these foreign natural substances. A membrane carrier phenomenon seems responsible but no common membrane carriers have been described. A few membrane proteins have been shown to be increased in these resistant cells but their exact function is unknown.

CELLULAR ACTIONS

Because of the quinone-containing structure of the anthracycline antibiotics, these agents were studied for redox properties in biological systems. With the appropriate redox potential of the anthracyclines, in the cell flavoproteins catalyze the reduction of the anthracycline to the semiquinone and hydroquinone state. Anthracyclines act as site specific free radical generating agents which through this mechanism and through the generation of secondary free radicals are cytotoxic.

As quinones, the anthracyclines can be reduced through a flavo-protein reductant, most likely either NADPA cytochrome P450 reductase or xanthine oxidase in the cell (Figure 3). These reductions are single electron reductions which generate the semiquinone form of the anthracycline antibiotics. This has been shown very clearly in EPR studies and in other types of research studies. The semiquinone of the

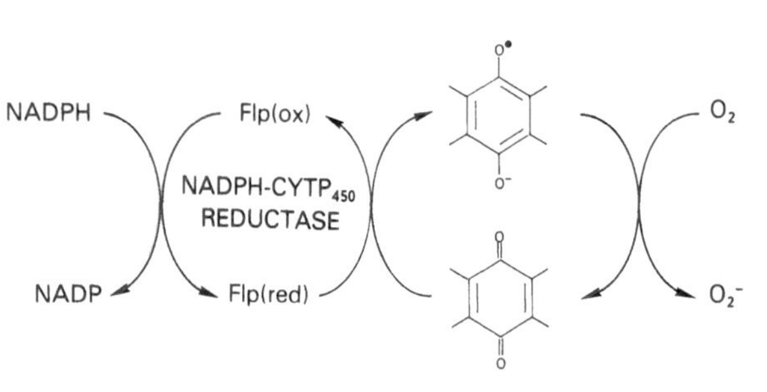

Figure 3. NADPA cytochrome P_{450} reductase.

anthracycline antibiotic is a very labile structure and quickly donates its electron to other acceptors, one of the most avid being molecular oxygen. When molecular oxygen is available, the anthracycline semiquinone is quickly depleted and the quinone structure is regenerated. The single electron donated to oxygen generates superoxide which is capable of reacting with other substances to generate other types of reacting oxygen components or other free radicals. If a free electron acceptor is not available, the reduced anthracycline will subsequently split at the glycocytic linkage point to generate the 7 deoxyaglycone and the sugar daunosamine as separate molecules. These reactions have been clearly described in both cellular and animal systems. These reactions occur in the cells and may occur at membranes where the flavoproteins are abundant such as in mitochondria microsomals and in the nuclear membrane. Because of the avidity of the anthracycline structure for DNA, it is proposed that an anthracycline free radical may bind rapidly to DNA after being activated and subsequently cause the DNA damage that has been described within cells through free radical breakage. This has been shown to occur in model systems and at present is one of the proposed mechanisms of toxicity and cytotoxicity for the anthracycline antibiotics.

TOXICITIES

Anthracyclines are very cytotoxic and display profound effects on tissues undergoing constant regeneration such as the GI tract, bone marrow, and hair follicles. During cellular replication in the S phase of the cell cycle, the cells are very susceptible to damage and cytotoxicity by anthracyclines. As a result, a major form of toxicity seen in patients is related to depression of bone marrow function. Depression of white blood counts and depression of platelet synthesis and anemia are direct results of toxic action. Vomiting, nausea, mucositis, diarrhea, and ulceration of the colon result from toxicity to the gastrointestinal tract. Partial or total alopecia occur because of the blockage of hair follicle growth. These are all temporary; and with the subsequent removal and excretion of the drug, these functions return to normal.

Associated with long-term anthracycline therapy and a cumulative dose of anthracyclines of about $550 \, mg/m^2$ has been the evolution of an unusual and pathonemonic type of heart toxicity. In this cardiomyopathy there is the destruction of cardiac myocytes with single cell drop-out and myofibril destruction and loss. When sufficient numbers of

myocytes are lost, failure of the heart muscle results. This is an irreversible process and is a major form of disappointment in cancer patients who are responding favorably with anthracycline therapy.

A significant clinical problem associated with the intravascular administration of anthracyclines is extravasation necrosis. This is a very destructive action which causes death of the tissues which have extracellular fluid contact with anthracycline producing subsequent necrosis, ulcer formation and delayed healing. Several studies have attempted to prevent this toxicity through different mechanisms, and it appears possible that antidotes which either split anthracyclines by free radical activation or ones which counteract free radical production may be the best type of antidote therapy.

CLINICAL USAGE

Doxorubicin and daunorubicin have evolved as important chemotherapeutic agents in the treatment of human malignancy. Clinical research in the mid 1960s indicated that daunorubicin was a very effective drug against adult and childhood acute leukemias. This sparked a remarkable interest in these agents since adult acute leukemia were especially difficult to treat effectively. Clinical trials with daunorubicin rapidly showed that both acute lymphocytic leukemia and acute myelogenous leukemia in both children and adults could be effectively treated to yield both a significant percentage of complete and partial remissions through the use of this single agent. Careful clinical evaluation of dosage regimens with daunorubicin increased the success rate by increasing remissions and reducing toxicity. Subsequently, the development of combined drug therapy for acute leukemias revealed that combinations of active drugs given at varying times and dosages could be more effective than a single drug. This development has continued with daunorubicin so that it is now used in combination with other active antileukemic drugs in the combination therapy of acute leukemias.

When doxorubicin became available in the late 1960s, clinical trials showed this anthracycline to be effective in the treatment of several types of solid tumors. With the development of combination therapy and new dosage regimens, doxorubicin has become a major anticancer therapeutic agent in the treatment of lymphomas, lung cancer, breast cancer, ovarian, gastric and other tumors.

Because of their chemical structure both doxorubicin and daunorubicin are administered parentally primarily through the intravenous route. Although dosage regimens have been examined thoroughly in clinical trials, recent evidence indicates that long-term infusion of doxorubicin may help in reducing the cardiotoxicity associated with cumulative dosing of these agents (see toxicity).

PHARMACOKINETICS – DISPOSITION AND METABOLISM

With the intravenous injection of doxorubicin or daunorubicin, there is very rapid uptake of these molecules into the cells of virtually every organ except brain. As a result, the

HUMAN METABOLISM OF DAUNORUBICIN

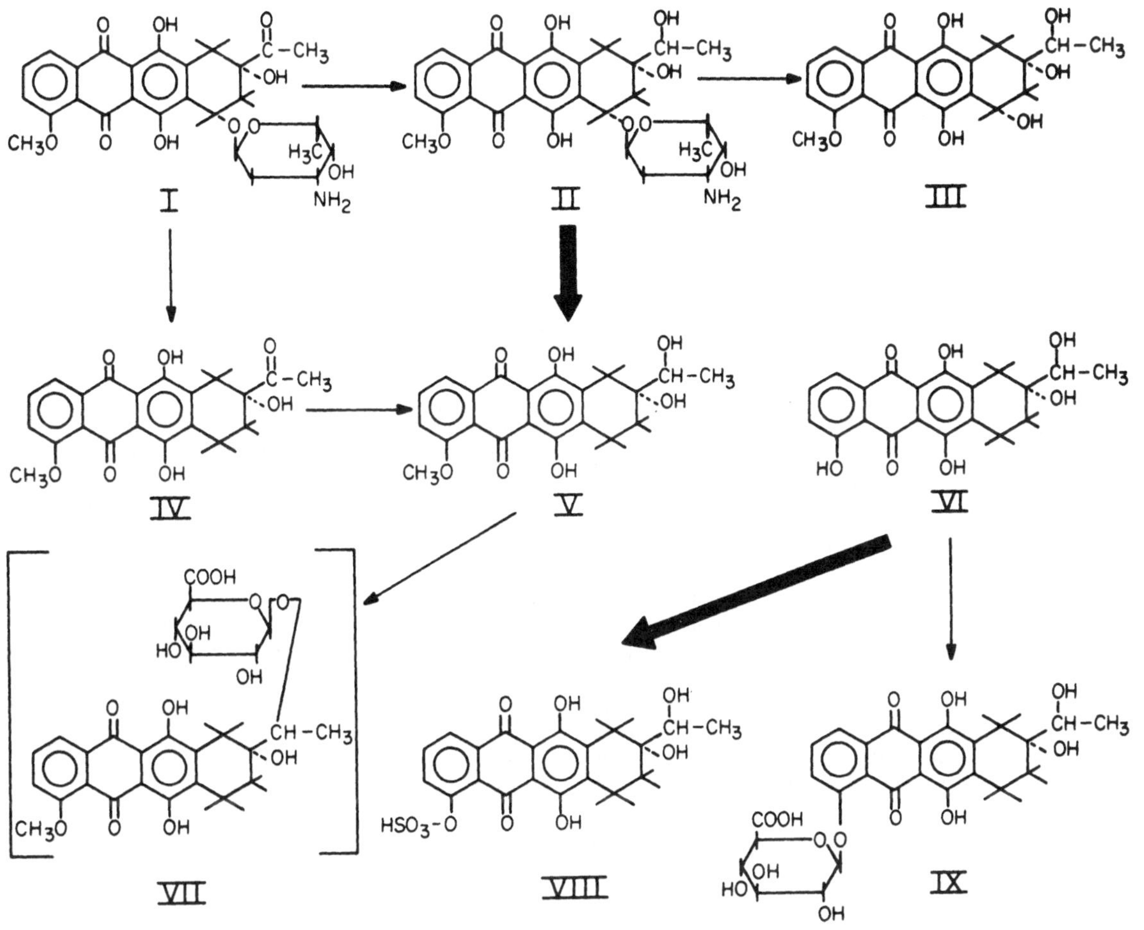

Figure 4.

plasma shows a rapid decrease in drug concentration as measured by a number of different techniques. After the initial rapid uptake into tissues, the distributive phase of the drug and metabolism occurs so that there is a gradual decline in plasma concentration over the next few hours giving way to a final phase of slow excretion and release from the tissues. The resulting plasma long half life approaches 30 hr with a significant degree of variation.

Tissue distribution of both drugs, doxorubicin and daunorubicin as studied in animals and acute studies in human autopsy tissues, shows a very rapid uptake of the drug, the parent molecule into lungs, liver and kidney with slower accumulation into heart muscle, gastrointestinal tract and skeletal muscle. With time, the concentration of drug or drug metabolites in liver and spleen tends to increase whereas other tissues show decrease in their drug concentrations. Tumor tissues show varying degrees of drug uptake depending on vascularity as well as the nature of the tumor cells. Uptake or retention into tumors does not exceed that with the average normal tissues.

In parallel with the tissue and plasma concentrations, the anthracyclines show initial outflow of drug through the kidney into the urine. This decreases rapidly. Simultaneously, with the increasing concentration of the drug in the liver, there is an increasing output of drug and metabolites through the biliary tract into the bile. As seen in both animals and humans, the urinary excretion is primarily of parent drug or of the primary alcohol metabolic product amounting to no more than about 10 to 15% of the administered agent over a period of a week. The biliary output, however, is significantly greater. Parent drug as well as several fluorescent metabolites are excreted for over a week into the biliary system. Most of the drug is excreted in the first and second day with rapid decline thereafter. Overall, approximately 50–60% of the administered drug is recovered in urine and biliary excretion. A significant amount of drug is not recovered; so these analytical techniques indicate either prolonged retention in tissues or metabolism to non-fluorescent species.

Extensive metabolism of the anthracyclines occurs in

mammalian species including humans, and how this metabolism is related to the mechanism of action and the toxicity of the anthracyclines is an important question (Figure 4). Neither drug is metabolized in the plasma. However, upon entry into cells, the anthracyclines are subject primarily to cytoplasmic enzymes known as the aldoketoreductases which can reduce the 13 keto substituent to a 13 hydroxy or alcohol product (Figure 4 I, II). This rapid reaction converts a significant portion of both doxorubicin and daunorubicin to their alcohol metabolites which retain both cytotoxicity and antitumor activity. The aldoketoreductases responsible for the production of the alcohol products are cytoplasmic enzymes that are constitutive and require NADPH for cofactor. They are a family of enzymes found in the cytoplasm of all cells including erythrocytes and platelets. These enzymes are known to be cytoplasmic converters of a number of keto and aldehyde drugs. Recent studies have shown that in aging individuals, the increased concentration of the alcohol products may relate to increased toxicity seen in elderly patients.

When the anthracyclines interact with the microsomal systems of cells, especially in kidney, liver or lung, additional transformations of the anthracycline drugs occur. The most important transformation involves the reductive glycolysis of the anthraquinone nucleus from the daunosamine sugar (Figure 4I, II, IV, V). This reaction has been studied in detail and involves flavoprotein reduction of the quinone structure to semiquinone and hydroquinone as described earlier in the reductive characteristics of the anthraquinone nucleus. Under suitable conditions in the cell, presumably where oxygen is limited, the anthracycline structure splits releasing 7-deoxyaglycone as a metabolite (Figure 4 IV, V). This highly hydrophobic product is metabolized through a number of steps to yield several other products leading way to conjugation reactions through sulfation or glucuronidation (Figure 4 V–VII, VI–VIII, VI–IX).

Although these metabolic reactions are numerous, additional reactions occur in cells with the anthracyclines since the metabolism of these substances leading to nonfluorescent metabolites has also been described.

SUMMARY

The discovery and development of the anthracycline antibiotics as anticancer drugs has been a major advance in the human endeavor to free mankind of disease. Although these drugs are imperfect, toxic, and have limited activity and utility, they have helped propel us toward our goal. The glimpses of success we have experienced in using them clinically lend hope to our cause.

REFERENCES

1. Arcamone F: *Doxorubicin, Anticancer Antibiotics*. Medicinal Chemistry Monograph Vol 17. Academic Press, New York, 1981
2. Arcamone F, Cassinelli G, Fantini G, Grein A, Orezzi P, Pol C, Spalla C: Adriamycin, 14-hydroxydanomycin, a new antitumor antibiotic from *S. peucetius* var. caesius. *Biotechnol Bioeng* 11:1101, 1969
3. Brockman H: Anthracyclinone Anthracycline, *Progress in the Chemistry of Organic Natural Products*, edited by Zechmeister L. Springer Verlag, Vienna, 1963
4. Gianni L, Corden BJ, Myers CE: *Annual Reviews in Biochemical Toxicology 5*, edited by Hodgson E, Bend JR, Philpot RM. Elsevier Biomedical, New York, 1983
5. Grein A, Spalla C, DiMarco H, Canevozzi G: Descrizione e classificazione di un attinomicete (Streptomyces peucetius sp. nova) produttore di una sostanza ad attivita antitumorale: la daunomicina. *Giorn Microbiol* 11:109, 1963
6. Naff MB, Plowman J, Narayanan VI: *Anthracycline Antibiotics*, edited by El-Khadem H. Academic Press, New York, 1982

11

ACTINOMYCIN

DAVID L. ANTON and PAUL A. FRIEDMAN

Actinomycins are antibiotics that were first isolated from cultures of *Streptomyces* in 1940 (36). Structurally they consist of a common phenoxazone ring chromophore, which imparts a bright red color to the compound, and two cyclic peptide lactone side chains of variable composition. The most potent and widely used of these is Actinomycin D which is often called dactinomycin (Figure 1). In addition to the naturally occurring actinomycins a large number of synthetic analogs with altered chromophores of cyclic peptides (19, 35) have been prepared (for a review see (7)).

Although originally isolated by their antibacterial action against gram positive bacteria, actinomycins soon were demonstrated to inhibit at very low concentrations the growth of DNA viruses and mammalian cells both in culture and in the intact animal (22). Gram negative bacteria are normally resistant to the antibiotic – a result of failure to transport actinomycin through the cell wall, since these organisms can be made sensitive by maneuvers that increase cell wall permeability. Most RNA viruses are not inhibited by actinomycin (22); those which are, such as influenza, are thought either to require cellular enzymes for replication or to replicate through an intermediate DNA, as is known to occur with the actinomycin sensitive RNA virus, Rous sarcoma virus.

MECHANISM OF ACTION

At low concentration actinomycin selectively inhibits DNA directed RNA polymerase both *in vivo* and *in vitro* (6, 16, 21). DNA replication and protein synthesis are also affected but only at much higher concentration (20). Initiation of

RNA synthesis by RNA polymerase occurs in the presence of actinomycin; it is the elongation step which is blocked (14, 17, 25, 28).

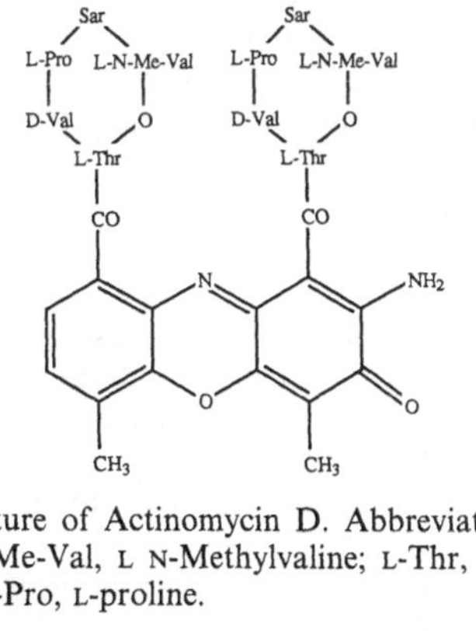

Actinomycin has been shown to bind tightly to duplex DNA. Complex formation can be demonstrated with a variety of techniques among which are: spectroscopic changes of the chromophore; decrease in the buoyant density of complexed DNA; increase in the melting temperature of complexed DNA (19). Complexes of actinomycin with either single stranded DNA or RNA or with DNA–RNA hybrids have not been observed (12). Maximal interaction occurs with synthetic DNA containing guanine or 2,6 diaminopurine, suggesting the importance of the 2-amino function of the purine for stable complex formation with actinomycin.

There is significant correlation of the biological activity of an actinomycin, its DNA binding ability, and its inhibition of RNA polymerase (23). From studies of a number of structurally modified actinomycins several functional groups have been shown to be essential for activity. These include the quinoidal oxygen, and the 3-amino group of the phenoxazone chromophore moiety and intact cyclic lactones of the pentapeptide side chains (24). Some changes in the amino acids markedly effect the conformation of the peptide and the activity of the antibiotic. Other amino acid changes result in only minor changes in activity (19, 22).

A model has been proposed for DNA binding based on crystallography of a complex formed between deoxyguanosine and actinomycin D (30, 31) (Figure 2). In this complex the phenoxazone ring intercalates between two G-C base pairs resulting in significant aromatic stacking interaction. The two pentapeptide lactone side chains project perpendicularly from either side of the plane of the chromophore. The peptides lie in the minor groove of the DNA helix. The 2-amino groups of the deoxyguanosine residues form specific hydrogen bonds to the carbonyl oxygen of the L-threonine residues of side chains. Weaker hydrogen bonds are evident from the N-3 ring nitrogen of deoxyguanosine and the NH of the same L-threonine. This structure is further stabilized by intramolecular hydrogen bonding between the two D-valines of the side chains. There are also numerous possibilities for hydrophobic and Van der Waals interactions.

This model of actinomycin binding most clearly explains its observed activity. In particular it emphasizes binding to G-C base pairs through hydrogen bond formation, and it is also consistent with observed changes in the polypeptide side chains. Furthermore, it is compatible with the observa-

Figure 1. Structure of Actinomycin D. Abbreviations used: Sar, Sarcosine; L-N-Me-Val, L N-Methylvaline; L-Thr, L-threonine; D-Val, D-valine; L-Pro, L-proline.

131

P.V. Woolley (ed.), Cancer management in Man: Biological Response Modifiers, Chemotherapy, Antibiotics, Hyperthermia, Supporting Measures
© 1989. Kluwer Academic Publishers, Dordrecht.

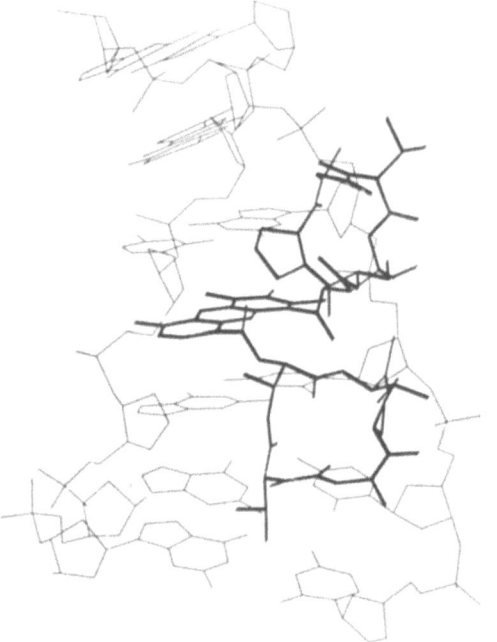

Figure 2. Actinomycin D binding to DNA. Model of Actinomycin D (in bold) binding to double stranded DNA (G_6:C_6) based on the coordinates in Sobell, H.M.; Tsai, C.; Jain, S.C.; and Gilbert, S.G.; *J Mol Biol*, **114**, 333–365, 1977

tion that RNA polymerase can initiate RNA synthesis, but elongation will be blocked when the enzyme, as it moves along the minor groove of the DNA template, encounters the cyclic peptides of actinomycin. DNA polymerase may be more resistant because it causes local denaturation of the DNA resulting in dissociation of the actinomycin (19).

ANTITUMOR ACTION

Actinomycin is highly toxic to all mammals, and this toxicity was initially thought to preclude its clinical use. However, further studies suggested that it might be used effectively as an antitumor agent with careful administration of the drug.

The most striking antitumor effect of actinomycin D in animals is the complete resolution of the Ridgeway osteogenic sarcoma of mice following a single non-lethal dose (27). Other experimental tumors of mice that are inhibited by the drug are sarcoma 180, Ehrlich carcinoma and Krebs-2 ascites carcinoma (3, 8, 33). Transplantable mammary adenocarcinoma is also treatable with actinomycin D; however, spontaneously developed adenocarcinomas are not (32). In rats actinomycin has been reported to inhibit Jensen sarcoma (9), human sarcoma 1 and human epithelioma 3 (17). Actinomycin is also effective against Rous sarcoma in chickens (10).

In man actinomycin D is highly effective in the treatment of gestational choriocarcinoma, and Wilms' tumor (unilateral nephroblastoma). In practice, the drug of choice for gestational choriocarcinoma is methotrexate; however, in the presence of renal or hepatic dysfunction or methotrexate

resistance, actinomycin is administered intermittently in large doses. Wilms' tumor is treated by surgical resection of the tumor followed by actinomycin D therapy in conjunction with radiation. In more advanced cases of Wilms' tumor actinomycin has been used in combination with vincristine and radiotherapy with improved results (4). Gonadal (primarily testicular) choriocarcinoma and mixed embryonal carcinomas have been successfully treated with actinomycin triple therapy with chlorambucil and methotrexate. Ewing's sarcoma and rhabdomyosarcoma of children also have been successfully treated with actinomycin alone and in combination with other agents or radiotherapy.

There is some evidence that both Hodgkin's and non-Hodgkin's lymphomas, and Kaposi's sarcoma are responsive to actinomycin (4).

PHARMACOLOGY AND TOXICITY

Actinomycin D is normally administered intravenously. Dosage schedules vary; a typical dosage schedule for gestational choriocarcinoma is 0.5 mg daily for five days. After a recovery period of 2 to 3 weeks dosing is repeated for 5 to 8 courses. The drug is rapidly removed from the plasma and accumulates in the tissue. Tissue distribution studies in the mouse, dog, monkey and rat indicate that liver, kidney, spleen and salivary gland accumulate actinomycin to the greatest extent; concentration is quite low in testis and brain (5, 26). Actinomycin D is not metabolized in animals and is excreted in both the urine and feces. A mean tissue half life in the dog has been estimated at 47 hours. Limited studies in humans show similar pharmacokinetics to those reported in animals. However, a small amount of actinomycin is converted to the monolactone, and there is prolonged excretion of the drug, with 30% being recovered in the urine and feces after 9 days (34).

Actinomycin D is much more toxic to dogs and monkeys (LD50 ≈ 0.01–0.02 mg/kg single injection) than to mice and rats (LD50 ≈ 0.6–1.2 mg/kg single injection) (27). Features of toxicity in the larger animals include gastrointestinal disturbances – vomiting, bloody diarrhea; in man nausea, anorexia, and vomiting occur within 4–5 hr after administration of the drug. Bone marrow depression and oral ulceration, other major toxicities are usually not evident until 2–4 days after a course of actinomycin and may not reach their maximum for one to two weeks. Depression of white blood cell and platelet production is the major dose limiting feature of actinomycin therapy (4).

DRUG RESISTANCE

Resistance to actinomycin D appears to result from decreased accumulation of the drug both in bacterial and mammalian systems (1, 2, 29). For example, in actinomycin-sensitive murine Ridgeway sarcoma cells initial actinomycin uptake was greater and retention prolonged compared to resistant sarcomas (27). For some resistant cells the nuclear membrane may be at least partially limiting; for example, resistant HeLa cells treated with hyper- or hypotonic media, resulting in damaged plasma membrane still did not accumulate actinomycin in the nucleoli (1).

REFERENCES

1. Biedler JL, Riehm H: Cellular resistance to actinomycin D in Chinese hamster cells *in vitro*, cross-resistance, radioautographic, and cytogenetic studies. *Cancer Res* 30:1174, 1970
2. Bosmann HB: Mechanism of cellular drug resistance. *Nature (Lond)* 233:566, 1971
3. DiPaolo JA, Moore GE, Niedbala TF: Experimental studies with actinomycin D. *Cancer Res* 17:1127, 1957
4. Frei E III: The clinical use of actinomycin. *Cancer Chemother Rep* 58:49, 1974
5. Galbraith WM, Mellett LB: Tissue disposition of ³H-actinomycin D (NSC-3053) in the rat, monkey and dog. *Cancer Chemother Rep* 59:1061, 1975
6. Goldberg IH, Rabinowitz M: Actinomycin D inhibition of nucleic acid dependent synthesis of ribonucleic acid. *Science* 136:315, 1962
7. Goldberg IH: Actinomycin D. In: *Antineoplastic and Immunosuppressive Agents*, Part II, edited by Sartorelli AC, Johns DG, Springer-Verlag, Berlin, 1975
8. Gregory FJ, Pugh LH, Hata T, Thielan R: The effect of actinomycin D on experimental ascitic tumors of the mouse. *Cancer Res* 16:985, 1956
9. Hackmann C: The effect of actinomycin on experimental tumors. *Ann NY Acad Sci* 89:361, 1960
10. Hackmann C, Schmidt-Kästner G: Über die cytostatische Wirkung verschiedener neuer biosynthetischer Actinomycine bei experimentellen Tumoren. *Z Krebsforsch* 61:607, 1957
11. Hamilton L, Fuller W, Reich E: X-ray diffraction and molecular model binding studies of the interaction of actinomycin with nucleic acids. *Nature (Lond)* 198:538, 1963
12. Haselkorn R: Actinomycin D as a probe for nucleic acid secondary structure. *Science* 143:682, 1964
13. Hurwitz J, Furth JJ, Malamy M, Alexander M: The role of deoxyribonucleic acid in ribonucleic acid synthesis. III. The inhibition of the enzymatic synthesis of ribonucleic acid and deoxyribonucleic acid by actinomycin D and proflavine. *Proc Natl Acad Sci USA* 48:1222, 1962
14. Hyman RW, Davidson N: Kinetics of the *in vivo* inhibition of transcription by actinomycin. *J Mol Biol* 50:421, 1970
15. Kessel D, Wodinsky I: Uptake *in vivo* and *in vitro* of actinomycin D by mouse leukemias as factors in survival. *Biochem Pharmacol* 17:161, 1968
16. Kirk J: The mode of action of actinomycin D. *Biochim Biophys Acta (Amst)* 42:167, 1960
17. Maitra U, Nakata Y, Hurwitz J: The role of deoxyribonucleic acid in ribonucleic acid synthesis. XIV. A study of the initiation of ribonucleic acid synthesis. *J Biol Chem* 242:4908, 1967
18. Merker PC, Teller MN, Palm JE, Wooley GW: Effect of actinomycin D on two human tumors growing in conditioned rats. *Antibiotics & Chemotherapy* 7:247, 1957
19. Muller W, Crothers DM: Studies on the binding of actinomycin and related compounds to DNA. *J Molec Biol* 35:251, 1968
20. Reich E: Actinomycin: correlation of structure and function of its complexes with purines and DNA. *Science* 143:684, 1964
21. Reich E, Franklin RM, Shatkin AJ, Tatum EL: Effect of actinomycin D on cellular nucleic acid synthesis and virus production. *Science* 134:556, 1961
22. Reich E, Goldberg LH: Actinomycin and nucleic acid function. In: *Progress in Nucleic Acid Research and Molecular Biology*, Vol. 3. Academic Press, New York, 1964
23. Reich E, Goldberg IH, Rabinowitz M: Structure activity correlations of actinomycins and their derivatives. *Nature (Lond)* 196:743, 1962
24. Reich E, Cerami A, Ward DC: In: *Antibiotics*, edited by Gottlieb D, Shaw PD, Springer-Verlag, New York, 1967
25. Richardson JP: The binding of RNA polymerase to DNA. *J Molec Biol* 21:83, 1966
26. Schwartz HS: *Sternburg and Philips in Actinomycin*, edited by Waksman SA. Interscience, New York 1968
27. Schwartz HS, Sodergren JE, Amboye RY: Actinomycin D – drug concentrations and actions in mouse tissues and tumors. *Cancer Res* 28:192, 1968
28. Sentenac A, Simon EJ, Fromageot P: Initiation of chains by RNA polymerase and the effects of inhibitors studied by a direct filtration technique. *Biochim Biophys Acta (Amst)* 161:299, 1968
29. Slotnick IJ, Sells BH: Actinomycin resistance in *Bacillus subtilis*. *Science* 146:407, 1964
30. Sobell HM: The stereochemistry of actinomycin binding to DNA. In: *Progress in Nucleic Acid Research and Molecular Biology*, Vol. 13A. Academic Press, New York, 1972
31. Sobell HM, Jain SC, Sakore TD, Nordman CE: Stereochemistry of actinomycin-DNA binding. *Nature New Biol* 231:200, 1971
32. Sugiura K: The effect of actinomycin D on a spectrum of tumors. *Ann NY Acad Sci* 89:368, 1960
33. Sugiura K, Stock CC, Reilly HC, Schmid MM: Studies in a tumor Spectrum VII. The effect of antibiotic on the growth of a variety of mouse, rat and hamster tumors. *Cancer Res* 18:66, 1958
34. Tattersall MHN, Sodergren JE, Sengupta DH, Trites, Modest EJ, Frei III E: Pharmacokinetic of actinomycin D in patients with malignant melanoma. *Clin Pharmacol Ther* 17:701, 1975
35. Waksman SA: *Actinomycin*. Interscience, New York, 1968
36. Waksman SA, Woodruff HB: Bacteriostatic and bactericidal substances produced by a soil actinomyces. *Proc Soc Exp Biol (NY)* 45:609, 1940

12

OTHER ANTITUMOR ANTIBIOTICS[1]

GARRETT R. LYNCH* and MONTAGUE LANE**

MITHRAMYCIN

Mithramycin, or aureolic acid, is an antitumor antibiotic derived from the species *Streptomyces plicatus*. At present, it is not a part of the therapeutic armamentarium of any specific malignancy. At one time, however, it played a significant role in the management of embryonal cell carcinoma of the testes. Currently, mithramycin is used chiefly in the treatment of cancer-related hypercalcemia.

Structure

The structure of mithramycin is shown in Fig. 1. Mithramycin is an aglycone chromomycinone which is attached to the three sugars, olivose, mycorose, and olise. The molecular weight of mithramycin is 1085.2 daltons (44).

Mechanism of action

Mithramycin binds to DNA in the presence of the magnesium cation and inhibits RNA synthesis without significantly affecting DNA or protein synthesis. Studies in the mouse ascites tumor 6CH3ED have been conducted, measuring the incorporation of phosphate-32P into DNA and RNA. There was marked inhibition of incorporation of phosphate-32P into the RNA of the tumor and liver, but no demonstrable effect upon incorporation of the isotope into tumor DNA (113). The maximal effect of RNA inhibition occurred within one hour. Like actinomycin D, DNA directed RNA synthesis seems to be affected. The guanine-cytosine base pairs appear to be the sites of DNA binding. The molecular mechanism of action of mithramycin does not appear to involve intercalation between base pairs (62). It appears that adenine deaminase is also inhibitited by the drug (37).

Disposition and fate

Pharmacologic studies to date have been quite limited due to the lack of a sensitive assay for mithramycin. Mithramycin is very poorly absorbed orally and is, therefore, given by the intravenous route. It is soluble in water and short chain alcohols. Tissue distribution studies in mice revealed peak accumulation of mithramycin in the kidney, lung and liver up to four hours after drug administration. It was detectable in the brain immediately after injection, but at no time thereafter (110). It penetrates the CSF, with blood and CSF levels of the drug being equivalent in four hours. Very little is known of the pharmacokinetics of mithramycin. Only one study was done in humans; this study involved a patient with glioblastoma (94). In this patient, the $T_1\frac{1}{2}$ was one hour and the $T_2\frac{1}{2}$ was twelve hours. Twenty-seven percent of the dose appeared in the urine in two hours, with an additional 27% appearing in the urine in thirteen hours. Studies to date have not elucidated if significant metabolism of mithramycin occurs.

Antitumor activity

1. *Animal data*

The introduction of mithramycin into animal systems revealed activity against P388 leukemia, with a 122% increase

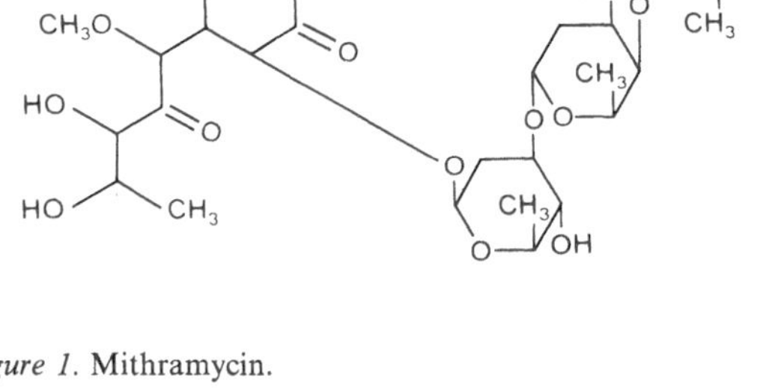

Figure 1. Mithramycin.

[1] Supported in part

[1] Supported in part by the Grady Goodpasture Grant and the E.R. Parkhurst Cancer Research Fund.

* Associate Professor of Medicine, Baylor College of Medicine, Chief, Medical Oncology, Ben Taub General Hospital, Houston, Texas.
** Professor of Pharmacology and Medicine, Head, Division of Clinical Oncology, Department of Pharmacology, Chief, Section of Medical Oncology, Department of Medicine, Baylor College of Medicine, Houston, Texas.

P.V. Woolley (ed.), Cancer management in Man: Biological Response Modifiers, Chemotherapy, Antibiotics, Hyperthermia, Supporting Measures vealed activity against P388 leukemia, with a 122% increase in survival noted over controls. Some activity was noted in Walker carcinosarcoma. Activity has also been noted against a transplantable glioma tumor in C57 black mice (59). No appreciable activity was noted in L1210 leukemia and B12 melanoma.

2. Clinical studies

Phase I–II studies have been conducted in several human tumors. Response rates have been reported as follows: non-Hodgkin's lymphoma (40%, 4/10 patients); adenocarcinoma of the colon (16%, 2/25 patients); breast carcinoma (16%, 5/34 patients); lung carcinoma (0%, 0/13 patients); and melanoma (15%, 2/13 patients). Isolated responses have also been noted in Ewing's sarcoma, ovarian carcinoma, prostate cancer, hepatoma and gastric carcinoma (63). A randomized trial in patients with malignant gliomas of mithramycin plus conventional therapy versus conventional therapy alone revealed no benefit for the addition of mithramycin (92). In all of the aforementioned studies, toxicity outweighed benefit.

The greatest antitumor activity of mithramycin is against embryonal cell carcinoma of the testes. A 47% response rate was demonstrated in twenty-three patients, including complete responses in five patients (60). Two of the complete responses were maintained over one year. These results were obtained with a schedule of 50 µg/kg/day by rapid IV infusion. Mithramycin was given every other day until toxicity was demonstrated. It was then held for greater than two weeks but not more than four weeks. This schedule was the most tolerable one with respect to toxicity. It involved close monitoring of LDH, BUN, PT and PTT; doses were held for PT > 15 seconds, LDH > 2500 IU, and BUN > 25 mg%. In the twenty-three patients initially treated on this schedule, there were no drug-related deaths. Other series utilizing this schedule revealed similar response rates and occasional long-term survivors. The alternate day treatment schedule has some basis in animal data (112). Studies of 32P incorporation into the RNA of liver and mouse glioma tissue demonstrated a marked difference in these two tissues in the recovery rate from the mithramycin-induced inhibition of RNA synthesis. Hepatic tissue rapidly recovered from the mithramycin effect, while the recovery of RNA synthesis in the glioma was delayed. This implied that an alternate day schedule of therapy may decrease toxicity while maintaining the antitumor effect. Very effective *cis*-platinum based regimens have replaced mithramycin in the therapeutic armamentarium of testicular cancer.

Hypocalcemic effect

Currently the major clinical use of mithramycin is in the treatment of tumor-related hypercalcemia. Mithramycin is able to inhibit osteoclast resorption of bone, via inhibition of RNA synthesis in osteoclasts. It is also able to block the hypercalcemic action of vitamin D (115). The effective hypocalcemic dose of mithramycin is lower than the standard antitumor dose. Patients often respond to a dose of 25 µg/kg given intravenously. Doses may be repeated every other day. Even with this schedule, renal function, hepatic function, coagulation parameters and the CBC must be followed very carefully. A study of mithramycin therapy in 89 cancer patients revealed normalization of the serum calcium after one intravenous injection in 56 patients, a significant but incomplete reduction of serum calcium in 30 patients, and no response in six patients (102). The hypocalcemic response is usually noted within 24 hours. In this study, patients with breast and kidney carcinoma responded better than patients with lung cancer, head and neck cancer, and multiple myeloma.

Toxicity

The high toxic-therapeutic ratio of mithramycin has prevented its widespread clinical use. Gastrointestinal toxicity, manifested as nausea, vomiting and diarrhea is not commonly seen with doses used to treat hypercalcemia, but is frequently seen with antineoplastic doses. A rash, facial flushing, and toxic epidermal necrolysis are also seen. Fever is noted in 15% of cases (89). A syndrome of sudden multiple arterial occlusions temporally associated with mithramycin therapy has also been described (76). The neurologic toxicity of mithramycin includes headache, drowsiness, depression and weakness. Hepatotoxicity, manifested as abnormal liver function tests, warrants monitoring the liver chemistries carefully, avoiding the drug in patients with altered hepatic function. Mithramycin can also be nephrotoxic; the dose should be attenuated or held in the presence of renal insufficiency. Clinically significant hypocalcemia and hypophosphatemia may be seen as a direct result of the toxic effect of mithramycin on osteoclasts.

The dose-limiting toxicity of mithramycin is hematologic. Myelosuppression, with thrombocytopenia predominating, is commonly seen, especially after prolonged courses of therapy. Leukopenia is not commonly noted. In one series of thirty-three patients with mithramycin, only seven of fifty-four courses of therapy were associated with a WBC < 5000 cells/mm³; no patients had a WBC < 3000 cells/mm³ (15). A unique hematologic syndrome is noted with mithramycin. It is manifested as thrombocytopenia, capillary fragility, and altered platelet function, with an inability of platelets to aggregate in the presence of ADP. Prolongation of PT, PTT, and the clotting time may be seen. Depletion of clotting factors II, V, VII and X are noted. A DIC syndrome can be seen with mithramycin therapy, even in the absence of depletion of liver dependent clotting factors. This hematologic syndrome is often unpredictable. It occurs in 5% of patients treated with a dose of 30 µg/kg/day for up to ten days. Hematologic parameters were monitored very carefully in a study of 41 patients treated with mithramycin; extensive testing was conducted in the eight patients who manifested bleeding (80). From the results of the study, the authors concluded that the etiology of mithramycin-induced hemorrhage was multi-factorial, with direct injury to the terminal vascular bed, quantitative and qualitative alteration of platelets, reduction of coagulation factors, and enhancement of fibrinolytic activity all noted. It was felt that the final common pathway in patients who bled was injury to the terminal vascular bed. It was also suggested that mithramycin therapy should be interrupted for any of the following: persistent epistaxis, marked facial flush and edema, bleeding time > 15 minutes, a platelet count < 50,000 cells/mm³, and significant increase in fibrinolytic activity. The dose of 50 µg/kg/day was felt to be excessive; it was recommended that doses of 25–35 µg/kg/day would produce equivalent therapeutic results with less hematologic toxicity. A 10% incidence of the syndrome is noted with higher doses of mithramycin or longer courses of therapy. The mortality from hemorrhagic diatheses in patients treated with mith-

MITOMYCIN C

Mitomycin C is one of several antibiotic and antineoplastic compounds isolated from *Streptomyces caespitasus*. It is isolated as blue crystals as a fermentation product of the actinomycete.

Chemistry

The structure of mitomycin appears in Fig. 2. Mitomycin C consists of a quinone A ring linked to an indole B group and 2 labile side chains. The side chains are a methoxyforma-mide and an azuridine ring. There are three potentially biological active sites on the mitomycin C molecule: the azuridine ring, the C-10 carbamate, and the dihydroquin-one. Mitomycin C has a molecular weight of 334. It is soluble in both aqueous and organic solvents (43).

Mechanism of action

The mechanism of action of mitomycin is not completely understood, although its antineoplastic effect is felt to be due to its ability to alkylate and cross link DNA (53). Mitomycin C is activated by reduction of the quinone ring. The quinone reduction requires an NADPH dependent quinone reductase system that causes spontaneous loss of the tertiary methoxy group (54). Subsequently, bond breaks in the azuridine ring result in the formation of carbonium ions, which alkylate the nucleophilic sites. In the process, a free radical semiquinone intermediate may form. The major site of DNA alkylation is the 6 oxygen of guanine. The multiplicity of reactive sites on DNA results in cross-linking. The steps in this reaction resulting in the formation of carbonium ions which react with DNA are shown in Fig. 3. A second effect of mitomycin C on DNA is to cause strand scission. This is mediated by free radical attack or by attempts to repair the alkylated sites of DNA (74). Of note, free radical scavengers, such as catalase or superoxide dismutase, can prevent strand breakage. In addition, after reduction, mitomycin C can form covalent bonds with nucleophilic groups on RNA and protein.

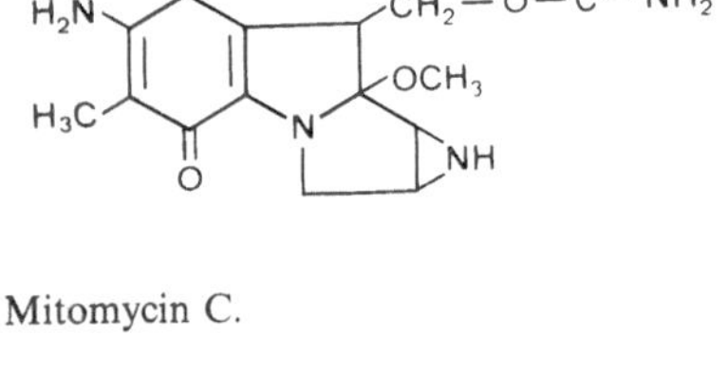

Figure 2. Mitomycin C.

In low doses, mitomycin C is selectively toxic to hypoxic cells. In high doses, superoxide radical formation occurs, and oxygenated and normal cells are damaged (61). Mitomycin C is both mutagenic and carcinogenic.

Disposition and fate

Mitomycin C has been administered by the oral, intraperitoneal, intrapleural, intravenous, intra-arterial, and direct perfusion routes. In man, mitomycin C is poorly absorbed orally, with the drug levels obtained being highly variable. Overall, the maximal concentration obtained by the oral route is 1/20 the maximal level obtained when mitomycin C is given intravenously (27). High local serum levels of mitomycin C are obtained when the drug is given by the intra-arterial or local perfusion routes. When given intraperitoneally, serum levels obtained in man exceed levels of drug obtained when given intravenously (26). Minimal drug is absorbed via the intravesical route, making mitomycin C an ideal drug for local therapy for superficial bladder cancer.

Mitomycin C is widely distributed. The highest concentrations of drug are found in the kidney, tongue, heart and lungs. High levels of mitomycin C have also been noted in ascites fluid. Mitomycin C does not penetrate the CNS (27).

Mitomycin C is rapidly cleared from the blood. The serum concentration at 80 minutes is only 10% of the maximal serum concentration obtained. Terminal half-lives of 50 and 42 minutes have been noted with single agent mitomycin C and when mitomycin C is given as part of a combination (31).

It is felt that the rapid clearance of mitomycin C is due to metabolism. Very little drug is found in the urine, with only 5.8% (range 2–15%) of a 20 mg intravenous dose excreted in the urine; glomerular filtration is responsible for the small amount of mitomycin C appearing in the urine (101). Mitomycin C is first activated by a reducing system utilizing NADPH and inactivated by liver, kidney and heart; inactivation is greatest under anaerobic conditions (100).

Antitumor activity

1. *Animal studies*

Animal studies have revealed a broad spectrum of activity. Mitomycin C was found to have activity against the Ehrlich carcinoma and the Yoshida sarcoma growing in ascites and subcutaneous tissue. Activity has also been noted in Dunning leukemia (IRC/741), Murphy lymphosarcoma, Walker carcinosarcoma 256, Jensen rat sarcoma, sarcoma 180, carcinomas 755, 63 and 1025 (55).

Studies from the original animal trials revealed that the safe starting dose for human use was 10 µg/kg/day and that doses exceeding 100 µg/kg/day would be toxic. A common regimen based on these data consisted of 50 µg/kg/day for 6 days; then the drug was given every other day until toxicity. Doses were repeated every 6–8 weeks. Problems with this schedule were that toxicity was cumulative and severe hematological toxicity was often not averted in spite of the fact that treatment was discontinued at the first sign of toxicity (33).

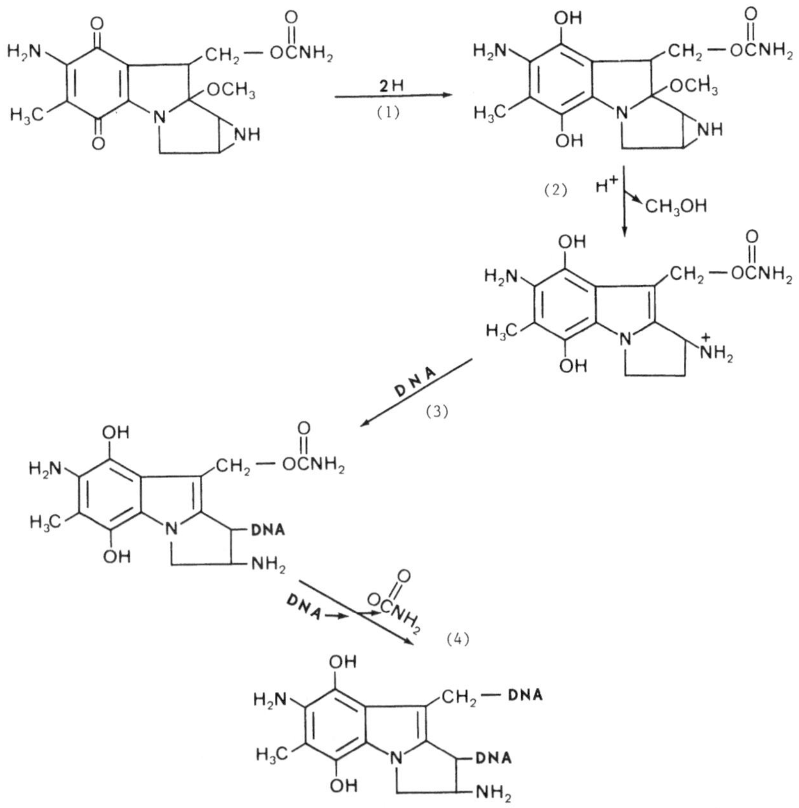

Figure 3. Steps in the reactions by which mitomycin C forms cross-linkages between DNA strands. In reaction (1), the quinone group is reduced. Subsequently (2), a methoxy group is lost and a carbonium ion is formed. The carbonium ion then reacts with a DNA guanine (3). A second carbonium ion is then generated which reacts with a guanine in another DNA strand. The two DNA strands may then form cross-linkages.

Studies involving Ehrlich ascites tumors revealed that intermittent therapy was as effective as daily therapy and was less toxic. This fact, as well as the unpredictable nature of the cumulative hematologic toxicity, led to the use of mitomycin C in intermittent bolus doses at 6–8 week intervals when used alone and in combination. The usual dose given on this schedule is 10–20 mg/m^2 (33).

Mitomycin C has been used in a number of clinical settings, both as single agent therapy and as part of combination chemotherapeutic regimens. To date, however, the exact role of mitomycin C is undefined.

2. Clinical studies

The initial human studies involving mitomycin C revealed 21/120 patients (17.5%) having an antitumor response. Responses were noted in the following tumors; breast (4/7), lung (1/15), colon (1/7), prostate (1/4), chronic myelogenous leukemia (1/2), chronic lymphocytic leukemia (1/1), rhabdomyosarcoma (2/4), Ewing's sarcoma (1/3), and unknown primary carcinoma (1/3). Of note, responses were not observed in the few patients with gastric, pancreatic, and uterine cervical carcinoma (55).

Subsequent studies better defined the activity of mitomycin C. Compiled single agent data in studies which utilized exact response criteria revealed significant single agent activity in the following tumors: gastric carcinoma 34.7% (26/75

patients), colon adenocarcinoma 18.5% (46/248 patients). pancreatic carcinoma 20.8% (11/53 patients), non-small cell lung carcinoma 16.9% (1,3/77 patients), head and neck cancer 20.9% (18/86 patients), and uterine cervix cancer 20% (4/20 patients) (26). The median duration of clinical response was of short duration in all of these studies, with a range of 6–16 weeks.

The role of mitomycin C in combination chemotherapy regimens for gastrointestinal neoplasms is controversial. The single agent activity of mitomycin C in gastrointestinal cancers has been reported to be 10–18%. In the early 1980's, a promising combination chemotherapy regimen of 5-fluorouracil, adriamycin and mitomycin C (FAM) was noted in patients with gastric and pancreatic carcinoma. An objective response rate in gastric adenocarcinoma of 42% was noted in the original study of 60 patients. The median duration of survival of responders was 12.5 months versus 3.5 months in nonresponders. Other investigators reported response rates of 42% and 55%, respectively, with prolongation of survival in responders (8, 41). Several trials utilizing the same regimen have been conducted in patients with adenocarcinoma of the pancreas. Response rates in series of 15–27 patients have been 37–48%, with median duration of survival of responders being 10.75–13.0 months (103). A regimen of streptozotocin, mitomycin C, and 5-fluorouracil produce similar results in pancreatic carcinoma (109).

The contribution of mitomycin C in FAM against gastric carcinoma is uncertain. A recent study compared 5-FU versus FA versus FAM in pancreatic and gastric carcinoma (29). Response rates and survival were equivalent in all arms, with the authors concluding that the combination regimens offered no advantage over single agent 5-FU. A large adjuvant study was conducted in patients with gastric carcinoma. No survival advantage was noted for the combination regimen, but toxicity was much greater, in large part due to the hemolytic uremia syndrome (38).

Mitomycin C is also used in the treatment of squamous cell carcinoma of the anus. 5-FU plus mitomycin C and radiation therapy has resulted in a higher cure rate in this disease, with subsequent preservation of the anal sphincter. The exact role of mitomycin C in this regimen is also undefined (16, 39, 77).

Mitomycin C has been used alone and in combination in adenocarcinoma of the breast. Response rates of 18% and 23%, respectively, have been observed in two series of 90 patients (24, 45), with response durations from 6–12 months. A combination of mitomycin C-vinblastine has produced a response rate of 27% in patients refractory to cytoxan, methotrexate, 5-fluorouracil, adriamycin and vincristine (64).

A single agent response rate of 20% has been noted in squamous cell carcinoma of the uterine cervix. A response rate of 93% was noted in one series of 15 patients treated with mitomycin C and bleomycin; these results could not be duplicated by others and was associated with a high incidence of pulmonary toxicity (79). A combination of mitomycin C, vincristine and bleomycin has produced a 37% response rate in this disease; responses to this regimen were of very short duration (5).

Mitomycin C has also been used to treat non-small cell lung carcinoma. Single agent response rates of 25% in adenocarcinoma and 13% in large cell carcinoma have been noted; these results were obtained in small series (95). Median duration of response for single agent mitomycin C in these studies was 17 weeks. Several combinations containing mitomycin C have been tried in non-small cell lung cancer; most of these series consisted chiefly of patients with adenocarcinoma. FOMI (5-FU, oncovin and mitomycin C) produced responses in 41% of 56 patients; response duration was 28 weeks (78). FAM produced a 30% response rate in adenocarcinoma of the lung; the responses were of 7 months median duration (94).

Although responses have been noted in other tumors, including sarcomas, head and neck cancer and chronic myelogenous leukemia, mitomycin C has not become a significant part of single agent or combination chemotherapy of these neoplasms.

Mitomycin C, when administered intravesically, is quite effective in treating low stage bladder carcinoma, with response rates of 72–83% noted (4). A complete response rate of 50% has been noted in one study of previously untreated patients, but only 31% of patients who received prior thiotepa had complete responses (85). In this trial, there has been no tumor recurrence at 12 months in 5 of the complete responders; 5 of the complete responders recurred within 6 months. Sixty-four percent of patients experienced no toxicity. The major toxicity encountered was bladder irritative symptoms; therapy was discontinued in 11% of patients

because of these symptoms. The dose of mitomycin C used in this study was 40 mg in sterile water given weekly for 8 weeks. No episodes of myelosuppression have been noted with intravesical mitomycin C.

Resistance to mitomycin C has been demonstrated in both human and animal tumors. It has been noted that remissions to mitomycin C given as a single agent are unusually brief. Although cell lines resistant to mitomycin C are resistant to alkylating agents, the converse is not true (26).

Toxicity

A number of common and unusual side effects have been noted with mitomycin C therapy. Anorexia, nausea and vomiting are the usual gastrointestinal toxicities; vomiting has been noted in 20–25% of patients receiving the drug. Diarrhea is noted in up to 10% of cases.

Skin and mucous membrane toxicities occur; alopecia and stomatitis occasionally have been observed. A maculopapular rash has been noted following intravesical and intravenous therapy. The most serious skin toxicity of mitomycin C is tissue necrosis secondary to extravasion of drug. Tissue necrosis may produce extensive ulceration and tendon damage; skin grafting is occasionally needed to treat mitomycin-induced injuries. Although no controlled data exists in humans on the treatment of extravasations, laboratory data suggests benefits from local injections of ascorbic acid or sodium thiosulfate (2, 51).

The dose limiting toxicity of mitomycin C is hematologic. Myelosuppression with mitomycin C is often prolonged and delayed, with the nadir occurring in 3–5 weeks; recovery generally takes 6–8 weeks, but may be longer. The degree and duration of myelosuppression may be cumulative, increasing with further courses of therapy. The white blood count and platelet count are affected more than the erythroid series. Hematologic toxicity in the original studies involving mitomycin C was related to the total dose; hematologic toxicity was rare below a total dose of 50 mg (45). With the currently used schedules of 10–20 mg/m^2, the median time to leukopenia was 3.5 weeks and to thrombocytopenia was 4.1 weeks. The duration of leukopenia was 1–2 weeks, while thrombocytopenia continued 2–3 weeks (40). This dose, given every 6–8 weeks, is associated with less hematologic toxicity. The mean total dose of responding patients was 99.8 mg. Fifty percent of patients experienced a WBC < 4000 cells/mm^3 and 70% experienced platelet counts < 90,000 cells/mm^3. The incidence of life-threatening toxicity or toxicity necessitating a discontinuation of therapy was low.

Nephrotoxicity has also been noted with mitomycin C therapy. Renal insufficiency, with rises in the serum creatinine, has been noted in 20% of cases. The renal failure may be reversible on discontinuing mitomycin C, but occasionally it is progressive. The pathologic lesion most commonly noted with mitomycin C-induced renal damage is glomerular sclerosis (40). Clinically significant renal failure associated with mitomycin C therapy is more commonly seen with the microangiopathic hemolytic anemia-renal failure syndrome.

A syndrome of microangiopathic hemolytic anemia and renal failure has been described in patients receiving mitomycin C (29, 56, 65, 85). Patients present with dyspnea, lethargy, and anemia. Renal insufficiency, usually progressive in nature, is present; fever, thrombocytopenia and neurological signs are often present. The syndrome is usually seen in patients who have been treated with mitomycin C for several months; it has, however, been noted after one course of mitomycin C and has developed after mitomycin C has been discontinued. At autopsy, little or no residual tumor has been noted in some patients who developed this syndrome. The incidence of this syndrome in patients receiving mitomycin C is unknown; in one series of over 100 patients treated with mitomycin C as part of the FAM regimen, 4 patients developed this clinical entity (65).

Renal pathology in patients with this syndrome revealed fibrin thrombi in afferent arterioles and glomerular loops. Onion skinning and fibrinoid necrosis are often noted in the arteriolar walls. Fibrin, red blood cell fragments and platelets have also been noted to be deposited in the walls of the renal arteries (65).

There is no effective therapy for the mitomycin C-related microangiopathic hemolytic anemia syndrome. Therapy with mitomycin C should be discontinued when this syndrome develops. Corticosteroids, plasmapheresis, dialysis and azathioprine have all been tried to no avail. Of note, patients often worsened following blood transfusions.

Interstitial pneumonitis has also been described with mitomycin C therapy (48, 83). Patients most often present with dyspnea and a nonproductive cough; chest pain may also be noted. The most common physical finding is the presence of basilar rales. Diffuse reticular infiltrates are the most common radiographic findings, although pleural effusions have been noted. Pathologic findings include diffuse alveolar septal edema, mononuclear cell infiltrates, and hypertrophy of the pulmonary lining cells. The mechanism of mitomycin associated pneumonitis is unknown. Patients may improve with discontinuation of mitomycin C therapy and corticosteroids. Concomitant therapy with vinca alkaloids may be associated with an increased risk of mitomycin C-associated pneumonitis.

Mitomycin C may be synergistic with adriamycin in causing cardiotoxicity. A study of patients receiving standard doses of mitomycin C after failing courses of adriamycin not exceeding $450 \, mg/m^2$ had an incidence of congestive heart failure of 15.3%, compared to an incidence of 3.4% of patients with similar characteristics who received adriamycin alone. The median time from the last adriamycin dose to the development of CHF was 8.5 months for patients treated with mitomycin C and adriamycin versus 1.5 months for patients treated with adriamycin alone. The significantly higher incidence of late congestive heart failure in the mitomycin C group implies that mitomycin C is potentially cardiotoxic (19).

Hepatic veno-occlusive disease has been noted in patients treated with very high doses of mitomycin C ($60–90 \, mg/m^2$) in association with autologous bone marrow transplantation. In this setting, where the normal dose limiting toxicity is overcome, hepatic veno-occlusive disease becomes the dose-limiting toxicity. Patients most often develop ascites, right upper quadrant abdominal pain and elevated liver function tests; on occasion, the patient may be asymptomatic. Pathologic findings consist of partial or complete occlusion of central or sublobular veins with edema and a con-

centric ring of reticular and collagen fibers. In one series of 29 patients treated with high dose mitomycin C and autologous bone marrow transplantation, clinical hepatic veno-occlusive disease was noted in 6/29 patients (24%) and pathologic disease was noted in the 4 patients with clinical disease who underwent autopsy (68). One of the 12 autopsied patients who had no symptoms of hepatic veno-occlusive disease had pathological evidence of this entity. There was a trend in the series for the incidence of veno-occlusive disease to increase with increasing dose levels. Patients previously treated with cytotoxic chemotherapeutic regimens had a higher incidence of this syndrome.

BLEOMYCIN

Bleomycin is a racemic mixture of antibiotics isolated from *Streptomyces verticilus*. It is a drug that is widely used in clinical cancer therapy, particularly in combination treatment programs.

Chemistry

The natural compounds contain copper bound in a coordination complex; however, the copper (CU II) compound does not have antitumor activity. The bleomycins with antitumor activity contain the ferrous ion. The bleomycins are sulfur containing polypeptides which are water soluble. The approximate molecular weight of these compounds is 1500. The various bleomycins differ only in their terminal amine groups. Chromatography has separated the bleomycins into two groups: A and B; these groups can be further divided into three fractions: A1-A6, A2, and B1-B2. The A2 subgroup accounts for 50% or more of most commercial preparations (9). The structure of bleomycin A2 is shown in Fig. 4.

Mechanism of action

The mechanism of action of bleomycin is the inhibition of DNA synthesis; RNA and protein synthesis are affected little, if at all. Bleomycin causes fragmentation of viral, bacterial, and animal cell DNA. Chromosomal changes are noted secondary to bleomycin, including gaps, fragments and deletions.

Bleomycin affects cells in the early S and G2 phases; progression of cells in G2 through the cell cycle is markedly delayed. Studies of cell cycle progression in Chinese hamster ovary cells revealed that mitosis (M) and the G2 phase were most susceptible to the effect of bleomycin. Mitosis was highly susceptible to the presence of bleomycin, with survival reduced to 2% in pure mitosis populations. Treatment of cells in the G2 phase was necessary to inhibit progression through the cell cycle. Interruption of transcriptional and translational processes in the G2 phase alters the synthesis or function of a division-specific protein that is necessary for the progression of cells from G2 to mitosis (6, 108).

Bleomycin acts on DNA to cause strand scission; the

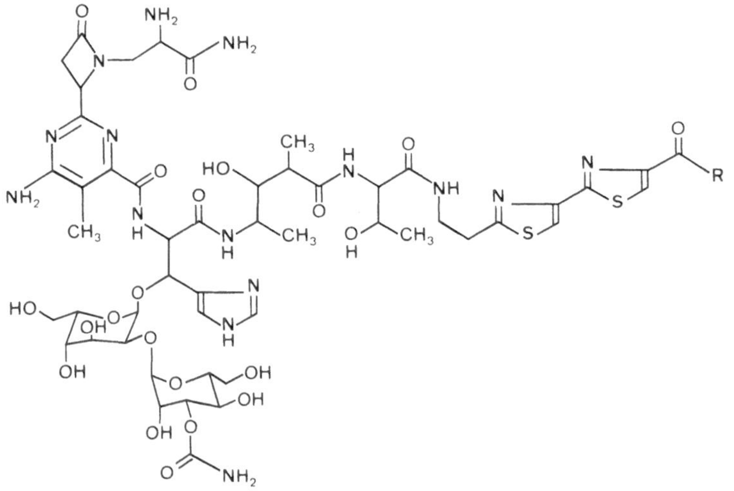

Figure 4. Bleomycin A$_2$.

degree of cytotoxicity correlates with the degree of strand scission noted. The strand scission is a direct effect of the bleomycin–DNA interaction (42, 73). The S tripeptide (aminoterminal tripeptide) of bleomycin binds to guanine bases of DNA. At saturation, one mole of bleomycin is bound for every 4–5 base pairs of DNA. The bithiazole rings of the S tripeptide are intercalated between the guanine–cytosine base pairs (86).

DNA cleavage is mediated via hydrolysis of the N-glycosidic bonds. The cleavage occurs at a specific site on the 3′ site of guanine, between guanine and the deoxyribose. Thymine is the chief product of DNA cleavage, especially at low bleomycin concentrations (104). The hydrolysis of the N-glycosidic bonds and subsequent thymine release results in single strand scission. Although double strand scission may occur, it does so at 1/10 the frequency of single-strand scission.

Of interest is the role of the ferrous ion (Fe II) in bleomycin cytotoxicity. Several studies have demonstrated an interaction between Fe II and bleomycin. The effect of bleomycin on DNA degradation has been shown to be enhanced in the presence of Fe II. DNA degradation by bleomycin is also enhanced by reducing agents under aerobic conditions (97).

Studies utilizing the reducing agent 2-mercaptoethanol revealed that bleomycin caused labeled DNA to become degraded to an acid labile form. It was felt that the role of the reducing agent was to convert trace metals from the oxidized to the reduced form. Fe II stimulates bleomycin activity in the absence of organic reducing agents, as well as in their presence. The same does not hold for the ferric ion, which stimulates bleomycin cytotoxicity only in the presence of a reducing agent (9). Fe II in the absence of bleomycin may cause degradation of DNA, but only to a minor extent. Of note, EDTA inhibits degradation of DNA by bleomycin, possibly by chelating Fe II. Studies have also demonstrated that under conditions in which DNA and bleomycin are active in DNA degradation, a complex is formed between the bleomycin and Fe II; the stability of the complex is oxygen sensitive (18).

Distribution and fate

Much of the pharmacology of bleomycin has been learned since radio-immunoassays of I-125 and Co-57-bleomycin have been developed (15). Bleomycin is widely distributed, with the highest levels noted in kidney, bladder, skin and lung. Very low to absent levels are noted in the brain, as bleomycin is unable to cross the blood-brain barrier (105).

Peak plasma levels of 1–10 million units/ml are noted with a 15 unit/m^2 intravenous bolus dose (1). After intramuscular injection, the peak plasma levels were 1/10 that of the bolus intravenous dose and were reached at 1 hour (82). Intracavitary administration of drug gives intracavitary levels that are 10 times higher than plasma levels; 45% of an intracavitary dose is absorbed systemically (2, 84).

The half-life of bleomycin after an intravenous bolus dose is 24 minutes for the first phase and between 2 and 4 hours for the second phase (22). A similar terminal half-life is noted after intramuscular injection. After continuous infusion of bleomycin, the terminal half-life post-infusion is three hours.

Bleomycin is cleared rapidly and excreted in the urine, with 45–70% of the drug appearing in the urine in a biologically active form in 24 hours (28). The remainder of the drug is felt to be metabolized. The best candidate for the mechanism of bleomycin metabolism is a bleomycin-inactivating enzyme that has been isolated from a mouse tumor line (106). The enzyme functions as an aminopeptidase, hydrolyzing the terminal aminoalanine portion of bleomycin.

Because the kidney is the major route of bleomycin excretion, the clearance of drug declines as renal function deteriorates and the plasma half-life is prolonged (28). Attempts to develop a dose attenuation schedule based on serum creatinine values have been unsuccessful, due to the variation in drug clearance among patients with similar serum creatinine values. Caution must be given in the use of this drug in patients with altered renal function. Doses of bleomycin are measured in units of antimicrobial activity. One unit consists of 1.2–1.7 mg of polypeptide protein.

Resistance to bleomycin has been noted in several animal cell lines and is felt to play a role in the short duration of activity seen in human tumors. In two resistant rat hepatoma cell lines, increased activity of an inactivating enzyme was noted; this activity was not increased in three resistant Chinese hamster ovary cell lines (13, 81). A bleomycin inactivating enzyme has also been noted in both normal and cancer cells. This enzyme has been partially purified from mouse liver (106). Minimal to no activity of this enzyme has been noted in lung and skin, accounting for increased toxicity of bleomycin in these tissues.

Altered membrane permeability may play a role in resistance to bleomycin. One bleomycin-resistant cell line showed sensitivity in the presence of the detergent Tween 80 (13).

Antitumor activity

1. *Animal studies*
Bleomycin is active against a variety of animal tumors, including Rous sarcoma virus-induced ascites, Friend's virus-induced ascites, Ehrlich ascites carcinoma, and a carbon tetrachloride-induced ascites hepatoma. Activity has also been demonstrated against Lewis lung carcinoma (9).

2. *Clinical studies*
Bleomycin has activity as a single agent and in combination therapy in a variety of malignancies. Although it is occasionally used as a single agent, its clinical use is chiefly as part of combination chemotherapy regimens.

Bleomycin is most commonly used as a single agent in squamous cell carcinoma of the head and neck. Single agent response rates have varied between 25–93%. Higher response rates are observed in patients with no prior radiation or chemotherapy. A compilation of trials in 576 patients revealed an overall response rate of 58% (9). However, careful analysis utilizing only objective criteria for response, revealed an overall response rate of 30%. The lower figure has been confirmed in other trials. Mean response duration was two months. Oral cavity lesions had the highest objective response rates. The response rate for bleomycin is similar to that for *cis*-platinum and methotrexate. However, the duration of response is longer with the other agents. Bleomycin has been used in combination chemotherapy in squamous cell carcinoma of the head and neck. Although objective response rates approaching 60% have been reported for these combinations, responses were of short duration and were associated with increased toxicity (36, 91).

In squamous cell carcinoma of the uterine cervix, an overall response rate of 21% was noted in a compilation of 78 cases in which bleomycin was given as a single agent (9). Responses were of short duration, with a mean response duration of 2.5 months (range 1–8 months). Bleomycin given by continuous intravenous infusion in carcinoma of the cervix resulted in a 38% response rate with a median response duration of 5.7 months (14). Combinations of bleomycin in cervical carcinoma have produced responses of 25–90%; the highest response rate was noted for mitomycin C, oncovin, and bleomycin (4). These combination series all involved small numbers of patients.

Bleomycin has been studied in small series of patients with carcinoma of the vulva and vagina. A 44% response rate was reported in one trial of 16 patients with vulvar and vaginal carcinoma (9).

In a series of 67 patients with squamous cell carcinoma of the penis, a complete plus partial response rate of 52% was noted (50).

Bleomycin plays a major role in the management of germ cell tumors. As a single agent bleomycin was associated with a response rate of 32% in 37 patients with testicular cancer. The duration of response was 1.5–2.0 months. Bleomycin is used in combination therapy of testicular carcinoma as part of the PVB (cis-platinum, velban, and bleomycin) or Einhorn regimen. This regimen produces a 70% complete remission rate and a 25–30% partial response rate (34). Of the patients achieving only a partial response, 19–20% were rendered disease-free after surgery. This regimen produces a 70% long-term disease-free survival and apparent cure rate. Regimens eliminating bleomycin have demonstrated a lower complete response rate.

Bleomycin also demonstrates some activity in squamous cell carcinoma of the skin. A US series revealed a 39% complete and partial response rate in 43 evaluable patients, with a median response duration of 2.8 months (9). Higher response rates have been noted in Japanese series (49).

Bleomycin has been used to treat Kaposi's sarcoma of both the classic and epidemic varieties. A 75% response rate has been noted for bleomycin in patients with the classic variety of Kaposi's sarcoma (107). In epidemic Kaposi's sarcoma, a combination of adriamycin, vinblastine, and bleomycin produced an 80% response rate in patients with fairly advanced disease (67). The toxicity rate for the combination was high, with 50% of patients experiencing opportunistic infections.

Bleomycin has also been evaluated in squamous cell carcinoma of the esophagus. Although a compilation series of 56 patients treated with bleomycin revealed a 54% response rate, most individual series have demonstrated response rates of only 15–20%, with response durations of only 3 months (57). Combination regimens involving bleomycin have given slightly higher response rates. A regimen of *cis*-platinum and bleomycin in patients with advanced measurable disease resulted in a 25% response rate; survival was only 4 months from the onset of chemotherapy (58). Chemotherapy with this regimen, when given preoperatively, has converted unresectable lesions into resectable tumors in rare cases.

Bleomycin has also been studied in squamous cell carcinoma of the lung. While worldwide series have reported overall response rates of 16%, US trials have demonstrated response rates of only 2–10% (9) that were of short duration. Bleomycin-containing combinations have given higher response rates, with little or no impact on survival (52, 71).

Bleomycin has been utilized extensively in patients with Hodgkin's disease and non-Hodgkin's lymphomas. US and European studies involving 198 patients yielded overall response rates of 44% with a 5% complete response rate (9,

36). When analyzed according to histologic type, the US trials demonstrated response rates of 43% for Hodgkin's disease, 47% for lymphocytic lymphoma, and 45% for large cell lymphomas. The duration of response was short lived for all types, being 3.1 months for Hodgkin's disease and lymphocytic lymphoma and 1.8 months for diffuse large cell lymphoma. The median total bleomycin dose for bleomycin responders was 225 units.

Bleomycin has been used extensively in combination chemotherapy of Hodgkin's disease. ABVD (adriamycin, bleomycin, vinblastine and DTIC) has been used in MOPP failures by a number of investigators. The original studies of ABVD conducted in Italy gave a 59% complete response rate, with a 27% 5-year disease free survival (38% for complete responders) (96). In the US, a 20–30% long term disease free survival has been noted with ABVD chemotherapy in MOPP failures (20). Other bleomycin-containing regimen such as B-CAVe (bleomycin, lomustine, doxorubicin, and velban) produced similar results (39). ABVD has been used alternating with MOPP as first line therapy for advanced Hodgkin's disease. The addition of the non-cross resistant ABVD combination alternating with MOPP improves the complete response rate to approximately 80% and improves the overall disease-free survival rate by an additional 10–15% (12).

Although bleomycin is used extensively in combination therapy for non-Hodgkin's lymphomas, its exact role is not clearly defined. In advanced diffuse large cell lymphomas, a regimen of BACOP (bleomycin, adriamycin, cytoxan, oncovin, prednisone), produced a 48% complete response rate in patients with advanced disease (99). Of the patients achieving complete remission, 84% remained disease-free beyond 2 years. Although similar results have been obtained with a regimen of CHOP-bleomycin, the response rate and survival rate did not differ from that utilizing CHOP alone (93). Bleomycin, velban and DTIC (BVD) may produce responses of 30% in patients with small and large cell lymphomas who fail first line chemotherapy. Responses to these regimens tend to be short lived.

Toxicity

Bleomycin is associated with some of the usual toxicities associated with chemotherapy, as well as toxicities that are unique to bleomycin. Bleomycin is only minimally myelosuppressive; this feature allows it to be used in full dosage in myelosuppressive combination chemotherapy protocols. In the original US trials of bleomycin, only 7/806 patients had significant thrombocytopenia or leukopenia (9). In one study of 172 patients, only 29% had WBC < 4500 cells/mm^3; the time to nadir was 12 days, with recovery by 16 days (43). In the same study, 48% of patients had platelet counts below 200,000 cells/mm^3; the nadir occurred by day 11 and the marrow recovered by day 17. The hemoglobin dropped in 58% of patients; the median decline, however, was only 16% from baseline. The median nadir of hemoglobin occurred by day 12 and recovery was by day 16. In this series, there was no need to attenuate drug doses due to hematologic toxicity; in this and in other series, there was no hematologic morbidity and mortality.

Anorexia, nausea, and vomiting occurs in 5–30% of cases; this is usually mild and of short duration. Diarrhea rarely occurs.

The dose limiting acute toxicity is mucositis. This is especially a problem with continuous intravenous infusion regimens. The presence of early mucositis is an immediate indication to discontinue therapy. The mucosal lesions often begin as linear white streaks on the lateral tongue surfaces. If they progress, severe limitation of oral intake may occur. Concomitant radiotherapy and bleomycin has resulted in life-threatening mucositis. Mucositis was noted in only 16% of patients treated with conventional dose intermittent therapy (47).

Fever is quite common with bleomycin, occurring in 20–50% of patients (90). Fever is most often noted on the day of therapy and is especially common after the first dose. Temperatures > 103°F have been noted in lymphoma patients. It has been suggested that bleomycin fever is due to the liberation of an endogenous toxin from host cells, probably leukocytes. In rabbits, a pyrogen is produced during the fever peak that can be transferred to other rabbits (45).

One of the most serious acute toxicities of bleomycin is an anaphylactoid reaction. This reaction is rare in solid tumor patients treated with bleomycin, the incidence being less than 1%; however, up to 6% (9/149) of patients with lymphoma develop this syndrome. The syndrome consists of hyperpyrexia, hypotension, bronchospasm, and occasionally, cardiac arrest. A review of four patients who developed this syndrome and later died revealed that they all had lymphomas, had doses of bleomycin exceeding 25 mg/m^2, and developed the reaction 6–15 hours after receiving bleomycin (69). The etiology of this reaction is elusive, as it does not meet the criteria of classic anaphylaxis. Endogenous pyrogen release is felt to be the etiology, although contamination of drug cannot be ruled out. Although this syndrome may resolve spontaneously, corticosteroids and antihistamines are recommended, as they can alleviate symptoms in a number of patients. It is currently recommended that patients with lymphomas who receive bleomycin should receive two 1-mg test doses of drug 24 hours apart. If no reaction is noted, then one can proceed with full doses of bleomycin.

Cutaneous toxicity is also a major problem with bleomycin therapy, developing in 50% of patients. The lack of a bleomycin-inactivating enzyme in the skin is felt to be reason why the integument is so sensitive to the effects of bleomycin. Numerous skin effects have been noted, with hyperpigmentation being the most common; hyperpigmentation is most common in skin creases, but may be diffuse. Characteristic linear streaks that are hyperpigmented commonly appear on the upper torso. Edema and erythema, especially of acral areas may occur. Rarely desquamation is noted. Although these changes are usually reversible, they remain permanently in a small percentage of patients (23). Raynaud's phenomenon may also complicate bleomycin therapy.

The most serious side effect of bleomycin is pulmonary toxicity. It may present as acute respiratory distress or chronic respiratory insufficiency. Although it may develop after one dose of bleomycin, it may likewise not become manifest until years after the last bleomycin dose.

The pathology of bleomycin-induced lung damage has been described in both light and electron microscopic studies (7). Light microscopy of lung tissue from patients with signs and symptoms of bleomycin pulmonary toxicity reveals intraalveolar amorphous and cellular debris, hyaline membranes, interstitial edema and fibrosis, a proliferation of atypical-appearing alveolar lining cells, and alveolar collapse. Electron microscopic studies have helped to elucidate these changes on an ultrastructural level. Alveolar spaces appear decreased in size and are occupied by cellular and amorphous debris; macrophages may be present ingesting the debris. Type I alveolar lining cells are markedly diminished to absent. Type II alveolar lining cells are increased in number; they exhibit marked variation in size and shape. These cells often have short microvilli, cytoplasmic edema, and disintegration of cellular lamellar bodies. Some of these cells are desquamated into the alveoli. The interstitium is edematous, with increased collagen; fibroblasts with collagen fibrils in their cytoplasm are present in the interstitium. The pulmonary capillary endothelium is normal.

It has been postulated that increased capillary permeability leads to interstitial and intraalveolar edema. Severe damage to the Type I alveolar lining cells lead to their disappearance. A proliferation of Type II alveolar cells ensues; the atypical Type II cells are impaired in their ability to produce surfactant, with alveolar collapse resulting. This proliferation of cells precludes absorption of intraalveolar and interstitial edema; this edematous material becomes organized and along with collagen production, results in diffuse fibrosis.

Although the exact site on the bleomycin molecule responsible for pulmonary toxicity is unknown, one investigator noted that the terminal amine substitute attached to the bithiazole group of the bleomycins could individually induce bleomycin lung toxicity when instilled into the trachea of mice (90). The terminal amine on B2 bleomycin was only a mild inducer of pulmonary damage. It was suggested that chemical modification of the terminal amine could possibly result in bleomycin analogues with less pulmonary toxicity.

The earliest clinical symptom of pulmonary toxicity is dyspnea on exertion; this may progress to dyspnea at rest and chronic respiratory insufficiency. Fever, chest pain, and a dry cough may be present. Although patients may present with acute symptoms of fever, cough, chest pain and shortness of breath, the more typical course is one of progressive dyspnea progressing in a subacute or chronic manner.

The earliest physical findings noted with bleomycin-induced pulmomary disease is coarse, basilar rales. In one series this occurred in 46% of patients treated with bleomycin; other series report a much lower incidence of this finding (11). Tachypnea, tachycardia and diminished breath sounds may occur. The paucity of physical findings often fails to reflect the severity of respiratory insufficiency.

Radiographically, the earliest finding is bibasilar alveolar-interstitial infiltrates. Later a pattern of diffuse interstitial fibrosis may be present. Occasionally, with the acute syndrome, fleeting alveolar infiltrates may be noted.

Although the arterial blood gases may reflect hypoxia, the earliest pulmonary function abnormality is a decline in the carbon monoxide diffusion capacity, especially when the total dose exceeds 240 units (72). It has been recommended that bleomycin be discontinued after a 50% decline in diffusion capacity. Late in the course of pulmonary toxicity, a decline in vital capacity and total lung capacity may be noted.

The incidence of bleomycin-induced lung toxicity has varied from study to study; an overall incidence of 5–10% has been noted. An analysis of 808 patients treated with bleomycin in the US revealed a 10.7% incidence of toxicity. Definite pulmonary toxicity was noted in 1.1% of patients, probable toxicity in 1.9%, unexpected autopsy findings of bleomycin toxicity in 2.0%, and questionable toxicity in 5.7%. In this study, the definite group had clinical toxicity with tissue documentation; the probable group had clinical findings without tissue documentation. Seven patients (1%) in this series had drug-induced pulmonary deaths (9).

When the doses at which pulmonary toxicity occurred were analyzed, it was noted that the incidence of pulmonary toxicity was relatively constant at doses lower than 400 units, being 3–5% at each 50 unit dose level. Above 400 units, the incidence of toxicity increased considerably. In the 450–549 unit range, 13% of patients experienced pulmonary toxicity; the incidence was 17% at doses greater than 550 units. Based on this data, it has been recommended not to exceed the 400 unit total dose.

Bleomycin must be used with caution in several clinical settings. Patients over age 70 tolerate bleomycin poorly; a dose of 300 units should not be exceeded in this population (25). In the animal model, older rats had less bleomycin-inactivating capacity than younger animals. Prior radiotherapy to the chest may increase the risk of bleomycin pulmonary toxicity (35). In addition, some studies have suggested that concomitant alkylating agent therapy may lower the total bleomycin dose at which pulmonary toxicity is seen. Patients with lymphomas who are receiving bleomycin appear to be especially prone to pulmonary toxicity at lower than normal doses.

Oxygen therapy greatly increases the risk of bleomycin pulmonary toxicity. Patients who have received bleomycin and are given high concentrations of oxygen, especially at the time of surgery or immediately postoperatively, are at increased risk for acute and chronic respiratory insufficiency (46). This increased sensitivity to high concentrations of inspired oxygen is felt to be due to increased formation of oxygen-derived free radicals which mediate pulmonary toxicity. The incidence of this toxicity can be greatly reduced by decreasing the FlO_2 to 24% and minimizing fluids administered at the time of surgery and in the immediate postoperative period.

REFERENCES

1. Alberts DS, Chen HSG, Liu R et al: Bleomycin pharmacokinetics in man. I. Intravenous administration. *Cancer Chemother Pharmacol* 1: 177, 1978
2. Alberts DS, Chen HSG, Mayersohn M et al: Bleomycin pharmacokinetics in man. II. Intracavitary administration. *Cancer Chemother Pharmacol* 2: 127, 1979
3. Argenta LC, Manderes EK: Mitomycin C extravasation injuries. *Cancer* 51: 1080, 1983
4. Baker LH: Study of mitomycin C in cervical cancer in the United States. In: *Mitomycin C: Current Status and New Developments*, pp. 159–162. Edited by SK Carter, ST Crooke. Academic Press, New York, 1979
5. Baker LH, Vaitkevicius VK: The development of an acute

intermittent schedule–mitomycin C. In: *Mitomycin C: Current Status and New Developments*, pp. 159–162. Edited by SK Carter, ST Crooke. Academic Press, New York, 77–82, 1979

6. Barranco SC, Humphrey RM: The effect of bleomycin on survival and cell progression in hamster cells *in vitro*. *Cancer Research* 31: 1218, 1971

7. Bedrossion CW, Luna MA, MacKay B et al: Ultrastructure of pulmonary bleomycin toxicity. *Cancer* 32: 44, 1972

8. Bitram JD, Dresser PK, Kozloff MF et al: Treatment of metastatic pancreatic and gastric adenocarcinoma with 5-fluorouracil, adriamycin, and mitomycin C (FAM) for advanced adenocarcinoma of the pancreas. *Cancer Treat Rep* 63: 2049, 1979

9. Blum RH, Carter SK, Agre K: A clinical review of bleomycin – a new antineoplastic agent. *Cancer* 31: 903, 1973

10. Bonadonna G, DeLena M, Monfordini S et al: Clinical trials with bleomycin in lymphomas and solid tumors. *Europ J Cancer* 8: 205–15, 1972

11. Bonadonna G: Chemotherapy of malignant lymphomas. *Semin Oncol* 12 (4 Suppl 6): 1, 1985

12. Bonadonna G, Vivini S, Bonfonte V et al: Alternating chemotherapy with MOPP/ABVD in Hodgkin's disease: updated results. *Proc Am soc Clin Oncol* 3: 254, 1984

13. Brabbs S, Warr JR: Isolation and characterization of bleomycin resistant clones of CHO cells. *Genet Res* 4: 269, 1979

14. Bracker RB, Johnson DE, van Eschenbach AC: Role of intravesical mitomycin C in the management of superficial bladder tumors. *Urology* 16: 11, 1980

15. Broughton A, Strong JE: Radioimmunoassay of bleomycin. *Cancer Res* 36: 1418, 1976

16. Bruckner HW, Spigelman MK, Mandel E et al: Carcinoma of the anus treated with a combination of radiotherapy and chemotherapy. *Cancer Treat Rep* 63: 395, 1979

17. Burger RM, Peisach J, Bumberg WE et al: Iron-bleomycin interaction with oxygen and oxygen analogues. Effects on spectra and drug activity. *J Biol Chem* 254: 10906, 1979

18. Burger RM, Horwitz SB, Peisach J et al: Oxygenated iron-bleomycin. A short-lived intermediate in the reaction of ferrous bleomycin with oxygen. *Biol Chem* 254: 12299, 1979

19. Buzdar AU, Legha SS, Tashima CK et al: Adriamycin and mitomycin C: Possible synergistic toxicity. *Cancer Treat Rep* 62: 1005, 1978

20. Cantrell J, Schein P, Winokur S et al: A cancer-related thrombotic microangiopathy: Natural history and therapy. *Proc Am Soc Clin Oncol* 2: 12, 1983

21. Case DC, Young CW, Lee BJH: Combination chemotherapy of MOPP-resistant Hodgkin's disease with B-CAVe following MOPP failure. *Cancer* 41: 1670, 1978

22. Chabner BA: Bleomycin. In: *Pharmacologic Principles of Cancer Treatment*, p. 381. Edited by B Chabner. WB Saunders Co, Philadelphia, 1982

23. Cohen IS, Mosher MB, O'Keefe EJ: Cutaneous toxicity of bleomycin therapy. *Arch Dermat* 107: 553, 1973

24. Creech RH, Catalano RB, Shah MK: An effective low dose mitomycin regimen for hormonal and chemotherapy refractory patients with metastatic breast cancer. *Cancer* 51: 1034, 1983

25. Crooke ST, Bradner WT: Bleomycin, a review. *Journ Med* 7: 333, 1976

26. Crooke ST, Bradner WT: Mitomycin C. A review. *Cancer Treatment Reviews* 3: 121, 1976

27. Crooke ST, Henderson M, Samson M et al: Phase I study of oral mitomycin C. *Cancer Treatment Rep* 60: 1633, 1976

28. Crooke ST, Light F, Broughton A et al: Bleomycin serum pharmacokinetics as determined by a radioimmunoassay and a microbiological assay in a patient with compromised renal function. *Cancer* 39: 1430, 1977

29. Cullinan SA, Moertel CG, Gleming TR et al: A comparison of three chemotherapeutic regimens in the treatment of advanced pancreatic and gastric carcinoma. *JAMA* 253: 2061, 1985

30. Curreri AR, Ansfield FJ: Mithramycin-human toxicology and preliminary therapeutic investigation. *Cancer Chemother Rep* 8: 18, 1960

31. denHartligh R, McVie JG, van Oort WJ et al: Pharmacokinetics of mitomycin C in humans. *Cancer Research* 43: 5017, 1983

32. Dinarello CA, Ward SB, Wolff SM: Pyrogenic properties of bleomycin (NSC-125066). *Cancer Chemother Rep* 57: 393, 1973

33. Doll DC, Weiss RB, Issell BF: Mitomycin C: Ten years after approval for marketing. *J Clinical Oncol* 3: 276, 1985

34. Einhorn LH, Donahue JP: *Cis*-diamminedichloroplatinum, vinblastine, and bleomycin chemotherapy in disseminated testicular cancer. *Ann Intern Med* 87: 293, 1977

35. Einhorn L, Krause M, Hornback N et al: Enhanced pulmonary toxicity with bleomycin and radiotherapy in oat cell lung cancer. *Cancer* 37: 2414, 1976

36. Ervin TJ, Weichselbaum RR, Miller D et al: Treatment of advanced squamous cell carcinoma of the head and neck with *cis*-platinum, bleomycin and methotrexate (PBM). *Cancer Treat Rep* 65: 787, 1981

37. Evans JT, Tritrach GL, Mittleman A: Mithramycin inhibition of adenosine deaminase activity. *Proc Am Soc Cancer Res* 20: 85, 1979

38. Fielding JW, Fagg SL, Jones BG et al: An interim report of a prospective, randomized controlled study of adjuvant chemotherapy in operable gastric cancer: British Stomach Cancer Group. *World J Surgery* 7: 390, 1983

39. Flam MS, John M, Lovalvo LJ et al: Definitive management of epithelial malignancies of the anal canal. A report of 12 cases. *Cancer* 51: 1378, 1983

40. Frank W, Osterberg AE: Mitomycin C. An evaluation of Japanese reports. *Cancer Chemother Rep* 52: 182, 1974

41. Gastrointestinal Tumor Study Group: A comparative clinical assessment of combination chemotherapy in the management of advanced gastric carcinoma. *Cancer* 49: 1362, 1961

42. Giloni L, Takeshita M, Johnson F et al: Bleomycin-induced strand scission of DNA: Mechanism of deoxyribose cleavage. *J Biol Chem* 256: 8608, 1981

43. Glaubiger D, Ramu A: Antitumor antibiotics. In: *Pharmacologic Principles of Cancer Treatment*, p. 407. Edited by B Chabner. WB Saunders Co, Philadelphia, 1982

44. Glaubiger D, Ramu A: Antitumor antibiotics. In: *Pharmacologic Principles of Cancer Treatment*, p. 140. WB Saunders Co, Philadelphia, 1982

45. Godfrey T: Mitomycin C in breast cancer. In: *Mitomycin C: Current Status and New Developments*, pp. 91–99. Edited by Sk Carter, ST Crooke. Academic Press, Orlando, Fla, 1974

46. Goldiner PL, Carlton P, Critovic E et al: Factors influencing post-operative morbidity and mortality in patients treated with bleomycin. *Br Med J* 1: 1664, 1978

47. Gottlieb JA: New drugs introduced into clinical trials. In: *Cancer Chemotherapy: Fundamental Concepts and Recent Advances*, pp. 79–98. Year Book Med Pub, Chicago, 1975

48. Gunstream SR, Seidenfield JJ, Sobonya RE: Mitomycin-associated lung disease. *Cancer Treat Rep* 67: 301, 1983

49. Ichikawa T: The clinical effects of bleomycin against squamous cell carcinoma and further developments. In: *Progress in Antimicrobial and Anticancer Chemotherapy*, Vol. 2, pp. 304–308. Univ. of Tokyo Press, Tokyo, 1970

50. Ichikawa T, Nakano I, Hirokowa I: Bleomycin treatment of tumors of the penis and scrotum. *J Urol* 102: 699, 1969

51. Ignoffo REJ, Friedman MA: Therapy of local toxicities caused by extravasation of cancer chemotherapeutic drug. *Cancer Treat Rev* 7: 17, 1980

52. Itri LM, Gralla RJ, Kelsen DP et al: *Cis*-platinum, vincris-

tine, and bleomycin in combination chemotherapy of advanced non-small cell lung cancer. *Cancer* 51: 1050, 1983

53. Iyer VN, Szybalski WA: A molecular mechanism of mitomycin C action: Linking of complimentary DNA strands. *Proc Natl Acad Sci* 50: 355, 1963

54. Iyer VN, Szybalski WA: Mitomycins and porfuromycins: Chemical mechanisms of activation and cross-linking of DNA. *Science* 145: 55, 1964

55. Jones R: Mitomycin C – A preliminary report of studies of human pharmacology and initial therapeutic trial. *Cancer Chemother Rep* 2: 3, 1985

56. Jones BJ, Newmann EE, Fielding JW et al: Intravascular hemolysis and renal impairment after blood transfusions in two patients on long-term 5-Fluorouracil and mitomycin C. *Lancet* 1: 1275, 1980

57. Kelsen D: Chemotherapy of esophageal cancer. *Seminars in Oncology* 11: 159, 1984

58. Kelsen DP, Cvitkovic E, Bains M et al: *Cis*-diamminedichloroplatinum (II) and bleomycin in the treatment of esophageal cancer. *Cancer Treat Rep* 62: 1941, 1978

59. Kennedy BJ, Sandberg-Wollheim M, Lolan M et al: Studies with tritiated mithramycin in C3H mice. *Cancer Res* 27: 1534, 1967

60. Kennedy BS: Mithramycin therapy in advanced testicular neoplasms. *Cancer* 26: 755, 1970

61. Kennedy KA, Rockwell S, Sartorelli AC: Preferential activation of mitomycin C to cytotoxic metabolites by hypoxic tumor cells. *Cancer Research* 40: 2356, 1980

62. Kiselera DA, Volkova NG, Stukacheve EA et al: Relationship between the structure and activity of antibiotics of the group of aureolic acid. Formation of complexes with DNA and suppression of RNA synthesis. *Mol Biol* 7: 741, 1974

63. Kolman S, Eisenstein R: Mithramycin in the treatment of disseminated cancer. *Cancer Chemother Rep* 32: 77, 1963

64. Konitis PH, Aisner J, vanEdhe DA et al: Mitomycin C and vinblastine chemotherapy in advanced breast cancer. *Cancer* 48: 1295, 1981

65. Kressel BR, Ryan KP, Duong AT et al: Microangiopathic hemolytic anemia, thrombocytopenia, and renal failure in patients treated for adenocarcinoma. *Cancer* 48: 1738, 1981

66. Krikorian JG, Portlock CS, Rosenberg SA: Treatment of advanced Hodgkin's disease with adriamycin, bleomycin, vinblastine and dacarbazine (ABVD). *Eur J of Clin Oncol* 18: 803, 1982

67. Laubenstein LJ, Krugel RL, Hynes KB et al: Treatment of epidemic Kaposi's sarcoma with VP-16 (Etoposide) and a combination of doxorubicin, bleomycin and vinblastine. *Proc Am Soc Clin Oncol* 2: 228, 1983

68. Lazarus HM, Gottfried MR, Herzig RH et al: Venoocclusive disease of the liver after high-dose mitomycin C therapy and autologous bone marrow transplantation. *Cancer* 49: 1789, 1982

69. Levy RL, Chiarillo S: Hyperpyrexia, allergic-type response, and death occurring with bleomycin administrations. *Oncology* 37: 316, 1980

70. Liu K, Mittleman A, Psroul EE et al: Renal toxicity in man treated with mitomycin C. *Cancer* 28: 1314, 1971

71. Livingston RB, Lee WH, Einhorn LH et al: BACON (bleomycin, adriamycin, CCNU, oncovin, and nitrogen mustard) in squamous cell lung cancer. *Cancer* 37: 1237, 1976

72. Lomis RL, Kuppinger MS, Ginsberg SJ et al: Role of single breath carbon monoxide diffusing capacity in monitoring the pulmonary effects of bleomycin in germ cell tumor patients. *Cancer Res* 39: 5076, 1979

73. Lown JW, Sim S: The mechanism of the bleomycin-induced cleavage of DNA. *Biochem Biophy Res Commun* 77: 814, 1976

74. Lown JW, Sim SK, Chen HH: Hydroxy radical production by free and DNA-bound aminoquinone antibiotics and its

role in DNA degradation. Electron spin resonance detection of hydroxy radicals by spin trapping. *Can J Biochem* 56: 1042, 1972

75. MacDonald JS, Schein PS, Wooley PV et al: 5-Fluorouracil, doxorubicin, mitomycin C (FAM) combination chemotherapy for advanced gastric cancer. *Ann Intern Med* 93: 533, 1980

76. Margileth D, Smith F, Lane M: Sudden arterial occlusion associated with mithramycin therapy. *Cancer* 31: 708, 1973

77. Michaelson RA, Magill GB, Quan SH et al: Preoperative chemotherapy and radiation therapy in the management of anal epidermoid carcinoma. *Cancer* 51: 390, 1983

78. Miller TP, MacMahon LJ, Livingston RB: Extensive adenocarcinoma and large cell undifferentiated carcinoma of the lung treated with 5-FU, vincristine and mitomycin C (FOMi). *Cancer Treat Rep* 64: 1241, 1980

79. Miyamoto T, Tarkabe Y, Watanabe M et al: Effectiveness of a sequential combination of bleomycin and mitomycin C on an advanced cervical cancer. *Cancer* 41: 403, 1978

80. Monto FW, Talley RW, Caldwell MJ et al: Observations on the mechanism of hemorrhagic toxicity in mithramycin (NSV-24559) therapy. *Cancer Res* 29: 697, 1969

81. Mujoki M, Ono T, Hori S et al: Binding of bleomycin to DNA in bleomycin-sensitive and resistant rat ascites hepatoma cells. *Cancer Res* 35: 2015, 1975

82. Oken MM, Crooke SK, Elson MK et al: Pharmacokinetics of bleomycin after intramuscular administration in man. *Cancer Treat Rep* 65: 485, 1981

83. Orwall ES, Kressling PJ, Patterson JR: Interstitial pneumonia from mitomycin. *Annals Int Med* 89: 352, 1978

84. Paladine W, Cunningham TJ, Sponzo R et al: Intracavitary bleomycin in the management of malignant effusions. *Cancer* 32: 1903, 1976

85. Pavey MD, Wiley EL, Abeloff MD: Hemolytic uremia syndrome associated with mitomycin therapy. *Cancer Treat Rep* 66: 457, 1982

86. Povirk LF, Hogan M, Dattagupta N: Binding of bleomycin to DNA: intercalation of the bithiazole rings. *Biochemistry* 18: 96, 1979

87. Pratt WB, Ruddon RW: The antibiotics. In *The Anticancer Drugs*, pp. 173–177. Edited by WB Pratt and RW Ruddon. Oxford University Press, New York, 1979

88. Prout GR, Griffin PP, Nochs BN et al: Intravesical therapy of low stage bladder carcinoma with mitomycin C: Comparison of results in untreated and previously treated patients. *J of Urology* 127: 1096, 1982

89. Purpora P, Ahern MJ, Shiverman N: Toxic epidermal necrolysis after mithramycin. *New England J of Med* 299: 1412, 1978

90. Raisfeld IH: Role of terminal substitution in the pulmonary toxicities of bleomycins. *Toxicol Appl Pharmacol* 57: 355, 1981

91. Randolph VL, Vallejo A, Spiro RH et al: Combination therapy of advanced head and neck cancer: Induction of remission with diamminedichloroplatinum (II), bleomycin, and radiation therapy. *Cancer* 41: 460, 1978

92. Ransohoff I, Martin BF, Medreh MN et al: Preliminary clinical study of mithramycin (NSC-24559) in primary tumors of the central nervous system. *Cancer Chemother Rep* 49: 51, 1965

93. Rodriquez V, Cabonilles F, Burgess MA et al: Combination chemotherapy (CHOP-BLEO) in the treatment of advanced (non-Hodgkin's) malignant lymphoma. *Blood* 49: 325, 1975

94. Rosi DR, Nogeline C, Brown B et al: 5-Fluorouracil, adriamycin and mitomycin C (FAM) chemotherapy for advanced adenocarcinoma of the lung. *Cancer* 48: 21, 1981

95. Samson MK, Comis RC, Baker LH et al: Mitomycin C in advanced adenocarcinoma and large cell carcinoma of the lung. *Cancer Treat Rep* 62: 163, 1978

96. Santoro A, Bonfonti V, Bonadonna G: Salvage chemotherapy with ABVD in MOPP-resistant Hodgkin's disease. *Ann Intern Med* 96: 139, 1982

97. Sausville EP, Peisach J, Horwitz SB: A role for ferrous ion and oxygen in the degradation of DNA by bleomycin. *Biochem and Biophys Res Commun* 73: 814, 1976

98. Sausville E, Stein R, Peisach J et al: Properties and products of the degradation of DNA by bleomycin. *Biochemistry* 18: 96, 1979

99. Schein PS, DeVita VT, Hubbard S et al: Bleomycin, adriamycin, cyclophosphamide, vincristine, and prednisone (BACOP): Combination chemotherapy in the treatment of advanced histocytic lymphoma. *Ann Intern Med* 63: 177, 1977

100. Schwartz HS: Pharmacology of mitomycin C. III. *In vitro* metabolism by rat liver. *J Pharmacol Exptl Ther* 136: 250, 1962

101. Schwartz HS, Phillips FS: Pharmacology of mitomycin C II. Renal excretion and metabolism by tissue homogenates. *J Pharmacol Exp Ther* 133: 335, 1961

102. Slayton RE, Shnider BI, Elias E et al: New approach to the treatment of hypercalcemia. The effect of short term treatment with mithramycin. *Clin Pharm and Therapeutics* 12: 833, 1971

103. Smith FD, Hoth DF, Levin B et al: 5-Fluorouracil, adriamycin, and mitomycin C (FAM) chemotherapy for advanced adenocarcinoma of the pancreas. *Cancer* 46: 2014, 1980

104. Takeshita M, Grollman AP, Ohtsubo E et al: Interaction of bleomycin with DNA. *Proc Natl Acad Sci USA* 75: 5983, 1978

105. Umezawa H, Takeuchi T, Hori S et al: Studies of the mechanism of anti-tumor effect of bleomycin on squamous cell carcinoma. *J Antibiot* 25: 409, 1972

106. Umezawa H, Hori S, Sawa T et al: A bleomycin inactivating enzyme in mouse liver. *Journal of Antibiotics* 27: 419, 1974

107. Vogel CL, Clements D, Wanume AK et al: Phase II clinical trials of BCNU and bleomycin in the treatment of Kaposi's sarcoma. *Cancer Chemo Rep* 57: 325, 1973

108. Wanatabe M, Takabe Y, Katoumata T et al: Effects of bleomycin on progression through the cell cycle of mouse L cells. *Cancer Research* 34: 2726, 1974

109. Wiggins RG, Woolley PV, MacDonald JS et al: Phase II trial of streptozotocin, mitomycin C and 5-fluorouracil (SMF) in the treatment of advanced pancreatic cancer. *Cancer* 41: 387, 1978

110. Woolley C, Pittillo RF: Microbiological assay and tissue distribution of mithramycin (NSC-24559) in mice. *Cancer Chemother Rep* 58: 311, 1974

111. Yagoda A, Mukhenji B, Young C et al: Bleomycin, an antitumor antibiotic. Clinical experience in 274 patients. *Ann Int Med* 77: 861, 1972

112. Yarbro JW, Kennedy BJ: A comparison of the rate of recovery from inhibition of RNA synthesis in mouse liver transplantable glioma. *Cancer Res* 27: 1779, 1967

113. Yarbro JW, Kennedy BJ, Barnum CP: Mithramycin inhibition of ribonucleic acid synthesis. *Cancer Res* 26: 36, 1966

114. Young RC: Gynecologic malignancies. In: *Cancer Chemotherapy*, pp. 340–375. Edited by HM Pinedo. Excerpta Medica, 1977

115. Zull JE, Czarnowska-Misztal E, DeLucca HF: On the relationship between vitamin D action and actinomycin-sensitive processes. *Proc Natl Acad Sci USA* 55: 177, 1966

13

PLANT ALKALOIDS: THE VINCA ALKALOIDS

M.C. CASTLE

INTRODUCTION

Although a large number of compounds from a wide variety of plants have been tested for antitumor activity, none has played a more vital role in cancer chemotherapy than the vinca alkaloids. These compounds are present in minute quantities in the plant *Catharanthus roseus* G. Don (*Vinca rosea* Linn.), commonly called the periwinkle. Although this plant contains in excess of fifty alkaloids, only two of these (vincristine and vinblastine) have become established as important cancer chemotherapeutic agents.

The antitumor activity of the vinca alkaloids was discovered independently and simultaneously by two groups of investigators who were testing extracts of *Vinca rosea* for purported hypoglycemic activity (2, 31). No hypoglycemic effects were demonstrated in these animal studies, but both groups noted that these plant extracts exhibited myelosuppressive activity and induced peripheral leukopenia. Subsequent isolation and characterization of the alkaloids in these plant extracts resulted in the identification of several compounds with antitumor activity. Of these, only vincristine and vinblastine have become established as therapeutic agents. Other vinca alkaloids with demonstrated antitumor activity include vinleurosine and vinrosidine, both of which have been abandoned due to excessive toxicity (13). Several semisynthetic derivatives have been prepared from the natural alkaloids and one of these (vindosine) has been introduced into clinical practice.

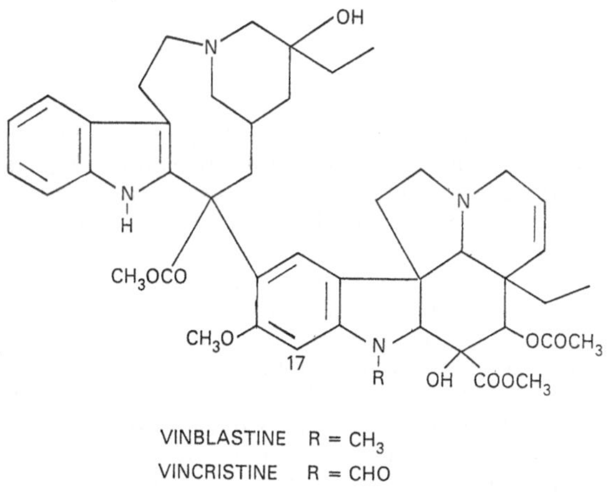

Vincristine (NSC-67574) was originally referred to as leurocristine and the salt form has the empirical formula $C_{46}H_{56}O_{10}N_4 \cdot H_2SO_4$. A commonly used abbreviation for this agent is VCR. Vinblastine (NSC-49842), frequently abbreviated as VLB or VBL, formally had the generic name vincaleukoblastine and has the empirical formula $C_{46}H_{58}O_9N_4 \cdot H_2SO_4$. Both are large molecules with quite similar but complex structures (see Fig. 1). Both compounds are composed of dimeric units: an indole nucleus (the catharanthine portion) and a dihydroindole nucleus (the vindoline portion). The two compounds are identical with the exception of the substituent attached to the nitrogen of the vindoline nucleus where vincristine possesses a formyl group and vinblastine has a methyl group. Both compounds are marketed as sulfate salts to enhance solubility and to minimize decomposition. Several of the structural features of these compounds are essential for antitumor activity (13).

Extensive reviews of the discovery, isolation and characterization of vinca alkaloids have been published (32, 35). Other plants alkaloids which have been investigated for antitumor activity have been reviewed elsewhere (14).

MECHANISM OF ACTION

Since the initial demonstration of the antitumor activity of vinca alkaloids a quarter of a century ago, these compounds have been intensively investigated in an attempt to establish the mechanism of action of their antitumor effects. Despite extensive evidence that the vinca alkaloids disrupt a wide variety of biochemical pathways and cellular events, the specific mechanism of action of these agents remains elusive. Among the biochemical effects which have been reported for the vinca alkaloids are the following: (1) Competition for transport of amino acids into cells; (2) Inhibition of purine biosynthesis; (3) Inhibition of synthesis of both RNA and DNA; (4) Inhibition of protein synthesis; (5) Interference with lipid metabolism; (6) Inhibition of glycolysis; (7) Alteration in the release of antidiuretic hormone, and (8) Inhibition of release of histamine by mast cells and enhanced release of norepinephrine. A complete review of these effects of the vinca alkaloids has been presented (13).

Despite the diversity of biochemical effects noted above, there is a general consensus that the vast majority of the biological effects produced by the vinca alkaloids are related directly or indirectly to their interactions with tubulin. These biological effects include arrest of mitosis, cytotoxicity, disappearance and disruption of microtubules, inhibition of

VINBLASTINE R = CH₃
VINCRISTINE R = CHO

Figure 1. Structure of vinca alkaloids.

147

P.V. Woolley (ed.), Cancer management in Man: Biological Response Modifiers, Chemotherapy, Antibiotics, Hyperthermia, Supporting Measures
© 1989. Kluwer Academic Publishers, Dordrecht.

the motility and phagocytotic activity of human polymorphonuclear leukocytes, anti-inflammatory activity, neurological toxicity, teratogenicity in laboratory animals, and inhibition of antibody formation (11). Several of these biological effects will be considered in more detail below.

In order to discuss the mechanism of action of the vinca alkaloids as antitumor agents, an understanding of the role of microtubules in cell division is essential. Microtubules, subcellular organelles present in all eukaryotic cells but not in prokaryotic cells, are associated with the shape of cells, with the movement of cells, and with the movement of components within cells (8). The steps involved in the formation of microtubules have been reviewed by Dustin (19). Briefly, this process begins with two globular proteins (alpha tubulin and beta tubulin) which come together to form a dimer. In several subsequent steps, these dimers form intermediate structures, protofilaments and finally a tubular structure which elongates to produce a microtubule. Microtubules can be disassembled into components and then reassembled into new microtubules. There is some evidence that these latter processes may be under the control of calmodulin (19).

Although their exact role in cell division is not fully understood, there seems little doubt that microtubules are essential to mitosis. As pointed out by Dustin (19), the spindle fibers are composed of microtubules. Microtubules are involved in the initial grouping of chromosomes and in the movement of these chromosomes toward poles in preparation for cell division. Microtubules also appear to play a role in the elongation of the cell just prior to the separation of the daughter cells.

The interaction of vinca alkaloids with microtubules results in changes which lead to disruption of mitosis with metaphase arrest. Under certain conditions, this arrest is reversible once the drug has been removed and cells may then proceed through the cell cycle. The disruption of microtubules of the mitotic spindle leads to an inability of the cell to segregate chromosomes correctly. The chromosomes become dispersed throughout the cytoplasm (exploded mitosis) or form unusual grouping (ball and star configurations). This appears to be the critical event leading to cell death. The vinca alkaloids are sometimes referred to as "spindle poisons". Other drugs which have a similar effect on the mitotic spindle include colchicine, griseofulvin and the podophyllotoxins, all of which bind at a different site than do the vinca alkaloids (49).

The vinca alkaloids bind to specific sites on tubulin and initiate a sequence of events which lead to disruption of the spindle apparatus. The microtubules become disassembled and the subunits form highly regular crystals which contain one mole of bound drug per mole of tubulin (6). As envisioned by Wilson [see (41)], the effect of the vinca alkaloids in the disassembly process is an indirect one. Microtubules are thought to be in a state of continuous change in which assembly of tubulin at one end causes elongation of the microtubule whereas disassembly at the opposite end shortens the chain. Vinca alkaloids bind to tubulin and prevent the polymerization of these subunits into microtubules but these drugs do not appear to affect the disassembly process. The net effect of these processes is dissolution of the microtubule and the formation of soluble tubulin.

To summarize, current evidence indicates that the vinca alkaloids bind to specific sites on tubulin and block the polymerization of tubulin into microtubules which compose the spindle apparatus of the cell. This disruption of microtubule formation eventually leads to inhibition of mitosis, metaphase arrest and death of the cell.

PHARMACOLOGICAL DISPOSITION

Precise knowledge of the pharmacokinetics, distribution, metabolism and excretion of vinca alkaloids has been hampered by deficiencies in the methodology required to isolate and quantitate the small amounts of these drugs present in most biological specimens. Those investigations which have been performed have utilized tritium-labeled alkaloid, bioassay with KG or L cell lines or radioimmunoassay techniques for quantitation. A variety of extraction and isolation procedures have also been utilized in an attempt to separate the parent compound from metabolic and decomposition products. It is perhaps not unexpected that numerous discrepancies exist in the reported results of these studies.

Although no definitive evidence has been presented concerning the degree of oral absorption of vinca alkaloids, there is a consensus that absorption by this route is unpredictable at best. Although adequate absorption after intraperitoneal administration has been demonstrated with vinblastine (3), this route is not used due to severe extravasation which occurs when these agents are present in high concentrations. There is also evidence that vinblastine is more toxic by the intraperitoneal route than when administered intravenously (32). As discussed in more detail below, these drugs are administered intravenously either by bolus injection or by continuous infusion.

The distribution of both vincristine and vinblastine has been investigated in several species of laboratory animals. Although there are differences in experimental design and in the reported results, some generalizations can be made. In the dog and the rat, the spleen concentrates vincristine to a greater extent than any other tissue studied (10, 36). In the monkey, the tissue with the highest concentration was the pancreas (20), a tissue which was not included in the studies with rats and dogs. There was general agreement among all of these studies that vincristine does not penetrate into the cerebrospinal fluid to any significant extent. Most of the vinblastine in the blood appears to be present in the buffy coat (21) and exists in a bound form with platelets (24). High concentrations of vinblastine have also been observed in leukocytes (16). Since all of these investigations were carried out with tritiated drugs, at least some of the measured radioactivity may have been products formed by tritium exchange including tritiated water.

The primary route of excretion for both vincristine and vinblastine in most species is in the feces via the bile. In the rat, only about 15 percent of the injected dose appears in the urine, mostly during the first 24 hours (10) whereas the mouse excretes more of the drug in the urine than in the feces (20). Approximately 60 percent of an injected dose of vincristine is excreted in the feces of rats within 24 hours and 70 percent within the first 72 hours. However, the portion of the injected dose excreted over these time intervals decreases with increasing dose (10). These investigations also demonstrated that over 25 percent of an injected dose of vincristine was excreted in the bile during the first 30 minutes. Similar results have been observed when vincristine is administered to humans. Urinary excretion accounts for about 10 percent of the injected dose (5, 39) while over 70 percent is excreted in the feces over a 72 hour period (5). Biliary excretion has been studied in one patient receiving vincristine for therapy of pancreatic carcinoma (26). Almost half of the injected dose was excreted during the first 24 hours with the bile and urine containing equal amounts.

The excretion of vinblastine has also been extensively investigated in several species. In humans, this alkaloid appears to be excreted much more slowly than vincristine in both the urine and the bile (40) although conflicting results have been reported (38). Using vinblastine labeled at different positions, these investigators found overall excretion rates to be 55 percent in the first study and 25 percent in the latter study covering a 72 hour period. These data seem to be in direct contrast to results with vincristine (see above) which suggest that most of this alkaloid is excreted within the first 24 hours. In the dog, vinblastine is excreted to a greater extent in the feces than in the urine (approximately 35 percent and 15 percent, respectively) over a nine day period (15). Most of the urinary excretion occurred in the first three days while fecal excretion remained relatively constant throughout

The metabolic fate of both vincristine and vinblastine has been investigated but little definitive information has been accumulated. This has been due partly to the complex structure and unstable nature of these agents. Some of the initial studies with tritiated vincristine were difficult to interpret due to a significant degree of degradation during extraction and thin-layer chromatographic analysis of biological specimens (37). Subsequent development of an analytical procedure employing high-performance liquid chromatography has provided a more efficient and more reliable technique for the analysis of vinca alkaloids and their metabolic and decomposition products (9). There appears to be a general agreement that vincristine is not extensively metabolized. Although significant amounts of other compounds have been isolated from the plasma, bile and urine of several species, most but not all of these products can be attributed to degradation processes (9, 37). In addition, attempts to demonstrate metabolism of vincristine by liver homogenates have not been successful (9).

At least one metabolic product (deacetylvinblastine) of vinblastine has been identified in both dog (12) and man (40). This metabolite, which may be as active as the parent compound, was detected in small quantities in the urine and stool. The site of this deacetylation reaction has not been established but is assumed to be the liver.

The pharmacokinetic behavior of all three alkaloids has been investigated by numerous groups, in several species, and employing widely different methodologies. The reported results are inconsistent and difficult to interpret. What is evident is that all three drugs are rapidly removed from the blood after intravenous administration. An initial plasma half-life of one to four minutes has been reported for all three alkaloids when administered by bolus intravenous injections to humans (5, 28, 29, 39, 40, 44, 45). The half-life of the second phase of plasma elimination has an even wider range of reported values (7 to 99 minutes) and the terminal

phase has been estimated to be between 3 and 26 hours.

In addition to the studies mentioned above involving bolus administration of vinca alkaloids, considerable data have also been obtained from studies in which these alkaloids were administered by continuous infusion over a period of several days (27, 34, 42). One of these studies (27) clearly demonstrated that continuous infusion maintained serum levels of vincristine which were above the therapeutic threshold for five days. Similar results have been reported with vinblastine (34, 50) and with vindesine (7).

TOXICITY

Although vincristine and vinblastine are capable of producing a wide variety of adverse reactions, there are marked differences in the incidence and severity of these toxic effects. There is currently no adequate explanation for these discrepancies but differences in the rate of uptake into cells and the formation toxic metabolites have been suggested. In general, the toxicity of these vinca alkaloids is most likely the result of their ability to bind to tubulin and disrupt microtubule formation (see section on Mechanism of Action above). This is probably not unexpected in view of the ubiquitous nature of microtubules.

One very important area in which there are major differences in toxicity between vinblastine and vincristine is bone marrow depression. Leukopenia is to be expected with the use of vinblastine with a nadir occurring five to ten days after the last dose of the drug. Both the extent and duration of leukopenia are dose-related and the white-cell count usually returns to normal in one or two weeks. Thrombocytopenia is not usually a problem with vinblastine unless other chemotherapeutic agents or radiation have been employed. Vincristine, on the other hand, is a particularly valuable agent in combination chemotherapy due to a lack of myelosuppression with conventional doses. Vincristine does not appear to have any consistent effect upon platelets when used in therapeutic doses. Thus bone marrow depression represents the dose-limiting factor in the clinical application of vinblastine but not of vincristine.

A prominent adverse reaction associated with all vinca alkaloids is neurological toxicity. The mechanism of this neurotoxicity is apparently related to properties of the vinca alkaloids discussed above: namely, the ability of these agents to bind to tubulin and disrupt the polymerization process which leads to the formation of microtubules. However, the toxicity of these agents to nervous tissue may be the result of different effects than the inhibition of mitosis and mitotic arrest which characterize their antineoplastic activity. The ubiquity of microtubules in eukaryotic cells and the marked affinity of tubulin for the vinca alkaloids predisposes a wide variety of functions to disruption in the presence of these agents. Among these processes are axoplasmic transport and secretory function which may represent the sites of action of the neurotoxicity of these drugs.

Although all three vinca alkaloids (vinblastine, vincristine and vindesine) produce qualitatively similar neurological toxicity, there are considerable quantitative differences in the neurologic sequelae [for reviews, see (25, 33, 43, 48)]. Vinblastine exhibits the least neurotoxicity of this group whereas this toxicity represents the dose-limiting effect with vincristine. Vindesine was originally thought to be free of neurotoxicity but clinical trials of this drug have established that it also is neurotoxic, albeit less so than vincristine.

It appears likely that almost every patient treated with vincristine will develop peripheral neuropathy to some extent. There is a fairly well-established progression of this neurotoxicity in most patients. The earliest manifestation of vincristine neurotoxicity is the loss of the Achilles tendon reflex which, though universal, may be asymptomatic (33). This may be followed by paresthesias in the hands and feet. If therapy with vincristine is continued, there may be a progression to muscle pain, weakness, difficulty in walking and sensory impairment. These neurotoxic effects are almost always symmetrical and may persist for weeks or months after discontinuation of the drug (33).

In addition to peripheral neuropathy, a less frequent complication of vincristine therapy is cranial neuropathy. Severe pain in the jaw (possibly related to effects on the trigeminal nerve) may occur soon after the initial dose of vincristine but usually does not persist with subsequent therapy (33). Ocular disturbances are also rare manifestations of vincristine toxicity. Mental changes such as depression, agitation, insomnia and hallucinations have been reported but the relationship of these to the administration of vincristine has not been established (43). There are numerous reports of seizures following administration of vincristine [see (33, 43)]. It is difficult to attribute this effect to a direct action of vincristine in view of the inability of this drug or its metabolites to enter the central nervous system (10, 28). Many of these seizures are probably attributable to factors such as intracranial metastases, infection, metabolic disturbances or other drug therapy. Seizures after vincristine therapy may also be associated with the well-documented ability of this drug to produce a syndrome of inappropriate antidiuretic hormone secretion leading to hyponatremia. This complication, which is apparently dose-related, may be due to an effect of the drug on the hypothalamus, neurohypophyseal tract or posterior pituitary (33).

Several toxic effects attributable to autonomic neuropathy are common with vincristine therapy. The most prominent of these are gastrointestinal disturbances including colicky abdominal pain, constipation and paralytic ileus. The presence of these symptoms is significant because they are usually the first indications of toxicity, preceding more serious toxic effects such as peripheral neuropathy. Paralytic ileus, though usually reversible, has resulted in several deaths (33). Urinary dysfunction and orthostatic hypotension have also been reported with vincristine therapy. Extensive electrophysiological and histological data have been accumulated from numerous investigations of the neuropathies produced by vincristine [see (33)].

Attempts to reverse or prevent the neurotoxicity of the vinca alkaloids have not been successful and treatment consists primarily of supportive care and adjustment of dosage. Folinic acid (leucovorin), but not folic acid, has been shown to protect mice against an otherwise lethal dose of vincristine (32). This approach has also been tried in several cases of vincristine overdose in humans but the results have not been encouraging. Anecdotal reports of effectiveness of this treatment have appeared (18) as well as conflicting published reports (22, 46). The effectiveness of folinic acid as an antidote for vincristine toxicity remains to be established.

Several agents have been employed in attempts to minimize paralytic ileus produced by the vinca alkaloids. Lactulose (23), caerulein (1, 4) and sincalide (30) have been used to stimulate bowel motility. While these agents appear to offer some benefit in the relief of gastrointestinal disturbances, their effects on the pharmacokinetics of vinca alkaloids have not been investigated. In view of the extensive biliary excretion and enterohepatic recirculation of vincristine and vinblastine, the use of bowel stimulants may reduce the half life of the vinca alkaloids.

The extravasation produced by the administration of vincristine has been treated with corticosteroid therapy (4). Although some steroids appear to reduce the cytotoxicity of vincristine (17), the anti-inflammatory activity of steroids may be responsible limiting tissue damage of these antineoplastic agents rather an inhibition of cytotoxicity.

REFERENCES

1. Agosti A, Bertaccini G, Paulucci R, Zanella E: Caerulein treatment for paralytic ileus. *Lancet* 1:395, 1971
2. Beer CT: The leukopenic action of extracts of *Vinca rosea*. *Brit Empire Cancer Campaign* 33:487, 1955
3. Beer CT, Richards JF: The metabolism of vinca alkaloids. Part II. The fate of tritiated vinblastine in rats. *Lloydia* 27:352, 1964
4. Bellone JD: Treatment of vincristine extravasation. *J Amer Med Assoc* 245:343, 1981
5. Bender RA, Castle MC, Margileth DA, Oliverio VT: Pharmacokinetics of ^{3}H-vincristine in man. *Clin Pharmacol Ther* 22:430, 1977
6. Bensch KG, Malawista SE: Microtubule crystals in mammalian cells. *J Cell Biol* 40:95, 1969
7. Bodey GP, Yap HY, Yap BS, Valdivieso M: Continuous infusion of vindesine in solid tumors. *Cancer Treatment Rev* 7:39, 1980
8. Bryan J: Biochemical properties of microtubules. *Fed Proc* 33:152, 1974
9. Castle MC, Mead JAR: Investigations of the metabolic fate of tritiated vincristine in the rat by high-pressure liquid chromatography. *Biochem Pharmacol* 27:37, 1978
10. Castle MC, Margileth DA, Oliverio VT: Distribution and excretion of ^{3}H-vincristine in man. *Cancer Res* 36:3684, 1976
11. Creasey WA: The vinca alkaloids. *Biochem Pharmacol Supplement* 2:217, 1974
12. Creasey WA, Marsh JC: Metabolism of vinblastine (VLB) in the dog. *Proc Amer Assoc Cancer Res* 14:57, 1973
13. Creasey WA: Vinca alkaloids and colchicine. In: *Antineoplastic and Immunosuppressive Agents*, Part II. Edited by Sartorelli AC, Johns DG. *Handbuch der Experimentellen Pharmakologie*, Vol. 38, Springer-Verlag, Berlin 1975, pp. 232–256
14. Creasey WA: Plant alkaloids. In: *Cancer 5: A Comprehensive Treatise*. Edited by Becker FF. Plenum Press, New York, 1977, pp. 379–425
15. Creasey WA, Scott AI, Wei CC, Kutcher J, Schwartz A, Marsh JC: Pharmacological studies with vinblastine in the dog. *Cancer Res* 35:1116, 1975
16. Creasey WA, Bensch KG, Malawista SE: Colchicine vinblastine and griseofulvin. Pharmacological studies with human leukocytes. *Biochem Pharmacol* 20:1579, 1971
17. Cutts JH: Protective action of diethylstilbestrol on toxicity of vinblastine in rats. *J Natl Cancer Inst* 41:919, 1968
18. Dyke RW: Treatment of vincristine overdose. *J Pediatr* 91:356, 1977
19. Dustin P: Microtubules. *Scientific Amer* 243:66, 1980

20. El Dareer, White VM, Chen FP, Mellett LB, Hill DL: Distribution and metabolism of vincristine in mice, rats, dogs and monkeys. *Cancer Treat Rep* 61:1269, 1977

21. Greenius HF, McIntyre RW, Beer CT: The preparation of vinblastine-4-acetyl-*t* and its distribution in the blood of rats. *J Med Chem* 11:254, 1968

22. Grush OC, Morgan SK: Folinic acid rescue for vincristine toxicity. *Clin Toxicol* 14:71, 1979

23. Harris AC, Jackson JM: Lactulose in vincristine-induced constipation. *Med J Aust* 2P:573, 1972

24. Hebden HF, Hadfield JR, Beer CT: The binding of vinblastine by platelets in the rat. *Cancer Res* 30:1417, 1970

25. Hildebrand J: *Lesions of the Nervous System in Cancer Patients*. Raven, New York, 1978, pp. 49–70

26. Jackson DV Jr, Castle MC, Bender RA: Biliary excretion of vincristine *Clin Pharmacol Ther* 24:101–7, 1978

27. Jackson DV, Sethi VS, Spurr CL, Williard VW, White DR, Richards F, Stuart JJ, Muss HB, Cooper MR, Homesley HD, Jobson VW, Castle MC: Intravenous vincristine infusion: Phase I trial. *Cancer* 48:2559, 1981

28. Jackson DV, Castle MC, Poplack DG, Bender RA: The pharmacokinetics of vincristine in the cerebrospinal fluid of subhuman primates. *Cancer Res* 40:722, 1980

29. Jackson DV, Sethi VS, Spurr CL, White DR, Richards F, Stuart JJ, Muss HB, Cooper MR, Castle MC: Pharmacokinetics of vincristine infusion. *Cancer Treat Rep* 65:1043, 1981

30. Jackson DV, Wu WC, Spurr CL: Treatment of vincristine-induced ileus with sincalide, a cholecystokinin analog. *Cancer Chemother Pharmacol* 8:83, 1982

31. Johnson IS, Wright HF, Svoboda GH: Experimental basis for clinical evaluation of antitumor principles derived from Vinca rosea Linn. *J Lab Clin Med* 54:830, 1959

32. Johnson IS, Armstrong JG, Gorman M, Burnett JP Jr: The vinca alkaloids: a new class of oncolytic agents. *Cancer Res* 23:1390, 1963

33. Kaplan RS, Wiernik PH: Neurotoxicity of antineoplastic drugs. *Seminars in Oncology* 9:103, 1982

34. Lu K, Yap HY, Loo TL: Clinical pharmacokinetics of vinblastine by continuous intravenous infusion. *Cancer Res* 43:1405, 1983

35. Neuss N, Johnso 1 IS, Armstrong JG, Jansen Jr CJ: The vinca alkaloids. In: *Advances in Chemotherapy*, Vol. 1. Edited by Goldin A, Hawking F, Schnitzer RJ. Academic Press, New York, 1964

36. Owellen RJ, Donigian DW: ³H-Vincristine: preparation and preliminary pharmacology. *J Med Chem* 15:894, 1972

37. Owellen RJ, Owens Jr AH, Donigian DW: The binding of vincristine, vinblastine and colchicine to tubulin. *Biochem Biophys Res Commun* 47:685, 1972

38. Owellen RJ, Hartke CA: The pharmacokinetics of 4-acetyl tritium vinblastine in two patients. *Cancer Res* 35:975, 1975

39. Owellen RJ, Root MA, Hains FO: Pharmacokinetics of vindesine and vincristine in humans. *Cancer Res* 37:2603, 1977

40. Owellen RJ, Hartke CA, Hains CO: Pharmacokinetics and metabolism of vinblastine in humans. *Cancer Res* 37:2597, 1977

41. Pratt WB, Ruddon RW: *The Anticancer Drugs*, Oxford University Press, New York, pp. 221–233, 1979

42. Rahmani R, Barbet J, Paul-Cano J: A ¹²⁵I-radiolabelled probe for vinblastine and vindesine radioimmunoassays: applica-

tions to measurements of vindesine plasma levels in man after intravenous injections and long-term infusions. *Clin Chim Acta* 129:57, 1983

43. Rosenthal S, Kaufman S: Vincristine neurotoxicity. *Ann Int Med* 80:733, 1974

44. Sethi VS, Kimball JC: Pharmacokinetics of vincristine sulfate in children. *Cancer Chemother Pharmacol* 6:111, 1981

45. Sethi VS, Jackson DV, White DR, Richards F, Stuart JJ, Muss HB, Cooper MR, Spurr CL: Pharmacokinetics of vincristine sulfate in adult cancer patients. *Cancer Res* 41:3551, 1981

46. Thomas LL, Braat PC, Somers R, Goudsmit R: Massive vincristine overdose: failure of leucovorin to reduce toxicity. *Can Treat Rep* 66:1967, 1982

47. Weber W, Nagel GA, Nager-Studer E, Albrecht E: Vincristine infusion: a Phase I study. *Cancer Chemother Pharmacol* 3:49, 1979

48. Weiss HD, Walker MD, Wiernik PH: Neurotoxicity of commonly used antineoplastic agents. *N Engl J Med* 291:75, 1974

49. Wilson L: Properties of colchicine binding protein from chick embryo brain. Interactions with vinca alkaloids and podophyllotoxin. *Biochemistry* 9:4999, 1970

50. Yap HY, Blumenschein GR, Keating MJ, Hortobagyi GN, Tashima CK, Loo TL: Vinblastine given as a continuous 5-day infusion in the treatment of refractory advanced breast cancer. *Cancer Treat Rep* 64:279, 1980

POSTSCRIPT

The recent review by Jackson (1) summarizes the clinical use of the vinca alkaloids. Considerable attention has been directed toward preventing, minimizing and reversing the neurotoxic effects of vincristine. Thiamine, vitamin B_{12}, folinic acid, pyridoxine, and glutamic acid have all been tried clinically but only glutamic acid has shown any benefit in reducing the neurotoxicity of vincristine. Greater success has been achieved in dealing with ileus, another major concern to the use of the vinca alkaloids. Improvement has been observed with sincalide (an analog of cholecystokinin) and with metoclopromide (a dopamine antagonist).

Improved clinical activity has been demonstrated with continuous infusion (as opposed to the usual bolus injection) of vinca alkaloids. Vincristine, vinblastine and vindesine have all undergone clinical trials in a variety of cancers and have produced encouraging results. In many of these studies, vinca alkaloid infusion was used in patients who were refractory to prior chemotherapy with other antitumor agents and to bolus administration of vinca alkaloids. Another approach has been to link vinca alkaloids to a monoclonal antibody in an attempt to increase delivery of the drug to the site of the tumor. These conjugates of vinca alkaloids are currently undergoing clinical trials. Finally, the observation that calcium-channel blockers reverse the development of resistance to the vinca alkaloids by tumor cells is being explored in a clinical setting.

POSTSCRIPT REFERENCE

Jackson DV: Vinca alkaloid chemotherapy. ISI Atlas of Science: Pharmacology 1:124, 1987

NON-ALKALOID NATURAL PRODUCTS AS ANTICANCER AGENTS

DAVID G.I. KINGSTON

INTRODUCTION AND SCOPE

Crude natural products have been used in the treatment of cancer since ancient times, but it is only in the last 30 years that serious scientific study of naturally occurring anticancer agents has been carried out. This work has resulted in the discovery of numerous antibiotics and alkaloids as effective clinically active anticancer agents, and these substances are discussed in other chapters of this volume. Large numbers of non-alkaloidal natural products have been discovered which have had promising activities in animal trials, but only a few of these compounds have shown clincial activity to date. The most useful compounds in this class are the podophyllotoxin derivatives VP16-213 (etoposide) and VM26 (teniposide), which have been the subject of extensive clinical studies and are now entering normal clinical practice. The bulk of this chapter is thus given over to a discussion of these two drugs, but later sections deal with some newer compounds which are still in development but which are candidates for clinical use in the future.

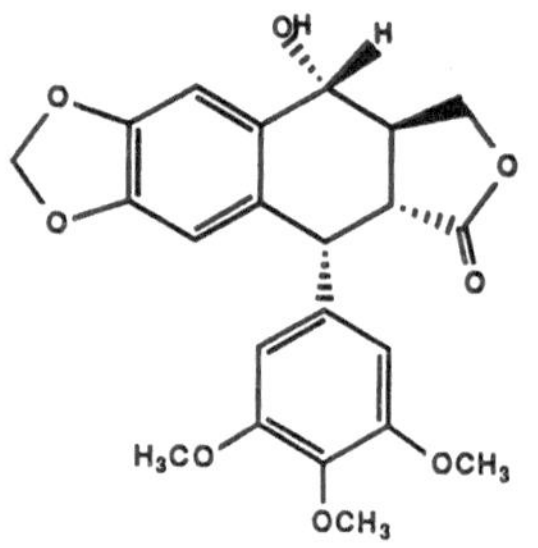

VP16-213 AND VM26

Introduction

The chemotherapy and pharmacology of the podophyllotoxin derivatives VP16-213 and VM26 has been discussed extensively in recent symposia (5, 7, 8, 16, 17, 30, 32). Since these symposia present convenient recent summaries of work on these compounds, many of the citations in this chapter will be to papers in symposia rather than to the original literature.

History

The dried roots and rhizomes of the North American plant *Podophyllum peltatum* Linnaeus, (the American mandrake or May apple) and of the related Indian species *Podophyllum emodi* Wallich have long been known to possess medicinal properties (21). The major active substance in podophyllin, which is the resin product obtained by extraction of the dried roots and rhizomes with ethanol, was shown to be the lignan lactone podophyllotoxin (**1**), although a variety of other lignans and lignan glycosides have been isolated from podophyllin. A review of the chemistry and pharmacology of podophyllin and its constituents summarizes develop-

Figure 1. Structural formula of podophyllotoxin (**1**).

ments to about 1957 (15). Podophyllotoxin itself is a potent antimitotic agent, but it proved to be too toxic to be useful in the treatment of human neoplasms. A variety of podophyllotoxin derivatives have been isolated from natural sources or prepared by partial synthesis, however, and the two cyclic acetals of 4'-demethylepipodophyllotoxin β-D-glucopyranoside known as VP16-213 (etoposide) and VM26 (teniposide) gave promising results in both *in vitro* and *in vivo* screening trials and were selected for clinical trials. These trials have proved the efficacy of these compounds in treating certain tumors. The remainder of this section will thus be concerned with these two compounds; information on the structures, chemistry, mode of action, and structure-activity relationships of other podophyllotoxin derivatives is contained in an excelllent recent review (18).

Chemistry

The chemical structures of VP16-213 and VM26 are shown in Fig. 2. They differ from podophyllotoxin in having a 4'-hydroxyl group instead of a 4'-methoxyl group, in having the epi configuration at the 4-position, and in having a substituted glucose residue at the 4-position. They differ from each other only in the nature of the substituent on the glucose ring: etoposide is the cyclic acetal prepared from 4'-demethylepipodophyllotoxin β-D-glucopyranoside and acetaldehyde (as its dimethyl acetal), while teniposide is the cyclic acetal prepared when 2-thiophenecarboxaldehyde replaces acetaldehyde (20). The two compounds are essentially insoluble in water, but are readily soluble in organic solvents such as chloroform.

P.V. Woolley (ed.), Cancer management in Man: Biological Response Modifiers, Chemotherapy, Antibiotics, Hyperthermia, Supporting Measures
© 1989. Kluwer Academic Publishers, Dordrecht.

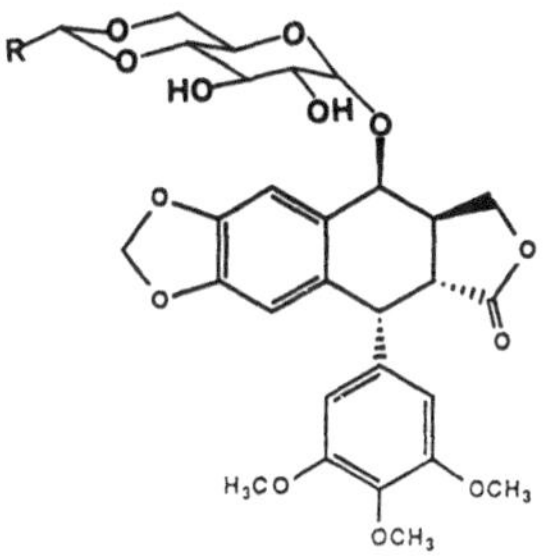

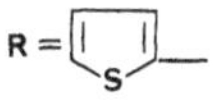

Figure 2. Structural formulae of the podophyllotoxin derivatives etoposide VP16-213 (**2**) and teniposide VM26 (**3**).

The chemistry and structure-activity relationships of VP16-213 have been reviewed (12), and it is concluded that there is a great deal of room for additional chemical work on the molecule. The lack of a practical synthetic route to the parent basic aglycone may be a barrier to this work, however.

Activity in *in vitro* and *in vivo* assay systems

In vitro activity of VP16-213 and VM26 has been shown against a number of cell lines (14, 20, 21). VP16-213 was active in P-815 murine mastocytoma with an ED_{50} of $0.031\,\mu g/ml$, while VM26 had an ED_{50} of $0.0048\,\mu g/ml$ in this system (20). Human lymphoid cells exposed to VP16-213 at $1.0\,\mu g/ml$ or VM26 at $0.1\,\mu g/ml$ for 24 hr have the major part of the population arrested with their DNA in the S part of the cell cycle (23). Other results suggest that VP16-213 arrests cells in the late S or G_2 phases of the cell cycle (14). In animal studies VP16-213 is generally more active than VM26; thus it gives an increase in survival time in the L1210 mouse leukemia system of 167%, while VM26 gives a 121% increase in the same system (20). In a comparative study of various dosage schedules in mice with L1210 leukemia, Dombernowsky and Wissen (11) concluded that VP16-213 was one of the most active drugs yet tested in the L1210 system.

In a discussion of the results of *in vitro* and *in vivo* assays, Rose and Bradner (44) point out that VP16-213 shows a broad-spectrum activity, but there is no correlation in activity for specific histologic types of neoplasms between species. Thus although VP16-213 shows excellent activity in the L1210 and P-388 leukemia assays, it is not particularly active in human leukemias. On the other hand, VP16-213 shows good activity in certain types of human lung carcinomas, but is only weakly active in the mouse lung carcinoma assays. This difference of response between species has also been observed with other antineoplastic agents.

Structure-activity studies and mechanism of action

In the initial search for podophyllotoxin derivatives with useful anticancer activity, a large number of modified podo-

phyllotoxins were prepared. Initial findings indicated that some podophyllotoxin derivatives such as podophyllinic acid ethylhydrazide (SP-1) did have some therapeutic activity but the most active derivatives prepared were those of the type exemplified by VP16-213 and VM26. Interestingly, the corresponding compounds in which the 4'-hydroxyl group is methylated (i.e., the epipodophyllotoxin derivatives) are much less active than the corresponding 4'-demethyl-epipodophyllotoxin derivatives. Of the many 4'-demethyl-epipodophyllotoxin β-D-glucopyranoside acetals prepared, VP16-213 showed the best activity in the L1210 *in vivo* system, while VM26 was one of the most active derivatives in the P-815 mouse mastocytoma cell assay. Changing the sugar moiety to galactose rather than glucose gave derivatives with lower activity (20). Various analogs of VP16-213 modified in the lactone ring have also been prepared, but they were uniformly less active than the parent compound (19).

The mode of action of the drugs VP16-213 and VM26 differs markedly from that of the parent compound podophyllotoxin. Podophyllotoxin is a potent inhibitor of microtubule assembly *in vitro*, and competitively inhibits colchicine binding to microtubules (18, 30). Because of this property, it arrests cells at mitosis by disrupting the equilibrium between tubulin polymer and tubulin dimer, thereby destroying the cytoskeletal framework for chromosome separation and arresting cell division at the mitotic stage of the cell cycle.

VP16-213 and VM26 appear to have a quite different mechanism of action. Both compounds arrest cells in the late S or G2 phase of the cell cycle, and have no effect on tubulin assembly. Instead, they induce single stranded breaks in HeLa DNA (VP16-213) or in the DNA in L1210 cells (VM26) (18, 43). They have also been shown to cause double-strand DNA breaks (31, 45). In the case of VM26, these breaks are predominantly double-stranded. It has been proposed (45) that VP16-213 and VM26 act as inhibitors of the DNA ligase activity of type II topoisomerases.

Pharmacology

Both compounds are only sparingly soluble in water, and are supplied for clinical use in nonaqueous formulations. VP16-213 is supplied in 5 ml ampules at a concentration of 20 mg/ml, while the VM26 ampules contain 10 mg/ml in a total of 5 ml. VP16-213 is also available for oral administration in 10 mg and 50 mg gelatin capsule formulations (16). VP16-213 is stable for at least 3 hr in various aqueous solutions, and is stable for up to 72 hr in aqueous dextrose or normal saline when its concentration does not exceed 0.25 mg/ml (5).

Dose schedules for VP16-213 are normally 300–600 mg/m^2 i.v. divided over 3 or 5 days and repeated every 3–4 weeks. For VM26 the schedule for adults is similar, but at a lower dose of 300 mg/m^2. The limiting toxicity in treatment with these drugs is myelosuppression, and hence a lower dose range is indicated for those patients whose bone marrow function has been compromised by prior radiotherapy or chemotherapy. For children, VM26 monotherapy is commonly used at a dose of 150–200 mg/m^2 weekly or 100 mg/m^2 twice weekly (16).

Studies on the clinical pharmacology of the drugs indicate

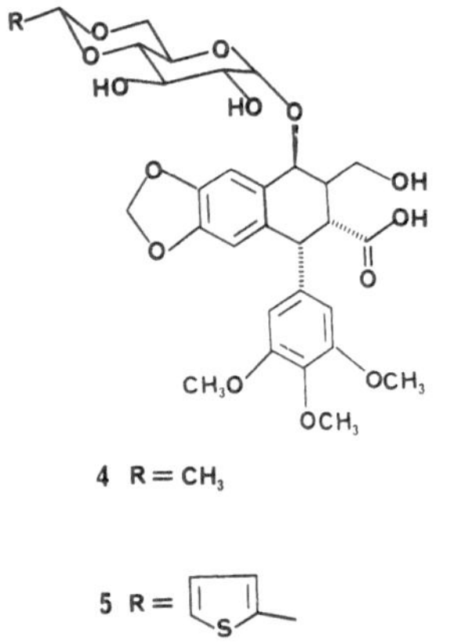

4   R = CH₃

5   R = [thienyl structure]

Figure 3. Structural formulae of the major urinary metabolites of VP16-213 (**4**) and VM26 (**5**).

that absorption from lipophilic capsules is erratic, but that absorption from oral solution and hydrophilic gelatin capsules is much better. Plasma levels of unchanged drug have been monitored both by thin layer chromatography and high performance liquid chromatography (HPLC), and these studies have shown that VP16-213 has a shorter terminal half-life than VM26. Both drugs are reported to have activity against intracranial neoplasms, with most work having been done on VM26. Only low levels of this drug have been found in the cerebrospinal fluid, however; typically these levels were 0.2–14.3% of the plasma levels found in the same patient (8).

Excretion of both drugs is primarily in the urine, with approximately 50% of the administered radioactivity being recovered in the urine within 72 hr of administration. Fecal excretion is variable, with amounts varying from 0–16% of the administered radioactivity being recovered in the feces of patients administered intravenous [³H]VP16-213. In the case of [³H]VM26, only 21% of the radioactivity recovered in the urine corresponded to unchanged drug, with the major metabolite being the ring-opened lactone 4'-demethyl-epipodophyllic acid-9-(4,6-O-ethylidene-β-D-glucopyranoside) (**4**). In the case of [³H]VP16-213, 67% of the urinary radioactivity was in the form of unchanged drug, and the major metabolite has been shown to be the acid **5** corresponding to the major metabolite of VM26 (1, 49). Reviews of the clinical pharmacology of VP16-213 in adults (9) and in children (13) have appeared.

Clinical single agent activity

The composite response rates for VP16-213 and VM26 have been compiled by Issell and this section is thus abstracted from his review (16).

VP16-213 is one of the most active single agents in small cell lung cancer with a composite single agent response rate of 40% in 262 patients, and a 6% complete response rate. VM26 has been less thoroughly evaluated in this cancer, but preliminary results show a 28% response rate with 8% complete responses in one trial.

For testicular cancer, response rates of up to 46% have been reported with VP16-213, and activity is retained even

in patients refractory to front-line combination therapy. VM26 has not been adequately tested in this situation.

Both VP16-213 and VM26 show activity against Hodgkin's disease and other malignant lymphomas, with especially encouraging results in treatment of diffuse histocytic lymphoma with VP16-213 in patients who had become refractory to front-line combination chemotherapy.

VP16-213 shows some activity against adult acute myelogenous leukemia, with a good response rate for patients with myelomonocytic and monocytic leukemia. VM26 and VP16-213 are both useful in pediatric leukemia, with VM26 showing activity against refractory acute lymphoblastic leukemia and VP16-213 against acute monocytic leukemia.

VP16-213 and VM26 both have meaningful activity in pediatric refractory neuroblastoma, with responses in up to 50% of the patients evaluated.

VM26 appears to have some activity in brain tumors, with responses in up to 35% of the patients evaluated; responses were seen in patients who were progressing on nitrosoureas. VP16-213 has some effect on breast cancer, with useful partial responses reported for 17% of heavily pretreated patients.

Finally, recent results (29) show that VP16-213 has activity against Kaposi's sarcoma associated with acquired immunodeficiency syndrome (AIDS); it is the most active single agent tested to date.

Clinical combination therapy

The drugs VP16-213 and VM26 are suitable candidates for combination therapy, since their toxicity is relatively low and they have unique modes of action. At this point, a number of combinations have been tested in experimental animals, but only a few are at the point where they are clinically useful. The most interesting situation to date is that of the combination of VM26 with cytarabine (ara C) in the treatment of refractory pediatric acute lymphoblastic leukemia. The drugs are reported to show a synergistic effect, and in one study 9 of 14 patients achieved complete remission after they had failed remission induction with standard therapy (42). VP16-213 has been used in combination with cisplatin for treatment of small cell lung cancer, non-small cell lung cancer, and refractory testicular cancer with encouraging results (16).

Toxicity

The two dose-limiting toxic effects of VP16-213 and VM26 are myelosuppression and gastrointestinal disturbances, with the former being the more important since the latter effect is usually easily controlled. Other toxicities include alopecia, and less commonly peripheral neuropathy and acute toxicities such as fever, chills, hypotension, and bronchospasm (16).

Conclusion

The modified podophyllotoxin derivatives VP16-213 and VM26 have demonstrated significant clinical activity in treatment of several tumors. VP16-213 shows particular promise in the treatment of small cell lung cancer and also shows pronounced activity in the treatment of testicular cancer, monocytic or myelomonocytic leukemia, non-Hodgkin's lymphomas, and hepatocellular carcinoma. VM26 has a role in the treatment of Hodgkin's disease, non-Hodgkin's lymphomas, neuroblastoma, and childhood acute lymphoblastic leukemia. It may also have efficacy in the treatment of primary brain tumors, although this is less certain. The current status of etoposide has been summarized by O'Dwyer and Wittes (34).

OTHER NATURALLY OCCURRING ANTICANCER AGENTS

As mentioned earlier, the epipodophyllotoxin derivatives VP16-213 and VM26 are the only non-alkaloid natural products from higher plants with clinical activity against cancer. The search for novel anticancer agents from plants and marine organisms is a continuing one, however, and the four compounds described below are representative of types of activity and structure that are being discovered.

Taxol

The novel diterpene derivative taxol (6) was discovered by Wani *et al.* (52). The drug shows confirmed activity in several animal systems, including the mouse leukemias L-1210, P-388, and P-1534, the B1 melanoma, B16 melanoma-carcinoma and the WA-256 carcinosarcoma. Taxol is of great interest from a pharmacological viewpoint, besides its mechanisms of action is quite unlike that of other anticancer agents. It completely inhibits division of exponentially growing HeLa cells at low concentration of drug, and it apparently does so by acting as a promoter of microtubule assembly (46). This is in contrast to other naturally occurring antimitotic agents such as colchicine and podophyllotoxin, which inhibit microtubule assembly. Taxol binds directly to polymerized tubulin, with saturation occurring at approximate stoichiometry with the tubulin dimer concentration (35). Some preliminary structure-activity correlations have been published (35) and it is shown that cytotoxicity and *in vitro* binding to microtubules require both an intact taxane ring and ester side chain at position C-13.

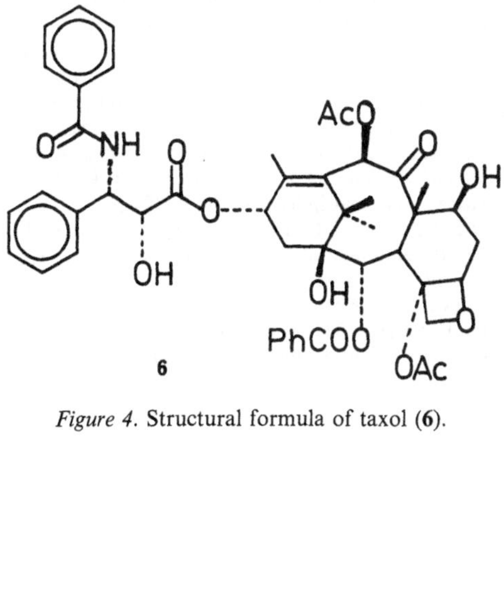

Acetylation at positions 2' and 7 results in loss of microtubule binding activity but not cytotoxicity.

The antitumor activity of taxol as tested at the National Cancer Institute has been summarized in a recent review (50). In addition, a series of novel taxol analogs having xylosyl substituents at position 7 has been reported (47) and a study of the ability of taxol and baccatin III derivatives to inhibit the disassembly of tubulin has appeared from the same group (28). The activity of 2- and 7-acetyltaxols has also been reported (33) and it is concluded that potentially either the 2'- or 7-substituents could be used to prepare taxol prodrugs. Studies on other taxol derivatives have shown that the oxetane ring is necessary for *in vitro* activity (22), and a partial synthesis of taxol starting from baccatin-III has been achieved (10).

The major difficulty in preparing taxol for clinical trial has been the development of a suitable formulation for the very lipophilic compound, but this difficulty was overcome with an emulsion formulation using a polyethoxylated castor oil as a surfactant. Taxol completed phase I clinical trials in March 1985, and is currently (1987) undergoing phase II trials. The results of three phase I trials have been reported (50); the dose-limiting toxicity of taxol is leukopenia, but other toxicities such as nausea and vomiting, stomitis, and various allergic type reactions are also observed.

Didemnins

The didemnins A-C are members of a new class of depsipeptides. They were isolated recently from a marine tunicate of the *Trididemnum* genus (39), and their structures were elucidated primarlily by mass spectrometry and nuclear magnetic resonance techniques (40). The structures of these compounds have recently been revised to 7–9, and their total synthesis has been accomplished (41). The most promising compound for development as an antitumor drug is didemnin B, which showed activity in the P388 leukemia assay in mice with T/C values up to 199, and a T/C of 160 against B16 melanoma (39, 40). The fact that didemnins A and C showed markedly different biological activities suggests that structure modification might provide useful activities in

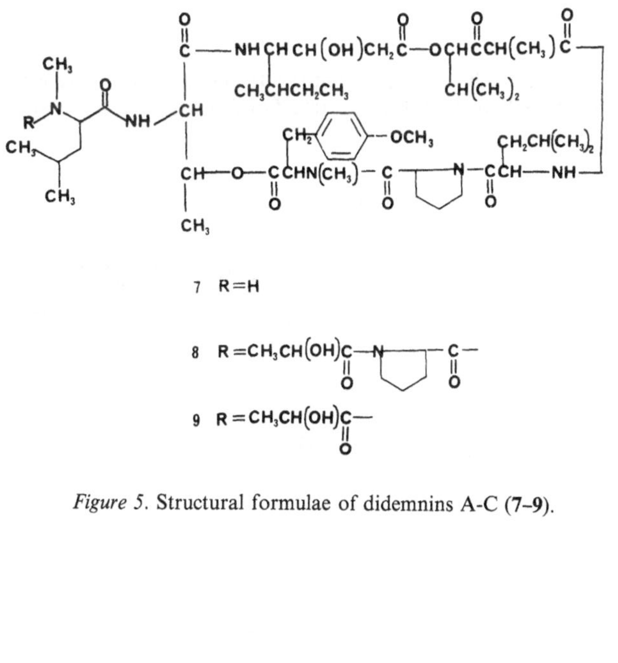

Figure 4. Structural formula of taxol (6).

Figure 5. Structural formulae of didemnins A-C (7–9).

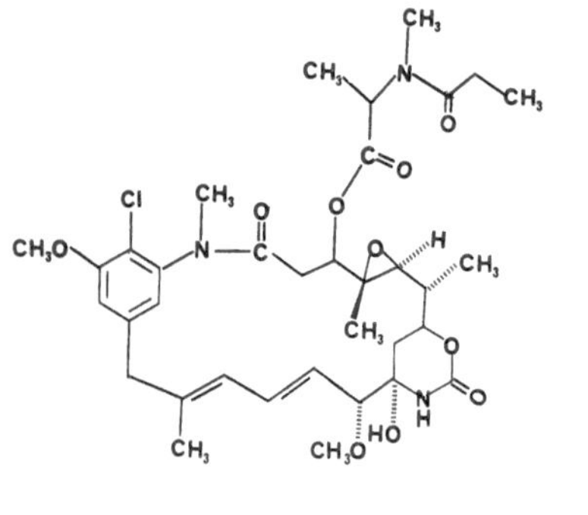

Figure 6. Structural formula of maytansine (**10**).

these compounds. Didemnin B (**8**) was 1987 ready to enter phase II clinical trials after successful completion of phase I trials (6).

Maytansine

Maytansine (**10**) is a novel ansa macrolide that was isolated from several *Maytenus* species by Kupchan and his co-workers (24); a number of related macrolides differing in the nature of the ester group at C-3 have also been isolated or prepared synthetically (25, 27, 51).

Maytansine was of great interest as an antileukemic drug because it was effective in animal models at very low doses ($< 25\,\mu g/Kg$) and has a wide effective dose range; the compound is a potent antimitotic agent (38). Structure-activity studies indicated that the C-3 ester is necessary for significant activity, while a free carbinolamide at C-9 is also advantageous for optimal activity (26). Regrettably, maytansine failed to show therapeutic activity in phase II clinical trials, even though it was tested in many different protocols, and clinical studies with this interesting compound have now been discontinued. Reviews on the chemistry and pharmacology of maytansine and the maytansinoids have appeared (48, 50).

Phyllanthoside

The novel glycoside phyllanthoside (**11**) was originally isolated by Kupchan from the tree *Phyllanthus acuminatus* and

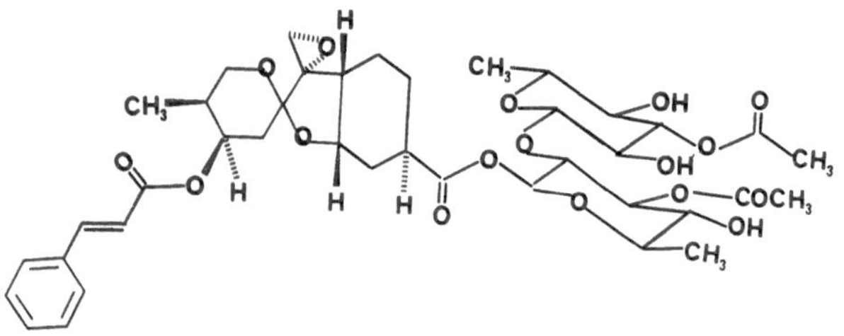

Figure 7. Structural formula of phyllanthoside (**11**).

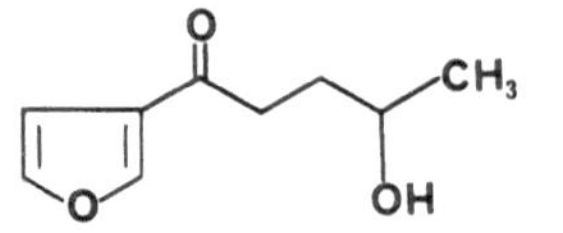

12

Figure 8. Structural formulae of 4-ipomeanol (**13**).

its structure partially elucidated (26). Subsequent work by Pettit and his co-workers has completed the structural elucidation and has uncovered the existence of several related glycosides named phyllanthostatins 1–3 (35, 36). Phyllanthoside has exhibited a curative level of activity against the murine B16 melanoma, and is presently in preclinical toxiclinical toxicology prior to consideration for eventual clinical trial (6).

4-Ipomeanol

The furan derivative 4-ipomeanol (**13**) was first isolated as the major component of a group of closely related toxic furans produced by the common sweet potato (*Ipomea batatas*) in response to infection by the fungus *Fusarium solani* (2, 3). 4-Ipomeanol and its congeners show lung toxicity in cattle. This toxicity has been shown to result from activation of the furan ring by a specific P-450 monooxygenase, generating a reactive electrophilic species which can then alkylate tissue (4). 4-Ipomeanol is under development at the National Cancer Institute as a lung specific antitumor agent and approval has been granted for phase I clinical trials (6).

REFERENCES

1. Allen LM, Marcks C, Creaven PJ: 4'-Demethylepipodophyllic acid-9-(4,6-D-ethylidene-β-D-glucopyranoside), the major urinary metabolite of VP16-213 in man. *Proc Am Assoc Cancer Res Am Soc Clin Oncol* 17: 6, 1976
2. Boyd MR, Burka LT, Harris TM, Wilson BJ: Lung-toxic furanoterpenoids produced by sweet potatoes (*Ipomoea batatas*) following microbial infection. *Biochim Biophys Acta* 337: 184, 1974
3. Boyd MR, Wilson, BJ: Isolation and characterization of 4-ipomeanol, a lung-toxic furanoterpenoid produced by sweet potatoes (*Ipomoea batatas*). *J Agric Food Chem* 20: 428, 1972
4. Boyd MR, Dutcher JS, Buckpitt AR, Jones RB, Statham CN: Role of metabolic activation in extrahepatic target organ alkylation and cytotoxicity by 4-ipomeanol, a furan derivative from moldy sweet potatoes: possible implications for carcinogenesis. In: *Naturally Occurring Carcinogens–Mutagens and Modulators of Carcinogenesis, Proceeding of the 9th International Symposium of The Princess Takamatsu Cancer Research Fund*, held in Tokyo, 1979, 399 pp
5. Canetta R, Hilgard P, Florentine S, Bedogni P, Lenaz L: Current development of podophyllotoxins. *Cancer Chemother Pharmacol* 7: 93, 1982
6. Cragg GM: Personal communication, 1987
7. Cavalli F: VP16-213 (Etoposide). A critical review of its activity. *Cancer Chemother Pharmacol* 7: 81, 1982
8. Creaven PJ: The clinical pharmacology of VM26 and VP16-213. A brief overview. *Cancer Chemother Pharmacol* 7: 133, 1982

9. Creaven PJ: The clinical pharmacology of etoposide (VP-16) in adults. In: *Etoposide (VP-16). Current Status and New Developments.* Edited by Issell BF, Muggia FM, Carter SK, pp. 103–115. Academic Press, New York, 1984

10. Denis JN, Greene AE, Guenard D, Gueritte-Voegelein F, Mangafal L, Potier F: A highly efficient, practical approach to natural taxol. *J Am Chem Soc* 110: 5917, 1988

11. Dombernowsky P, Nissen NI: Schedule dependency of the anti-leukaemic activity of the podophyllotoxin derivative VP16-213 (NSC 141540) in L1210 leukaemia. *Acta Path Microbiol Scand [A]* 81: 715, 1973

12. Doyle TW: The chemistry of etoposide. In: *Etoposide (VP-16). Current Status and New Developments.* Edited by Issell BF, Muggia FM, Carter SK, pp. 15–32. Academic Press, New York, 1984

13. Evans WF, Sinkule JA, Hutson PR, Hayeo FA, Rivera G: The clinical pharmacology of etoposide (VP16-213) in children with cancer. In: *Etoposide (VP-16). Current Status and New Developments.* Edited by Issell BF, Muggia FM, Carter SK, pp. 117–125. Academic Press, New York, 1984

14. Grieder A, Maurer R, Stahelin H: Effect of an epipodophyllotoxin derivative (VP16-213) on macromolecular synthesis and mitosis in mastocytoma cells *in vitro. Cancer Res* 34: 1788, 1974

15. Hartwell JL, Schrecker AW: The chemistry of podophyllum. *Fortschr Chem Org Naturst* 15: 83, 1958

16. Issell BF: The podophyllotoxin derivatives VP16-213 and VM26. *Cancer Chemother Pharmacol* 7: 73, 1982

17. Issell BF, Maggia FM, Carter SK (Eds): *Etoposide (VP-16). Current Status and New Developments.* Academic Press, New York, 1984

18. Jardine I: Podophyllotoxins. In: *Anticancer Agents Based on Natural Product Models.* Edited by Cassady JM, Douros JD, pp. 319–351. Academic Press, New York, 1980

19. Jardine I, Strife RJ, Kozlowski J: Synthesis, 470-MHz ¹H-NMR spectra, and activity of delactonized derivatives of the anticancer drug etoposide. *J Med Chem* 25: 1077, 1982

20. Keller-Juslén C, Kuhn M, Von Wartburg A, Stahelin H: Synthesis and antimitotic activity of glycosidic lignan derivatives related to podophyllotoxin. *J Med Chem* 14: 936, 1971

21. Kelly MG, Hartwell JL: The biological effects and the chemical composition of podophyllin. A review. *J Natl Cancer Inst* 14: 967, 1954

22. Kingston DGI, Magri NF, Jitrangsri C: Synthesis and Structure – activity relationships of taxol derivatives as anticancer agents. In: *New Trends in Natural Products Chemistry 1986.* Edited by Atta-ur-Rahman and LeQuesne PW. Elsevier Science Publishers B.V., Amsterdam 1986

23. Krishan A, Paika K, Frei E III: Cytofluorometric studies on the action of podophyllotoxin and epipodophyllotoxins (VM26, VP16-213) on the cell cycle traverse of human lymphoblasts. *J Cell Biol* 66: 521, 1975

24. Kupchan SM, Komoda Y, Court WA, Thomas GJ, Smith RM, Karim A, Gilmore CJ, Haltiwanger RC, Bryan RF: Maytansine, a novel antileukemic ansa macrolide from *Maytenus ovatus. J Am Chem Soc* 94: 1354, 1972

25. Kupchan SM, Branfman AR, Sneden AT, Verma AK, Dailey RG Jr, Komoda Y, Nagao Y: Novel maytansinoids. Naturally occurring and synthetic antileukemic esters of maytansinol. *J Am Chem Soc* 97: 5294, 1975

26. Kupchan SM, Lavoie EJ, Branfman AR, Fei BY, Bright WM, Bryan RF: Phyllanthocin, a novel bisabolane aglycon from the antileukemic glycoside, phyllanthoside. *J Am Chem Soc* 99: 3199, 1977

27. Kupchan SM, Sneden AT, Branfman AR, Howie GA, Rebhun LI, McIvor WE, Wang RW, Schnaitman TC: Structural requirements for antileukemic activity among the naturally occurring and semisynthetic maytansinoids. *J Med Chem* 21: 31, 1978

28. Lataste H, Sénilh V, Wright M, Guénard D, Potier P: Relationships between the structures of taxol and baccatin III derivatives and their *in vitro* action on the disassembly of mammalian brain and *Physarum* amoebal microtubules. *Proc Natl Acad Sci USA* 81: 4090, 1984

29. Laubenstein LJ, Krigel RL, Odajnyk CM, Hymes KB, Friedman-Kien A, Wernz JC, Muggia FM: Treatment of epidemic Kaposi's sarcoma with etoposide or a combination of doxorubicin, bleomycin, and vinblastine. *J Clin Oncol* 2: 1115, 1984

30. Loike JD: VP16-213 and podophyllotoxin. A study on the relationship between chemical structure and biological activity. *Cancer Chemother Pharmacol* 7: 103, 1982

31. Long BH, Brattain MG: The activity of etoposide (VP16-213) and teniposide (VM-26) against human lung tumor cells *in vitro*: cytotoxicity and DNA breakage. In: *Etoposide (VP-16). Current Status and New Developments.* Edited by Issell BF, Muggia FM, Carter SK, pp. 63–86. Academic Press, New York, 1984

32. Macbeth FR: VM26: Phase I and II studies. *Cancer Chemother Pharmacol* 7: 87, 1982

33. Mellado W, Magri NF, Kingston DGI, Garcia-Arenas R, Orr GA, Horwitz SB: Preparation and biological activity of taxol acetates. *Biochem Biophys Res Commun* 124: 329, 1984

34. O'Dwyer PJ, Wittes RE: Etoposide (VP16-213) current status and new directions. In: *Etoposide (VP-16). Current Status and New Developments.* Edited by Issell BF, Muggia FM, Carter SK, pp. 345–355. Academic Press, New York, 1984

35. Parness J, Kingston DGI, Powell RG, Harracksingh C, Horwitz SB: Structure-activity study of cytotoxicity and microtubule assembly *in vitro* by taxol and related taxanes. *Biochem Biophys Res Commun* 105: 1082, 1982

36. Pettit GR, Cragg GM, Gust D, Brown P: The isolation and structure of phyllanthostatins 2 and 3. *Can J Chem* 60: 544, 1982

37. Pettit GR, Cragg GM, Gust D, Brown P, Schmidt JM: The structures of phyllanthostatin 1 and phyllanthoside from the Central American tree *Phyllanthus acuminatus* Vahl. *Can J Chem* 60: 939, 1982

38. Remillard S, Rebun LI, Howe GA, Kupchan SM: Antimitotic activity of the potent tumor inhibitor maytansine. *Science* 189: 1002, 1975

39. Rinehart KL Jr, Gloer JB, Hughes RG Jr, Renis HE, McGovren JP, Swynenberg EB, Stringfellow DA, Kuentzel SL, Li LH: Didemnins: antiviral and antitumor depsipeptides from a caribbean tunicate. *Science* 212: 933, 1981

40. Rinehart KL Jr, Gloer JB, Cook JC Jr, Mizsak SA, Schaill TA: Structures of the didemnins, antiviral and cytotoxic depsipeptides from a caribbean tunicate. *J Am Chem Soc* 103: 1857, 1981

41. Rinehart KL Jr, Kishore V, Bible KC, Sakai R, Sullins DW, Li KM: Didemnins and tunichlorin: novel natural products from the marine tunicate *Trididemnun solidum. J Nat Prod* 51: 1, 1988

42. Rivera G, Dahl GV, Bowman WP, Avery TL, Wood A, Aur RJ: VM26 and cytosine arabinoside combination chemotherapy for initial induction failures in childhood lymphocytic leukemia. *Cancer* 46: 1727, 1980

43. Roberts D, Hilliard S, Peck C: Sedimentation of DNA from L1210 cells after treatment with 4'-demethylepipodophyllotoxin-9-(4,6-O-2-thenylidene-β-D-glucopyramoside) of 1-β-D-arabinofuranosylcytosine or both drugs. *Cancer Res* 40: 4225, 1980

44. Rose WC, Bradner WT: *In vivo* experimental antitumor activity of etoposide. In: *Etoposide (VP-16). Current Status and New Developments.* Edited by Issell BF, Muggia FM, Carter SK, pp. 33–47. Academic Press, New York, 1984

45. Ross W, Wozmak A, Smallwood S, Yalowich JC: DNA damage by VP-16: mechanism and relationship to cytotoxicity. In:

158   *David G.I. Kingston*

Etoposide (VP-16). Current Status and New Developments. Edited by Issell BF, Muggia FM, Carter SK, pp. 49–61. Academic Press, New York, 1984

46. Schiff PB, Fant J, Horwitz SB: Promotion of microtubule assembly *in vitro* by taxol. *Nature* 277: 665, 1979
47. Sénilh V, Blechert S, Colin M, Guénard D, Picot F, Potier P, Varenne P: Mise en évidence de nouveaux analogues du taxol extraits de *Taxus baccata. J Nat Prod* 57: 131, 1984
48. Smith CR Jr, Powell RG: Chemistry and pharmacology of the maytansinoid alkaloids. In: *Alkaloids: Chemical and Biological Perspectives. Vol. 2.* Edited by Pelletier SW, pp. 149–204. John Wiley and Sons, New York, 1984
49. Strife RJ, Jardine I, Colvin M: Analysis of the anticancer drugs VP16-213 and VM26 and their metabolites by high performance liquid chromatography. *J Chromatogr* 182: 211, 1980
50. Suffness M, Cordell GA: Antitumor alkaloids. In: *The Alkaloids. Chemistry and Pharmacology. Vol. 25.* Edited by Brossi A, pp. 1–369. Academic Press, New York, 1985
51. Wall ME, Wani MC: Antineoplastic agents from plants. *Ann Rev Pharmacol Toxicol* 17: 117, 1977
52. Wani MC, Taylor HL, Wall ME, Coggon P, McPhail AT: Plant antitumor agents. VI. The isolation and structure of taxol, a novel antileukemic and antitumor agent from *Taxus brevifolia. J Am Chem Soc* 93: 2325, 1971

15

HYPERTHERMIA

MARK W. DEWHIRST

This chapter will provide a brief overview of the biologic rationale for the use of hyperthermia in cancer therapy, a review of the current clinical literature and a discussion on areas for future research. Readers interested in further details about this form of therapy are referred to several recent books and monographs (13, 31, 37, 38, 57, 61, 63, 67, 68, 88, 92).

BIOLOGICAL RATIONALE

There are several biologic effects observed when tissues are raised to temperatures in the range of 39–50°. These effects form a strong biologic rationale for the use of hyperthermia in cancer therapy:

(1) Temperatures above 41.5°C are cytotoxic, with the rate of cell kill being dependent on temperature (14).

(2) The cytotoxicity may be more prominent in cells which are at a low pH and pO_2; a condition often seen in tumors but uncommon in normal tissues (85).

(3) Hyperthermia may preferentially act in tumor tissues because it causes microcirculatory collapse at lower temperatures in tumors than in normal tissues (85).

(4) Tumor microcirculation is vasodilated and generally unable to respond to hyperthermia, whereas normal tissues can vasodilate providing a mechanism for cooling. This difference tends to lead to preferential tumor heating during hyperthermia treatment (95).

(5) Hyperthermia is known to be synergistic with radiotherapy and a variety of chemotherapeutic drugs, including nitrogen mustards, cisplatin, adriamycin, nitrosoureas and mitomycin-c (31).

Since the rate of cell kill by hyperthermia is dependent upon temperature and time, it is theoretically possible to compare the relative effectiveness of different time temperature combinations. The relationship is most readily demonstrated by utilizing an Arrhenius plot. In an Arrhenius plot the rate of cell kill is plotted as a function of temperature. Roughly speaking, the rate of cell kill doubles for every 1°C above 43°C and reduces by a factor of 4–6 for every 1°C drop below 43°C (21, 83). This relationship has been shown to exist *in vitro* and *in vivo*, for a variety of tumor and normal tissues. Formulations of time-temperature equivalency, based on the Arrhenius relationship have been proposed, to form the basis for a clinically useful estimate of treatment effectiveness (or dose) (21, 83). The use of the word "dose" for these conversions has been somewhat misleading since they do not refer to a physical quantity (22). More importantly, there are several assumptions inherent in their current use, which could make their validity questionable, without appropriate modifications.

One of the largest modifiers of hyperthermia sensitivity is thermotolerance (acquired resistance to hyperthermic cell kill) (31). Thermotolerance can develop as a result of long heat treatments (> 3 hours) at temperatures less than 43°C or from treatment at hyperthermic temperatures, followed by a return to normothermia. The kinetics of thermotolerance development and rate of its decay are dependent on the time and temperature of the initial exposure. This phenomenon could reduce the effectiveness of fractionated hyperthermia, especially when the intertreatment interval is less than 72 hours (60).

A somewhat opposite effect can occur in so called "step-down" heating. In this case, temperatures are brought above 43°C and subsequently dropped to temperatures below 43°C. When this happens, the slope of the Arrhenius plot does not change below 43°C, as described previously, but remains at a factor 2 drop in rate of cell kill for every 1°C drop in temperature below 43°C. Thus, when step down heating occurs clinically, temperatures less than 43°C can be more effective than would be predicted from the time-temperature equivalency calculations. (35).

Three other factors which can alter the slope or position of the Arrhenius plot are pH, the resting temperature of the tissue prior to heating and the combination with radiotherapy (12, 23, 69).

It should be noted that although the slopes of the Arrhenius plots for various tissues are similar, the absolute heat sensitivity varies considerably. For example, muscle, fat and skin are relatively heat resistant while brain and liver are relatively heat sensitive (19).

In addition to the factors defined above, the current time-temperature equivalency calculations do not provide information on potentially important interactions that may occur at sublethal but supranormal temperatures (39–41.5°C). For example, temperatures between 39 and 41.5°C may improve tumor blood flow and oxygenation, thereby increasing radiosensitivity (62, 85). In addition they are known to inhibit repair of sublethal radiation damage. Furthermore, when hyperthermia is combined with some chemotherapeutic drugs, such as melphalan, cytoxan and cisplatin, synergism in terms of cell kill is observed even though temperatures between 39 and 41.5°C are not cytotoxic by themselves (31).

The ultimate usefulness of time-temperature equivalency calculations will be dependent upon future research which

P.V. Woolley (ed.), Cancer management in Man: Biological Response Modifiers, Chemotherapy, Antibiotics, Hyperthermia, Supporting Measures
© 1989. Kluwer Academic Publishers, Dordrecht.

will delineate how to make appropriate modifications of the basic Arrhenius relationship to account for the various modifiers discussed above (21, 22, 83).

In spite of the problems encountered currently in quantitating thermal "dose" the biologic rationale for its use is quite strong. The enthusiasm from the biologists has carried over into the clinical as well. The human studies which have been done to date have shown rather impressive tumor response rates without significant toxicity. Overgaard (70) recently reviewed the world's literature and found that nearly 11,000 human patients had been treated with hyperthermia in the past ten years. The most impressive subgroup were those patients where paired nodules were treated – one with radiotherapy alone and the second with hyperthermia and radiotherapy. This subgroup numbered several hundred. The encouraging fact was that the complete response rates for the combined therapy group were consistently 1.5 to 2 times higher than the radiotherapy alone controls. This was in spite of considerable variation in method and dose of radiotherapy and techniques of hyperthermia delivery. The question which remains largely unanswered at this time, however, is whether the improvement in response rates will affect cure rates. Development of clinical trials to answer this question have been slow, largely because of a lack of equipment which can reliably and predictably heat target tumor tissues without harming adjacent normal tissues. As will be shown in a later section, nonuniform intratumoral temperatures have a significant prognostic effect in clinical hyperthermia. Thus, many investigators have been reluctant to initiate phase III testing in potentially curable patients until improvements in hyperthermia delivery and monitoring can be made (16, 70). In the next section, the most commonly used hyperthermia devices will be discussed, with an emphasis on the strengths and weaknesses of each.

PHYSICAL TECHNIQUES OF HYPERTHERMIA

There are two challenges in hyperthermia engineering today. The first is to be able to measure temperature in heated tissues and the second is to be able to deliver power to a given target volume reliably and predictably.

Hyperthermia delivery devices can be conveniently categorized into those which are designed to heat locally, regionally and systemically. Local hyperthermia techniques have included external microwave applicators (29, 39, 40, 56, 72), ultrasound (18, 20, 50, 56), small magnetic induction coils (2, 6, 32, 33, 42, 47, 48), and capacitive radiofrequency techniques. Implantable microwave antennae (90), metallic needles conducting radiofrequency currents (localized current field LCF) (18) and ferromagnetic techniques (86) have also been investigated for their potential usefulness in local hyperthermia. Typically, these techniques have been used for treatment of peripherally accessible lesions. Interstitial techniques have also been investigated for their usefulness in treating deep seated sites, such as pelvis (54, 96) and brain (53). The external beam techniques have been restricted to superficial lesions because of their limited depth of penetration. For example, for 915 MHz microwaves, the maximum depth that can be heated is 4 cm. Plane wave ultrasound may do somewhat better, but is still probably limited to a maximum of 6–7 cm (63). A second limit to many external micro-

wave and ultrasound techniques is an inability to control applied power spatially. As mentioned earlier, the temperature in homogeneities which develop during hyperthermia have significant prognostic importance. Therefore, devices which have the capability of controlling power in individual parts of the heated volume should help to improve the temperature uniformity and the effectiveness of this therapy. Devices of this type are being developed currently and it is hoped that they will begin to solve this problem. Spatial temperature control is already somewhat achievable with interstitial microwave antennae (53) and with the LCF technique (5). A third, rather novel, approach to the problem has been the development of ferromagnetic implants, which undergo a curie point transition in the desired temperature range. When the seeds are placed in an inductive magnetic field, eddy currents develop in them leading to resistive heating. However, once the curie point temperature is reached, they lose their magnetic properties and cease to heat. The adjacent tissues subsequently heat by thermal conduction. With proper implantation techniques, it is theoretically possible to achieve very uniform heating with this technique, despite wide variations in tumor blood perfusion, a major avenue for heat loss and temperature inhomogeneity during hyperthermia (55, 86).

REGIONAL HEATING TECHNIQUES

The depth of heating with single external beam applicators is limited. Thus, for deep seated lesions, alternative methods have been devised which generally are capable of applying power to a relatively large region of the body, such as the pelvis or abdomen. With these techniques, one relies largely upon the commonly encountered sluggish tumor blood flow to result in preferential tumor heating, relative to surrounding normal tissue.

Regional hyperthermia has been investigated utilizing techniques involving magnetic induction at 13.56 MHz (63), cophasic microwave arrays (91) and capacitively coupled radiofrequency techniques (41). Comparisons have been made between the magnetic induction techniques and the cophasic array, on a theoretical and clinical basis. In general, neither device is capable of heating all the tumor volume in many deep seated lesions, although the annular cophasic array tends to do better (26, 82, 89). Less work has been done thus far, to document the capacitive of technique, and it has not been directly compared with the other two regional heating techniques on an experimental or theoretical basis. It is known, however, that heating of superficial fat layers is a potentially serious limitation and cannot be overcome when fat exceeds 3 cm depth (41).

A variety of methods have been utilized for induction of whole body hyperthermia. They have included hot wax, water suits, arteriovenous shunts and radiant heating devices (58). Recent advances in anesthetic management and methods of hyperthermia induction have reduced the systemic toxicity of this procedure (11, 81), although its efficacy has yet to be documented fully (79). One potential advantage of total body hyperthermia is a reduction in the magnitude of temperature gradients. Thus, it may be of use in combination with radiotherapy, in addition to its potential as an adjuvant to chemotherapy. However, systemic temperatures cannot safely exceed 42°C. Thus, direct heat cytotoxicity will be less of a factor with this form of therapy than is observed with local and regional techniques.

Monitoring of the efficacy and safety of hyperthermia treatment is dependent upon the measurement of temperature. The importance of temperature monitoring has been demonstrated in a number of clinical reports (4, 15, 17, 52, 64, 94). However, thermometry in clinical hyperthermia is problematic, because it is necessarily invasive. No accurate method for measuring temperature noninvasively is available (8). Development of noninteractive sensors has greatly improved the accuracy of measurement in microwave and radiofrequency fields (9), but patient tolerance and practicality limit the number of thermometers which can be placed. The recent development of multijunction thermometers (93) and pull back techniques (25) have increased the amount of information which can be gained from a single catheter placement. However, even more information will be needed to generate complete three-dimensional temperature fields. The problem may ultimately be solved by combining limited invasive temperature measurements with heat transfer modelling (82).

CLINICAL RESULTS

Heat alone

The clinical effects of heat alone have been recently summarized by Meyer (57). In general, heat alone is of limited usefulness, since complete responses are infrequent and regrowth is common.

Heat and radiotherapy

Most of the clinical experience which has been obtained thus far with hyperthermia has been with peripherally accessible lesions. This has been true because the development of safe and practical methods of heating deep seated tumors has been relatively slow. The clinical data has been recently reviewed (70, 73). Much has been learned from this initial experience, although the majority of patients have not been evaluable for long-term tumor control.

Several institutions have reported on patients with two or more lesions where one lesion served as a radiotherapy alone control (70, 73). In all series reported the response rates of those lesions receiving the combined therapy was superior to the controls, usually by a factor of 1.5–2. In addition, these results have been obtained without significant enhancement of normal tissue effects, from radiotherapy or hyperthermia itself. More recently, the encouraging results obtained for initial response have been shown to hold true for long-term tumor control (4, 84). In both studies, control lesions received tolerance dose radiotherapy alone with small doses per fraction. The failure rate in the control lesions was higher, but no thermal enhancement in late radiation effects was observed in those sites that received the combination therapy. Thermal enhancement in early and late radiation effects has been observed in other reports, with the severity being dependent upon the radiation dose per fraction and the sequence used between hyperthermia and radiotherapy.

When hyperthermia was given immediately after radiotherapy with doses per fraction of 4–5 Gy, enhancement in normal tissue effects was observed (3, 71). These results are in agreement with extensive data in murine models which have investigated sequencing. Minimization of normal tissue effects was seen when hyperthermia followed radiotherapy by 2–3 hours (66).

In summary, the results from the paired lesions studies have demonstrated that the combination therapy is superior to radiotherapy alone for palliative treatment of recurrent or metastatic lesions. Consequently, the modality is rapidly developing as an adjuvant treatment option in general radiotherapy practice. Hyperthermia systems are now commercially available for external and interstitial treatment of the above mentioned lesions. In one sense, it is encouraging to see the general employment of this modality, since it can offer effective therapy. However, there are many factors which influence its effectiveness and safety; work is continuing to elucidate these factors further. Some of these factors are discussed below.

Perhaps the most influential factor influencing therapy effectiveness and safety is the temperature gradient which develops during hyperthermia treatment. Temperature gradients were first demonstrated to be clinically important in murine systems (27, 97). Clinically, this was verified in pet animal tumors by Dewhirst *et al* (17) when they demonstrated a significant correlation between minimum monitored tumor temperature and prognosis for tumor control. Several human clinical reports have substantiated the importance of temperature gradients as well (4, 52, 64). It is clear that in most clinical situations it is not possible to heat all of the tumor volume. Unfortunately, because of the limited thermometry which is currently available, it is not feasible to determine how much a tumor volume must be heated to achieve a maximal effect. Therefore, it is very difficult to document when adequate therapy has been delivered (15). These results emphasize the need for development of improved thermometry systems, which may ultimately rely partially on heat transfer modelling (82). Quality assurance in hyperthermia therapy is further complicated by factors which relate to patient tolerance of the therapy and the experience of the personnel involved in therapy delivery. Furthermore, techniques for therapy documentation and verification of reproducibility are still under development (65). Several studies have demonstrated that radiotherapy dose influences the efficacy of the combined modality (28, 52, 64, 71, 94). Thus, when previously irradiated lesions are being treated it is necessary to deliver a dose which is as close to tolerance as possible. When previously unirradiated lesions are treated, conventionally fractionated tolerance doses are probably indicated (73). One reported advantage of thermoradiotherapy over radiotherapy alone has been its ability to control relatively large tumors. However, even with this form of therapy, tumor response rates tend to drop with increasing tumor volume (4, 17, 64). Two factors are probably responsible for this phenomenon. Firstly, larger tumors probably have more clonogenic cells in them, thus requiring more optimal hyperthermia. Secondly, larger tumors are more difficult to heat. This difficulty may, in large part, be reflective of inadequate hyperthermia devices (17, 74).

Three other factors which will probably play a role in

hyperthermia treatment efficacy are the timing between hyperthermia fractions, the number of fractions delivered and optimization of the combination with fractionated radiotherapy. Protocols are underway in a number of institutions to define these parameters but currently data are just not available (73). It should be emphasized that the clinical data which is currently available has been gained from phase I–II testing. Phase III testing has not been done in human patients to date and this must be done to confirm whether hyperthermia will be an effective adjuvant form of therapy for potentially curable patients (16, 70, 73).

Hyperthermia and chemotherapy

Progress in the clinical utilization of hyperthermia and chemotherapy has not been as rapid or as extensive as with radiotherapy. Thus, its value in this setting is less well defined (43). Rationale for its use lies in the following observations: (1) It is synergistic with a variety of chemotherapeutic drugs, including nitrogen mustards such as cytoxan and melphalan, cisplatin, adriamycin mitomycin-c (31) and lonidamine (70). (2) It makes some drugs, not normally thought of as chemotherapeutic agents, cytotoxic. Examples of these types of agents include Actinomycin D (31), Lidocaine (98) and thiopental (80). (3) Its combination with local or regional hyperthermia could potentiate its effects in the region of tumor, while reducing systemic toxicity.

Perhaps the most impressive series of clinical reports published thus far have involved low temperature (40–41.4°C) limb perfusion combined with melphalan for the treatment of limb sarcomas and melanomas (7, 87). These investigators have had the longest clinical experience with the use of hyperthermia and chemotherapy. Therefore, it has been possible to assess long-term control and survival. The results for advanced loco-regional disease have been reported to be superior to historical controls involving perfusion with melphalan at normothermia. For example, Stehlin (87) reported 5-year survival rates for stage IIIA melanoma to be 22% and 76.7% for perfusion alone and combined with hyperthermia, respectively. It is unfortunate, that these studies were not randomized prospective trials. Therefore, it has been difficult to make a definitive statement about this procedure, relative to more conventional forms of therapy. Recently, however, results of a randomized prospective trial were reported in which hyperthermic limb perfusion, used as a postoperative procedure, was compared to surgery alone (24). Statistically significant improvements in local control rates were observed for all stages of loco-regional disease (I, II, III) with the addition of hyperthermic limb perfusion with melphalan.

The rationale for the use of whole body hyperthermia in combination with chemotherapy lies in its potential to treat refractory disseminated solid malignancies and other forms of systemic malignancy. The question which must be addressed, however, is whether this type of treatment can be given without causing significant systemic toxicity. There is some evidence from murine models that a therapeutic gain is possible through manipulation of sequencing between drug administration and induction of hyperthermia (1, 36). Alterations in pharmacokinetics during hyperthermia due to changes in the rates of metabolism and/or biodistribution

may provide mechanisms for exploiting this combination to achieve therapeutic gain (36, 59, 78).

The clinical studies which have been published to date investigating total body hyperthermia and chemotherapy have focused largely on physiologic effects and defining toxicities. Nevertheless, some tumor response information has been provided. For example, Pettigrew and collaborators (46, 75, 76, 77) observed objective responses in 11/13 patients treated with heat and chemotherapy. Larkin (44, 45) reported a 43% response rate in 72 patients treated with a variety of disseminated solid malignancies. Historically the toxicity of the hyperthermia procedure itself has limited a more rapid development of this technique. Recent advances in method of anesthetic management (11) and techniques for hyperthermia induction (81) have renewed interest in this technique. It remains to be seen, however, whether the procedure will be of clinical value.

SUMMARY

It is clear that there is a strong biologic rationale for the use of hyperthermia in combination with chemo- and radiotherapy. The clinical results which have been obtained thus far confirm that the modality has clinical utility.

In future years, studies must concentrate on optimization of the use of heat with other modalities, especially in regard to sequencing and time-dose fractionation. In addition, the true test of hyperthermia; namely demonstration that it can result in increased tumor control rates without significant elevation of toxicity, has not been demonstrated in randomized studies. Such studies will be greatly facilitated by continued development in hyperthermia delivery and monitoring devices.

REFERENCES

1. Alberts DS, Peng Y, Chen HSG et al: Therapeutic synergism of hyperthermia cis-platinum in a mouse tumor model. *JNCI* 65: 455, 1980
2. Antich PP, Tokita N, Kim JH et al: Selective heating of cutaneous human tumors at 27.12 MHz. *IEEE Trans MIT* 26: 569, 1978
3. Arcangeli G, Cividalli A, Nervi A, Creton F: Tumor control and therapeutic gain with different schedules of combined radiotherapy and local external hyperthermia in human cancer. *Int J Radiation Oncology Biol Phys* 9: 1125, 1983
4. Arcangeli G, Arcangeli G, Guerra A, Lovislo G, Cividalli A, Marino C, Mauro F: Tumor response to heat and radiation: Prognostic variables in the treatment of neck node metastases from head and neck cancer. *Int J Hyperthermia* 1: 207, 1985
5. Astrahan MA: A localized current field hyperthermia system for use with 192 iridium implants. *Med Phys* 9: 419, 1982
6. Carnochon P, Jancar MP, Jones CH: The assessment of RF inductive applicators suitable for clinical hyperthermia. *Br J Cancer* 45: 25, 1982
7. Cavaliere R, Mondovi B, Moricca G et al: Regional perfusion hyperthermia. In: *Hyperthermia in Cancer Therapy*. Edited by FK Storm. Boston, GK Hall Medical Publishers, pp 369, 1983
8. Cetas TC: Will thermometric tomography become practical for hyperthermia treatment monitoring? *Cancer Res* 44: 4805, 1984
9. Cetas TC: Thermometry and thermal dosimetry. In: *Hyper-*

thermic Oncology, Vol. 2. Edited by J. Overgaard. Taylor and Francis, London, pp. 91–112, 1985

10. Corry PM, Spanos WJ, Tilchen EJ et al: Combined ultrasound and radiation therapy treatment of human superficial tumors. *Radiology* 145: 165, 1982

11. Cronau LS, Bourke DL, Bull JM: General anesthesia for whole body hyperthermia. *Cancer Res* 44: 4873, 1984

12. Culver PS, Gerner EW: Temperature acclimation and specific cellular components in the regulation of thermal sensitivity of mammalian cells. *NCI Mongr* 61: 99, 1982

13. Dethlefsen LA (ed): *Third International Symposium*: Cancer therapy by hyperthermia, drugs, and radiation. NCI, Mongr 61, 1982

14. Dewey WC, Freeman ML: Rationale for use of hyperthermia in cancer therapy. *Ann NY Acad Sci* 335: 372, 1980

15. Dewhirst MW, Sim DA: The utility of thermal dose as a predictor of tumor and normal tissue responses to combined radiation and hyperthermia. *Cancer Res* 44: 4772, 1984

16. Dewhirst MW, Sim DA: Estimation of therapeutic gain in clinical trials involving hyperthermia and radiotherapy. *International Journal of Hyperthermia* 2: 165, 1986

17. Dewhirst MW, Sim DA, Sapareto S, Connor WG: The importance of minimum tumor temperature in determining early and long term responses of pet animal tumors to heat and radiation. *Cancer Res* 44: 43, 1984

18. Doss JD, McCabe CW: A technique for localized heating in tissue: An adjunct to tumor therapy. *Med Instrum* 10: 16, 1976

19. Fajardo LP: Pathologic effects of hyperthermia in normal tissue. *Cancer Research* (suppl) 44: 4826, 1984

20. Fessenden P, Lee ER, Anderson TL, Strohbehn JW, Meyer JL, Samulski TV, Marmor JB: Experience with a multitransducer ultrasound system for localized hyperthermia of deep tissues. *IEEE Trans Biomed Eng* 31: 126, 1984

21. Field SB, Morris CC: The relationship between heating time and temperature: Its relevance to clinical hyperthermia. *Radiotherapy and Oncology* 1: 179, 1983

22. Gerner EW: Definition of thermal dose biological isoeffect relationships and dose for temperature induced cytotoxicity. In: *Hyperthermic Oncology, Vol 2*. Edited by J Overgaard. Taylor and Francis, London, pp 245–252, 1985

23. Gerweck LE, Richards B: Influence of pH on the thermal sensitivity of cultured human glioblastoma cells. *Cancer Res* 41: 845, 1981

24. Ghussen F, Nagel K, Groth W, Muller JM, Stutzer H: A prospective randomized study of regional extremity perfusion in patients with malignant melanoma. *Ann Surg* 200: 764, 1984

25. Gibbs FA: Thermal mapping in experimental cancer treatment with hyperthermia: Description and use of a semi-automated system. *Int J Radiation Oncology Biol Phys* 9: 1057, 1983

26. Gibbs FA: Regional hyperthermia, a clinical appraisal of non-invasive deep heating methods. *Cancer Res* 44: 4765, 1984

27. Gibbs FA, Peck JW, Dethlefsen LA: The importance of intratumor temperature uniformity in the study of radiosensitizing effects of hyperthermia *in vivo*. *Rad Res* 87: 187, 1981

28. Gillette EL: Clinical use of thermal enhancement and therapeutic gain for hyperthermia combined with radiation or drugs. *Cancer Res* 44: 4826, 1984

29. Guy AW, Lehmann JF, Stonebridge JB et al: Development of a 917-MHz direct-contact applicator for therapeutic heating of tissues. *IEEE Trans. MIT* 26: 550, 1978

30. Hafstrom L, Hugander A, Jonsson P, Westling H, Ehrsson H: Blood leakage and melphalan leakage from the perfusion circuit during regional hyperthermic perfusion for malignant melanoma. *Can Treat Rep* 68: 867, 1984

31. Hahn GM: *Hyperthermia and Cancer*. New York, Plenum Press, 1982

32. Hand JW, Ledda JL, Evans NTS: Considerations of radiofrequency induction heating for localized hyperthermia. *Phys Med Biol* 27: 1016, 1982

33. Hand JW, Ledda JR, Evans NTS: Temperature heating in tissues subjected to local hyperthermia by RF induction heating. *Br J Cancer* 45: 31, 1982

34. Henle KJ, Leeper DB: The modification of radiation damage in CHO cells by hyperthermia at 40 and 45°C. *Rad Res* 70: 415, 1977

35. Henle KJ, Dethlefsen LA: Time-temperature relationships for heat-induced killing of mammalian cells. *Ann NY Acad Sci* 335: 234, 1980

36. Honess DJ, Bleehen NM: Thermochemotherapy with cis-platinum, CCNU, BCNU, chlorambucil and melphalan on murine marrow and two tumors: therapeutic gain for melphalan only. *Br J Rad* 58: 63, 1985

37. Hornback N, Shupe R: *Hyperthermia and Cancer: Human Clinical Trial Experience*. CRC Press, Boca Raton, FL. 1984, 2 volumes

38. Jain RK, Gullino PM (eds): *Thermal Characteristics of Tumors: Applications in Detection and Treatment*. Ann NY Acad Sci 335: 1980

39. Kantor G, Cetas TC: A comparative heating pattern study of direct contact applicators in microwave diathermy. *Radio Sci* 12: 111, 1977

40. Kantor G, Whitters DM, Greiser JW: The performance of a new direct contact applicator for microwave diathermy. *IEEE Trans MIT* 26: 563, 1978

41. Kato H, Hiraoka M, Nakajima T, Ishida T: Deep-heating characteristics of an RF capacitive heating device. *Int J Hyperthermia* 1: 15, 1985

42. Kim JH, Hahn EW, Tokita N et al: Local tumor hyperthermia in combination with radiation therapy. *Cancer* 40: 161, 1977

43. Landberg T: Hyperthermia and cancer chemotherapy. In: *Hyperthermic Oncology, Vol. 2*. Edited by J Overgaard. Taylor and Francis, London, pp. 169–180, 1985

44. Larkin JM: A clinical investigation of total-body hyperthermia as cancer therapy. *Cancer Res* 39: 2252, 1979

45. Larkin JM, Edwards WJ, Smith DE et al: Systemic thermotherapy: Description of a method and physiologic tolerance in clinical subjects. *Cancer* 40: 3155, 1977

46. Law HT, Pettigrew RT: Heat transfer in whole-body hyperthermia. *Ann NY Acad Sci* 335: 298, 1980

47. Lehmann JF, Guy AW, DeLateur BJ et al: Heating patterns produced by short-wave diathermy using helical induction coil applicators. *Arch Phys Med Rehabil* 49: 193, 1968

48. Lehmann JF, DeLateur BJ, Stonebridge JB: Selective muscle heating by shortwave diathermy with a helical coil. *Arch Phys Med* 50: 117, 1969

49. Lehmann JF, Guy AW, Stonebridge JB et al: Evaluation of a therapeutic direct-contact 915-MHz microwave applicator for effective deep-tissue heating in humans. *IEEE Trans MIT* 26: 556, 1978

50. Lele PP: Physical aspects and clinical studies with ultrasonic hyperthermia. In: *Hyperthermia in Cancer Therapy*. Edited by FK Storm. Boston, GK Hall Medical Publishers, pp. 333–367, 1983

51. Lowenthal JP (ed): Hyperthermia in cancer treatment. *Cancer Res* 44: Suppl, 1984

52. Luk KH, Pajak TF, Perez CA, Johnson RJ, Connor N, Dobbins T: Prognostic factors for tumor response after hyperthermia and radiation. In: *Hyperthermic Oncology* Vol. 1. Edited by J Overgaard. Taylor and Francis, London, pp. 353–356, 1984

53. Lyons BE, Britt RH, Strohbehm JW: Localized hyperthermia in the treatment of malignant brain tumors using an interstitial microwave antenna array. *Biomed Engineering* 31: 53, 1984

54. Manning MR, Cetas TC, Miller RC, Oleson JR, Connor WG and Gerner EW: Results of a phase I trial employing hyperthermia alone or in combination with external beam or interstitial radiotherapy. *Cancer* 29: 205, 1982

55. Matloubieh AY, Roemer RB, Cetas TC: Numerical simulation of magnetic induction heating of tumors with ferromag-

netic seed implants. *IEEE Trans Biomed Eng* 31: 227, 1984

56. Mendecki J, Friedenthal E, Botstein C et al: Therapeutic potential of conformal applicators for induction of hyperthermia. *J Microwave Power* 14: 761, 1978

57. Meyer JL: The clinical efficacy of localized hyperthermia. *Cancer Res*: 44: 4745, 1984

58. Milligan AJ: Whole body hyperthermia induction techniques. *Cancer Res* 44: 4869, 1984

59. Mimnaugh EG, Waring RW, Sikic BI, Magin RL, Drew R, Litterst CL, Gram TE, Guarino AM: Effect of whole body hyperthermia on the disposition and metabolism of adriamycin in rabbits. *Cancer Res* 38: 1420, 1978

60. Nielsen OS, Overgaard J: Influence of time and temperature on the kinetics of thermotolerance in L_1A_2 cells *in vitro*. *Cancer Res* 42: 4190, 1982

61. Nussbaum GH (ed): *Physical Aspects of Hyperthermia*, New York, American Institute of Physics, Inc., 1982

62. O'Hara MD, Hetzel FW, Avery K: Mild (40°C) microwave hyperthermia and tumor oxygenation (meeting abstract). Thirty-third Annual Meeting of the Radiation Research Society, May 5–9, 1985, Los Angeles, CA p. 59, 1985

63. Oleson JR, Dewhirst MW: Hyperthermia: An overview of current progress and problems. *Current Problems in Cancer* 8: 1983

64. Oleson JR, Sim DA, Manning MR: Analysis of prognostic variables in hyperthermia treatment of 163 patients. *Int J Radiation Oncology Biol Phys* 10: 2231, 1984

65. Oleson JR, Dewhirst MW, Duncan D, Engler M, Thrall D: Temperature gradients: Prognostic and dosimetric implications. In: *Proc of IEEE Conference of EMBS, IEEE*, New York, 1985

66. Overgaard J: The biological basis for clinical treatment with combined hyperthermia and radiation. In: *Prog in Radio-Oncology II*. Edited by KH Karcher. New York, Raven Press, 415–423, 1982

67. Overgaard J (ed): *Hyperthermic Oncology*, Vol. 2. Taylor and Francis, London, 1985

68. Overgaard J (ed): *Hyperthermic Oncology*, Vol. 1, Taylor and Francis, London, 1984

69. Overgaard J: Time-temperature relationship for hyperthermic cytotoxicity and radiosensitation: Implications for a thermal dose uit. In: *Hyperthermic Oncology, Vol. 1*. Edited by J Overgaard, Taylor and Francis, pp. 191–194, London, 1984

70. Overgaard J: Rationale and problems in the design of clinical studies. In: *Hyperthermic Oncology, Vol. 2*. Edited by J Overgaard, Taylor and Francis, London, pp. 325–340, 1985

71. Overgaard J, Overgaard M: A clinical trial evaluation of the effect of simultaneous or sequential radiation and hyperthermia in the treatment of malignant melanoma. In: *Hyperthermic Oncology, Vol. 1*. Edited by J Overgaard. Taylor and Francis, London, pp. 383–386, 1984

72. Paglione R, Sterzer F, Mendecki J et al: 27 MHz ridged waveguide applicators for localized hyperthermia treatment of deep-seated malignant tumors. *Microwave J* 14: 71, 1981

73. Perez CA, Meyer JL: Clinical experience with localized hyperthermia and irradiation. In: *Hyperthermic Oncology, Vol. 2*. Edited by J Overgaard. Taylor and Francis, London, pp. 181–198, 1985

74. Perez CA, Nussbaum G, Emami B, Von Gerichten D: Clinical results of irradiation combined with local hyperthermia. *Cancer* 52: 1597, 1983

75. Pettigrew RT, Galt JM, Ludgate CM et al: Clinical effects of whole body hyperthermia in advanced malignancy. *Br Med J* 4: 679, 1974

76. Pettigrew RT, Galt CM, Ludgate CM et al: Circulatory and biochemical effects of whole-body hyperthermia. *Br J Surg* 61: 727, 1974

77. Pettigrew RT, Ludgate CM, Gee AP et al: Whole-body hyper-

thermia combined with chemotherapy in the treatment of advanced human cancer. In: *Cancer Therapy by Hyperthermia and Radiation*. Edited by C. Streffer. Baltimore and Munich, Urban & Schwarzenberg, pp. 337–339, 1978

78. Riviere JE, Page RL, Dewhirst MW, Tyczkowska K, Thrall DE: Effect of hyperthermia on cis-platinum pharmacokinetics in normal dogs. *Int J Hyperthermia* 2: 351, 1986

79. Robins HI: Role of the whole body hyperthermia in the treatment of neoplastic disease: Its current status and future prospects. *Cancer Res* 44: 4878, 1984

80. Robins HI, Dennis WH, Slattery JS, Lange TA, Yatvin MB: Systemic lidocaine enhancement of hyperthermia-induced tumor regression in transplantable murine tumor models. *Can Res* 43: 3187, 1983

81. Robins HI, Dennis WH, Neville AJ, Shecterle LM, Martin PA, Grossman J, Thomas E, Neville SR, Gillis W, Rusy BF: A nontoxic system for 41.8°C whole-body hyperthermia: Results of phase I study using a radiant heat device. *Cancer Res* 45: 3937, 1985

82. Roemer RB, Cetas TC: Applications of bioheat transfer simulations in hyperthermia. *Cancer Res* 44: 4788, 1984

83. Sapareto SA, Dewey WC: Thermal dose determination in cancer therapy. *Int J Radiation Oncology Biol Phys* 10: 787, 1984

84. Scott RS, Johnson RJR, Story KV, Clay L: Local hyperthermia in combination with definitive radiotherapy: Increased tumor clearance, reduced recurrence rate in extended follow-up. *Int J Radiation Oncology Biol Phys* 10: 2119, 1984

85. Song CW, Lokshina A, Rhee JG, Patten M, Levitt SH: Implication of blood flow in hyperthermic treatment of tumors. *Biomed Engineering* 31: 9, 1984

86. Stauffer PR, Cetas TC, Fletcher AM, DeYoung DW, Dewhirst MW, Oleson JR, Roemer RB: Observations on the use of ferromagnetic implants for inducing hyperthermia. *Biomed Engineering* 31: 76, 1984

87. Stehlin JS, Giovanella BC, Delpolyi PD, Anderson RF: Eleven years experience with hyperthermic perfusion for melanoma of the extremities. *World J Surg* 3: 305, 1979

88. Storm FK (ed): *Hyperthermia in Cancer Therapy*. Boston, GK Hall Medical Publishers, 1983

89. Strohbehn JW: Calculation of absorbed power in tissue for various hyperthermia devices. *Cancer Res* 44: 4781, 1984

90. Strohbehn JW, Bowers ED, Walsh JE, Douple EB: An invasive microwave antenna for locally-induced hyperthermia for cancer therapy. *J Microwave Power* 14: 339, 1979

91. Turner PF: Deep heating of cylindrical or elliptical tissue masses. *NCI Monogr* 61: 493, 1982

92. Vaeth JM (ed): Hyperthermia and radiation therapy, chemotherapy in the treatment of cancer. *Frontiers of Radiation Therapy and Oncology*, Vol. 18, 1984

93. Vaguine VA, Christensen DA, Lindley JH, Walston TE: Multiple sensor optical thermometry system for application in clinical hyperthermia. *Biomed Engineering* 31: 168, 1984

94. Van der Zee J, van Rhoon GC, Wike-Hooley JL, and Reinhold HS: Clinically derived dose effect relationship for hyperthermia given in combination with low dose radiotherapy. *Brit J Radiol* 58: 243, 1985

95. Voorhees WD, Babbs CF: Hydralazine enhanced selective heating of transmissible venereal tumor implants in dogs. *Europ J Cancer Clin Oncol* 18: 1027, 1982

96. Vora N, Forell B, Joseph C, Lipsett J, Archambeau JD: Interstitial implant with interstitial hyperthermia. *Cancer* 50: 2518, 1982

97. Wallen AC, Michaelson SM, Wheeler KT: Temperature and cell survival variability across 9L subcutaneous tumors heated with microwaves. *Rad Res* 85: 281, 1981

98. Yatvin M, Clifton K, Dennis W: Hyperthermia and local anesthetics: Potentiation of survival of tumor-bearing mice. *Science* 205: 195, 1979

For postscript see end of Volume, p. 247.

16

CURRENT ADVANCES IN BMT* FOR CANCER TREATMENT

DAHLIA V. KIRKPATRICK and LILIAN DELMONTE

LIST OF ABBREVIATIONS

AL	acute leukemia
ALL	acute lymphoblastic leukemia
ANLL	acute non-lymphocytic leukemia
AP	acute phase
ASTA-Z	mephosphamide
BCNU	carmustine
BMT	bone marrow transplantation
BP	blast phase (blast crisis)
CGL	chronic granulocytic leukemia (see CML)
CML	chronic myelocytic leukemia (see CGL)
CP	chronic phase
CP-1	first chronic phase
CP-2	second chronic phase
CR	complete response: 100% regression of all measurable lesions
CR-1	first complete remission
CR-2	second complete remission
CR-3	third remissions
CT	chemotherapy
DMSO	dimethyl sodium dioxide
DTIC	dacarbazine
EBV	Epstein-Barr virus
4-HC	4-hydroperoxycyclophosphamide
GvHD	graft-versus-host disease
GvL	graft-versus-leukemia
HCL	hairy cell leukemia
HD	Hodgkin's disease
MAb	monoclonal antibody
NHL	non-Hodgkin's lymphoma
PR	parital response: $\geq$ 50% regression of all measurable marrow
RT	radiotherapy
SBA	soybean hemagglutinin
SCLC	small cell lung carcinoma (oat cell carcinoma)
TBI	total body irradiation
VP-16	etoposide

INTRODUCTION

Bone marrow transplantation (BMT) has become an accepted form of treatment for acute leukemia, aplastic anemia, and severe combined immunodeficiencies, and has recently become an alternative treatment for solid tumors, particularly lymphoma. The purpose of BMT is to repopulate the hemopoietic and lymphoid system following eradication of malignant cells with extremely high doses of chemotherapy (CT) and/or radiotherapy (RT) and, hopefully, to inhibit progression of the malignant process.

In the clinical situation, three types of BMT are possible: (1) Autologous BMT, using the patient's stored bone marrow; (2) syngeneic BMT, using identical twin donor marrow; or (3) allogeneic BMT, using marrow from related or unrelated individuals (Table 1). Allogeneic BMT is done primarily using intact marrow from genetically matched siblings or, occasionally, using T lymphocyte-depleted marrow from a genetically mismatched parent or other close relative.

The difficulty of finding genetically matched donors, and the high risk of graft-versus-host disease (GvHD) and fatal interstitial pneumonitis, even with the best of matches, has led to the exploration of autologous BMT as a viable alternative for allogeneic BMT. Unfortunately, it is becoming increasingly apparent that the autologous approach may be less effective than the allogeneic approach for achieving durable suppression of malignant disease (Table 1).

Prior to marrow infusion, the patient is usually put into remission using CT and RT. Immunosuppressive conditioning is required only in the allogeneic situation (Table 1).

GRAFT-VERSUS-HOST DISEASE

Graft-versus-host disease (GvHD) has been a major complication for the transplant recipient, and continues to be so in spite of recent attempts using monoclonal antibodies (MAbs) to deplete the marrow of T cells (15, 42). Other T

Table 1. Complication risk in bone marrow transpantation (BMT).

Donor:recipient match	Immunosuppression before BMT	Risk of GvHD	Risk of relapse	Risk of fatal pneumonitis
Allogeneic	+	+	+	+ + +
Syngeneic (Twin)	−	−	+ + +	+
Autologous	−	−	+ + +	+

* Bone marrow transplantation.

165

P.V. Woolley (ed.), Cancer management in Man: Biological Response Modifiers, Chemotherapy, Antibiotics, Hyperthermia, Supporting Measures
© 1989. Kluwer Academic Publishers, Dordrecht.

cell depletion techniques, notably the soybean lectin, have been highly successful in limiting the severity of GvHD, but have resulted in a higher rate of rejection and relapse (15).

GRAFT-VERSUS-LEUKEMIA

In 1965, Mathe *et al.* (90) observed that CT could reduce the tumor burden of mice bearing L1210 leukemia by no more than 5 logs at best. Thus, when early trials with BMT failed to achieve lasting therapeutic effects in cancer patients, this was generally thought to reflect a failure of the pre-BMT conditioning regimens to extirpate all malignant cells.

More recently, improvements in transplant technology have led to long-term survival in 20–60% of patients with acute lymphoblastic leukemia (ALL) transplanted in first or second remission (CR-1 or CR-2) (30, 142), and 50–60% of patients with acute non-lymphocytic leukemia (ANNL) transplanted in first remission (CR-1) (141) or CR-2 (31). This has led to the widespread assumption that the efficacy of BMT in acute leukemia is related to improved anti-leukemic efficacy of the high doses of CT and RT administered to condition the patient for BMT.

A factor that may contribute to the antileukemic efficacy of allogeneic BMT is graft-versus-leukemia (GvL) reactivity, a phenomenon first proposed by Barnes (7) and Mathe *et al.* (90), and then later by Bortin *et al.* (14) who observed that development of GvHD in mice engrafted with genetically matched allogeneic marrow was frequently associated with an increased tumor cure rate. The GvL hypothesis proposes that destruction of residual leukemia cells during the post-transplant period may be effected by the GvHD process itself, or by antibodies to alloantigens (minor histocompatibility antigens and/or leukemia-associated antigens) expressed by engrafted donor lymphocytes.

In man, the concept of GvL activity was supported by a study by Weiden (145). He documented a low relapse rate in patients with chronic GvHD, and a high relapse rate in recipients of syngeneic (identical twin) transplants. He documented disease-free survival vs leukemic relapse in 46 syngeneic marrow recipients. One-hundred seventeen allogeneic sibling marrow recipients developed only low-grade or no GvHD, and 49 allogeneic sibling marrow recipients developed moderate to severe acute GvHD or chronic GvHD. Survival was 50% at 2 years for patients with grade II–IV acute GvHD, as compared with 25% for those with grades O–I acute GvHD. Patients who developed chronic GvHD without prior acute GvHD had an 80% survival at 2 years. Thus, the likelihood of achieving a remission lasting two years appeared to be significantly higher for allogeneic transplant recipients with moderate to severe GvHD than for those with only mild GvHD or no GvHD.

In 1985, Gale and Champlin (45) reviewed the leukemic relapse rates reported by various centers for a total of 370 marrow transplant recipients conditioned with the same CT/RT regimen. Thirty-one had received marrow from a monozygotic twin; 339, marrow from a matched allogeneic sibling. The actuarial relapse rate among the twin marrow recipients was 59%, while that among sibling allograft recipients was 18% – a highly significant difference. The authors proposed that the high relapse rate in the twin situation might be due to the absence of GvHD, while the low relapse

rate in the allogeneic situation might reflect GvHD-associated GvL reactivity. Ongoing clinical investigations are aimed at manipulating GvHD in marrow allograft recipients to exploit this apparent antileukemic effect.

SECONDARY MALIGNANCIES AFTER BMT

Secondary malignancies occur with a greater frequency in marrow transplant recipients than in the general population.

Canine studies have suggested that such malignancies arise as a consequence of the high dose of total body irradiation (TBI) used in conditioning the recipient for BMT (27). Among 153 healthy dogs who received marrow auto- or allografts, the incidence of malignancies developing over a median period of 33 months was five times greater when their conditioning regimen included TBI than when their conditioning regimen consisted of CT (cyclophosphamide and myleran) without TBI.

While cytogenetic studies have shown that in man most leukemic recurrences after BMT are of host cell origin, about 5% of recurrences do occur in donor cells. In a retrospective analysis of almost 2000 marrow allograft recipients, Deeg *et al.* (28) documented 20 secondary malignancies occurring within 2 months to 5 years after transplantation. All but one (a patient with aplastic anemia) had been transplanted for hemopoietic malignancy. All but three had received TBI (8.0–15.75 Gy) as part of their conditioning regimen. Six of the 20 patients with secondary malignancies had recurrence of leukemia in donor-type cells, eight developed lymphoproliferative malignancies (four of donor-type, three of host-type, and one of undetermined origin), and six developed solid tumors.

Epstein–Barr virus (EBV) associated lymphoma or lymphoproliferative disease in donor-derived cells has been reported in two recipients of marrow treated with monoclonal antibody (MAb) (89) and recipients of donor marrow depleted of T cells prior to transplantation (126). In a survey of 33 BMT recipients with leukemic relapse, Schubach *et al.* (127) identified secondary lymphoproliferative malignancies in the five patients whose cells contained the EBV genome or expressed the viral antigen, but not in the other 28 patients who were EBV-negative. This observation is consonant with the widely-held hypothesis that oncogenic viruses may play a role in the development of secondary malignancies in BMT recipients. The investigators concluded that the etiology of secondary malignancies in human BMT recipients is probably multifactorial, and may include TBI, immunosuppression, and transformation of donor cells by a viral oncogene or by viral transfection.

HIV infection and marrow transplantation

Following BMT the immune response is altered and many patients are unable to mount normal antibody responses. In the early post transplant period HIV infections are difficult to document because many patients are unable to produce specific antibodies to HIV. These patients should be evaluated for HIV antigen and the polymerase chain reaction test for HIV should be used in lieu of the HIV antibody test.

Studies of infants infected with HIV have demonstrated

that some of these infants are negative on the antibody test but have now shown to be infected with the virus by the polymerase chain reaction (84).

BMT has been attempted without success for HIV. A twin transplant was performed by Hassett, Zaroulis et al (66) however; the recipient failed to attain immune reconstitution. The donor cells probably became infected with the virus and the patient's condition ultimately deteriorated. Although BMT has been successful in reconstituting congenital severe combined immunodeficiency the patient with acquired immunodeficiency has a viral vector which is capable of transfecting the immunocompetent cells of the donor. Transplantation of normal cells into a host with an immunosuppressive virus is doomed to fail unless a satisfactory antiviral agent is available.

BMT FOR ACUTE LEUKEMIAS

Allogeneic BMT for acute leukemia

In initial studies, Thomas and colleagues (137) established that 15% of patients who had terminal acute leukemia (AL) resistant to all standard therapies, could achieve long-term survival with BMT. These observations in poor risk patients prompted the investigators to consider using BMT earlier in the course of the disease.

Acute nonlymphocytic leukemia (ANLL)

The dismal prognosis for CT-treated patients with early acute non-lymphocytic leukemia (ANLL) – a median survival of one year (see (111)) – and the equally dismal outlook for patients transplanted in the late course of their disease

(137), prompted investigators to explore allogeneic BMT for early ANLL. The Seattle group (124, 141) reported that transplantation for ANLL in CR-1 increases the survival rate to approximately 60%, and is associated with a high early mortality but a dramatic reduction of the relapse rate to 15–21% (Table 2). These data demonstrated that some BMT-associated risks relate directly to the patient's physical condition and remission status at transplantation.

Encouraged by these results, several cancer centers initiated prospective randomized trials comparing the therapeutic efficacy of CT followed by allogeneic BMT and CT with the efficacy of CT alone for ANLL. While about 50% of adults were found to achieve long-term survival when transplanted in CR-1 (140, 141), it remains controversial whether this is a significant improvement over results with CT alone (22). Occasional late relapses have occurred in the transplant arm of these studies and has led to some to recommend BMT in early 1st relapse or 2nd remission in the older patient.

For children and young adults, the situation is more clear-cut. Data from four centers in the U.S. (31, 43, 78, 125) and the Royal Marsden Hospital in England (111, 112) have documented a two-year median survival rate as high as 77–80% for children transplanted in early stage ANLL (Table 2). A recent report from the Children's Cancer Study Group clearly shows a statistically significant advantage for BMT in a large group of patients (63).

At this point in time, it appears that BMT in CR-1 may prove to be the treatment of choice for children. The indicatiion is less clear in adults with ANLL.

Timing of BMT for optimal disease-free survival of patients with ANLL remains to be determined. The high morbidity and mortality during the early post-transplant period (47), particularly in the older patient, is a risk factor that requires careful reassessment within the context of this question.

Table 2. Results of allogeneic BMT for children with ANLL in first remission.

BMT center	Number of patients	Age	Complete remission	Disease-free survival	Relapse rate	Non-leukemic death rate
Memorial Sloan-Kettering Cancer Center (1)	13	1–19 years	78%	3 years	4%	17%
Fred Hutchinson Cancer Center (2)	38	0.8–17 years	66%	3.5 years	21%	15%
City of Hope (3)	10	0–19 years	80%	10 months	20%	0%
University of Minnesota (4)	17	6–28 years	77%	2 years	17%	17%
Royal Marsden Hospital, London (5)	9	8–20 years	77%	2 years	11%	11%

1. Dinsmore R, Kirkpatrick D, Flomenberg N, *et al.*: Allogeneic bone marrow transplantation for patients with acute non-lymphocytic leukemia. *Blood* 63:649, 1984
2. Sanders JE, Thomas ED, and the Seattle Marrow Transplant Group: Marrow transplantation for children with acute nonlymphoblastic leukemia in first remission: An update. *Blood* 66:460, 1985
3. Forman SF, Spruce WE, Farbstein MJ, *et al.*: Bone marrow ablation followed by allogeneic marrow grafting during first complete remission of acute nonlymphocytic leukemia. *Blood* 61:439, 1983
4. Kersey JH, Ramsay NKC, Kim T, *et al.*: Allogeneic bone marrow transplantation in acute nonlymphocytic leukemia: A pilot study. *Blood* 60:400, 1982
5. Powles RL, Morgenstern G, Clink HM, *et al.*: The place of bone marrow transplantation in acute myelogenous leukemia. *Lancet* 1:1047, 1980

The Memorial Sloan Kettering Cancer Center (MSKCC) transplant group found (31) that patients with ANLL who are transplanted in CR-2 are doing as well as patients with ANLL transplanted in first remission. In contrast, the Seattle Bone Marrow Transplant Group (135) has reported that patients transplanted in first relapse of ANLL are enjoying longer disease-free survival than those transplanted in CR-2. It is difficult to explain why patients transplanted in relapse should do better than patients transplanted in remission. Patients in early first relapse normally have had less exposure to CT than patients in CR-2, and may therefore have disease that has not yet become refractory to CT.

The increased risk for post-transplant complications such as veno-occlusive disease, congestive heart failure, and hepatic damage, must be taken into consideration when using agents such as anthracyclines and cytosine arabinoside to induce a second remission prior to BMT. This is a major consideration when contemplating BMT in CR-2.

In spite of recent progress in chemotherapeutic management of ANLL, more than 50% of these patients relapse with CT, whereas only 8–20% relapse after BMT (84). Consequently, BMT is being considered as an alternative therapy for ANLL in first relapse.

Acute lymphoblastic leukemia (ALL)

Until recently, BMT for acute lymphoblastic leukemia (ALL) in children in remisssion was considered highly controversial because of excellent response rate (90%) to CT (90). It soon became apparent that patients with ALL who relapsed while on CT have very poor prognosis, even if a second remission is attained, and that patients with ANLL transplanted in CR-1 have good prognosis. This finding raised interest in the use of BMT for ALL. While most investigators would not transplant ALL in CR-1, some have proposed transplanting CR-1 patients with Philadelphia chromosome-positive ALL (117).

In the early 1980s, two reports appeared in the literature, comparing therapeutic responses of children with ALL in CR-2 to allogeneic BMT and CT (Table 3). Johnson *et al.* (75) reported that 8 of 24 allogeneic marrow recipients but none of 32 CT-treated patients were surviving 3–6 years in unmaintained CR. Woods *et al.* (150) observed comparable responses: 43% of allografted but only 5% of CT-treated children remained free of disease at 36 months. These two studies demonstrated that BMT is indicated for ALL in CR-2.

Leukemic relapse remains the principal reason for failure of BMT in ALL. The Seattle Group (139, 142), who conditioned their patients with 120 mg/kg of cyclophosphamide followed by 10 Gy total body irradiation (TBI), reported a greater than 50% relapse rate during the first year for patients with ALL, regardless of whether they were transplanted in CR-2 or in subsequent remission. Moreover, they found no survival advantage for patients transplanted in CR-1. Others (151, 155), using similar pretransplant conditioning regimens, have observed a comparable relapse rate. Recently Butturini (20) reviewed the outcome of BMT in 871 patients with childhood ALL reported to the International Bone Marrow Transplant Registry. In these patients, the major reason for transplant failure was leukemic relapse, irrespective of whether patients were transplanted in CR-1, CR-2 or later remission.

In contrast, the MSKCC marrow transplant group (30), using an alternative approach to the standard pre-BMT RT/CT regimen, achieved dramatic reduction of the first year relapse rate and an increase in the projected disease-free survival of patients transplanted in early ALL. They conditioned a series of 52 patients with hyperfractionated TBI (13.2 GY given in 11 doses of 1.2 Gy over a 4-day period) followed by 120 mg/kg of cyclophosphamide. Twenty-two of the patients were transplanted in CR-2, and had a projected disease-free survival of 62%. Twenty-two of the patients were transplanted in CR-3, and had a projected disease-free survival of 26%. These data suggest that allogeneic BMT for ALL can be effective when done in early remission, but still has a poor outcome when done in late disease (CR-3) or relapse.

BMT for ALL in CR-1 is still very controversial, because of the high success rate of CT for patients at this early stage

Table 3. Comparison of allogeneic chemotherapy for children with ALL in CR-2.

Cancer center	Patients (no.)	Age (yrs)	CR (%)	BM* Relapse (%)	3-year Survival #	Follow-up (mos)	Patients (no.)	Age (yrs)	Chemotherapy** CR (%)	Relapse (%)	3-year survival (mos)	Follow-up (mos)
Fred Hutchinson Cancer Center (1)	24	4–16	60	60%	33%	36–72	21	4–16		100	0%	36
University of Minnesota (2)	15	4–22	58	58%	33%	36–72	23	4–22		95	5%	36

* Transplanted in CR-2 to CR-4
** Treated in CR-2
# Disease-free survival

1. Johnson FL, Thomas ED, Clark BS, *et al.*: A comparison of marrow transplantation to chemotherapy for children with acute lymphoblastic leukemia in second or subsequent remission. *New Engl J Med* 305:846, 1981
2. Woods WG, Nesbitt NE, Ramsay NKC, *et al.*: Intensive therapy followed by bone marrow transplantation for patients with acute lymphocytic leukemia in second or subsequent remission. Determination of prognostic factors (a report from the University of Minnesota bone marrow transplant team. *Blood* 6:1182, 1983

of disease, and because of the difficulty in selecting poor-risk patients. Three transplant groups have initiated BMT for ALL in CR-1, but the patient population is heterogeneous and the follow-up is quite short. The Seattle Group (134) reported 32% disease-free survival, with a median follow-up of 38 months. The European Group for BMT (155) reported 64% survival at 19 months' median follow-up. The City of Hope group (128) reported 60% survival after 30 months' follow-up. The disparity in these results may reflect either differences in patient characteristics (e.g., age, disease subtype, extramedullary relapse) or in pre-transplant therapies. It is much too early to draw conclusions as to the value of BMT for ALL patients in CR-1.

Autologous BMT for acute leukemias

Autologous BMT for AL is still considered by some to be experimental. One of the earliest trials of autologous BMT for ALL, using marrow purged MAb J-5 to delete CALLA-positive leukemic B cells, was done by the Boston Children's Hospital transplant group (9, 120). Eight of 24 patients transplanted in CR-2 or CR-3 remained in CR for a median period of 16+ months (range: 4–44 months). More recently, Burnett (19) reported survival rate of 50% or better among 12 adult patients with ANLL in CR-1 given untreated marrow autografts. This is an excellent response, when one considers the high early mortality among adults receiving allogeneic BMT. Long-term follow-up is needed to determine if these results will hold up.

CHRONIC LEUKEMIAS

Chronic myelogenous leukemia

Over the past 80 years, no major advances have been made in the treatment of chronic myelogenous leukemia (CML) with CT. Myleran, used since the 1950s because of its relatively selective myelodepressive effect, and hydroxyurea, the two standard drugs used in chronic phase CML, did not significantly prolong survival. Multidrug combinations can frequently induce remission, but these are usually short-lived. Recent trials of interferon in chronic phase CML suggest that this lymphokine may be useful in inducing a peripheral blood remission. However, interferon has no effect on the accelerated phase of the disease (84).

There have been promising case reports of plicamycin (mithramycin) inducing remissions in blast phase patients, but the follow-up is too short in the majority of patients (81).

Syngeneic (Twin) BMT
Between 1974 and 1982, the Seattle transplant team treated 34 patients with CML with syngeneic BMT. There was only one long-term survivor among the first group of eight patients, all of whom were transplanted in blast phase (BP) (see (38, 39)). In contrast, eight of 12 subsequent patients, who were transplanted in chronic phase (CP), survived for a median period of 30 months (range: 21–65 months) without cytogenetic evidence of disease (41). At the Hammersmith Hospital in London, two patients given twin marrow

for CML in accelerated phase (AP), have remained free of disease for over three years (50). These observations have led to the conclusion that prolonged arrest of CML progression can occur independently of GvHD-associated GvL activity.

Autologous BMT
Concurrently with attempts at treating CML with syngeneic BMT, the Seattle group (17, 18) and the Hammersmith Hospital group (49) explored the usefulness of myeloablative high-dose CT/RT followed by reinfusion of untreated autologous marrow collected in CP or blood collected in BP, respectively, for treating patients in BP. Another rationale for this approach was the extreme resistance of patients in BP to sublethal CT and RT. The majority of patients (47/57) showed rapid hematologic engraftment, but median duration of CR-1 was only 15 weeks (range: 2–152 weeks). Clearly, this approach offers little benefit for treating CML in blast crisis, possibly due to persistence of leukemic cells in the autologous marrow.

Intensive CT or splenic RT alone can induce transient suppression of Ph^1-positive hemopoiesis in a small number of patients. This observation suggests the usefulness of autologous marrow or blood harvested in CP for restoring Ph^1-negative (presumably non-leukemic) hemopoiesis in CML patients following intensive myeloblative CT. It remains to be determined whether this phenomenon reflects merely prolonged transitory reestablishment of normal hemopoietic cell population, or whether it reflects an actual antitumor activity of the engrafted autologous marrow.

Allogeneic BMT
A number of transplant groups have treated patients with CML with allogeneic BMT (21, 47, 87, 130). The 1985 report of the International Bone Marrow Transplant Registry (see (47)) projected a three-year disease-free survival rate of 63% for 199 patients transplanted in CP, 36% for 146 patients transplanted in AP, and 12% for 146 patients transplanted in BP. The risk of relapse within 3 years of BMT was projected at 11% for patients transplanted in CP, and 41% for those transplanted in AP or BP (47). Patients allografted early in first CP appear to have a better chance for 3-year survival (95%) than those allografted late in first CP (130). Results with patients transplanted in BP have been uniformly poor.

There is still considerable controversy as to whether splenectomy prior to BMT is necessary. In two studies (27, 48), it appeared that splenectomy did not improve the outcome. Subsequent studies have suggested that transfusion requirements and engraftment following BMT may be improved by prior splenectomy, but that the incidence of GvHD may be increased (10).

HAIRY CELL LEUKEMIA

Hairy cell leukemia (HCL) is a rare variant of chronic lymphocytic leukemia seen predominantly in older individuals. About one half of these patients respond to splenectomy, and require no further treatment until disease progresses. Those who fail splenectomy may respond to a limited number of modalities such as chlorambucil (53), androgens (88), or leukapheresis (152). The most promising investigational agents for inducing remissions in this disease appear to be alpha interferons (72, 114, 116), and pentostatin (2-deoxycoformycin) (132).

Syngeneic BMT, following conditioning with high-dose CT (cyclophosphamide, dimethyl myleran) and TBI, has been used successfully in a 47 year-old male patient who has remained free of evidence of disease for six years (23). This suggests that BMT might be a potentially curative therapeutic modality that should be explored further in patients who fail standard therapy.

SOLID TUMORS

More than one half of solid tumors of childhood are now curable by combination CT (83). Many adult tumors – including testicular carcinoma, teratomas, and breast cancer – are also responding well to currently used combination CT. However, certain tumors – such as neuroblastoma Stage IV, metastatic malginant melanoma, lymphomas (particularly B cell lymphomas), Ewing's sarcoma, rhabdomyosarcoma Stage IV, and metastatic retinoblastoma – remain a serious challenge to the oncologist. Despite excellent initial response to CT and RT, patients relapse rapidly. Many clinicians feel that some of these patients might be salvaged with extremely high doses of CT and RT. However, the myelotoxocity of most effective agents limits this approach.

BMT rescue has always been an attractive therapeutic option. Currently, several cancer centers are exploring this treatment modality as a means for permitting wider applicability of high-dose CT. Autologous BMT has the advantage of avoiding the high risk of fatal GvHD and greatly reducing the incidence of fatal viral infections that plague recipients of allogeneic BMT, and of circumventing the problem of finding a genetically matched parent marrow donor. Nevertheless, the usefulness of autologous BMT remains questionable for patients with malignant invasion of the marrow.

The chemotherapeutic agent that has been found most appropriate for pretransplant conditioning in patients with solid tumors is high-dose melphalan. Its principal toxicity is to the marrow. Unlike cyclophosphamide, melphalan has the advantage not being included in standard protocols for most solid tumors other than myeloma. Therefore, the majority of solid tumors are not likely to have developed resistance to melphalan.

In addition to melphalan, numerous new drug combinations are being evaluated in solid tumors. Of these, the combination of thioTEPA with cyclophosphamide is probably the most effective for conditioning preparatory to autologous BMT (147). ThioTEPA has had limited use in standard therapy of solid tumors because of its severe myelotoxicity. The advantage of using ThioTEPA for cytoreduction preparatory to BMT is that most patients have not received this drug, and that most refractory solid tumors are sensitive to combinations incorporating this drug. The list of tumours responding to thioTEPA is impressively long: It includes breast cancer, small cell lung cancer, and colon cancer.

In the light of these findings, many investigators are now re-evaluating old therapeutic agents, withdrawn from the clinic because of unacceptable myelotoxicity, for potential use for cytoreduction prior to BMT.

A variety of chemical, immunologic, and physical methods have been explored to purge the marrow of tumor cells *in vitro* prior to autologous BMT (Fig. 1). This offers an exciting therapeutic potential: It is possible to treat marrow *in vitro*, without significantly affecting its hemopoietic repopulation *in vivo*. It has been reported that autologous BMT accelerates the rate of recovery from CT-induced myelosuppression (2, 54, 86). However, in some patients hemopoietic recovery following transplantation of stored autologous marrow has been exceedingly slow and incomplete, irrespective of whether the marrow has been 'purged' or left untreated prior to cryopreservation (35, 116). Thus, this problem is probably a consequence of the cryopreservation methodology. Recent improvements in cryopreservation (see (69)) may help resolve this problem.

Marrow 'purging' techniques

Chemical 'purging'
Two cyclophosphamide metabolites – 4-hydroperoxycyclophosphamide (4-HC) and mephosphamide (ASTA-Z) – and a derivative podophylline – etoposide (VP-16) – are being looked at in both the laboratory and the clinic. ASTA-Z has the advantage of being much more stable in its crystalline form than 4-HC, but the disadvantage of only preventing cells from entering DNA synthesis, rather than killing them as 4-HC does.

At dose levels used *in vitro* in most clinical laboratories to 'purge' marrow preparatory to autologous BMT, 4-HC (100 μg/ml) and ASTA-Z (80 μg/ml) inhibit growth of leukemia cells as well as growth of 90–95% of morphologically recognizable precursor cells (32, 123, 129), while VP-16 (20 μg/ml) has the advantage of sparing about 40% of normal myeloid precursor cells while killing the majority of leukemic cells (121). However, since patients given marrow purged with 4-HC and ASTA-Z have good hemopoietic regeneration, in spite of the absence of morphologically identifiable myeloid precursors, and since more clinical data is available on engraftment with 4-HC and ASTA-Z-purged marrow than on engraftment of VP-16-purged marrow (56, 76, 129), most investigators continue to use 4-HC and ASTA-Z in clinical trials.

Immunologic 'purging'
In ongoing clinical trials, tumor-specific heterologous antibodies of monoclonal antibodies (MAb) are being used *in vitro* to 'purge' residual malignant cells from marrow prior to autologous BMT. Most investigators are using complement to destroy antibody-coated tumor cells (see (8, 95, 96, 115)). Others are exploring the usefulness of immunotoxins, i.e., MAbs conjugated with ricin chain-A. The advantage of this approach is that, after the antibody moiety binds to specific receptors on the tumor cell surface, the immunotoxin complex is internalized into the cytoplasm where the toxin inhibits protein synthesis. Several ricin-conjugated anti-T cell MAbs have been used to 'purge' malignant T cells from marrow prior to autologous BMT (56, 74), or to prevent GvHD by 'purging' normal T cells from normal donor marrow prior to allogeneic BMT (15, 144).

The advantage of immunologic 'purging' of marrow is that this method is tumor cell-specific and far less toxic to normal hemopoietic and lymphoid progenitor cells *in vitro* than currently used chemical 'purging' agents. The disadvantage is that unbound substances such as ricin or cross-reactive antibodies could potentially be toxic to the patient, unless the treated marrow is washed adequately prior to infusion. Furthermore, in the clinical setting, immunologic 'purging' has not been found to be superior to chemical 'purging' with regard to the rate of hemopoietic recovery following autologous BMT (9).

The increasing availability of MAbs against a wide variety of human leukemias and solid tumors, and the unique tumor specificity of such MAbs, appears to offer an unique tool for selectively ablating residual tumor cells during remission. Serotherapy with MAbs has been attempted in a limited number of patients resistant to standard therapies, and has been reported to be effective primarily for clearing circulating tumor cells. Using anti-idioptypic MAbs, Miller and colleagues (92, 93) have induced regression of malignant infiltrates of skin and lymph nodes of some patients with B cell or T cell NHL. One case achieved prolonged CR. However, such responses to MAbs are the exception rather than the rule. For this reason, the most widespread application of MAbs has been for ablating of residual tumor cells from marrow *in vitro*.

Marrow 'purging' with MAbs has proved disappointing, because its effectiveness is limited by cross-reactivity of some MAbs with normal cells, ineffective complement-mediated lysis of MAb-coated cells, and factors such as antigenic modulation of malignant cells. For example (see (119)), the J5 MAb is reactive with ALL cells and lymphoma cells from most patients with CALLA-positive lymphoblasts but is, unfortunately, cross-reactive with differentiated granulocytes, renal glomerular cells, and renal proximal tubule epithelium. Other MAbs such as Leu I and T101 react with both normal and malignant cells of the T lineage. Their usefulness for ablating residual leukemic T cells from remission marrow of patients with T-cell ALL is under clinical investigation.

Physical 'purging' methods are also being explored. In 1981, Helson and Reisner (pers. comm.) found that soybean hemagglutinin (SBA) binds neuroblastoma cells *in vitro* permitting physical separation from hemapoietic cells. SBA *in vitro* treatment also removes a number of normal cell populations from the marrow, leaving a cell concentrate greatly enriched for hemopoietic progenitor cells, lymphoid progenitor cells, and natural killer cells. However, the usefulness of 'purging' with SBA is limited by the fact that it only reduces the tumor load of marrow or blood by one log.

Attempts to 'purge' marrow using MAb-coated magnetic microspherules are under laboratory investigation. Although this technique appears attractive in principle, its eventual clinical applicability is questionable, since it only reduces the tumor load by about 2 logs '*in vitro*' (77).

Clinical outcome of autologous BMT

The early mortality during the first month following autologous BMT reported in most published studies varies from 6–15%, and is due primarily to complications of CT conditioning prior to BMT. It is noteworthy that while as many as 95% of recipients of autologous marrow develop infections, particularly viral infections (herpes zoster, cytomegalovirus, EBV), only a small number of these infections prove fatal (10, 57).

Most investigators are agreed that the primary value of autologous BMT is repopulation of the hemopoietic system following myeloablation. This permits the use of extremely high and potentially curative doses of certain CT agents, and extends the therapeutic range of other agents that could not previously be used because of dose-limiting myelotoxicity. Autografted patients may additionally benefit from the presence of traces of DMSO in the marrow inoculum (24). DMSO is used as a cryopreservative, and is diluted but not washed out of the thawed marrow before transplantation. Since DMSO is a differentiating agent, it may promote residual tumor cells into marrow inoculum and thus render them less malignant.

HEMATOLOGIC TUMORS

Hodgkin's disease

Hodgkin's disease (HD) is one of the tumors most sensitive to RT and CT. About 68% of patients with Stage III B and IV B HD treated with combination CT/RT remain disease-free beyond 10 years (29). Of those who relapse, about 50% can still respond to CT and achieve long-term survival.

A small number of HD patients who relapse repeatedly on CT have poor prognosis, and are candidates for BMT. Goldstone (52) reviewed the experience of nine European centers, and described the response of 29 patients autotransplanted for HD in relapse. These patients had failed initial CT/RT as well as multiple salvage regimens. There was a 57% rate of CR but, unfortunately, a 21% rate of cytoreduction-related death. The duration of disease-free survival and rate of relapse were not given.

Fay *et al.* (37) achieved CR in 9 of 14 patients given autologous BMT for HD in relapse. The median follow-up was not stated.

The M.D. Anderson Hospital marrow transplant group (73) autografted 16 poor-risk patients for refractory or relapsed HD. Twelve patients had progressed on salvage CT; four had relapsed after completing salvage CT. One half of the patients had extranodal disease in sites including lung, bone, pleura, kidney, liver, and thyroid. The majority (60%) also had constitutional 'B' symptoms. Six of the 16 patients achieved CR. Three remained in continuous remission for a median period of 15 months, two died in CR of interstitial pneumonia, and two relapsed.

In order to assess the value of autologous BMT in HD, one must evaluate the initial stage of the patients at presentation, and the extent of disease at relapse. At present, these data are not readily evaluable, except in the study of Jagannath *et al.* (73). The chronically relapsing HD patient who has been heavily treated appears to relapse just as readily after BMT as after CT.

Non-Hodgkin's lymphomas

Non-Hodgkin's lymphomas (NHL) are a heterogeneous group of diseases with different clinical courses.

Low-grade forms of NHL run a very indolent course. The median survival for this type of patient is 11 years, even when CT is delayed (70, 110, 122). Although the majority of patients run an indolent course, a few develop disease progression to a high grade malignancy.

Patients with intermediate-grade or high-grade NHL such as diffuse histiocytic lymphoma and Burkitt's lymphoma have aggressive disease, with a relapse rate in excess of 50% with standard therapies (83, 109, 154). Relapsing patients are candidates for BMT in CR-2.

Since many of these patients will not achieve a CR-2, several ongoing studies are designed to harvest the autologous marrow in CR-1. The patient is then offered the option of undergoing autologous BMT in CR-1, as part of the consolidation phase of treatment, or receiving the autograft in CR-2 (56, 60, 104).

Gorin's preliminary data on 12 patients with poor prognosis nodular lymphoma showed a 75% response rate, based on median follow-up of 27 months (56). This high response rate is not surprising, since nodular lymphoma usually has a better prognosis than diffuse histiocytic lymphoma.

Fay *et al.* (37) reported that of 51 patients with poor-prognosis NHL, 25 of whom had relapsed diffuse histiocytic lymphoma, 13 (51%) achieved CR with autologous BMT. Although the follow-up was very short (2–49 months), and the data thus still preliminary, duration of response already appears to be longer than on standard CT.

Of 81 patients with NHL who received marrow autografts at nine European cancer centers, 73% achieved CR (52). BMT-related mortality was as low as 6%. Unfortunately, 35% of the complete responders relapsed. The best outcome – 68% survival – was reported to have occurred in those patients who received their autografts while in CR. This survey is difficult to evaluate, since the classification of the NHLs and the duration of follow-up was not stated.

African Burkitt's lymphoma responds well to combination CT. However, the subtype of Burkitt's lymphoma seen in American and European patients is very poorly amenable to standard CT/RT, is the most rapidly progressive solid tumor in man, and has a relapse rate as high as 80% (153). Despite significant advances in CT for this disease (154), most clinicians tend to consider this the most troublesome of the NHLs.

Patients with relapsed Burkitt's lymphoma, who have been treated extensively with CT or CT/RT, have an extremely poor prognosis with a survival expectancy of only a few months. Treatment failure is due primarily to incomplete ablation of the malignant clone, and development of resistance to CT. It is noteworthy that even relapsed Burkitt's lymphoma frequently is very sensitive to high-dose cyclophosphamide (97). Possibly, autologous BMT will permit the use of this drug at a dose high enough to overcome apparent resistance.

O'Leary *et al.* (98) reported that three of six patients allografted for relapsed Burkitt's lymphoma have remained in continuous unmaintained CR for over 1-1/2, 2, and 6 years, respectively. Similarly, Philip *et al.* (104, 105), reviewing results of 37 patients given autologous BMT for relapsed Burkitt's lymphoma at various centers, reported that 25 patients achieved CR, and that 10 responders have remained in unmaintained remission for up to 5 years or longer.

The follow-up period of allogeneic BMT for NHL is sufficiently long to indicate that its use in CR-2 may prove to be superior to that of standard CT (1, 98). Autologous

BMT for NHL is still investigational, but the morality of these procedure is sufficiently low to justify using marrow harvested in CR-1 for autografting in CR-2. The potential benefit of both allogeneic and autologous BMT is high enough to warrant referral for transplantation for NHL in CR-2.

Multiple myeloma

Limited success has been achieved in a small number of patients treated for far advanced multiple myeloma with chemoradiotherapy followed syngeneic (40, 99), or autologous (101) BMT rescue. Although all patients engrafted and appeared to be free of disease, as judged by disappearance of myeloma proteins and detectable myeloma cells for 1–2 years, most eventually relapsed.

The unsatisfactory results achieved so far with BMT, and the advanced age of most myeloma patients under consideration for BMT, makes it difficult to recommend this treatment modality for multiple myeloma.

AUTOLOGOUS BMT FOR NON-HEMATOLOGIC TUMORS

Autologous BMT for non-hematologic tumors is still experimental. Limited success has been achieved with this modality in children with neuroblastoma or Ewing's sarcoma, and in adults with malignant melanoma and small cell carcinoma of the lung. It has also been tried in several other tumors.

Childhood tumors

Neuroblastoma
The clinical outcome of neuroblastoma is linked to the patient's age and disease stage at diagnosis. Neuroblastoma diagnosed in infants younger than one year has a basically benign course. Older children with early (Stages I and II) disease have excellent prognosis with CT, more than 50% surviving over five years after multimodal therapy (83).

Unfortunately, more than one half of the patients present with advanced disease. While many will achieve complete remission on conventional chemotherapy, only about 10% will remain free of disease for two years. The other 90% will relapse repeatedly and have a life expectancy of less than eight months (83).

Over the past seven years, BMT has been used successfully in small numbers of patients with Stage IV neuroblastoma (4, 5, 6, 34, 57, 60, 67, 68). Some groups have explored supralethal high-dose CT, with or without TBI, followed by rescue with BMT (primarily, autologous) for treating over 80 of these high-risk patients. It is of special interest that advanced disseminated neuroblastoma is sensitive to high-dose melphalan, since the disease is notoriously resistant to conventional therapies.

A variety of methods have been explored for 'purging' the marrow of neuroblastoma cells. Most groups have been using the cyclophosphamide analogs 4-HC or ASTA-Z which, unlike their parent compound, do not require oxidation by hepatic microsomal enzymes to the active alkylating species.

Recently, good results have been reported, using autologous marrow 'purged' with agents that have high affinity for neuroblastoma cells, such as hydroxydopamine/ascorbic acid, SBA, or MAbs conjugated with magnetic microspheres (61, 67, 143). Hydroxydopamine/ascorbic acid reduces the tumor cell load by 2–3 logs *in vitro* (61). SBA can only affect a one log neuroblastoma cell reduction; but it also concentrates the marrow, allowing for more effective subsequent ablation of the remaining tumor cells with monoclonal antibodies (6).

Most groups have achieved sustained disease-free periods with an average duration of about two years in more than 30% of their patients (see (6, 57, 61)), whereas one group (68) reported a mean duration of CR of only 6 months in 10 similarly-treated patients.

The best results with autologous BMT for advanced stage neuroblastoma were reported in two French groups (65, 104). Of 15 patients treated by Hartmann *et al.* (67), 7 who were transplanted in PE failed to respond, whereas 5/8 (63%) patients transplanted in CR responded and are still in CR at 29–54 months. Phillip (1985) (104) transplanted 56 consecutive patients (14 in CR, 40 in PR), using melphalan/vincristine/TBJ as the preparative regimen, and achieved an overall disease-free survival of 39% after a median follow-up period of 24 months post-BMT (up to 32 months post-diagnosis). These results are impressive, in the light of an expected survival time of less than 10% for patients treated with standard chemotherapy. A more recent protocol using high dose chemotherapy and no RT reported a 50% survival rate (11). If comparable results can be achieved in larger patient series, the high-dose CT/RT approach might be considered for children with advanced neuroblastoma in CR-1.

Ewing's sarcoma

Children with early stage Ewing's sarcoma have an excellent prognosis for 5-year survival with multimodal CT/RT therapy (83). Patients with advanced disease at diagnosis also respond readily to CT, but tend to relapse just as readily. Bone marrow involvement is rare.

High-dose melphalan or cyclophosphamide/TBI followed by autologous BMT has been reported to achieve CR in over one half of the children with relapsed or therapy-resistant Ewing's sarcoma (25, 33, 58, 68). However, duration of response in the majority of the patients has been disappointingly brief – only 2–6 months. The best results were those of Cornbleet *et al.* (25) and Graham-Pole *et al.* (58), who achieved CR lasting 12–13 months in two children.

Other childhood tumors

Children early Wilms' tumor, retinoblastoma, and rhabdomyosarcoma can be cured with combination surgery/CT/RT (83). For Wilms tumor with favorable histology, even stage IV disease responds to standard therapeutic modalities. Autologous BMT has been tried in a small number of children with poor prognosis Wilms' tumor, retinoblastoma, and rhabdomyosarcoma, but results to date have not been encouraging (16, 34, 68).

ADULT TUMORS

Malignant melanoma

There are no adequate therapies for managing metastatic malignant melanoma. Metastatic disease is not amenable to either surgery or RT, but frequently responds to chemotherapeutic agents such as BCNU, DTIC, or melphalan. However, responses tend to be brief, and the outcome is generally fatal within 6–7 months. Autologous BMT is under investigation as a possible salvage modality for these patients.

To date, approximately 100 patients with Stage IV metastatic malignant melanoma have been treated at various centers with intensive CT (BCNU, melphalan) followed by rescue with autologous BMT harvested during remission of metastatic disease (see (68)). Although the overall initial complete and partial response rate has been good (45% and 73%, respectively), disease recurred within 10–16 weeks. Among 48 patients treated with a combination of BCNU and melphalan, followed by autologous BMT, 63% had objective response, but only 10% had a disease-free survival of one year or more (36, 68, 79).

Small cell carcinoma of the lung

Small cell lung carcinoma (SCLC, oat cell carcinoma) accounts for approximately 25% of the new cases of lung cancer in the US each year. Localized disease will metastasize rapidly to the liver and brain. Metastases are often present at diagnosis. Left untreated, SCLC is fatal within three months (94). SCLC differs from the other types of lung cancer in that up to 90% of the cases will respond initially to CT, but that the responses are generally brief. Median survival with optimal current CT is 10 months. Only 4–16% of CT-treated patients achieve long-term survival (94).

The exquisite sensitivity of these tumors to chemotherapy, and their propensity to spread, has resulted in the selection of patients with SCLC for autologous BMT.

Harper *et al.* (62) reviewed the results of intensive CT with autologous BMT rescue in 77 untreated patients from four centers and 61 relapsed patients from five other centers. Thirty-eight of the 77 newly diagnosed patients (49%) achieved CR, whereas only six of the 61 relapsed patients (10%) had confirmed CR. The duration of unmaintained remission was short (median: 9 months). Follow-up, even in the best studies, was also short (42–74 weeks). Only one center, M.D. Anderson Hospital, reported a high response rate (69%) for newly diagnosed patients, but disease-free survival was highly variable (8–47 months) (133).

Other investigators (71, 135) used late CT intensification followed by autologous BMT rescue, but found that it conferred no clinical benefit.

These results are not encouraging. Autologous BMT does prolong life, but at the present time does not appear to offer any advantage for the management of SCLC. Studies with other CT combinations may prove to be more promising, since these tumors do show transitory responses to many CT agents.

Breast cancer

There is considerable controversy regarding the optimal approach to management of metastatic breast cancer. Median survival from time of diagnosis with metastatic breast cancer is 18 months. While a number of alkylating agents produce responses in this disease, adequate dose escalation is prevented by myelotoxicity, and no cures can be achieved. This has led to a limited number of clinical trials using autologous BMT rescue to permit administration of more intensive CT.

In Phase I trials, only 11 of 58 patients (19%) at 11 centers achieved CR with high-dose CT followed by autologous BMT (see (103)). Duration of follow-up to date has been inadequate to determine effects on survival.

In another study, 16 heavily pretreated patients with metastatic breast cancer were given late intensification therapy with high-dose mitomycin-C followed by autologous BMT rescue (136), but achieved only brief partial remissions.

In a recent phase I trials with thioTEPA followed by autologous BMT show impressive albeit brief partial remissions in about 72% of patients with advanced breast cancer (147).

At present, no single agent therapy is satisfactory. Further studies are needed to identify the most effective CT combinations.

Other adult solid tumors

Autologous BMT has been attempted for a variety of other CT-resistant solid tumors in adults (see (68, 107)). Responses have been primarily partial and of short duration. Hence, the high response rates listed in the table do not reflect disease-free survival.

In one recent study of 18 patients with high-grade gliomas (predominantly brain stem tumors) treatment with high-dose carmustine conditioning followed by autologous BMT resulted in a median survival of 17.5 months from diagnosis, and a projected 22% survival rate of more than 27 months (149). This is a striking improvement of the median survival time of 3 months seen in conventionally treated patients.

PERSPECTIVES

Current results support the use of BMT for hematologic malignancies. The selection of the appropriate patients for BMT remains an area that is highly controversial.

In the younger patient, allogeneic BMT has been accepted

Table 4. Responses of some solid tumors to intensive chemotherapy with autologous BMT rescue.

| Tumor | Pre-BMT Chemo-therapy | Number of patients | Response | | | | Source |
			CR	PR	Rate	Duration (mos)	
Ovarian cancer	Melphalan	7	1	3	57%	3–18+	(1)
Germ cell cancer	Melphalan	6	1	3	67%	2–21+	(1)
Gastrointestinal cancer	BCNU	9	1	1	22%	5–24	(1)
Colon cancer	Melphalan	7	1	3	57%	2–3	(1)
Sarcoma	BCNU or melphalan	11	1	3	36%	1–9	(1)
Testicular cancer	Multiple	15	2	7	60%	0.7–28	(2)
Teratocarinoma	VP-16 and/or HDM-200	3	0	0	0%	–	(3)
Glioblastoma/ astrocytoma	BCNU and/or VP-16	47	23		49%	1–71+	(4)

1. Herzig RH, Phillips GL, Lazarus HM, *et al.*: Intensive chemotherapy and autologous bone marrow transplantation for the treatment of refractory malignancies. *Proc 1st Internatl Symp on Autologous Bone Marrow Transplantation*, pp. 197–202. Edited by KA Dicke, G Spitzer, AR Zander. UT MD Anderson Hospital and Tumor Institute, Houston, Texas, 1985.
2. Biron P, Philip T, Maraninchi D, *et al.*: Massive chemotherapy and autologous bone marrow transplantation in progressive disease of nonseminomatous testicular cancer. *Proc 1st Internatl Symp on Autologous Bone Marrow Transplantation*, pp. 203–210. Edited by KA Dicke, G Spitzer, AR Zander. UT MD Anderson Hospital and Tumor Institute, Houston, Texas, 1985.
3. Kolb HJ, Ledderose G, Hartenstein R, *et al.*: Autologous bone marrow transplantation in patients with advanced teratocarcinoma *Proc 1st Internatl Symp on Autologous Bone Marrow Transplantation*, pp. 211–217. Edited by KA Dicke, G Spitzer, AR Zander. UT MD Anderson Hospital and Tumor Institute, Houston, Texas, 1985.
4. Wolf NS, Phillips GL, Fay JW, *et al.*: High-dose chemotherapy with autologous bone marrow transplantation for primary tumors of the central nervous system: Phase II and II studies of the Southeastern Cancer Study Group. *Proc 1st Internatl Symp on Autologous Bone Marrow Transplantation*, pp. 255–259. Edited by KA Dicke, G Spitzer, AR Zander. UT MD Anderson Hospital and Tumor Institute, Houston, Texas, 1985.

as a reasonable therapy for ANLL in CR-1 and CR-2, and is now being established as the treatment of choice for ALL in CR-2, and NHL in CR-2.

In the older patient, the indication for allogeneic BMT is not as clear-cut. Early mortality associated with GvHD and interstitial pneumonia dampen the enthusiasm for this approach. The elimination of the problem of GvHD, and the marked reduction of interstitial pneumonia during the early post-transplant period, make autologous BMT attractive for the older patient. However, increased risk of relapse with autologous BMT is the price paid for reduction of mortality during the early post-transplanted period.

For tumors other than NHL, autologous BMT is being explored as a means of permitting delivery of very high doses of CT. The finding of appropriate chemotherapeutic agents and dosage schedules is the task of future studies. Until these regimens have been found, indications for high dose CT followe by autologous BMT remain unresolved. While reports of 'good' responses are numerous, few of the responses are complete, and duration of response is generally brief. Partial responders have residual disease, even after intensive CT/RT and, despite BMT rescue for myelotoxicity, are ultimately destined to die from their disease. Consequently, long-term disease-free survival remains elusive.

REFERENCES

1. Appelbaum FR, Deiseroth AB, Graw RG, et al.: Prolonged complete remission following high dose chemotherapy of Burkitt's lymphoma in relapse. *Cancer* 41:1059, 1978
2. Appelbaum FR, Herzig G, Graw RG, et al.: Accelerated hemopoietic recovery following the infusion of cyropreserved autologous bone marrow in human. *Exp Hematol* 7 (Suppl 5):297, 1979
3. Appelbaum FR, Dahlberg S, Thomas ED, et al.: Bone marrow transplantation or chemotherapy after remission induction for adults with acute nonlymphoblastic leukemia. A prospective comparison. *Ann Int Med* 101:581, 1984
4. August C, Elkins W, Evans A, et al.: Metastatic neuroblastoma (M/NBL) managed by supralethal therapy and bone marrow reconstitution (BMRC). Results of a four-institution Children's Cancer Study Group pilot study. *Proc 3rd Conf Adv Neuroblastoma Res* May, 1984 (abstr)
5. August C, Serota FT, Koch PA, et al.: Treatment of advanced neuroblastoma with supralethal chemotherapy, radiation and allogeneic or autologous marrow reconstitution. *J Clin Oncol* 2:609, 1984 (abstr)
6. August CS, Elkins WL, Burkey E, et al.: Treatment of advanced metastatic neuroblastoma with supralethal chemotherapy. In: *Autologous Bone Marrow Transplantation*, pp. 167–171. Edited by KA Dicke, G Spitzer, AR Zander. UT MD Anderson Hospital and Tumor Institute at Houston, 1985
7. Barnes DWA, Corp MJ, Loutit JE, Neal FE: Treatment of murine leukemia with x-rays and homologous bone marrow. *BR Med J*, 626, 1956
8. Bast RC Jr, Di Fabritiis P, Maver C, et al.: Application of monoclonal antibodies to autologous bone marrow transplantation. *13th Int Congr Chemother*, Vienna. SS76, 1983
9. Bast RC Jr, Sallan SE, Reynolds C, et al.: Autologous bone marrow transplantation for CALLA-positive acute lymphoblastic leukemia: An update. In: *Autologous Bone Marrow Transplantation*, pp. 3–6. Edited by KA Dicke, G Spitzer, AR Zander. UT MD Anderson Hospital and Tumor Institute at Houston, 1985
10. Baugham ASJ, Worsley AM, McCarthy DM, et al.: Hematological reconstitution and severity of graft versus host disease after bone marrow transplant for chronic granulocytic leukemia: The influence of previous splenectomy. *Brit J Haematol* 56:445, 1984
11. Bernard JL, Philip T, Zucker JM, et al.: 91 successive BMT in advanced neuroblastoma. *ASCO/AACR 24th Ann Meetg Prog*, 1988
12. Biron P, Philip T, Maraninchi D, et al.: Massic chemotherapy and autologous bone marrow transplantation to progressive disease of nonseminomatous testicular cancer. In: *Proc 1st Conf on Autologous Bone Marrow Transplantation*, pp. 203–210. Edited by KA Dicke, G Spitzer, AR Zander. UT MD Anderson Hospital and Tumor Institute at Houston, 1985
13. Blume K, Beutler E, Bross KJ, et al.: Bone marrow ablation and allogeneic marrow transplantation in acute leukemia. *New Engl J Med* 302:1041, 1980
14. Bortin MM, Truit RL, Rimm A: Graft versus leukemia reactivity induced by alloimmunization without augmentation of graft versus host reactivity. *Nature* 281:490, 1979
15. Brenner MK, Grob JP, Prentice HG: The use of monoclonal antibodies in graft versus host disease prevention. *Haematologia (Budap)* 19(3):167, 1986
16. Brun del Re G, Baumgartner C, Bleher EA, et al.: Autologous bone marrow transplantation in the treatment of advanced malignant tumors in children and adolescents. *Folia Haematol (Leipzig)* 111:243, 1984
17. Buckner CD, Clift RA, Fefer A, et al.: Treatment of blastic transformation of chronic granulocytic leukemia by high dose cyclophosphamide, total body irradiation and infusion of cryopreserved autologous marrow. *Exp Hematol* 2:138, 1974
18. Buckner JC, Stewart P, Clift RA, et al.: Treatment of blastic transformation of chronic granulocytic leukemia by chemotherapy, total body irradiation, and infusion of cryopreserved autologous marrow. *Exp Hematol* 6:96, 1978
19. Burnett AK: Prolonged survival in patients with acute myeloid leukemia in first remission following autologous bone marrow transplantation. In: *Proc 1st Conf on Autologous Bone Marrow Transplantation*, pp. 7–10. Edited by KA Dicke, G Spitzer, AR Zander. UT MD Anderson Hospital and Tumor Institute, Houston, Texas, 1985
20. Butturini A, Rivera GK, Bortin JJ, Gale RP: Which treatment for childhood acute lymphoblastic leukaemia in second remission? *Lancet* Feb 21; 1(8530):429, 1987
21. Champlin R, Ho W, Arenson E, et al.: Allogeneic bone marrow transplantation for chronic myelogenous leukemia in chronic or accelerated phase. *Blood* 60:1038, 1982
22. Champlin RE, Ho WG, Gale RP, et al.: Treatment of acute myelogenous leukemia. A prospective controlled trial of bone marrow transplantation versus consolidation chemotherapy. *Ann Intern Med* 102:285, 1985
23. Cheever MA, Fefer A, Greenberg PD, et al.: Treatment of hairy cell leukemia with chemoradiotherapy and identical twin bone marrow transplantation. *New Engl J Med* 307:479, 1982
24. Collins SJ, Ruscetti FK, Gallagher RE, et al.: Terminal differentiation of promyelocytic leukemic cell induced by diemthyl-sulfoxide and other polar compounds. *Proc Natl Acad Sci USA* 75:2458, 1978
25. Cornbleet MA, Corringham REJ, Prentice HG, et al.: Treatment of Ewing's sarcoma with high-dose melphalan and autologous bone marrow transplantation. *Cancer Treat Rep* 65:241, 1981
26. Cunningham I, Gee T, Dowling M, et al.: Results of treatment of Ph + chronic myelogenous leukemia with an intensive treatment regimen (L-5 protocol). *Blood* 53:375, 1979

27. Deeg HJ, Prentice R, Fritz TE, et al.: Increased incidence of malignant tumors in dogs after total body irradiation and marrow transplantation. *Int J Radiat Oncol Biol Phys* 9:1505, 1983

28. Deeg HJ, Sanders J, Martin P, et al.: Secondary malignancies after marrow transplantation. *Exp Hematol* 12:660, 1984

29. DeVita V, Canellos G, Hubbard S, et al.: Chemotherapy of Hodgkin's disease (HD) with MOPP: A 10 year progress report. *Proc Am Soc Clin Oncol* 17:269, 1976 (abstr)

30. Dinsmore R, Kirkpatrick D, Flomenberg N, et al.: Allogeneic bone marrow transplantation for patients with acute lymphoblastic leukemia. *Blood* 62:381, 1983

31. Dinsmore R, Kirkpatrick D, Flomenberg N, et al.: Allogeneic bone marrow transplantation for patients with acute non-lymphocytic leukemia. *Blood* 63:649, 1984

32. Douay FK, Gorin NC, Najman A, et al.: Continuous bone marrow culture: Sensitivity to chemotherapeutic agents of probable pluripotential stem cells. Application to autologous bone marrow transplantation. *Exp Hematol* 11 (Suppl 14):7, 1983 (abstr)

33. Douer D, Champlin RE, Ho WG, et al.: High dose combination therapy and autologous bone marrow transplantation in resistant cancer. *Am J Med* 71:973, 1981

34. Ekert H, Ellis WM, Waters KD, et al.: Autologous bone marrow rescue in the treatment of advanced tumors of childhood. *Cancer* 49:603, 1982

35. Fabian I, Douer D, Wells JR, et al.: Cryopreservation of the human stem cell. *Exp Hematol* 10:119, 1982

36. Fay JW, Levine NM, Phillips GL, et al.: Treatment of metastatic melanoma with intensive 1,3-BIS(2-chloroethyl)-1-nitrosourea (BCNU) and autologous marrow transplantation (AMX). *Proc Am Assoc Cancer Res* 22:532, 1981 (abstr)

37. Fay JW, Phillips GL, Herzig GP, et al.: Treatment of refractory malignant lymphoma with intensive chemoradiotherapy and autologous marrow transplantation. *Exp Hematol* 11(5):406, 1985 (abstr)

38. Fefer A, Cheever MA, Thomas ED, et al.: Disappearance of Ph'-positive cells in four patients with chronic granulocytic leukemia after chemotherapy, irradiation and marrow transplantation form an identical twin. *New Engl J Med* 300:333, 1974

39. Fefer A, Cheever MA, Greenberg PD, et al.: Treatment of chronic granulocytic leukemia with chemoradiotherapy and transplantation of marrow from identical twins. *New Engl J Med* 306:63, 1982

40. Fefer A, Greenberg PD, Cheever MA, et al.: Treatment of multiple myeloma (MM) with chemoradiotherapy and identical twin bone marrow transplantation (BMT). *Proc Am Sco Clin Oncol* 1:C-731, 1982 (abstr)

41. Fefer A, Cheever MA, Greenberg PD, et al.: Bone marrow transplantation (BMT) for acute leukemia in patients with identical twins: improved results with BMT in complete remission (CR). *Proc Annu Meet Am Soc Clin Oncol* 2:C-708, 1983 (abstr)

42. Filipovich AH: Progress in broadening the uses of marrow transplantation: donor availability. *Vox Sang* 51 Suppl 2:95, 1986

43. Forman SF, Spruce WF, Farbstein MJ, et al.: Bone marrow ablation followed by allogeneic marrow grafting during first complete remission of acute nonlymphocytic leukemia. *Blood* 61:439, 1983

44. Gale RP, Kay Humphrey, Rimm A, Bortin M: Bone marrow transplantation for Acute Leukemia in first remission. *Lancet* 8:10, 1982

45. Gale RP, Champlin RE: How does bone marrow transplantation cure leukemia? *Lancet* 7:28, 1984

46. Gee AP, Graham-Pole J, Boyle MDP: Purging bone marrow for autologous transplantation – Are methods for monitoring the elimination of tumor cells reliable? *Exp Hematol* 11 (Suppl 14):7, 1983 (abstr)

47. Goldman JM, for the Advisory Committee of the International Bone Marrow Transplant Registry. *Blood* 66 (Suppl 1):251a, 1985 (abstr)

48. Goldman JM, Baugham A: Application of bone marrow transplantation in chronic granulocytic leukemia. *Clin Hematol* 12:739, 1983

49. Goldman JM, Catovsky D, Galton DAG: Reversal of blast-cell crisis in CGL by transfusion of stored autologous buffy-cold cells. *Lancet* 1:437, 1978

50. Goldman JM, Johnson SA, Catovsky D, et al.: Identical twin marrow transplantation for patients with leukemia and lymphoma. *Transplantation* 31:140, 1981

51. Goldman JM, Catovsky D, Goolden AWG, et al.: Buffy coat autografts for patients with chronic granulocytic leukaemia in transformation. *Blut* 42:149, 1982

52. Goldstone AH: Autologous bone marrow transplantation for non-Hodgkin's lymphoma: The preliminary European experience. In: *Proc 1st Internatl Symp on Autologous Bone Marrow Transplantation*, pp. 67–74. Edited by KA Dicke, G Spitzer, AR Zander. UT MD Anderson Hospital and Tumor Institute, Houston, Texas, 1985

53. Golomb HM, Schmidt K, Iman JW: Chlorambucil therapy of twenty-four post-splenectomy patients with progressive hairy cell leukemia. *Sem Oncol* 11:502, 1984

54. Gorin NC, Najman A, Salmon C, et al.: High dose combination chemotherapy (TACC) with and without autologous bone marrow transplantation for the treatment of acute leukaemia and other malignant diseases. *Eur J Cancer* 15:1113, 1979

55. Gorin NC, Najman A, Van der Akker J, et al.: Disappearance of Philadelphia chromosome after autologous bone marrow transplantation for treatment of chronic myeloid leukaemia in acute crisis. *Lancet* 1(8262):44, 1982 (Letter)

56. Gorin NC, Duay FK, Jansen GA, et al.: Preclinical study of immunotoxin T101: Absence of cytotoxicity against hemopoietic progenitor stem cells. Application to *in vitro* therapy prior to autologous bone marrow transplantation. *Exp Hematol* 11 (Suppl 14):6, 1983 (abstr)

57. Graham-Pole J: Transplantation for patients with neuroblastoma. *Proc 1st Internatl Symp on Autologous Bone Marrow Transplantation*, pp. 173–182. Edited by KA Dicke, G Spitzer, AR Zander. UT MD Anderson Hospital and Tumor Institute, Houston, Texas, 1985

58. Graham-Pole J, Lazarus HM, Herzig RH, et al.: High-dose melphalan therapy for the treatment of children with refractory neuroblastoma and Ewing's sarcoma. *Am J Pediatr Hematol Oncol* 6:17, 1984

59. Gulati SC, Helson L, Langleben A, et al.: Therapy of disseminated neuroblastoma with intensive therapy and autologous stem cell rescue. *SIOP* 14:25, 1982 (abstr)

60. Gulati SC, Fedorciw B, Gopal A, et al.: Autologous stem cell transplant for poor prognosis diffuse histiocytic lymphoma. In: *Proc 1st Internatl Symp on Autologous Bone Marrow Transplantation*, pp. 75–81. Edited by KA Dicke, G Spitzer, AR Zander. UT MD Anderson Hospital and Tumor Institute, Houston, Texas, 1985

61. Gulati S, Helson L, et al.: Presented orally at the International Autologous Transplant Meeting, Parma, Italy, 1985

62. Harper PG, Souhami RL, Spiro SG, et al.: A review of the use of very high dose chemotherapy in small cell carcinoma of the lung. *Proc 1st Internatl Symp on Autologous Bone Marrow Transplantation*, pp. 141–148. Edited by KA Dicke, G Spitzer, AR Zander. UT MD Anderson Hospital and Tumor :Institute, Houston, Texas, 1985

63. Harris R, Feig S, Coccia P, et al.: All in second remission – A CCSG study of maintenance chemotherapy vs marrow transplantation. In: *Progress in Bone Marrow Transplantation*, pp. 91–92. Alan R Liss, New York, 1987

64. Hartmann O, Kalifa C, Bayle C, et al.: Treatment of stage IV neuroblastoma with high-dose chemotherapy regimens and autologous bone marrow transplantation. *Proc Third Conf Adv Neuroblastoma Res*, 1984 (abstr)

65. Hartmann O, Kalifa C, Benhamou E, Patte C, Flamant F, Jullien C, Beaujean F, Lemerle J: Treatment of advanced neuroblastoma with high-dose melphalan and autologous bone marrow transplantation. *Cancer Chemother Pharmacol* 16(2):165, 1986

66. Hassett JM, Zaroulis CG, Greenberg ML, Siegal FP: Bone-marrow transplantation in AIDS. *N Engl J Med* 1983; 309:11–665

67. Helson L, Gulati S, O'Reilly R, et al.: Autologous bone marrow transplantation (ABMT) in neuroblastoma (NBL). *Proc Third Conf Adv Neuroblastoma Res*, 1984 (abstr)

68. Herzig RH, Phillips GL, Lazarus HM, et al.: Intensive chemotherapy and autologous bone marrow transplantation for the treatment of refractory malignancies. In: *Proc 1st Internatl Symp on Autologous Bone Marrow Transplantation*, pp. 197–202. Edited by KA Dicke, G Spitzer, AR Zander. UT MD Anderson Hospital and Tumor Institute, Houston, Texas, 1985

69. Hill RS, Buskard NA, Still BJ, et al.: Studies of cryopreservative methods for human bone marrow. In: *Proc 1st Internatl Symp on Autologous Bone Marrow Transplantation*, pp. 273–279. Edited by KA Dicke, G Spitzer, AR Zander. UT MD Anderson Hospital and Tumor Institute, Houston, Texas, 1985

70. Horning SJ, Rosenberg SA: The natural history of initially untreated low-grade non-Hodgkin's lymphoma. *N Engl J Med* 311:1471, 1984

71. Ihre DC, Lichter AS, Deisseroth AB, et al.: Late intensive combined modality therapy with autologous bone marrow infusion in extensive stage small cell lung cancer. *Proc Am Assoc Clin Oncol* 2:198, 1983 (abstr C-774)

72. Jacobs AD, Champlin RE, Golde DW: Recombinant alpha-2-interferon for hairy cell leukemia. *Blood* 65:1017, 1985

73. Jagannath S, Dicke KA, Spitzer G, et al.: Role of autologous transplantation in Hodgkin's disease. In: *Proc 1st Internatl Symp on Autologous Bone Marrow Transplantation*, pp. 83–86. Edited by KA Dicke, G Spitzer, AR Zander. UT MD Anderson Hospital and Tumor Institute, Houston, Texas, 1985

74. Jansen FK, Blythman HE, Carriere D, et al.: Immunotoxins: Hybrid molecules combining high specificity and potent cytotoxicity. *Immunologic Rev* 62:185, 1982

75. Johnson FL, Thomas ED, Clark BS, et al.: A comparison of marrow transplantation to chemotherapy for children with acute lymphoblastic leukemia in second or subsequent remission. *New Engl J Med* 305:846, 1981

76. Kaizer H, Stuart RK, Colvin M, et al.: Autologous bone marrow transplantation in acute leukemia: A pilot study utilizing *in vitro* incubation of autologous marrow with 4-hydroperoxycyclophosphamide (4HC) prior to cryopreservation. *Proc Am Soc Clin Oncol* 22:483, 1981 (abstr)

77. Kemshead JT, Ugelstad J, Rembaum A, et al.: Monoclonal antibodies attached to microspheres containing magnetic compounds, used to remove neuroblastoma cells from bone marrow taken for autologous transplantation. *Proc XIVth Mett Internatl Soc Ped Oncol*, Bern, Switzerland, 1982, P-14

78. Kersey JH, Ramsay NKC, Kim T, et al.: Allogeneic bone marrow transplantation in acute nonlymphocytic leukemia: A pilot study. *Blood* 60:400, 1982

79. Knight WA III: Autologous bone marrow transplantation for human solid tumors. *Tex Med* 80:50, 1984

80. Kolb HJ, Ledderose R, Hartenstein B, et al.: Autologous bone marrow transplantation in patients with advances teratocarcinoma. In: *Proc 1st Internatl Symp on Autologous Bone Marrow Transplantation*, pp. 211–217. Edited by KA

Dicke, G Spitzer, AR Zander. UT MD Anderson Hospital and Tumor Institute, Houston, Texas, 1985

81. Koller C, Miller D: Preliminary observations on the therapy of myeloid blast phase of chronic granulocytic leukemia with plicamycin and hydroxyurea. *NE Journal of Medicine* 315:23, 1986

82. Korbling M, Burke P, Braine H, et al.: Successful engraftment of blood-derived normal hemopoietic stem cells in chronic myelogenous leukemia. *Exp Hematol* 9:684, 1981

83. Lanzkowsky P (ed): *Pediatric Oncology*. McGraw-Hill Book Co, New York, 576 pp., 1982

84. Laure F, Rouvioux C, et al.: Reduction of HIV-1 DNA in infants and children by means of the polymerase chain reaction. *Lancet* 2: 538–541, 1988

85. Lister TA, Ronatiner AZS: The treatment of acute myelogenous leukemia in adults. *Sem Hematol* 19:172, 1982

86. McElwain JJ, Hedley DW, Burton G, et al.: Marrow auto-transplantation accelerated haematological recovery in patients with malignant melanoma treated with high dose melphalan. *Brit J Cancer* 40:72, 1979

87. McGlave PB, Kim TH, Hurd DD, et al.: Successful allogeneic bone marrow transplantation for patients in the accelerated phase of chronic granulocytic leukemia. *Lancet* 2(8299):625, 1982

88. Mage M, Gee TS, Arlin Z, et al.: Androgen therapy in post-splenectomy patients with hairy cell leukemia. *Blood* 58 (Suppl 1):145a, 1981 (abstr)

89. Martin PJ, Shulman HM, Schubach WH, et al.: Fatal Epstein–Barr virus associated proliferation of donor B cells after treatment of acute graft versus host disease with a murine anti-T cell antibody. *Ann Int Med* 10:310, 1984

90. Mathe G, Amiel JL, Schwarzenberg L: Adoptive immunotherapy of acute leukemia: Experimental and clinical results. *Cancer Res* 25:1525, 1965

91. Miller DR: Acute lymphoblastic leukemia. *Ped Clin North America* 27:269, 1980

92. Miller RA, Levy R: Response of cutaneous T-cell lymphoma to therapy with hybridoma monoclonal antibody. *Lancet* 2:226, 1981

93. Miller RA, Maloney DG, Warnke R, et al.: Treatment of B cell lymphoma with monoclonal anti-idiotype antibody. *New Engl J Med* 306:517, 1982

94. Minna JD, Higgins GA, Glatstein EJ: In: *Cancer: Principles and Practice of Oncology*, pp. 396–474. Edited by V de Vita Jr, S Hellman, S Rosenberg. JB Lippincott, Philadelphia, 1983

95. Nadler LM, Takavorian T, Botnick L, et al.: Anti-B1 monoclonal antibody and complement in treatment of autologous bone marrow transplantation for relapsed B-cell non-Hodgkin's lymphoma. *Lancet* 2(8400): 427, 1984

96. Netzel B, Rodt H, Haas RJ, et al.: Immunologic conditioning of bone marrow for autotransplantation in childhood acute lymphoblastic leukemia. *Lancet* 2: 1330, 1980

97. Nkrumah FK, Perkins I: Burkitt's lymphoma in Ghana: Clinical features and response to chemotherapy. *Int J Cancer* 17: 445, 1976

98. O'Leary M, Ramsay NK, Nesbit ME Jr, et al.: Bone marrow transplantation for non-Hodgkin's lymphoma in children and young adults. A pilot study. *Am J Med* 74: 497, 1983

99. Osserman EF, DiRe LB, Sherman WH, et al.: Identical twin marrow transplantation in multiple myeloma. *Acta Haematol (Basel)* 68(3): 215, 1982

100. Owens AH Jr: Effect of graft versus host disease on the course of L1210 leukemia. *Exp Hematol* 20: 43, 1970

101. Ozer H, Han T, Nussbaum-Blumenson A, et al.: Allogeneic bone marrow transplantation and idiotype (ID) monitoring in multiple myeloma. *Proc Am Soc Ca Res* 25: 161, 1984 (abstr)

102. Papa G, Arcese W, Mauro FR, Bianchi A, Alimena G,

DeFelice L, Isacchi G, Pasqualetti D, Malagnino F, Purpura M, et al.: Standard conditioning regimen and T-depleted donor bone marrow for transplantation in chronic myeloid leukemia. *Leuk Res* 10(2): 1469, 1986

103. Peters WP: Autologous bone marrow support in treating breast cancer. In: *Proc 1st Internatl Symp on Autologous Bone Marrow Transplantation*, pp. 189–195. Edited by KA Dicke, G Spitzer, AR Zander. UT MD Anderson Hospital and Tumor Institute, Houston, Texas, 1985

104. Philip T, Biron P, Maraninchi D, et al.: Massive chemotherapy with autologous bone marrow transplantation in 50 cases of non-Hodgkin's lymphoma with poor prognosis. In: *Proc 1st Internatl Symp on Autologous Bone Marrow Transplantation*, pp. 89–107. Edited by KA Dicke, G Spitzer, AR Zander. UT MD Anderson Hospital and Tumor Institute, Houston, Texas, 1985

105. Philip T, Biron P, Philip M, et al.: Burkitt's lymphoma and autologous bone marrow transplantation: An overview. In: *Proc 1st Internatl Symp on Autologous Bone Marrow Transplantation*, pp. 109–115. Edited by KA Dicke, G Spitzer, AR Zander. UT MD Anderson Hospital and Tumor Institute, Houston, Texas, 1985

106. Philip T, Bernard JL, Zucker JM, Pinkerton R, Lutz P, Bordigoni P, Plouvier E, Robert A, Carton R, Philippe N, et al.: High-dose chemoradiotherapy with bone marrow transplantation as consolidation treatment in neuroblastoma; an unselected group of stage IV patients over 1 year of age. *J Clin Oncol* Feb 5(2): 266, 1987

107. Phillips GL: Current clinical trials with intensive therapy and autologous bone marrow. In: *Recent Advances in Bone Marrow Transplantation*, pp. 567–597. Edited by RP Gale. Alan R Liss, Inc, New York, 1983

108. Phillips GL, Herzig RH, Lazarus HM, et al.: Treatment of resistant malignant lymphoma with cyclophosphamide, total body irradiation and transplantation of cryopreserved autologous marrow. *New Engl J Med* 310:1557, 1984

109. Portlock CS, Rosenberg SA: Chemotherapy of the non-Hodgkin's lymphomas. The Stanford experience. *Cancer Treat Rep* 61: 1049, 1977

110. Portlock CS, Rosenberg SA: No initial therapy for stage III and IV non-Hodgkin's lymphomas of favorable histologic types. *Ann Intern Med* 90: 10, 1979

111. Powles RL, Morgenstern G, Clink HM, et al.: The place of bone marrow transplantation in acute myelogenous leukemia. *Lancet* 1: 1047, 1980

112. Powles RL, Palu G, Raghavan D: The curability of acute leukemia. In: *Topical Reviews in Haematology*, pp. 186–219. Edited by S Roath. London, John Wright, 1980

113. Pritchard J, McElwain TJ, Graham-Pole J: High-dose melphalan with autologous marrow for treatment of advanced neuroblastoma. *Brit J Cancer* 45: 86, 1982

114. Quesada JR, Reuben JR, Manning JT, et al.: Alpha interferon for the induction of remission in hairy cell leukemia. *N Engl J Med* 310: 15, 1984

115. Ramsay N, LeBien T, Nesbit M, et al.: Autologous bone marrow transplantation for patients with acute lymphoblastic leukemia in second or subsequent remission: Results of bone marrow treated with monoclonal antibodies BA-1, BA-2, and BA-3 plus complement. *Blood* 66: 508, 1985

116. Ratain MJ, Golomb HM, Vardiman JW, et al.: Treatment of hairy cell leukemia with recombinant alpha-2 interferon. *Blood* 65: 644, 1985

117. Reece DE, Buskard NA, Hill RS, Fryer CJ, Naiman SC, Phillips GL: Allogeneic bone marrow transplantation for Philadelphia-chromosome positive acute lymphoblastic leukemia. *Leuk Res* 10(4): 457, 1986

118. Reiffers J, Vezon G, Bernard P, et al.: Hemopoietic stem cell autografting for chronic granulocytic leukemia in transformation. *Exp Hematol* 11 (Suppl 13): 148, 1983

119. Ritz J: Use of monoclonal antibodies in autologous and allogeneic bone marrow transplantation. *Clin Hematol* 12: 813, 1983

120. Ritz J, Bast RC, Clavell LA, et al.: Autologous bone marrow transplantation in CALLA positive acute lymphoblastic leukaemia after *in vitro* treatment with J5 monoclonal antibody and complement. *Lancet* 2: 60, 1982

121. Rizzoli V, Caramatti C, Mangoni L: The effect of 4-hydroperoxycyclophosphamide (4HC) and VP-16-213 on leukemic and normal myeloid progenitor cells. *Exp Hematol* 11 (Suppl 14): 9, 1983 (abstr)

122. Rosenberg SA: The low-grade non-Hodgkin's lymphomas: Challenges and opportunities. *J Clin Oncol* 3: 299, 1985

123. Rowley SD, Stuart RK: 4-hydroperoxycyclophosphamide (4-HC) effects on human pluripotent stem cells (CFU-GEMM) *in vitro*. *Exp Hematol* 11 (Suppl 14): 8, 1983 (abstr)

124. Sanders JE, Thomas ED, the Seattle Marrow Transplant Group: Marrow transplantation for children with acute nonlymphoblastic leukemia in first remission. *Blood* 66: 460, 1985

125. Sanders JE, Thomas ED: Marrow transplantation for children with acute nonlymphoblastic leukemia in first remission. *Med Pediatr Oncol* 9(5): 423, 1981

126. Schubach WH, Hackman R, Neiman PE, et al.: A monoclonal immunoblastic sarcoma in donor cells bearing Epstein–Barr virus genomes following allogeneic marrow grafting for acute lymphoblastic leukemia. *Blood* 60: 180, 1982

127. Schubach WH, Miller G, Thomas ED: Epstein–Barr virus genomes are restricted to secondary neoplastic cells following bone marrow transplantation. *Blood* 65: 535, 1985

128. Scott EP, Forman SJ, Spruce WE, et al.: Bone marrow ablation followed by allogeneic bone marrow transplantation for patients with high-risk acute lymphoblastic leukemia during complete remission. *Transplant Proc* 15: 1395, 1983

129. Siena S, Castro-Malaspina H, Gulati SC, et al.: Effect of *in vitro* purging with 4-hydroperoxycyclophosphamide (4-HC) on the hemopoietic microenviromental elements of human bone marrow. *Blood* 65: 655, 1985

130. Speck B, Bortin MM, Champlin R, et al.: Allogeneic bone-marrow transplantation for chronic myelogenous leukemia. *Lancet* 1(8378): 665, 1984

131. Spiegel Robert J: Intron A (Interferon Alfa-26): Clinical Overview and Future Directions. Seminars in Oncology 13: 3 Suppl 2, 1986

132. Spiers ASD, Parekh SJ, Bishop MB: Hairy cell leukemia: Induction of complete remission with pentostatin (2′-deoxycoformycin). *J Clin Oncol* 2: 1336, 1984

133. Spitzer G, Valdivieso M, Farha P, et al.: Bone marrow support in limited small cell bronchogenic carcinoma. In: *Proc 1st Internatl Symp on Autologous Bone Marrow Transplantation*, pp. 155–160. Edited by KA Dicke, G Spitzer, AR Zander. UT MD Anderson Hospital and Tumor Institute, Houston, Texas, 1985

134. Stewart P, Sanders J: Marrow transplantation for acute lymphoblastic leukemia in first remission. *Proc 13th Internatl Cancer Congr, Seattle*, UICC, Abstr 794, 1982

135. Syman M, Humblet Y, Bosly A, et al.: Treatment of small cell lung cancer with non-cross-resistant induction and intensive consolidation chemotherapy and autologous marrow transplantation: A randomized study. In: *Proc 1st Internatl Symp on Autologous Bone Marrow Transplantation*, pp. 161–165. Edited by KA Dicke, G Spitzer, AR Zander. UT MD Anderson Hospital and Tumor Institute, Houston, Texas, 1985

136. Tannir N, Spitzer G, Dicke K, et al.: Phase I–II study of high-dose mitomycin with autologous bone marrow transplantation in refractory metastatic breast cancer. *Cancer Treat Rep* 68: 805, 1984

137. Thomas ED, Buckner CD, Banaji M, et al.: One hundred

patients with acute leukemia treated by chemotherapy, total body irradiation, and allogeneic bone marrow transplantation. *Blood* 49: 511, 1977

138. Thomas ED, Buckner CD, Clift RA, et al.: Marrow transplantation for acute nonlymphoblastic leukemia in first remission. *New Engl J Med* 301: 597, 1979

139. Thomas ED, Sanders JE, Flournoy N, et al.: Marrow transplantation for patients with acute lymphoblastic leukemia in remission. *Blood* 54: 468, 1979

140. Thomas ED: Marrow transplantation for marrow failure or leukemia. *Compr Ther* 6(7): 69, 1980

141. Thomas ED, Clift RA, Buckner CD: Marrow transplantation for patients with acute nonlymphoblastic leukemia who achieve first remission. *Cancer Treat Rep* 66: 1463, 1982

142. Thomas ED, Sanders JE, Flournoy N, et al.: Marrow transplantation for patients with acute lymphoblastic leukemia: A long-term follow-up. *Blood* 62: 1139, 1983

143. Treleaven JG, Gibson FM, Uglestad J, et al.: Removal of neuroblastoma cells from bone marrow with monoclonal antibodies conjugated to magnetic microspheres. *Lancet* 1: 70, 1984

144. Uckun FM, Azemove SM, Myers DE, Vallera DA: Anti-CO2 (T, p50) intact ricin immunotoxins for GVHD-prophylaxis in allogeneic bone marrow transplantation. *Leuk Res* 10(2): 145, 1986

145. Weiden PL, Flournoy M, Thomas ED, et al.: Antileukemic effect of graft-versus-host disease in human recipients of allogeneic marrow grafts. *New Engl J Med* 300: 1068, 1979

146. Wells JE, Billing R, Herzig R, et al.: Autotransplantation after *in vitro* immunotherapy of lymphoblastic leukemia. *Exp Hematol* 7: 164, 1979

147. Williams SF, Bitran JD, Kaminer L, Westbrook C, Jacobs R, Ashenhurst J, Robin E, Purl S, Beschorner J, Schroeder C, et al.: A phase I–II study of bialkylator chemotherapy, high-dose thiotepa, and cyclophosphamide with autologous bone marrow reinfusion in patients with advanced cancer. *J Clin Oncol* Feb 5(2): 260, 1987

148. Wolf NS, Phillips GL, Fay JW, et al.: Transplantation for primary tumors of the central nervous system: Phase II and III studies of the Southeastern Cancer Study Group. In: *Proc 1st Internatl Symp on Autologous Bone Marrow Transplantation*, pp. 255–259. Edited by KA Dicke, G Spitzer, AR Zander. UT MD Anderson Hospital and Tumor Institute, Houston, Texas, 1985

149. Wolff SN, Phillips GL, Herzig GP: High-dose carmustine with autologous bone marrow transplantation for the adjuvant treatment of high-grade gliomas of the central nervous system. *Cancer Treat Rep* 71(2): 183, 1987

150. Woods WG, Nesbit NE, Ramsay NKC, et al.: Intensive therapy followed by bone marrow transplantation for patients with acute lymphocytic leukemia in second or subsequent remission. Determination of prognostic factors (a report from the University of Minnesota bone marrow transplant team). *Blood* 6: 1182, 1983

151. Woods WG: Supportive care for children with cancer. Guidelines of the Childrens Cancer Study Group. Prevention of graft-vs. host disease. *Am J Pediatr Hematol Oncol* 6(3): 283, 1984

152. Yam LT, Klick JC, Mielke CH: Therapeutic leukapheresis in hairy cell leukemia: Review of literature and personal experience. *Sem Oncol* 11: 493, 1984

153. Ziegler JL: Burkitt's lymphoma. *Med Clin No Amer* 61: 1073, 1977

154. Ziegler JL: Management of Burkitt's lymphoma: An update. *Cancer Treat Rev* 6: 95, 1979

155. Zwann FE, Hermans J, Berrett AJ, et al.: Bone marrow transplantation for acute lymphoblastic leukemia. A survey of the European Group for Bone Marrow Transplantation (E.G.B.M.T.). *Blood* 58: 33, 1984

HEMATOLOGIC SUPPORT OF THE PATIENT WITH MALIGNANCY

JOHN C. PHARES

INTRODUCTION

Patients with malignancy frequently develop significant degrees of compromised bone marrow function and increased loss and utilization of the formed elements of the blood as a consequence of the disease process. Surgical therapy frequently results in the external loss of blood components and significant suppression of bone marrow function occurs as the result of medical therapy for the malignancy. The availability of hematologic supportive therapy in the form of transfusion of blood products has, over the past several years, in conjunction with overall improved medical support, made it possible to deliver more effective antitumor therapy and palliative support to these patients. Modern transfusion techniques and practices now provide effective temporizing measures for use during the treatment of patients with a wide variety of malignancies.

COMPONENT THERAPY

The history of transfusion of blood and blood products is an old concept dating to the seventeenth century however, it was not until the 1900's with the discovery of blood groups by Landsteiner that it became possible to consider using blood transfusions in man to any significant extent. Widespread use of transfusions did not occur until the 1940's when the concepts of blood banking and blood preservation were developed, in part, due to the stimulus of World War II (54). In the ensuing years, as the techniques of blood collection and preservation improved, the concepts and the use of component therapy evolved. The patient has available to him a large number of blood components which can be utilized in a selective manner to meet his individual needs and requirements. It is now possible to administer red cells, platelets, granulocytes, plasma, and plasma components selectively to replace the specific components needed by the patient. The appropriate dose can now more easily and safely be given and at the same time a limited resource can more efficiently and effectively be utilized. Whole blood rarely is the product of choice.

*Head, Hematology Division, Department of Internal Medicine, Naval Hospital, Bethesda, Maryland 20814, U.S.A. The opinions expressed are the private ones of the author and are not to be construed as official or reflecting the views of the Navy Department, of the Naval Service at large or the Department of Defense.

RISKS OF TRANSFUSION THERAPY

Transfusion therapy, although widely used and relatively safe, is not without significant risks. The incidence of transfusion reactions has been estimated as occurring with a frequency of 1 to 20%, however, accurate figures are difficult to obtain. In 1975 the Food and Drug Administration required the reporting of fatal reactions and initial figures would suggest that in the United States, 30 to 40 fatal transfusion reactions occur yearly among recipients of nearly 12 million units of blood (50). Meticulous blood banking techniques, procedures and controls and careful clinical care minimize these risks however, adverse reactions, as with all medical interventions, continue to be present and the clinician must be aware of the potential risks and be able to recognize their occurrence. The risk-benefit ratio of transfusions must not be lost sight of.

Adverse reactions to transfusion of blood and blood products may be classified into immune mediated reactions and those unrelated to immune mechansism.

Hemolytic transfusion reactions

Immediate. Immediate hemolytic transfusion reactions fortunately are among the less common of the various transfusion reactions. Although this problem was responsible in large part for the lack of widespread use of transfusion therapy, until the discovery of the blood group antigens by Landsteiner, it has progressively become a more infrequent problem. In an early series reported in 1942, the incidence was noted to be one in 541 transfusions and in a more recent series was recorded as one in 6,232 transfusions with a mortality rate of 17% (55). Other series have reported mortality rates for hemolytic transfusion reactions to be as high as 50%.

The mechanism of hemolysis is immune in nature with either naturally occurring (anti A; anti B) antibodies or acquired isoantibodies being responsible for the hemolysis in asssociation with complement. The mechanism by which the antibodies and complement produce hemolysis has not been clearly defined. Factors which influence the degree of hemolysis and its clinical consequences include the antigen to which the antibodies are directed, the class and subclass of the antibodies, antibody affinity, antibody titer and the volume of blood transfused.

The signs and symptoms of a hemolytic transfusion reactions are variable in severity. In some individuals the reac-

P.V. Woolley (ed.), Cancer management in Man: Biological Response Modifiers, Chemotherapy, Antibiotics, Hyperthermia, Supporting Measures
© 1989. Kluwer Academic Publishers, Dordrecht.

tion may pass all but unnoticed while in others it may be fulminant in nature with the variability being due to those factors previously mentioned as well as the individuals underlying state of health and consciousness. Symptoms of a severe hemolytic reaction include fever, chills, anxiety, back pain, chest tightness, dyspnea, hypotension, urticaria, nausea, vomiting, diarrhea, bleeding, renal failure, jaundice and hemoglobinuria. The frequency of these various signs and symptoms varies depending upon the series reported, however, fever tends to be one of the more frequent occurrences in most series.

The bleeding diathesis associated with a hemolytic transfusion reaction may be manifest by oozing from venapunctures, operative sites and mucous membranes and may progress to generalized fulminant bleeding. The bleeding disorder has the characteristics of generalized dissemination intravascular coagulation. The DIC is triggered by the activation of the coagulation sequence both by thromboplastic substances released from the lysed red cells and by antigen-antibody complexes.

The renal failure association with transfusion reactions was long thought to be the result of free hemoglobin in the plasma and its subsequent precipitation in the renal tubules or due to a direct toxic effect of the hemoglobin on the renal tubules. This has been shown not to be the case with the demonstration that stroma-free hemoglobin does not lead to renal failure (57, 58). It has been shown that incompatable hemoglobin free red cell stroma is capable of inducing renal failure (62). It now appears that the renal failure is a consequence of antigen-antibody complex formation resulting in DIC and vasomotor disturbances induced by these factors (27).

The activation of the coagulation system and the development of DIC results in the formation of intravascular fibrin deposits within the kidney. In addition, the activation of Hageman Factor (FXII) results in the formation of vasoactive kinins. The antigen-antibody complexes also activate the complement cascade which may cause release of histamine and serotonin. These substances are likely responsible for hypotension and the secondary release of catecholamines seen in association with transfusion reactions with renal vasoconstriction being the end result. The combination then of the renal vasoconstriction, hypotension and renal vascular fibrin deposition is renal failure.

Current recommendations for the management of immediate hemolytic transfusion reactions although unproven in clinical trials are based upon the aforementioned pathophysiological mechanisms and are aimed primarily at the prevention of renal failure. These measures include correcting hypotension, maintaining urine output and control of DIC with heparin.

Delayed. Delayed hemolytic transfusion reactions were first recognized in 1957 with the incidence apparently increasing. The incidence of delayed hemolytic transfusion reactions of one per 4,000 units of blood transfused has been reported in one series. The apparent increasing incidence can probably be attributed to increased sensitivity of testing methods and awareness of the entity (47).

The etiology, like that of immediate hemolytic transfusion reactions, is antibody formation, usually an isoantibody, with subsequent red blood cell destruction. The responsible antibody in most cases goes undetected at the time of transfusion due to its low titer and the lack of sensitivity of the screening procedures used but increases in titer significantly post transfusion via an anamnestic response.

In general delayed hemolytic transfusion reactions are of a lesser degree of severity than immediate hemolytic transfusion reactions. However, renal failure may develop (46) and all the severe manifestation seen with immediate hemolytic reaction may occur (56).

Leukocyte antibodies

Febrile transfusion reactions are the most common of all transfusion reaction accounting for up to 80% of all non-hemolytic transfusion reactions (31). These reactions are characterized by the onset of fever usually within 1/2 to 2 hours following the initiation of a transfusion, however, the onset of fever may be delayed up to 24 hours with resolution over the next several hours (74). These febrile reactions are relatively benign, however, on occasion may be severe. It is now generally accepted that the vast majority of such reactions are due to antibodies directed against white cell and platelet antigens (4). The white cell antibodies may be either leukoagglutinins or lymphocytotoxic antibodies. The majority of the antibodies are induced by either prior transfusion or pregnancy and patients requiring repeated transfusion over a prolonged period of time are at the greatest risk of developing this type of transfusion reaction. Although the most common reaction is isolated fever, on occasion pulmonary symptoms may develop in association with pulmonary infiltrates which occur in association with the finding of leukoagglutinins (71).

Febrile transfusion reactions for the most part may be managed with antipyretics, antihistamines and steroids. If reactions are particularly severe leukocyte poor red cell preparations such as buffy coat poor red cells, washed red cells or frozen-thawed red cells may be considered. A recently available alternative to such preparations is to use a leukocyte filter, an in-line device through which the blood is passed at the time of transfusion.

Platelet antibodies

Platelets have been shown to contain multiple antigens including HLA antigens, ABO antigens and platelet specific antigens (74). The existence of these antigens and resulting antibody formation accounts for the development of febrile transfusion reactions, post transfusion purpura and poor response to platelet transfusions. Post transfusion purpura is characterized by the development of severe thrombocytopenia, usually about one week following a transfusion (63). Such reactions usually occur in individuals who have had a prior pregnancy or to whom multiple prior transfusions have been given. In most instances reported the affected individuals lack PL_A1 antigen, an antigen found in 98% of the population (1, 63). Although it is felt that an antibody directed against this antigen is responsible for the destruction of platelets, the mechanism involved is unclear (4). Other platelet associated antigens may play a role in development of the thrombocytopenia and it has been suggested that the disorder may be more heterogeneous (77). Exchange transfusion (11), plasmapheresis (1) and steroids (72) have been utilized successfully in treating this disorder.

A much more common problem associated with platelet antigens and antibodies is encountered in the administration of platelets to which the recipient becomes refractory. Allo-immunization is manifest as a poor platelet incremental increase post transfusion as well as impaired control of thrombocytopenic hemorrhage by platelet transfusions.

Graft versus host disease

Graft versus host disease has long been recognized as a common complication of bone marrow transplantation. This disorder is due to the engraftment of donor lymphocytes and is manifest by skin rashes, abnormal liver function and gastrointestinal symptoms. More recently, graft versus host disease has been recognized as occurring in a variety of individuals following blood transfusion. These have included patients with congenital immunodeficient syndromes, neonates receiving intrauterine or exchange transfusion (53) and patients with hematologic malignancies (5, 13, 16, 21, 59). Donor lymphocytes which are responsible for this disorder may be found in virtually all blood component preparations and thus in a subgroup of patients receiving transfusion, the potential for graft versus host disease exists, although the incidence is unknown. The occurrence of graft versus host disease has led some to recommend prophylactic irradiation of blood components used for transfusion in selected patients although firm guidelines for this are lacking. Studies have been conducted which indicate that the functional qualities of the formed elements of the blood are not significantly impaired by 5,000 rads of radiation, a dose which significantly impairs tritiated thymidine uptake by lymphocytes (9), a measure of their proliferative potential.

Antibodies against plasma components

Approximately one in 800–900 (38, 39, 41, 70) healthy individuals are deficient in or have markedly diminished quantities of IgA. Approximately 20–25% of such individuals have anti-IgA antibodies, many of which appear to occur spontaneously (38, 70) although prior transfusion and sensitization have occurred in some individuals. The transfusion of small quantities of IgA into such individuals, via an antigen antibody reaction, may result in a severe anaphylactic reaction.

Antibodies directed against other plasma components have been identified including antibodies against other immunoglobulins which have the potential for causing allergic reactions. The allergic reactions noted earlier are due to antibodies in the transfused recipient directed against transfused material. Another mechanism for allergic reactions is the infusion of antibodies contained in the donor material. Antibodies may be transfused which subsequently may mediate allergic reactions when the recipient is challenged with the antigen to which the antibodies are directed (4).

Allergic reactions, most commonly urticarial in nature, although as with IgA may have a specific etiology identified

frequently occur in which the specific etiologic factor cannot be identified.

Nonimmune mediated transfusion problems

Nonimmune mediated problems associate with transfusion include metabolic disturbances associated with transfusion, mechanical/physical problems and disease transmission by transfusion.

Metabolic. Blood and its components are collected in the majority of instances in a citrate solution. Citrate phosphate dextrose (CPD), a commonly used solution, contains 3.2 g of citric acid and 25.8 g of sodium citrate per liter of solution with 14 milliliters of the solution being used per 100 milliliters of blood collected (74). Thus, a blood recipient may receive substantial quantities of citrate. If the rate and quantity of blood and thus the quantity of citrate infused is great enough, or citrate metabolism is impaired, citrate intoxication with its primary manifestation being due to hypocalcemia may occur. This results in muscular tremors, electrocardiographic changes, arrhythmias and diminished cardiac output. Such hypocalcemia may be rapidly reversed by the administration of calcium. This, however, is infrequently needed, as citrate is metabolized rapidly. It has been suggested that calcium is rarely needed until the infusion rate approximates 1 liter over a ten minute period of time or in exchange transfusions being performed more rapidly than an exchange over a two hour period of time (4).

Stored red cells over a period of time release potassium into the extracellular fluid and the potential exists for infusion of significant quantities of potassium. Modern storage techniques tend to minimize this however, and rarely does this present significant problems. Problems are most likely to occur in patients receiving massive transfusions in the setting of impaired renal function or with extensive tissue damage.

One unit of red blood cells contains approximately 250 mg of iron. As the daily excretion of iron is limited to approximately 1 to 2 mg of iron, regular transfusions of red blood cells soon result in the net gain of iron and iron overload. The rapidity at which iron is accumulated depends not only on the quantity transfused but also on the patient's bone marrow erythroid mass. In individuals with erythroid hyperplasia iron absorption is significantly greater than in individuals with hypoplastic erythropoiesis. The transfused individual with active but ineffective erythropoiesis will develop clinically significant iron overload at a much more rapid pace than comparably transfused individuals with diminished erythropoiesis. The excess iron becomes deposited in tissues resulting in their dysfunction with signs and symptoms of overload occurring as the body's iron stores approach 25 g (74), an amount present in approximately 100 units of blood. Iron chelation therapy which to date has been used most extensively in thalessemia offers a means of retarding and/or preventing iron overload.

Nonmetabolic. Circulatory overload with the development of congestive heart failure and pulmonary edema may develop with the rapid transfusion of large quantities of blood, particularly in individuals with compromised cardiac function. Signs and symptoms which include cough, chest pain, dyspnea, cyanosis and chest discomfort may develop during or up to 24 hours after a transfusion. The risk of this occurrence can be minimized by the use of slow infusion rates, component therapy and, on occasion, exchange transfusion to avoid intravascular volume expansion.

Hypothermia, with significant lowering of body temperature, may occur with the transfusion of large quantities of blood and may predispose to cardiac arrhythmias. Blood may be warmed to prevent this but overheating of the blood must be avoided as hemolysis may occur.

The transmission of diseases by blood and blood products poses significant risks to patients requiring transfusion therapy. The most common transfusion transmitted disease is viral hepatitis. Viral hepatitis infection may be hepatitis A, hepatitis B or hepatitis non-A, non-B with recent information suggesting that 80 to 90% of post transfusion hepatitis is of the non-A, non-B type. It has been suggested that a portion of transfusion related hepatitis is caused by infectious agents not yet identified (20). The risk of developing hepatitis from the transfusion of blood obtained from volunteer donors is approximately 1% per unit transfused with approximately 20% of patients becoming icteric from the hepatitis (14).

A number of other infectious diseases including malaria, syphilis, leishmaniasis, trypanosomiasis, toxoplasmosis, microfilariae, cytomegalovirus and Epstein-Barr Virus may be transmitted by blood transfusion (14).

Bacterial contamination of blood, most commonly with staphylococci and diphtheroids, may occur, usually as the result of improper techniques of collection and handling of blood and rarely as the result of unsuspected bacteremia in donors (13).

The transmission of acquired immunodeficiency syndrome by transfusion has been reported (15). With the subsequent availability of a screening test for HIV antibody blood banks have instituted screening for the antibody to the causative agent of this disorder. The incidence of transfusional transmission of HIV is not known with certainty but has been estimated to occur at a frequency of 1:40,000 to 1:1,000,000(4) (See also postscript of chapter 19, Volume VI, p. 189.)

Tumor cell infusion

Tumor cells have been demonstrated to be present in the peripheral circulation of patients with neoplasms. One might expect that the potential exists for the transfusion of viable tumor cells, via blood obtained from blood donors with unsuspected neoplasms, into recipients with resulting grafting of these cells and the development of tumors in susceptible individuals, a situation analogous to the development of graft versus host disease due to transfusion of viable lymphocytes. This to date has not been reported in humans. The lack of its occurrence may be related to the number of factors. Transfused cells may be rejected as foreign and in the vast majority of instances this would be expected. Tumor cells collected and transfused may not be viable, either due to their inherent characteristics or due to an irrepairable damage inflicted upon them by the collection process and storage techniques used in blood banking. It has

been reported that the vast majority of tumor cells in the circulation are rapidly cleared without the development of metastases and that their presence in the blood is not in itself sufficient for metastases to occur (8). In experimental animals the dose of tumor inoculum needed to transplant tumors suggests that the number of cells introduced is an important variable and it is not unlikely that if viable tumor cells are transfused they are in insufficient quantities to engraft. It has also been shown that clumps of tumor cells are more likely to result in metastatic tumor formation than single cells. In animal models, the majority of circulating tumor cells are single (43). The anticoagulant in which donor blood is collected would be expected to cause cell dispersion and if tumor clumps were present, to perhaps result in their being dissociated into either smaller clumps or single cells. Other factors undoubtedly also are of importance.

RED BLOOD CELL TRANSFUSION

The primary function of the red cell is to carry oxygen to the tissues of the body. The oxygen carrying capacity of normal blood is 1.34 ml of oxygen per gram of hemoglobin and therefore with a normal hemoglobin concentration, approximately 20 ml (1.34 ml O_2/gram hemoglobin × 15 gr hemoglobin/100 ml blood = 20 ml O_2 per 100 ml of blood) of oxygen may be transported by 100 ml of blood. As anemia develops the oxygen carrying capacity of the blood decreases, however, tissue oxygenation is not impaired proportionally to the decrease in hemoglobin as compensatory mechanism become operative. As anemia develops red cell 2,3 diphosphoglycerate increases which results in a shift in the hemoglobin-oxygen dissociation curve with a decreased affinity of the hemoglobin for oxygen thus enhancing tissue oxygen delivery. Other compensatory mechanisms to prevent tissue hypoxia include a redistribution of blood flow to oxygen sensitive organs and an increase in cardiac output. In addition, other responses such as an increase in respiratory activity occur. This type of response, however, does little to increase oxygen delivery as blood leaving the pulmonary veins contains nearly 100% saturated hemoglobin. This type of response, in fact, may increase the oxygen requirements due to an increase in muscular activity associated with increasing respirations. Thus, rather than acting as compensatory mechanisms, this type of response may aggravate the situation and be responsible for such symptoms as dyspnea.

The signs and symptoms of anemia result not only from tissue hypoxia due to decreased oxygen delivery but also frequently and to a greater extent from activation of compensatory mechanisms and the underlying disease process. The rapidity at which anemia develops plays a significant role in the development of symptoms. Individuals who rapidly become anemic tend to be more symptomatic than those in whom the anemia is slowly progressive or chronic in nature. For example, patients with severe but chronic anemia such as individuals with Sickle Cell Disease and those with severe megaloblastic anemia of insidious onset have remarkably fewer symptoms compared to those individuals with rapidly progressive anemias as may be seen in acute bone marrow suppression due to, among other factors, cancer chemotherapy.

Transfusion with red blood cells offers an effective means of rapidly alleviating anemia and its signs, symptoms and consequences. A variety of blood products are available by which red cells may be delivered to the patient requiring such treatment. Whole blood may be utilized, however, seldom is the product of choice. The plasma contained in the product usually is not needed by the patient and in fact, due to volume considerations, frequently is undesirable. In addition, the use of whole blood poorly utilizes a limited resource which may be fractionated into components, a much more effective and wise utilization of blood. Red cell rich preparations, most commonly prepared by centrifugation of whole blood, are the usual preferred product. In such preparations of packed red blood cells approximately 80% of the plasma has been removed with the resulting hematocrit of the preparation being in the range of 60 to 90. Leukocyte poor red cell preparations are available and may be indicated for a small subset of patients requiring transfusion, such as in individuals who have demonstrated significant reactions to leukocytes. Leukocyte poor preparations have been prepared in a number of ways including sedimentation with removal of the leukocyte buffy coat, centrifugation, filtration, saline washing of red cells and freezing and thawing of blood.

The decision to use red cells for transfusion frequently is taken somewhat lightly. The primary indications for red cell transfusions are to restore and/or maintain blood volume in the prevention of/or treatment of hypovolemic hemorrhagic shock and to restore the oxygen carrying capacity of the blood in patients with significant degrees of anemia in whom the total blood volume may not be markedly diminished.

In hypovolemia or hemorrhagic shock the volume of blood to be transfused cannot with any degree of reliability be estimated based upon the patient's hemoglobin or hematocrit as in acute blood loss these values do not acutely reflect the degree of volume depletion. With acute hemorrhage the hematocrit falls only after a time of equilibration which may require several days (2) before a stable value is reached. The treatment thus of hemorrhagic shock depends much more on the estimate of the volume of blood lost utilizing clinical parameter such as tachycardia, pulse pressure, absolute blood pressure, orthostatic changes in blood pressure, venous pressure and cardiac output. The interpretation of these parameters is much easier in previously healthy patients suffering hemorrhage than in individuals with significant underlying disease such as a malignancy and those receiving a variety of drugs which may alter the physiologic response to acute volume depletion.

The administration of red cells to patients with more subacute or chronic forms of anemia may more reliably be guided by the hemoglobin and hematocrit levels. However, the degree of anemia at which transfusion is considered must be highly individualized.

The decision to institute transfusion therapy in nonhemorrhagic, non-hypovolemic anemia must take into account a number of variables and considerations. One must consider not only the hemoglobin level but also the symptoms associated with the anemia or the likelihood of the development of symptoms. Individuals with relatively severe but stable anemia tolerate their low red cell mass remark-ably well as evidenced by patients with Sickle Cell Anemia who may frequently be managed without transfusion, whereas patients with more acute lowering of the red cell mass may be quite symptomatic. Therefore the duration as well as the degree of anemia must be considered.

Younger patients are likely to tolerate a significant degree of anemia well whereas older individuals with compromised cardiac function are more likely to develop symptoms of tissue hypoxia such as angina pectoris. Therefore the threshold for transfusion may be influenced by the patient's age and known or estimated cardiac reserve as well as other physiologic factors.

Another consideration is the etiology of anemia and the likelihood of either reversibility or improvement with some measure other than transfusion. Or conversely whether one might expect the anemia to become progressively worse. One would be more included to avoid transfusions in patients with, for example, pernicious anemia in whom treatment can be expected to result in a rather rapid improvement as opposed to individuals with severe and prolonged bone marrow suppression due to cancer chemotherapy in whom one might expect worsening of the anemia and significantly delay in improvement occurring.

Therefore, the decision to institute transfusions in nonhemorrhagic anemia should be based not only on the degree of anemia but also consideration must be given to its etiology, chronicity and expected course as well as the status of the patient and their estimated or demonstrated tolerance for a decreased red cell mass.

PLATELET TRANSFUSIONS

It has long been recognized that thrombocytopenia is a common cause of significant bleeding. Bleeding is frequently contributed to by the coexistence of other factors such as the presence of other coagulation defects, fever and infection. However, the platelet count remains a significant independent variable. The frequency of hemorrhage and its clinical severity is closely related to the platelet count. In one study (25) of patients with leukemia thrombocytopenic hemorrhage of varying severity was observed to occur on 92% of the days during which the platelet count was less than 1,000 in contrast to its being noted on only 8% of the days when the platelet count was between 50,000 and 100,000. Severe hemorrhage occurred at a lower frequency, but again could be correlated in a very similar manner with the degree of thrombocytopenia, with such hemorrhage occurring about 5% of the time with platelet levels greater than 100,000 and increasing to 33% with platelet counts less than 1,000. Gross hemorrhage defined as gross hematuria, melena or hematemesis occurred rarely at platelet counts greater than 20,000. In another study, looking at patients with aplastic thrombocytopenia, fecal blood loss was utilized as a measure of the relationship between bleeding and platelet count (67). Again the relationship between bleeding and platelet count was demonstrated. It was found that at platelet counts of greater than 10,000 stool blood loss was no greater than in normal subjects, at counts of 5–10,000 blood loss was slightly increased and at counts less than 5,000 markedly elevated fecal blood loss was noted.

Although the platelet count is an important predictor of

the chances of hemorrhage, other factors are of significance. The etiology of the thrombocytopenia is important. The aforementioned data is operative primarily in hypoproliferative thrombocytopenias. In thrombocytopenia due to immune destruction of platelets (ITP) the chances of bleeding are usually less than in patients with comparable platelet counts due to defective production. This relationship has been graphically demonstrated by the correlation of bleeding times and platelet counts (29). Here it was demonstrated that the bleeding time and platelet count were inversely related in patients with hypoproliferative thrombocytopenias. However, in patients with ITP and those in whom rapid recovery of bone marrow function following chemotherapy was occurring the bleeding time was shorter than in those with hypoproliferative thrombocytopenias and comparable platelet counts.

Conversely, bleeding time and clinical hemorrhage may be greater than might be expected based upon the platelet count if a coexistent congenital or acquired platelet function abnormality is present or other coagulation defects are present. Multiple drugs, aspirin being a prime example, alter platelet function and thus predispose to thrombocytopenic hemorrhage out of proportion to the platelet count. This has been demonstrated both via bleeding time (29) and fecal blood loss (67). Concurrent uremia, disseminated intravascular coagulation and infection likewise have the potential for exacerbating thrombocytopenic bleeding.

As early as 1910 (18) the ability of transfused platelets to elevate platelet counts and improve hemostasis was recognized. However, many years elapsed before platelet transfusions were investigated or utilized to any significant extent.

With the advent of modern blood banking techniques and the availability of platelets for transfusion, control of thrombocytopenic hemorrhage has become possible. The effectiveness of platelet transfusions in raising the platelet count and in controlling thrombocytopenic hemorrhage has been repeatedly demonstrated (10, 23, 24). With the utilization of platelet transfusions hemorrhage as a cause of death in patients with leukemia has become less frequent (32) decreasing from 67% in the preplatelet transfusion era to 38% following the availability and use of platelet transfusions.

An extension of the therapeutic effectiveness of platelet transfusions in controlling hemorrhage has been the prophylactic use of platelets to prevent hemorrhage in severely thrombocytopenic patients not actively bleeding. The utility of platelet transfusions given prophylactically in preventing hemorrhage has been shown (24) where the number of days with bleeding was reduced in prophylactically transfused patients in comparison with historical controls. Other reports have confirmed this (60) including randomized trials (35, 49). Various recommendations as to use of prophylactic platelet transfusions have emerged including maintaining the platelet count via transfusion above 20,000 (23) and initiating transfusion only when the platelet count is less than 5,000 (67).

These recommendations are operative primarily in those disorders with diminished platelet production. The etiology of thrombocytopenia must be considered when contemplating prophylactic platelet transfusions. Patients with hypoplastic thrombocytopenia are the primary candidates for platelet transfusions given in a prophylactic manner. In those disorders involving platelet destruction such as disseminated intravascular coagulation, immune thrombocytopenia and drug related thrombocytopenias mediated via immune mechanisms, prophylactic platelet transfusions are not generally of value as platelet survival is markedly diminished and thus the effectiveness of transfused platelets is severely compromised. Nevertheless, therapeutic platelet transfusions in individuals with this type of disorder with life threatening hemorrhage may be of value.

The prophylactic use of platelet transfusions, although widely accepted and utilized is not without some degree of controversy, however, with this controversy relating primarily to the development of antibodies and refractoriness to platelet transfusions.

The effectiveness of the prophylactic transfusions of platelets in preventing hemorrhage in most instances has been correlated with the ability to obtain and maintain post transfusion incremental increases in platelet counts.

The frequency of transfusion and the quantity of platelets transfused to achieve this desirable effect is variable. Freireich reported that 4 units of platelet rich plasma per square meter of body surface area administered twice weekly would maintain the platelet count above 20,000 most of the time with platelet concentrations being 80 to 90% as effective (23). Another study (60) suggested that a dose of 3 platelet concentrates per 100 lb of body weight was sufficient as a prophylactic dose in noninfected patients. In this study the majority of patients received transfusions on a daily basis. There are multiple factors which may alter the effectiveness of prophylactic transfusions and dictate altering the use of, schedule of and the quantity of platelets transfused. In patients with decreased platelet production there is a modest decrease in platelet recovery and survival when compared to normal individuals (65). In patients with malignancy and particularly leukemia the decreases are more marked (66) and thus patients with leukemia may require significantly greater quantities of platelets given more frequently to obtain a desired effect than patients with aplastic anemia. Fever and infection may in a similar manner decrease the effectiveness of transfused platelets both in post transfusion incremental increases in platelet counts and survival of transfused platelets.

Compounding the problem of effectiveness of prophylactic platelet transfusions in preventing hemorrhage is the quality of the infused platelet and endogenous factors which may affect the platelet function. Storage techniques for platelets to be transfused have long been recognized as an important variable in altering platelet recovery, viability and functional integrity. Storage temperature plays a significant role in platelet yield, viability and function and currently storage at room temperature in the majority of instances appears preferable to refrigeration (65, 74). Potential exists for transfusion of functionally deficient platelets due to acquired defects in the donor platelets. Perhaps the most prominent concern in this area is donor use of aspirin which results in irreversible platelet function defects and thus would be expected to significantly compromise the effectiveness of platelets obtained from such a donor. Also compromising the effectiveness of transfused platelets are recipient factors. As was noted earlier fever, infection and malignancy alter yield and survival of transfused platelets. A significant number of drugs are known to affect platelet function and more are being identified. Patients requiring platelet transfusion very frequently require such platelet function suppressing drugs and are at greater risk for bleeding than would be anticipated if only platelet counts were considered. The concurrent existence of other disorders, for example uremia, in the recipient may likewise compromise the function of infused platelets.

A significant continuing problem in the field of platelet transfusion and one which requires further study is the development of refractoriness to platelet transfusions. This results in transfusion reactions, diminished survival of transfused platelets and most importantly the inability of platelet transfusions to control thrombocytopenic hemorrhage. Alloimmunization with antibodies directed against platelet antigens is in large part responsible for the development of refractoriness to platelet transfusions. The relationship has been shown to exist between the number of transfusions and the likelihood of developing refractoriness to transfusion. Shulman in 1966 (64) reported the relationship between the number of transfusions and the frequency of occurrence of detectable antibodies. In patients receiving less than 10 transfusions only 5% had detectable antibodies, whereas in patients receiving greater than 100 transfusions 80% had developed antibodies. Eys in 1978 reported a progressive decrease in the effectiveness of platelet transfusions to elevated platelet counts and control hemorrhage which was related to the number of prior transfusions (19). Adequate incremental rises in platelet counts occurred in 57% of patients who had received less than 3 prior transfusions and only in 9% of patients who had received more than 30 prior transfusions. The ability to control hemorrhage was similarly affected with hemorrhage being controlled in 62% of the patients who had received fewer than 3 prior transfusions while it was controlled in less than 10% of patients who had received greater than 20 prior transfusions. Such data would suggest the use of prophylactic platelet transfusions may compromise the ability to control thrombocytopenic hemorrhage at a future date and requires one to be thoughtful in the use of prophylactic platelet transfusions.

Several strategies have been employed and reported in addressing the problem of sensitization to transfused platelets with the resulting refractoriness to platelet transfusions. These have included using family members as platelet donors, using HL-A identical family members as donors (75), using HL-A compatible unrelated donors (44, 76), using HL-A compatible leukocyte poor platelet preparations (33) and utilizing single donors rather than multiple random donors as the source of platelets to be transfused (26). Although these approaches have been shown to be of value, further work is required to solve the problem of alloimmunization and the development of refractoriness to platelet transfusion.

A recent study (6) has more systematically analyzed factors contributing to poor incremental responses in platelet counts to platelet transfusions and while recognizing that further work is required adds to our understanding of the issues. The factor of major importance identified was HLA antibody grade. Of lesser importance were the presence of platelet-specific antibodies, the concurrent use of antibacterial antibiotics, the grade of clinical bleeding and the patient's temperature. The number of prior red cell, platelet and granulocyte transfusions, the presence of infection, age,

blood group, diagnosis, sex, pretransfusion platelet count, prior pregnancies and the use of concurrent antineoplastic drugs did not have a demonstrable effect upon the efficacy of platelet transfusions.

Additional strategies reported to be of use in preventing and/or managing refractoriness to platelet transfusions include measurement of lymphocytotoxic antibody titers (42), leukocyte depletion of transfused blood products (52, 68), ABO and HLA crossmatching of platelets (30) and the use of intravenous gamma globulin in high doses (78).

GRANULOCYTE TRANSFUSIONS

Infection is a common problem and major cause of death in patients with granulocytopenia of a variety of etiologies and frequently is encountered in patients with malignancy with decreased granulocyte counts being the result of both the disease process and its treatment with radiation and chemotherapy. The risk of infection is roughly proportional to the granulocyte count (7). At granulocyte counts greater than 1,000 the incidence of infection is not significantly increased above that seen in patients with normal granulocyte counts but progressively increases as the granulocyte count falls below 1,000. The incidence and severity of infections relate not only to the absolute granulocyte count but also to the duration of the granulocytopenia, increasing with more prolonged granulocytopenia. The overall status of the immune system likewise contributes with infection being more likely with concurrent immune suppression.

The potential usefulness of the transfusion of leukocytes in neutropenic infected patients was suggested in the 1960's when granulocytes from patients with chronic myelogenous leukemia were transfused into leukopenic patients (48). Subsequently, several trials utilizing granulocytes obtained by continuous flow centrifugation and filtration leukopheresis were conducted and suggested the efficacy of such transfusions in infected neutropenic patients (17, 28, 45). Randomized trials utilizing granulocytes collected by continuous flow centrifugation (34, 69) and filtration leukophoresis (3, 37) likewise suggested the efficacy of granulocyte transfusions in patients with sepsis. Some conflicting data, however, exists and at least one trial failed to document a benefit of transfusion of granulocytes into patients with neutropenia and fever (22).

The precise role and indications for granulocyte transfusions in the treatment of infected neutropenic patients is not well defined. Generally, leukocyte transfusions are considered for patients with severe neutropenia with documented infections, unresponsive to appropriate antibiotics. In deciding to initiate granulocyte transfusions, in addition to the above, consideration should also be given to the type and severity of infection, expected duration of the neutropenia and the overall status of the patient (35).

Granulocyte transfusions, in addition to their use as an adjunct to antibiotic treatment of infections in neutropenic patients, have been utilized in a prophylactic setting in severely neutropenia patients. The apparent ability of prophylactic granulocyte transfusions to decrease the incidence in infection has been shown (12), however, survival of patients so treated was not significantly improved. By contrast another study (73) failed to demonstrate a statistically significant improvement in infection rate among patients treated with prophylactic transfusions and moreover noted an increased incidence of pneumonia and cytomegalovirus infection and showed, like the prior study, no survival benefit to prophylactic use of granulocytes. In addition, prophylactic transfusions of granulocytes have been demonstrated to be associated with increased numbers of transfusion reactions, fevers, pulmonary infiltrates and refractoriness to platelet transfusion as the result of alloimmunization (61).

The role of granulocyte transfusions in support of neutropenic patients is changing and is likely to continue to change. The current trend has been one of using granulocyte transfusions infrequently. Improvements in antibiotic therapy and changes in the treatment strategies of malignancies are likely to alter the requirement for granulocyte support and dictate that the indications for the use of granulocytes be reevaluated. In addition potential future improvements in the collection and storage of granulocytes may likewise alter their effectiveness and thus the indications for their use.

REFERENCES

1. Abramson N, Eisenberg PD, Aster RH: Post-transfusion purpura: immunologic aspects and therapy. *N Engl J Med* 291:1163, 1974
2. Adamson J, Hilman RD: Blood volume and plasma protein replacement following acute blood loss in man. *JAMA* 205:63, 1968
3. Alavi JB, Root RK, Djerassi I, Evans AE, Gluckman SJ, MacGregor RR, Guerry D, Schreiber AD, Shaw JM, Koch P, Cooper RA: A randomized clinical trial of granulocyte transfusions for infection of acute leukemia. *N Engl J Med* 296:706, 1977
4. Barton JC: Non hemolytic, non infectious transfusion reactions. *Seminars in Hematology* 18:95,1981
5. Betzhold J, Hong R: Fatal graft-versus-host disease after a small leukocyte transfusion in a patient with lymphoma and varicella. *Pediatrics* 62:63, 1978.
6. Bishop JF, McGrath K, Wolf MM, Mathews JP, De Luise T, Holdsworth R, Yuen K, Veale M, Whiteside MG, Cooper IA, Szer J: Clinical factors influencing the efficacy of pooled platelet transfusions. *Blood* 71:383, 1988
7. Bodey GP, Buckley M, Sather YS, Freireich EJ: Quantitative relationships between circulating leukocytes and infections in patients with acute leukemia.*Ann Intern Med* 64:328, 1966
8. Butler TP, Gullino PM: Quantitation of cell shedding into efferent blood of mammary adenocarcinoma. *Cancer Research* 35:512, 1975
9. Button LN, DeWolf WC, Newburger PE, Jacobson MS, Kevy SV: The effects of irradiation on blood components. *Transfusion* 21:419, 1981
10. Cavins JA, Farber S, and Roy AJ: Transfusion of fresh platelet concentrates to adult patients with thrombocytopenia. *Transfusion* 8:24, 1968
11. Cimo PL, Aster RH: Post-transfusion purpura. *N Engl J Med* 287:290, 1972
12. Clift RA, Sanders JE, Thomas ED, Williams B, Buckner CD: Granulocyte transfusions for the prevention of infection in patients receiving bone marrow transplants. *N Engl J Med* 298:1052, 1978
13. Cohen D, Weinstein H, Mihm M, Yankee R: Nonfatal graft-versus-host disease occurring after transfusion with leukocytes and platelets obtained from normal donors. *Blood* 53:1053, 1979

14. Conrad ME: Disease transmissible by blood transfusion: viral hepatitis and other infectious disorders. *Seminars in Hematology* 18:122, 1981
15. Curran JW, Lawrence DN, Jaffe H, Kaplan JE, Zyla LD, Chamberland M, Weinstein R, Lui KJ, Schonberger LB, Spira TJ, Alexander WJ, Swinger G, Ammann A, Solomon S, Auerbach D, Mildvan D, Stoneburner R, Jason JM, Haverkos HW, Evatt BL: Acquired immunodeficiency syndrome (AIDS) associated with transfusions. *N Engl Med* 310:6° '984
16. Dinsmore RE, Straus DJ, Pollack MS, Woodruff JM, Garrett TJ, Young CW, Clarkson BD, Dupont B: Fatal-graft-versus-host disease following blood transfusion in Hodgkin's disease documented by HLA typing. *Blood* 55;831, 19XX
17. Djerassi I, Kim JS, Suvansi J: Filtration leukopheresis: principles and techniques of harvesting and transfusion of filtered granulocytes and monocytes. *Proceedings of the International Symposium on Leukocyte Separation and Transfusions*. London, England, New York, Academic Press, 1974
18. Duke WW: The relation of blood platelets to hemorrhagic disease: descriptive of a method for determining the bleeding time and coagulation time and report of three cases of hemorrhagic disease relieved by transfusion. *JAMA* 55:1185, 1910
19. Eys JV, Thomas D, Olivos B: Platelet use in pediatric oncology: a review of 393 transfusions. *Transfusion* 18:169, 1978
20. Feinstone SM, Kapikian AZ, Purcell RH, Alater HJ, Holland PV: Transfusion-associated hepatitis not due to viral hepatitis type A or B.*N Engl J Med* 292:767, 1975
21. Ford JM, Cullen, MH, Lucey JJ, Tobias JS, Lister TA: Fatal-graft-versus-host disease following transfusion of granulocytes from normal donors. *Lancet* 1167, 1976
22. Fortuny IE, Bloomfield CD, Hadlock DC, Goldman A, Kennedy BJ, McCullough JJ: Granulocyte transfusion: a controlled study in patients with acute nonlymphocytic leukemia. *Transfusion* 15:548, 1975
23. Freireich EJ: Effectiveness of platelet transfusion in leukemia and aplastic anemia. *Transfusion* 6:50, 1966
24. Freireich EJ, Kliman A, Gaydos LA, Mantel N, Frei E: Response to repeated platelet transfusion from the same donor. *Ann Intern Med* 59:277,1963
25. Gaydos LA, Freireich EJ, Mantel N: The quantitative relation between platelet count and hemorrhage in patients with acute leukemia.*N Engl J Med* 266:905, 1962
26. Gmur J, von Felten A, Osterwalder B, Honegger H, Hormann A, Sauter C, Deubelbeiss K, Berchtold W, Metaxas M, Scali G, Frick PG: Delayed alloimmunization using random single donor platelet transfusions: a prospective study in thrombocytopenic patients with acute leukemia. *Blood* 62:473, 1983
27. Goldfinger D: Acute hemolytic transfusion reactions – a fresh look at pathogenesis and considerations regarding therapy. *Transfusion* 17:85, 1977
28. Graw RG Jr, Herzig G, Perry S, Henderson ES: Normal granulocyte transfusion therapy of septicemia due to gram-negative bacteria. *N Engl J Med* 287:367, 1972
29. Harker LA, Slichter SH: The bleeding time as a screening test for evaluation of platelet function. *N Engl J Med* 287:155, 1972
30. Heal JM, Blumberg N, Masel D: An evaluation of cross-matching, HLA, and ABO matching for platelet transfusions to refractory patients. *Blood* 70:23, 1987
31. Heinrich D, Mueller-Eckhardt C, Stier W: The specificity of leukocyte and platelet alloantibodies in sera of patients with non-hemolytic transfusion reactions. *Vox Sang* 25:442, 1973
32. Hersh EM et al.: Causes of death in acute leukemia. *JAMA* 193:105, 1965
33. Herzig RH, Herzig GP, Bull MI, Decter JA, Lohrmann HP, Stout F, Yankee RA, Graw RG Jr: Correction of poor platelet transfusion responses with leukocyte-poor HLA-A-matched platelet concentrates. *Blood* 46:743, 1975
34. Herzig RH, Herzig GP, Graw RG Jr, Bull MI, Ray KK:

Successful granulocyte transfusion therapy for gram-negative septicemia. *N Engl J Med* 296:701, 1977

35. Higby DJ, Burnett D: Granulocyte transfusions: current status. *Blood* 55:2, 1980

36. Higby DJ, Cohen E, Holland JF, Sinks L: The prophylactic treatment of thrombocytopenic leukemic patients with platelets: a double blind study. *Transfusion* 14:440, 1974

37. Higby DJ, Yates JW, Henderson ES, Holland JF: Filtration leukopheresis for granulocyte transfusion therapy. *N Engl J Med* 292:761, 1975

38. Holt PDJ, Tandy NP, Anstee DJ: Screening of blood donors for IgA deficiency: a study of the donor population of South-West England. *J Clin Path* 30:1007, 1977

39. Huestis DW: Anti-IgA in blood donors. *Transfusion* 16:289, 1976

40. Hutchin P: History of blood transfusion: a tercentennial look. *Surgery* 64:685, 1968

41. Koistinen J: Selective IgA deficiency in blood donors. *Vox Sang* 29:192, 1975

42. Lee EJ, Schiffer CA: Serial measurement of lymphocytotoxic antibody and response to nonmatched platelet transfusions in alloimmunized patients. *Blood* 70:1727, 1987

43. Liotta LA, Kleinerman J, Saidel GM: The significance of hematogenous tumor cell clumps in the metastatic process. *Cancer Research* 36:889, 1976

44. Lohrmann HP, Bull MI, Decter JA, Yankee RA, Graw RG: Platelet transfusions from HL-A compatible unrelated donors to alloimmunized patients. *Ann Intern Med* 80:9, 1974

45. McCredie KB, Freireich EJ, Hester JP: Leukocyte transfusion therapy for patients with host-defense failure. *Transplant Proc* 5:1285, 1973

46. Meltz DJ, David DS, Bertles JF, deCiutiis AC: Delayed hemolytic transfusion reactions with renal failure. *Lancet* 1348, 1971

47. Moore SB, Taswell HF, Pinedia AA, Sonnenberg CL: Delayed hemolytic transfusion reactions. *Amer Jour Clin Path* 74:94, 1980

48. Morse EE, Freireich EJ, Carbone PP: The transfusion of leukocytes from donors with chronic myelocytic leukemia to patients with leukopenia. *Transfusion* 6:183, 1966

49. Murphy S, Koch PA, Evans AE: Randomized trial of prophylactic vs. therapeutic platelet transfusion in childhood acute leukemia. *Clin Research* 24:379A, 1976

50. Myhre BA: Fatalities from blood transfusion. *JAMA* 244:1333, 1980

51. National Institutes of Health Consensus Development Conference Statement: Perioperative Red Cell Transfusion. Vol. 7, Number 4, June 27–29, 1988

52. O'Donnell I, Nowicki B, Hill LR: Prevention of refractoriness using filtered blood products. *Blood* 71:1402, 1988

53. Parkman R, Mosier D, Umansky I, Cochran W, Carpenter CB, Rosen FS: Graft versus host disease after intrauterine and exchange transfusion for hemolytic disease of the newborn. *N Engl J Med* 290:359, 1974

54. Parpat AK: Whole blood preservation. *J Clin Invest* 26:641, 1947

55. Pineda AA, Brzica SM, Taswell HF Jr: Hemolytic transfusion reaction, recent experience in a large blood bank. *Mayo Clin Proc* 53:378, 1978

56. Pineda AA, Taswell HF, Brzica SM Jr: Delayed hemolytic transfusion reaction, an immunologic hazard of blood transfusion. *Transfusion* 18:1, 1978

57. Rabiner SF, Helbert JR, Lopas H, Friedman LH: Evaluation of stroma-free hemoglobin solution for use as a plasma expander. *J Exp Mex* 126:1127, 1967

58. Relihan M, Litwin MS: Effects of stroma free hemoglobin solution on clearance rate and renal function. *Surgery* 71:395, 1972

59. Rosen RC, Huestis DW, Corrigan JJ Jr: Acute leukemia and granulocyte transfusion: fatal graft-versus-host reaction following transfusion of cells obtained from normal donors. *Journ Ped* 93:268, 1978

60. Roy AJ, Jaffe N, Djerassi J: Prophylactic platelet transfusions in children with acute leukemia: a dose response study. *Transfusion* 13:283, 1973

61. Schiffer CA, Aisner J, Daly PA, Schimpff SC, Wiernik PH: Alloimmunization following prophylactic granulocyte transfusion. *Blood* 54:766, 1979

62. Schmidt PJ, Holland PV: Pathogenesis of the acute renal failure associated with incompatible transfusion. *Lancet* 2:1169, 1967

63. Shulman NR, Aster RH, Leitner A *et al.*: Immunoreactions involving platelets. Post-transfusion purpura due to a complement-fixing antibody against genetically controlled platelet antigen: a proposed mechanism for thrombocytopenia and its relevance in "autoimmunity" *J Clin Invest* 40:1597, 1961

64. Shulman NR: Immunological considerations attending platelet transfusion. *Transfusion* 6:39, 1966

65. Slichter SJ: Controversies in platelet transfusion therapy. *Ann Rev Med* 31:509, 1980

66. Slichter SJ, Harker LA: Hemostasis in malignancy. *Ann NY Acad Sci* 230:252, 1974

67. Slichter SJ, Harker LA: Thrombocytopenia: mechanisms and management of defects in platelet production. *Clinics in Haematology* 7:523, 1978

68. Van Prooijen HC, Riemens TI, Akkerman JW: Clinical experience with transfusion of leukocyte-poor platelet concentrates prepared by filtration with prostacyclin. *Blood* 70:243, 1987

69. Vogler WR, Winton EV: A controlled study of the efficacy of granulocyte transfusions in patients with neutropenia. *Am J Med* 63:548, 1977

70. Vyas GN, Perkins HA, Yang YM, Basantani GK: Healthy blood donors with selective absence of immunoglobulin A: prevention of anaphylactic transfusion reactions caused by antibodies to IgA. *J Lab Clin Med* 85:838, 1975

71. Ward HN: Pulmonary infiltrates associated with leukoagglutinin transfusion reactions. *Ann Intern Med* 73:689, 1970

72. Weisberg JL, Linker CA: Prednisone therapy of post-transfusion purpura. *Ann Intern Med* 100:76, 1984

73. Winston DJ, Ho WG, Gale RP: Prophylactic granulocyte transfusions during chemotherapy of acute non-lymphocytic leukemia. *Ann Intern Med*: 94:616, 1981

74. Wintrobe MM, Lee GR, Boggs DR, Bithel TC, Foerster J, Athens JW, Lukens JN: *Clinical Hematology* Eighth Edition, Philadelphia, Lea & Febiger, 1981

75. Yankee RA, Grumet FC, Rogentine GN: Platelet transfusion therapy. *N Engl J Med* 281:1208, 1969

76. Yankee RA, Graff KS, Dowling R, Henderson ES: The selection of unrelated compatible platelet donors by lymphocyte HL-A matching. *N Eng J Med* 288:760, 1973

77. Zeigler Z, Murphy S, Gardner FH: Post-transfusion purpura: a heterogeneous syndrome. *Blood* 45:529, 1975

78. Zeigler ZR, Shadduck RK, Rosenfeld CS, Mangan KF, Winklestein A, Oral A, Ramsey GE, Duquesnoy RJ: High-dose intravenous gamma globulin improves responses to single-donor platelets in patients refractory to platelet transfusion. *Blood* 70:1433, 1987

18

THE SPHYGMOCHRON FOR CHRONOBIOLOGIC BLOOD PRESSURE AND HEART RATE ASSESSMENT IN CANCER PATIENTS

JULIA HALBERG, GERMAINE CORNÉLISSEN, FRANZ HALBERG, FRANCINE HALBERG AND ERNA HALBERG

INTRODUCTION

Chronobiometry (11, 15), a subdiscipline of chronobiology*, serves, among other uses, for cardiovascular assessment of a cancer patient. This approach is advocated for everyone, in order to obtain individualized reference standards in health. The assessment of a reliable chronobiologic mean (the **m**idline-**e**stimating **s**tatistic **o**f **r**hythm, briefly the MESOR) is particularly pertinent in the case of heart rate for patients with cancer who are treated with doxorubicin, where it can serve as a gauge of cardiotoxicity. The purpose of this chapter is to introduce the chronobiologic approach to the measurement of blood pressure and heart rate and to distinguish it from any conventional 24-hour ambulatory monitoring. The 24-hour profile (carried out without chronobiologic analyses) is a valuable yet incomplete substitute for the conventional casual spotchecks, currently practiced for convenience rather than at pertinent times.

CASUAL MEASUREMENTS

In measuring blood pressure, a conventional approach seeks to identify values that are too high or too low with respect to time-unspecified reference standards (35, 39). This *conventional* inquiry based on casual spotchecks can be questioned as wasteful (18). Indeed, the outcome of large-scale clinical trials such as the Australian Therapeutic Trial in Mild Hypertension (see 18 for discussion) reflects the status quo. Out of nearly 2,000 individuals in this study who received a placebo, 48% responded to this 'treatment', most of them within less than a year. This fact renders that 'office-hypertension' or 'white-coat hypertension' associated with the excitement of visits to a physician's office leads to the entry into large-scale studies of many false positive cases (5, 18, 38, 39). Taking '**the**' blood pressure at health fairs or in shopping centers is a put-on (18). The physician can consult at least the personal and familial history of high blood pressure and/or related disease.

The placebo effect in studies such as the Australian trial (18) may be contributed in part by a substantial error in diagnosis, not only at the outset of a study (false positives entering the study), but also by false negative diagnoses contributing to the outcome at the completion of a study.

The outcome is somewhat less ambiguous in those studies relying on endpoints such as morbidity and mortality; yet in these cases as well, the uncertainty associated with the diagnosis at the entry into the study may greatly complicate or even invalidate the outcome (18). Whether individuals who respond to stimuli such as a physical examination by blood pressure elevation are at an increased risk remains a matter for further chronobiologic research. Such individuals may already reveal an alteration of dynamic rhythm characteristics as a harbinger of subsequent MESOR-hypertension (17, 127).

Ambulatory blood pressure monitoring, ABPM

Indications for ambulatory blood pressure monitoring have been restricted to special groups of patients, notably those with 'borderline hypertension' for whom office and home measurement disagree markedly. Certain basic questions have been raised before recommending ABPM for routine diagnostic use in the clinical setting. Among these questions, Weber, notwithstanding earlier chronobiologic contributions (3, 39), points to the difficulty of interpreting the data ABPM generates (38). The computation of mean values and the inspection of a single 24-hour record, which can hardly predict a given pattern's uncertainty on subsequent days, indeed may be improved by computing the percentage of measurements above some arbitrary limit as an assessment of load (38). Critical limits should, however, be adjusted to account for the predictable variability in blood pressure. Moreover, visual inspection alone cannot resolve sensitive parameters that may be informative in their own right. Restriction of monitoring to 24 hours and to special categories of individuals, a useful first step, may lead *a priori* to an as-yet indeterminate number of false negative and false positive diagnoses and should be replaced by more general and extensive chronobiologic approaches discussed below. Since chronobiologic methodology will also focus on a rhythm alteration more broadly, cost-effectiveness may thereby be improved, rather than violated. The objective clarification of this point is an urgent matter of research.

Chronobiology

Chronobiologists advocate, for everyone, cancer patients included, both automatic monitoring and the interpretation of (even single time-specified and) serial measurements in

---

* Chronobiology is the study (*logos*) of time (*chronos*) in the fabric of life (*bios*), characterized by rhythms, defined as algorithmically validated, reproducibly recurring dynamics (11).

P.V. Woolley (ed.), Cancer management in Man: Biological Response Modifiers, Chemotherapy, Antibiotics, Hyperthermia, Supporting Measures
© 1989. Kluwer Academic Publishers, Dordrecht.

the light of time-varying reference standards. Monitoring for at least 48 hours, if possible, is advocated since two 24-hour profiles can have means which differ substantially (4, 18). Special chronobiologic methods serve for analyses beyond the computation of conventional means (over 24 hours and separately for the day and the night spans), standard deviations and coefficients of variation, the inspection of data for the determination of the peak and the nadir, and a comparison of all values with time-unspecified limits such as 140/90 mm Hg. Chronobiologic analyses yield new endpoints that allow predictions with estimates of the uncertainties involved (3, 4, 5, 7, 11, 15, 17, 18, 25, 27, 36).

Parametric and non-parametric endpoints

Some of the new endpoints are inferential statistical *parameters*: an improved 24-h mean, the MESOR; the amplitude (half the total predictable difference between high and low values); the acrophase (an indication of the times when high values are more likely to occur overall); and the period. Confidence intervals provide some measure of uncertainty, while 90% prediction limits (chronodesms) serve as reference limits for dynamic characteristics of change. The MESOR is superior to the arithmetic mean as a location index when measurements are unequally spaced. For equally-spaced measurements, the MESOR is identical to the mean, yet when the data are characterized by a rhythm, the MESOR has a smaller uncertainty than that of the arithmetic mean. For the individual patient, the effect of a treatment may be rigorously validated by a MESOR test, when a comparison of means by a t-test fails to achieve this task. Nonparametric features of numerical integration over time include time-tension products reflecting the extent of any excess (or deficit), the time when excess (or deficit) is most likely to occur and the duration of elevation (or deficit) within a 24-h day. These endpoints are obtained by a comparison of the patient's profile with reference chronodesms also serving for the interpretation of single time-specified measurements (18).

The sphygmochron

There are charts called the long and short form of the 'sphygmochron' (sfig' ● mo ● kron). **Sphygm** denotes a relation to the circulation – a sphygmomanometer is the device used to measure blood pressure – and **chron** (from *chronos*) refers to a rigorous evaluation over time. The sphygmochron is a computer-prepared comparison of a given individual's data with those of clinically healthy individuals of the same age and gender (peers), if not with earlier data of the same subject. The reference data base is summarized as time-specified ranges or regions for single values or rhythm parameters, which can involve more components (harmonics) than the 24- and 12-h cosine curves, the most prominent features in the circadian waveform of most individuals.

A computer helps to fill out the sphygmochron, using the blood pressure and heart rate measurements collected over at least two full days, and for longer spans if necessary. The computer calculates the circadian rhythm parameters and

any measure of excess or deficit. These characteristics indicate, for the individual patient, whether values or the characteristics computed from them are within the time-varying peer group limits or outside these chronodesms. Values outside the chronodesms are of interest as an estimate of the amount of time and the extent to which an individual's blood pressure or heart rate will be deviant, perhaps as a function of chemotherapy, increasing the risk of health problems. The 24-hour time-tension product assessing excess should be less than 50 mm Hg × h over 24 hours. If this is not the case, interventions should be recommended in order to achieve this goal.

The sphygmochron can help the physician prescribe timing as well as dosing. Medication can be taken in such a way as to lower blood pressure or heart rate at the times when the individual would have high values, if left untreated. This timing of treatment not only makes the medication more effective, it also avoids reducing the blood pressure at times when it is already low, leading to the dizziness many people experience when taking medication for high blood pressure. A follow-up sphygmochron can be completed while one takes medication, often allowing the physician to prescribe the timing of drugs in order to reduce or reschedule dosages and help prevent undesirable or harmful side-effects. Timing antihypertensive treatment is particularly indicated in the case of amplitude-hypertension (18, 27) or when insufficient conventional treatment by drugs reduces the MESOR but enlarges the amplitude, the extent of predictable variation (18).

A sphygmochron should be used routinely

Cancer patients, among others, might appear to be well-treated for high blood pressure, yet have (undetected) undesirably high pressures or fast heart rates at odd times. Alternatively, one may be overtreated by antihypertensive medication when actually much less medication is needed, if given at the right time.

To summarize, features of the chronobiologic approach include: 1. monitoring all rather than a select group of individuals to obtain individualized reference standards; 2. starting monitoring early in life, preferably at birth (17, 18); 3. monitoring over at least a 48-h span; 4. interpreting the record by reference to chronobiologic standards relying on living healthy peers.

The following clinical case serves for the purpose of illustrating the application of chronobiologic methodology, including a demonstration of tests of statistical significance applicable to the given patient, as a step toward rendering the art of treatment into a science. With the availability of ambulatory monitors, the test for statistical significance of a change in blood pressure or heart rate should always be considered, in addition to the also-indispensable consideration of clinical significance.

CLINICAL CASE

A 39-year-old woman, diagnosed ∼ 1.5 years earlier to have elevated blood pressure, was treated daily (in the morning) for this condition with 12.5 mg of spironolactone and

Table 1. Cardiovascular profiles of a 39-year-old woman treated for metastatic breast cancer and high blood pressure*

Profile #	Date (Aug. 1982)	Cosinor results				
		MESOR ± SE		Amplitude	(95% Cl)	Acrophase (95% Cl) ($360° \equiv 24\,h; 0° = 00^{00}$)
Systolic BP						
1	1–2	123.9 ± 0.9	11.9		(9.5, 14.4)	−270° (−258, −282)
2	7–8	114.2 ± 0.9	8.2		(5.6, 10.9)	−230° (−213, −248)
3	20–21	116.6 ± 0.8	13.6		(11.5, 15.8)	−276° (−268, −285)
Diastolic BP						
1	1–2	79.3 ± 0.6	8.2		(6.5, 9.8)	−249° (−237, −261)
2	7–8	72.1 ± 0.7	7.5		(5.3, 9.7)	−195° (−179, −211)
3	20–21	76.2 ± 0.7	9.7		(7.7, 11.6)	−291° (−279, −304)
Heart rate						
1	1–2	76.6 ± 0.7	6.8		(4.8, 8.8)	−211° (−195, −228)
2	7–8	78.2 ± 0.9	12.3		(9.8, 14.8)	−213° (−202, −224)
3*	20–21	85.8 ± 0.7	6.4		(4.6, 8.3)	−261° (−246, −277)

* Blood pressure (BP) in mm Hg; heart rate in beats/min. N of measurements are 102, 85 and 85 for profiles 1, 2 and 3, respectively. State 5 months after removal of the left breast and adjuvant chemotherapy, including a total of 300 mg of doxorubicin. Three around-the-clock profiles are summarized above, one 15 and another 22 days after the last oncologic combination treatment, Rxo (with 50 mg [cardiotoxic] doxorubicin, 500 mg cytoxan and 1.5 mg vincristine) and a third profile 3 days after another course of the same Rxo. The patient received concomitant daily treatment with 12.5 mg of spironolactone and 12.5 mg of hydrochlorothiazide, continued unchanged throughout span investigated. P from zero-amplitude test for rhythm detection < .001 in each (not shown). For inter-profile changes see Table 2.

12.5 mg hydrochlorothiazide (one-half tablet of 25 mg/ 25 mg of Aldactazide). In March 1982, she underwent a left mastectomy for a biopsy-proven infiltrating ductal carcinoma. At the time of surgery, 5 of 16 lymph nodes contained metastatic tumor, with the same histology as the breast neoplasm. In August 1, 1987, after having received a cumulative dose of 300 mg doxorubicin, the patient's blood pressure and heart rate were monitored at 10-minute intervals with a room-restricted instrument, manufactured by Nippon Colin Ltd. (Komaki, Japan), connected to a personal computer in the patient's home. Around-the-clock profiles obtained on several occasions were analyzed by chronobiologic methods.

Table 1 shows the circadian characteristics of blood pressure and heart rate for 3 consecutive profiles. A rhythm is demonstrated in each case. The model accounts for from 30 to over 50% of the total variation. Tests of changes in the circadian characteristics, shown in Table 2, reveal a decrease in blood pressure MESOR between the first and third profiles. This decrease is statistically significant but is not necessarily relevant to a dose modification, since infradian variations can bring about statistically significant changes as well. This comment also applies to a statistically significant increase in the circadian amplitude of heart rate between the first and the second profile, followed by an increase in heart rate MESOR, Figure 1. The statistical significance of a change, while it is a *sine qua non* for rigorous inferences, is not in itself a sufficient condition for biologic significance. The latter must be judged in a broader context of earlier data.

Since an increased circadian amplitude of blood pressure can be a harbinger of a MESOR increase (27), the question may be raised whether similar changes in heart rate may have been associated with the known cardiotoxicity of doxorubicin (5). The increase in the circadian amplitude of heart rate occurs, however, with a relatively long lag after the last doxorubicin treatment on July 17, and hence could be an infradian change. By contrast, the MESOR increase in the profile on August 20 occurs rather soon after doxorubicin treatment on August 17. This increase is statistically significant, as shown in Table 2 and could well be a harbinger of cardiotoxicity. Accordingly, the doxorubicin-containing treatment was replaced by methotrexate and 5-fluorouracil. By the time of the change in therapy, however, the damage to the patient's heart was apparently irreversible. A switch to other, presumably non-cardiotoxic therapy notwithstanding, the patient died ~5 months later of congestive heart failure.

This clinical case demonstrates the feasibility, by 1982, of chronobiologic cardiovascular home monitoring prompting modifications of the treatment. It is recommended that the cardiovascular monitoring of cancer (and other) patients receiving potentially cardiotoxic treatment be implemented by ambulatory monitoring at the outside and followed longitudinally (rather than only by 48-hour profiles, as in Fig. 1) for the early detection of cardiotoxicity (5) and a timely change in medication, if need be. Such longitudinal monitoring is the more important since it can assess the extent of spontaneous change in a given subject. In the clinical case discussed herein, if we restrict our attention to the three profiles compared in Tables 1–2, one is certainly led to believe that the MESOR increase was a result of cardiotoxicity (5). Figure 1, however, shows a broader picture. It reveals a lower heart rate MESOR after discontinuance of the doxorubicin-containing treatment, on September 9, as anticipated. On September 11 and again on September 25, however, following a different, presumably non-cardiotoxic treatment, a large heart rate MESOR is again seen. In this case, it cannot be decided whether, on September 25 and October 4, one is dealing with an expression of congestive

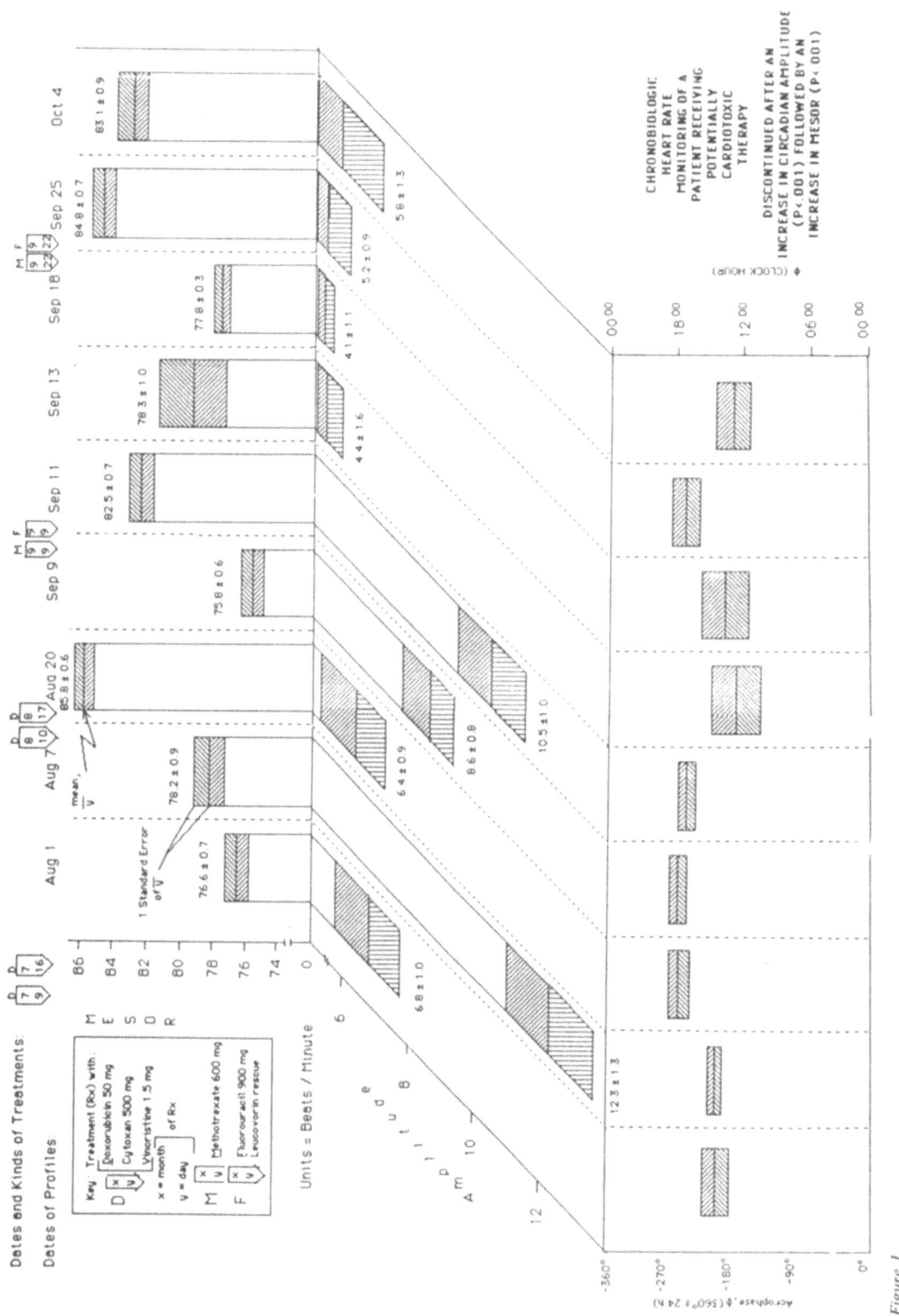

Figure 1.

heart failure or with a spontaneous variation. Had one had serial MESORs in longitudinal studies with around-the-clock monitoring, each day from the start of treatment, one could have tested statistically whether a given change in a rhythm characteristic (MESOR, amplitude or acrophase) was within or outside the limits of individualized standards of infradian variation. In such prospective studies, the changes in MESOR may be much more reliably interpreted on an individualized basis. Miniaturized instrumentation for such purposes is within the state of the art, even if it is not commercially available. Such instrumentation will be required if death from the cardiotoxic chemotherapy is to be prevented by timely action. Results such as those in Table 1 and 2 should be routinely given on the back of follow-up sphygmochrons, to assess the time course of a condition, as in this case, and in particular the success or failure of a given treatment.

TASKS AHEAD

Very often in medicine and more so in facing a patient with coexisting disease conditions, such as the infiltrating ductal carcinoma and high blood pressure in the clinical case discussed above, a variety of medical issues have to be addressed. In this particular case, the cardiotoxicity of the previously prescribed doxorubicin, apart from the *fait accompli* of prior treatment for an elevated blood pressure, was the clinical problem that needed attention as much as the cancer treatment itself. Under the circumstances, little could be done. A diagnostic reevaluation of the 'hypertension' or of finer points such as a question of free-running vs. synchronization of the circadian cardiovascular rhythms (11, 20) was beyond the scope of a consultation, nor was there any opportunity to consider chronotherapy for high blood pressure (6, 40) or of cancer (21).

A broader perspective of the tasks on hand is the more important. One should consider what could have been done by treatment initiated earlier and chronobiologically. One may ask what research must focus on in order to eventually prevent both disease conditions. For prevention as well as treatment, rhythms with several frequencies have been found to be relevant in the clinical case in this chapter, as in the other contributions on approaches by chronobiology to cancer in this book (5, 9, 29, 30). Today, circadian rhythms start to be emphasized and exploited. But optimization

according to infradian rhythms should also become practical in medicine.

From a chronoepidemiologic viewpoint, the circannual amplitude of prolactin and TSH have been related to the risk of developing breast cancer (19, 37) and the circannual amplitude of aldosterone to cardiovascular disease risk (19). These results stem from international studies of clinically healthy women of 3 age groups studied around-the-clock in each season. The circannual amplitude of plasma prolactin is low and that of plasma TSH is high in women at high risk of developing breast cancer (19). In adult women with fibrocystic disease of the breast, also characterized by an increased risk of developing breast cancer, there is also a damping of the circannual amplitude of plasma prolactin (37).

A model of the murine carcinogenesis, related to the prolactin secreted abundantly by an ectopic pituitary, initiated by the gland removed from its proximal neurohumoral coordination in the *sella turcica*, is interesting, since it implies that local neuroendocrine interactions are critical. Ectopic pituitary-induced carcinogenesis in the mouse breast can be reversed by no more than the addition of a hypothalamus to the ectopic pituitary (16, 21). The 'replace' approach is thus selective, since the entire brain is not required for the reversal. Hormonal cycles may be involved in these processes of early carcinogenesis and neurohumoral factors may interact in a partial or complete reversal.

From a clinical viewpoint, a given treatment may be more or less effective, depending on the circannual stage. This has been shown to be the case for oncostatic agents such as doxorubicin and cisplatin (13) as well as for cyclosporine, a drug acting upon immunity, a function also pertinent to a patient's response to cancer therapy. Lentinan, a potential immunomodulator, can modify, in either direction, the host's response to a subsequent cancerous growth (8). Depending on the circadian-circaseptan pattern of its administration, lentinan enhances or delays the growth of a subsequently implanted myeloma; and this effect depends further on the stage of circannual rhythms at treatment time. In the context of multifrequency interactions, it is interesting that some aspects of the circadian cell cycle also undergo circannual changes (31, 34). Recent results from studies on immunology and shifts of the circadian synchronizer have shown that apart from optimizing the circadian stage of treatment, benefits could be derived from repeatedly changing treatment times. Such a strategy may benefit the host by spread-

---

Figure 1. **Clinical case**. Changes in rhythm characteristics of heart rate of a patient receiving cardiotoxic treatment for metastatic breast cancer. Interpretation is difficult, notwithstanding the statistical significance of the changes occurring among the first 3 profiles shown in Table 2. The contribution of infradian rhythms cannot be ruled out. Admittedly with *a posteriori* reasoning, one may be tempted to see an increase in the circadian amplitude preceding the increase in MESOR on August 20, that could be discussed as a possible harbinger of cardiotoxicity by virtue of its occurrence promptly after the administration of cardiotoxic treatment. Results of follow-up heart rate monitoring of the patient in six additional profiles suggest that caution is warranted. It can be seen that changes occur not only before but also after discontinuation of the cardiotoxic treatment. A lasting cumulative role of the prior cardiotoxic treatment cannot be ruled out. The patient's conditioned response to a treatment that previously constituted a cardiotoxic

and other burden also comes to mind.

For statements that are valid on an individualized basis, it is important to assess spontaneous fluctuations. In this clinical case, monitoring was started so late that the changes shown in this figure cannot be separated from a trend toward congestive heart failure, which eventually killed the patient. If the spontaneous rhythmic changes could have been monitored for several months earlier, starting at least at the onset of treatment, their extent could have provided an individualized reference standard to assess treatment effects. If so, ambulatory monitoring with chronobiologic assessment, as here advocated, could have overcome a traditional dilemma in clinical treatment. Long-term monitoring (perhaps with miniaturized devices inplanted at the time of diagnosis, once these will be developed) remains the long-term goal of a chronbiologic approach to the cancer patient.

Table 2. Test of equality of rhythm characteristics in 3 blood pressure and heart rate profiles of a 39-year-old woman treated for metastatic breast cancer and high blood pressure*

Parameter(s)	df	F	P
Systolic blood pressure			
August 1–2/20–21, 1982			
MESOR, M	(1, 180)	39.05	< 0.001
amplitude, A	(1, 181)	1.07	0.302
acrophase, ϕ	(1, 175)	0.74	0.392
(A, ϕ)	(2, 181)	1.16	0.315
(M, A, ϕ)	(3, 181)	12.88	< 0.001
August 7–8/20–21, 1982			
MESOR, M	(1, 157)	3.90	0.050
amplitude, A	(1, 156)	9.84	0.002
acrophase, ϕ	(1, 121)	17.01	0.001
(A, ϕ)	(2, 164)	18.63	< 0.001
(M, A, ϕ)	(3, 164)	14.96	< 0.001
Diastolic blood pressure			
August 1–2/20–21, 1982			
MESOR, M	(1, 171)	10.62	0.001
amplitude, A	(1, 170)	1.30	0.256
acrophase, ϕ	(1, 179)	20.09	< 0.001
(A, ϕ)	(2, 181)	12.89	< 0.001
(M, A, ϕ)	3, 181)	11.58	< 0.001
August 7–8/20–21, 1982			
MESOR, M	(1, 163)	15.41	0.001
amplitude, A	(1, 162)	2.04	0.155
(A, ϕ)	(2, 164)	39.84	< 0.001
(M, A, ϕ)	(3, 164)	34.93	< 0.001
Heart rate			
August 1–2/7–8, 1982			
MESOR, M	(1, 169)	2.25	0.135
amplitude, A	(1, 164)	11.76	0.001
acrophase, ϕ	(1, 165)	0.02	0.886
(A, ϕ)	2, 181)	6.16	0.003
(M, A, ϕ)	(3, 181)	5.33	0.002
August 7–8/20–21, 1982			
MESOR, M	(1, 152)	49.73	< 0.001
amplitude, A	(1, 152)	14.01	< 0.001
acrophase, ϕ	(1, 146)	19.86	< 0.001
(A, Pf)	(2, 164)	19.01	< 0.001
(M, A, ϕ)	3, 164)	31.36	< 0.001
August 1–2/20–21, 1982			
MESOR, M	(1, 181)	91.68	< 0.001
amplitude, A	(1, 181)	0.07	0.795
acrophase, ϕ	(1, 181)	14.3	< 0.001
(A, ϕ)	(2, 181)	9.27	0.001
(M, A, ϕ)	(3, 181)	40.37	< 0.001

* See footnote to Table 1.

ing defense mechanisms allowing not only for 'killing the last cell' (2), but what may be even more important, for the first cell kill.

A basis for dramatic interindividual differences (in a population) in proneness to cancer may be found in the intra-individual spectrum of host rhythms already mapped at all levels of organization pertinent to carcinogenesis. The cell cycle (31, 34), the immune surveillance of the cell cycle (2, 26), and the neuroendocrine feedsidewards modulating defense (20), are pertinent. Rhythm stages are critical for all these functions. They also affect a patient's response to treatment, both from a therapeutic viewpoint (9, 12) and from the viewpoint of toxic side effects (5, 21, 23). Rhythm stages have also been shown to be critical for carcinogenesis, for instance in the case of the circadian susceptibility to DMBA (21, 24). As noted earlier, rhythm stages have even been shown to be important to determine the risk of developing breast cancer and other diseases. The hours of changing resistance have been amply documented in different laboratories (14, 28, 32, 33). The response to whole-body irradiation, i.e., the dose that kills 50% of the animals in 30 days (LD_{30}^{50}), also changes drastically as a function of the host's circadian timing (10, 28), as does the nonlethal body weight loss associated with exposure to partial body irradiation. Chronorisk, as a concept, may well apply to carcinogenic, much lower doses of radiation, as it does to a host of other agents. This is the more likely since the circadian stage dramatically determines the outcome of chemical carcinogenesis (24). The concept of chronorisk is thus found to be critical at all stages, not only treatment but also induction and promotion, and even earlier.

This state of affairs leads us to ask whether early chronorisk assessment may not be utilized with an aim of prevention. To turn back to blood pressure, differences in the dynamics of blood pressure may already be detected at birth. A larger circadian and circaseptan amplitude characterizes babies with a positive as compared to those with a negative family history of high blood pressure. The two groups may differ even in their circannual modulations of the circadian blood pressure amplitude and MESOR (17, 18). Chronorisk may be formulated as a constellation of unfavorable acrophases in circadian rhythmic risk factors. Circannual rhythms modulate circadian rhythms not only in the newborn but even during pregnancy (18).

Chronobiology also aims at a timely prevention. The late John J. Bittner (discoverer of the first mammalian breast cancer agent, or virus) already emphasized, that genetic and acquired endocrine features were critical aspects of mammary carcinogenesis, interacting with the agent which bore his name (1). Intuitively, he anticipated the description of intermodulation among several frequencies characterizing rhythms that may coordinate certain natural killer cell subpopulations that patrol at the level of the cell cycle. Bittner made a major discovery by an astute observation of what happened when the progeny of mice of an inbred strain with a high breast cancer incidence were foster-nursed by animals of a strain with a low such incidence. The animals were mostly free of breast cancer. Just as Bittner's weaning experiments have been reproduced innumerable times, so a spectrum of rhythms is now amply documented (14, 32, 33). The external biologic response modifiers can and should exploit the spontaneous rhythmic changes in host response (2, 22).

Chronorisk characterizes organisms throughout life, before a cancerous process is induced, at initiation and thereafter. Endeavors to reduce such risk may be started very early in life. In the ectopic pituitary in the mouse, chronorisk can be largely reversed. Future chronobiologists are challenged to achieve the same result in human beings. The five chapters on chronobiology are dedicated to the memory of John J. Bittner, who built the first chronobiology laboratory, at the University of Minnesota.

ACKNOWLEDGEMENT

The clinical case presented in this chapter was originally summarized by us with Prof. David Kiang and Mr Robert Kelsey for the Proceedings of the 1st World Conference on Clinical Chronobiology, held in Monte Carlo, Monaco, March 17–20, 1988.

SUPPORT

U.S. Public Health Service (GM-13981 and HL-40650); Colin Medical Instruments (Komaki, Japan); Hoechst Italia Foundation (Milan, Italy); Medtronic Inc. (Minneapolis, MN, USA); Dr. h.c.Dr.h.c. Earl Bakken & Dr. Betty Sullivan Funds.

REFERENCES

1. Bittner JJ: *Texas Rep Biol Med* 10: 160–166, 1952.
2. Carandente F, Dammacco F, Halberg F (eds.) Chronoimmunomodulation by an Antimicrobial Agent, 1989. Chronobiologia 15, #1 & 2, 194 pp., 1988.
3. Carandente F, Halberg F (eds.) Chronobiology of Blood Pressure in 1985. Chronobiologia 11, #3, 152 pp., 1984.
4. Cornélissen G: In: Chronobiotechnology and Chronobiological Engineering, Scheving LE, Halberg F, Ehret CF, eds., Martinus Nijhoff, Dordrecht, The Netherlands, pp. 241–261. (See also pp. 262–269, 270–277, 278–281, 282–288, 289–298, 299–303, 304–309, and 310–317.) 1987
5. Cornélissen G, Halberg F: In: This series, HE Kaiser (ed.), Volume IX, AL Goldson (ed.), pp. 103–133, Dordrecht, Kluwer Academic Publishers, 1989.
6. Güllner HG et al.: The Lancet, p. 527, 1979.
7. Haen E, Halberg F: Deutsches Ärzteblatt 82: 3837–3948, 1985.
8. Halberg E, Halberg F: Chronobiologia 7: 95–120, 1980.
9. Halberg Francine, et al.: this volume.
10. Halberg F: *Cold Spr Harb Symp quant Biol* 25: 289–310, 1960.
11. Halberg F: *Ann Rev Physiol* 31: 675–725, 1969.
12. Halberg F: Guest Lecture, Proc 30th Ann Cong Rad, January 1977, Post-Graduate Institute of Medical Education and Research, Chandigarh, India.
13. Halberg F: In: Cellular Pacemakers, D.O. Carpentered, John Wiley & sons Inc., New York, pp. 261–297, 1982.
14. Halberg F: *Am J Anat* 168: 543–594, 1983.
15. Halberg F, Bingham C: Proc. Biopharmaceutical Section, Am Statistical Assn, Chicago, Illinois, pp. 11–32, 1987.
16. Halberg F, et al.: *Proc Soc exp Biol (N.Y.)* 102: 650–654, 1959.
17. Halberg F, et al.: *Postgrad Med* 79: 44–46, 1986.
18. Halberg F, et al.: Chronobiology of humanblood pressure. Medtronic Continuing Medical Education Seminars, 4th ed., 242 pp., 1988.
19. Halberg F, et al.: In: Neoplasms – Comparative Pathology of Growth in Animals, Plants and Man, H Kaiser ed., Williams and Wilkins, Baltimore, pp. 553–596, 1981.
20. Halberg F, et al.: *Circulation* 34: 715–717, 1966.
21. Halberg F, et al.: In: Proc. XIV Int Cong Therapeutics, Montpellier, France, L'Expansion Scientifique Française, pp. 151–196., 1977.
22. Halberg F, Halberg E: In: Pharmacokinetic Basis for Drug Treatment, LZ Benet, N Massoud, JG Gambertoglio eds., Raven Press, New York, pp. 221–248, 1984.
23. Halberg F, et al.: Experientia (Basel) 29: 909–934, 1973.
24. Halberg F, et al.: In: Biomathematics and Cell Kinetics, AJ Valleron and PDM Macdonald eds., Elservier/North-Holland Biomedical Press, Amsterdam, pp. 175–190, 1978.
25. Halberg F, Reale L, Tarquini B (eds.) Proc. II Int Symp on Chronobiologic approach to social medicine (Florence, Oct. 2, 1984). Istituto Italiano di Medicina Sociale, Rome, 1986. (See pp. 65–104, 345–366, 395–394, 417–426, 557–568, 569–574.)
26. Halberg F, et al.: In: Advances in Immunopharmacology, J Hadden L, Chedid P, Dukor F, Spreafico D, Willoughby eds., Pergamon Press, Oxford, pp. 463–478, 1983.
27. Halberg J, et al.: *Int J Chronobiol.* 7: 17–64, 1980.
28. Haus E, et al.: In: Space Biology, Tobias CA, Todd P eds., Academic Press, New York/London, 1974, pp. 435–474.
29. Hermida RC, Halberg F: this volume a.
30. Hermida RC, Halberg F: this volume b.
31. Lærum OD, et al.: *Chronobiology int.* 5: 19–35, 1988.
32. Pauly JE: *Am J Anat.* 168: 365–388, 1973.
33. Scheving LE: Endeavour 35: 66–72, 1976.
34. Sletvold O, et al.: *Mechanisms of Ageing and Development* 42: 91–104, 1988.
35. Strasser T: *J Hypertension* 4: 383–386, 1986.
36. Tarquini B (ed.) Social Diseases and Chronobiology: Proc. 3rd Int Symp Social Diseases and Chronobiology, Florence, Italy, Nov. 29, 1986, Societá Editrice Esculapio, Bologna. (See pp. 113–122, 123–128, 129–133, 135–144, 145–151, 209–220, 221–224, 225–233, 373–380 and 471–476.) 1987
37. Tarquini B, et al.: *Am J Med.* 66: 229–237, 1979.
38. Weber MA: *Mayo Clin Proc.* 63: 1151–1153, 1988.
39. Weber MA, et al.: In: Scheving LE, Halberg F, Ehret CF (eds.) Chronobiotechnology and Chronobiological Engineering. Martinus Nijhoff, The Netherlands, pp. 270–277, 1987.
40. Zaslavskaya R, et al.: Abstract III Int Symp 'Social Diseases and Chronobiology', Florence, November 29, Tarquini B, Vergassola R eds., p. 79, 1986.

19

NUTRITIONAL SUPPORT OF CANCER PATIENTS DURING CANCER PROGRESSION

TAKAO OHNUMA

Cachexia and malnutrition are among the major causes of morbidity in patients with progressive cancer. The causes of cancer-related malnutrition are multifold, and can be conveniently divided into 3 interrelated groups; anorexia, mechanical obstruction of the alimentary tract and metabolic derangements (57).

Anorexia is known to be induced by abnormalities in taste sensation (21) as well as metabolic abnormalities shown in cancer patients and in animal studies (2, 18, 42, 69, 79, 81, 83).

Food intake is impaired in cancer patients when tumors interfere mechanically with the anatomic structure and function of the gastrointestinal tract. Thus, tumors of the oropharynx, esophagus, stomach, pancreas, liver and peritoneum can compromise oral intake. Ascites and intestinal obstructions are often the initial manifestations of ovarian carcinoma. Malabsorption syndrome secondary to infiltration of the intestine by cancer, particularly lymphomas, has been described (64).

Metabolic derangements considered to be causally related to the pathogenesis of cancer cachexia are as follows (57):

(a) The elaboration of pharmacologically active tumor byproducts. Among the nonhormonal tumor byproducts affecting cell metabolism, the polypeptide isolated by Sylven appears to be important in relation to cachexia (80).

(b) Selective parasitism of the host by the tumor in the form of successful competition for substrates with limited availability (49, 53). Chemical analysis has failed, however, to convincingly demonstrate unusual shifts of any nutrient into the tumor (74).

(c) The systemic energy-losing cycle, dependent on an interplay of tumor glycolysis and host glyconeogenesis (28). High rates of glucose utilization with production of lactic acid are characteristic features of the neoplastic cell. Lactic acid so produced may be utilized for energy purposes by other tissues or transported to the liver for resynthesis to glucose. This cyclic metabolic pathway, in which glucose is converted to lactic acid by glycolysis and then reconverted to glucose in the liver, is referred to as the Cori cycle. Glucose to lactate in cancer cells yields 2 ATPs, whereas lactate to glucose in the liver requires 6 ATPs. Therefore, the cancer cell is an energy parasite. A significant increase in the Cori cycle was shown in cancer patients with progressive weight loss as compared to those without weight loss (32). Expendable protein stores appear inappropriate consumed for this purpose (67).

(d) Hypogonadism or low testosterone levels in male patients (12, 30, 66). Abnormally low levels of male hormone were described in patients with advanced cancer and correlated with weight loss and adverse outcome.

(e) Certain aspects of cachexia might be mediated by immunologic reaction (10). It is known that many patients with advanced cancer have anergic reactions to recall antigens. It is possible that the factors that produce cancer cachexia overlap those with immunologic disturbances. In cachectic animals a hypertriglyceridemic state is frequently seen and this was shown to be due to the production of cachectin, a protein secreted from macrophages, which causes systemic suppression of enzyme lipoprotein lipase (4). Recently a high degree of homology was found between the N-terminal sequence of mouse cachectin and the N-terminal sequence for human tumor necrosis factor (3). These observations may open new areas of research relating to cancer and cachexia.

(f) Complications from the treatment of cancer add to cancer cachexia. Therapeutic modalities such as systemic chemotherapy, radiation to the head and neck or abdomen may produce stomatitis, vomiting, diarrhea and a further decrease in appetite through the weeks of treatment and thereafter. Analgesic medications produce lethargy and decreased physical activity. This iatrogenically produced decrease in caloric intake accelerates the deterioration of the nutritional status in these patients.

Patients with anorexia from decreased physical activity, concomitant infection and toxicities to the alimentary tract from radio- and chemotherapy are clinically managed symptomatically for maintenance of nutritional status and quality of life (26). Such management includes the use of mouthwash for stomatitis, frequent small volume feedings, antiemetics, antibiotics, providing a dining room atmosphere and/or oral and parenteral nutritional supplement.

It would be ideal to reverse cancer-related malnutrition by correcting the underlying biochemical and/or immunological mechanisms (5). Very few attempts, however, have been made to correct the cancer-related malnutrition by correcting the proposed metabolic derangements.

Hydrazine sulfate, an inhibitor of an enzyme, phosphoenolpyruvate carboxykinase, was shown to interrupt gluconeogenesis in animals (65). This observation led to the clinical studies of hydrazine in attempts to prevent or reverse cancer-related cachexia and weight loss (see (c) above) (13, 29, 43, 78). Recent randomized studies have shown that hydrazine sulfate-treated patients had significant improvements in abnormal glucose tolerance, decrease in the rate of total glucose production and maintenance of body weight (13). It is, therefore, possible to prevent cachexia by using

196

P.V. Woolley (ed.), Cancer management in Man: Biological Response Modifiers, Chemotherapy, Antibiotics, Hyperthermia, Supporting Measures
© 1989, Kluwer Academic Publishers, Dordrecht.

hydrazine sulfate or related compounds. Whether hydrazine sulfate improves the survival of cancer patients or improves the tolerance or the efficacy of therapeutic intervention remains to be established.

Beneficial effects from anabolic steroid hormones have been reported in patients undergoing chemotherapy (14, 77). It is unclear, however, whether abnormalities in hypogonadism was corrected in these patients (see (d) above). In attempts to correct androgen abnormalities a randomized clinical trial was carried out to test whether supplements of nandrolone decanoate can influence the outcome of chemotherapy. Although the treated group experienced less weight loss (with borderline statistical significance) whether correction of gonadal function was made has not been demonstrated (14).

For the correction of cancer-related malnutrition enteral and parenteral administration of nutrient solutions has been widely carried out. The role of nutritional support in cancer patients during tumor progression should, however, be considered at several different levels.

Parenteral nutritional support in cancer patients with obstructions of the gastrointestinal tract, gastrointestinal fistula, evisceration and intraabdominal infection appears justified during and after surgery (7, 19). Although strong data is lacking, parenteral nutritional support is considered beneficial in these patients who have not been eating for at least 10 days or have lost more than 10% of their usual body weight (22, 48).

A number of nonrandomized studies claimed benefit from parenteral nutrition in cancer patients requiring surgery. Such benefit included maintenance of body weight and positive nitrogen balance, maintenance of immune status and increased wound healing. However, such claims have not been uniformly substantiated by randomized studies.

Available randomized studies asking questions of what impact the parenteral nutrition will have on the outcome of surgery are summarized in Table 1. Although 4 of 7 randomized studies claimed benefit from parenteral nutritional support it ranged from improved wound healing to decreased infection, decrease in major complications to decrease in mortality. All of these reports were, however, isolated observations and none were reproducibly significant. Indeed, Dionigi and Dominioni (22) observed an increase in the rate of major complications among patients treated with parenteral nutrition. Such adverse effects of parenteral nutrition were also reported by Brister *et al* who found, in a retrospective analysis, more pulmonary infection and longer hospital stay (9).

Only after compiling 28 published randomized studies, Klein *et al* felt that total parenteral nutrition might be useful when used preoperatively in patients with gastrointestinal tract cancer (40). Total parenteral nutrition significantly reduced major surgical complications and operative mortality in pooled population. Recently a randomized study between total parenteral nutrition and elemental diet administered by needle-catheter jejunostomy was carried out in patients who had undergone pancreatico-biliary surgery (6). Both routes of treatment provided adequate nutritional support. The latter group compared favorably with significant cost efficiency. More importantly, there has so far been no evidence that nutritional support improved survival of cancer patients after surgery as a group (68, 89). These observations indicate that indiscriminatory use of parenteral nutritional support is not justified as an adjuvant for surgery in patients with cancer.

Similar discrete considerations are needed for the nutritional support of cancer patients during radiotherapy and chemotherapy.

Pretreatment weight loss and low serum albumin in cancer patients often spell out short survival and poor tolerance to chemotherapy. Nutritional support for improvements in the performance status of cancer patients seemed possible (17, 60). Since response rates to chemotherapy and performance status were positively correlated (38, 50), nutritional support to improve the performance status and response rate was considered logical. Likewise, malnutrition and an increased rate of infection in children with malignant neoplasms have been correlated (34). Thus, the idea of nutritional support to improve malnutrition and prevent therapy-related infection seemed reasonable. Indeed, early uncontrolled trials did claim that nutritional support lessened the side effects of radiotherapy and chemotherapy while improving the outcome of therapy (16, 18). These initial observations led to extensive evaluation of nutritional support in cancer patients during therapeutic intervention and a number of prospective randomized trials were carried out.

Table 2 summarizes the results of available randomzied studies asking the question of whether parenteral nutrition influences tumor response and survival from chemotherapy and/or radiotherapy. In contrast to earlier expectations, none of these studies showed that parenteral nutrition in the currently available form could augment the response rate or survival of patients treated with radiotherapy and/or chemotherapy. In addition, reports have appeared indicating that parenteral nutritional support was detrimental. Thus, Shamberger *et al* showed that patients with parenteral nutrition had a significantly lower duration of response (72). Nixon *et al* found that patients treated with parenteral nutrition had shorter survival (56).

Available randomized studies questioning the role of nutritional support in ameliorating therapy-induced toxicities are summarized in Table 3. Although earlier studies reported favorable effects from parenteral nutritional support (35, 76), more recent studies failed to show that the support can decrease gastrointestinal, hematological and/or infectious complications of radiotherapy and/or chemotherapy. Weiner *et al* have reported that parenteral nutritional support produced considerable complications of its own which included mechanical difficulties with the catheter leading to discontinuation of nutritional support, subclavian vein thrombosis, sepsis, fluid overload, hyponatremia and hyperglycemia (87). Although parenteral nutrition groups had higher granulocyte nadirs, the difference was considered to be caused by fever and infection associated with parenteral nutritional support rather than any nutritional effect on granulopoiesis. They suggested that further studies must have a significant rationale for adjunctive use to justify the potential risk (87).

Parenteral nutrition was reported to be beneficial in children with leukemia and lymphoma who were treated with intensive chemotherapy and radiotherapy followed by autologous bone marrow transplantation. Patients who received prophylactic total parenteral nutrition engrafted donor cells

Table 1. Effects of nutritional support on surgery (randomized studies).

Senior author (year)	Tumor type	Time of support	Type of support	No. of patients	Complication	Survival	Reference
Holter (1977)	Gastrointestinal cancer	Peri	PN C[a] C[b]	30 26 28	No differences in rate of major or minor complications or mortality	NA	33
Moghissi (1977)	Esophageal cancer	Peri	PN C	10 5	PN group had no weight loss, wound healing was faster	NA	51
Heatley (1979)	Esophageal and gastric cancer	Pre	PN C	38 36	Pn group had less wound infection. No differences in anastomatic leakage or death rate	NA	31
Lim (1981)	Esophageal cancer	Pre	PN C[c]	10 10	Anastomatic leakage (1/10 *vs* 4/10), wound infection (3/10 *vs* 5/10) and operative mortality (1/10 *vs* 2/10) were higher in control	NA	45
Sako (1981)	Head and neck cancer	Pre or Post	PN C	30 32	No differences in major complication operative mortality 2/34 *vs* 0/32	60%/12 mos 86%/12 mos ($p = 0.01$)	68
Thompson (1981)	Gastrointestinal cancer	Peri	PN C[a] C[b]	12 9 20	No differences in major complications. Mortality 0/12 *vs* 0/9 *vs* 2/10	NA	82
Muller (1982)	Gastrointestinal cancer	Pre	PN C	66 59	PN group had less major complications and less mortality. No differences in the rate of wound infection or pneumonia	NA	54
Yamada (1983)	Gastric cancer	Post	PN C	11 12	PN group had increased disease-free intervals	73%/3 yr[e] 58%/3 yr	89
			PN[d] C[d]	18 16	PN group had increased disease-free intervals	55.6%/3 yr[e] 36.4%/3 yr	
Dionigi (1985)	Esophageal cancer	Peri	PN C	11 10	PN group had more major postoperative complications	NA	22
Silverman (1985)	Gastrointestinal cancer	Pre	PN C	66 59	PN group had less major postoperative complications and mortality	NA	75
Jensen (1985)	Rectal cancer	Peri	PN C	10 10	PN group had less major complications (1/10 *vs* 6/10, $p < 0.05$)	NA	36

PN: parenteral nutrition; C: control; NA: not available.
[a] Weight loss more than 10 lbs.
[b] Weight loss less than 10 lbs.
[c] Feeding gastrostomy.
[d] Treated with 5-fluorouracil.
[e] Differences are not significant.

Table 2. Effects of nutritional support on tumor response and survival from chemotherapy and/or radiotherapy (randomized studies).

Senior author (year)	Tumor type	Treatment	Type of support	No. of patients	Response	Survival	Comment	Reference
Issell (1978)	Squamous cell carcinoma of the lung	CT & IT	PN C	13 13	4 PR/13 1 PR/13	NA	Differences in response rates, NS	35
Valerio (1978)	Adenocarcinoma or transitional carcinoma of the abdomen	RT	PN C	11 9	5 PR/11 3 PR/9	NA	Differences in response rate, NS	85
Douglas (1978)	GI malignancy	RT[a]	EN C	13 17		*pancreas* 9.4 *vs* 9.5 mos *stomach* 14.5 *vs* 7.0 mos *colorectal* 15.4 *vs* 14.8 mos		25
Solassol (1979)	Ovarian carcinoma	RT	PN C	42 39		*median* 9.0 mos 8.3 mos	Differences in survival, NS	76
Van Eys (1980)	Childhood neoplasms	CT	PN C	10 9	NA NA	*outcome* 80% alive 78% alive	Differences in survival, NS	86
Kinsela (1981)	Pelvic or abdominal malignancy	RT	PN C	17 15	NA NA	*16 mos followup* 53% alive 53% alive		39
Nixon (1981)	Colorectal cancer	CT	PN C	20 25	*> 25% response* 3/20 3/25	*median* 79 days 308 days	Control patients lived longer; response rate NS	56
Jordan (1981)	Adenocarcinoma of the lung	CT	PN C	41 24	*CR + PR* 8/30 7/18	*median* 21.5 weeks[a] 28 weeks[b] 40 weeks		37
Popp (1981)	Lymphoma	CT	PN C	20 21	NA NA	69%/2 yr 66%/2 yr		63
Samuels (1981)	Testicular	CT	PN C	16 14	63% CR 79% CR	72%/2 yr 77%/2 yr		70
Valdivieso (1981)	Small cell carcinoma of the lung	CT & RT	PN C	21 28	85% CR 59% CR	71%/1 yr 55%/1 yr	Differences in response rate and survival, NS	84
Donaldson (1982)	Childhood malignancy	CT ± Adj CT	PN C	12 13	NA NA	*during study* 92% 92%		24
Ghavimi (1982)	Childhood malignancy	RT & CT	PN C	11 14	NA NA	*alive* 73% 71%		27
Levine (1982)	Sarcomas	CT or CT + RT Some with ABMT	PN C	14 18	No difference	48%/2 yr 64%/2 yr	Differences in survival, NS	44
Serrou (1982)	Small cell carcinoma of the lung	CT	PN C	19 20	10 CR/19 9 CR/20	73%/1 yr 68%/1 yr	Differences in response and survival, NS	71
Shamberger (1984)	Sarcoma	CT ± RT some with AMBT	PN C	14 18	*Response* 10/14 12/14	*2 yr 3 yr* 25% 12% 43% 43%	Duration of response significantly lower in PN group	72
Clamon (1985)	Small cell carcinoma of the lung	CT & RT	PN C	59 62	24 CR, 20 PR/50 26 CR, 32 PR/60	No difference	Differences in response rate, NS	15

CT: chemotherapy; IT: immunotherapy; RT: radiotherapy; ABMT: autologous bone marrow transplants; PN: parenteral nutrition; EN: enteral nutritional; C: control; PR: partial response; CR: complete response; NS: statistically not significant.
[a] Chemotherapy and nutritional support given together.
[b] Nutritional support prior to chemotherapy.

Table 3. Effects of nutritional support on chemotherapy and/or drug of radiation-induced toxicities (randomized studies).

Senior author (year)	Tumor type	Treatment	Type of support	No. of patients	Toxicities GI	Hematological	Infection	Comment	Ref.
Bounous (1975)	Abdominal and pelvic malignancy	RT	EN C	9 9	NA	(–)	NA	Less lymphocyte drop in EN group	5
Issell (1979)	Squamous carcinoma of the lung	CT (IT)	PN C	13 13	NA	(↑)[a]	NA	[a] After 1st course only, no changes after 2nd & 3rd course	35
Solassol (1979)	Ovarian carcinoma	RT	PN C	42 39	(↑)	NA	NA		76
Van Eys (1980)	Childhood neoplasms	CT	PN C	10 9	NA	NA	Infect(–)[b] Sepsis(↑)[b]	[b] Included non-randomized patients (total 36)	86
Nixon (1981)	Colorectal carcinoma	CT	PN C	20 25	N & V (–)	(–)	NA	PS (–)	56
Jordan (1981)	Adenocarcinoma of the lung	CT	PN C	41 24	N & V (–)	(–)	(–)	PN group had additional complications (hyperglycemia)	37
Popp (1981)	Lymphoma	CT	PN C	15 18	NA	(–)	NA	Tolerance to dosage (–)	62
Samuels (1981)	Testicular	CT	PN C	16 14	(–)	(–)	(↓)[c]	[c] PN group had more infectious complications; PN group had no weight loss	70
Valdivieso (1981)	Small cell carcinoma of the lung	CT & RT	PN C	21 28	N & V (–) mucositis (↓)[d]	(–)	(–)	[d] Days with mucositis was longer in PN group; Weight (↑); Immunological status (↑)	84
Donaldson (1982)	Childhood malignancy	RT (± CT)	PN C	12 13	N & V (–) bowel movement (–)	NA	NA	Nutritional status (↑)	24
Gharimi (1982)	Childhood malignancy	RT & CT	PN C	11 14	N & V (–) bowel movement (↓)	(↓)[e]	(↓)[f]	[e] Days with WBC < 1500/μl 52 vs 11 [f] Days with fever 110 vs 37	27
Serrou (1982)	Small cell carcinoma of the lung	CT	PN C	19 20	NA	(–)	(–)	BW (–)	71
Lioudice (1983)	Gynecologic malignancy	RT	PN(± MP) EN(± MP)	12 12	Absorption study (↑)	NA	NA	Radiographic score (↑)	46
Shamberger (1983)	Sarcomas	CT ± RT ± ABMT	PN C	12 15	NA	(–)	(–)		72
Clamson (1985)	Small cell carcinoma of the lung	CT RT	PN C	59 62	NA	(↑)[g]	(↓)	[g] Granulocyte nadir 600 vs 350/μl but PN group had more febrile episodes. See Ref. 87	15
Weiner (1985)	Small cell carcinoms of the lung	CT RT	PN C	54 62	Mucositis (–) N & V (–) Diarrhea (↓)	(–)[h]		[h] Same data as Ref. 15 and reanalyzed	87
							(↓)[i]	[i] More than 50% of patients in PN group developed PN related complications (see Table 4)	

(–), No differences in severity and/or incidence and/or length of complications between study group and control; (↑), study group had favorable effect; (↓), study group had detrimental effects; CT, chemotherapy; RT, radiotherapy; IT, immunotherapy; ABMT, autologous bone marrow transplantation; PN, parenteral nutritional support; EN, enteral nutritional support; C, control; NA, not available; PS, performance status; N & V, nausea and vomiting; BW, body weight; MP, methylprednisone.

Table 4. Complications from parenteral nutrition.

Complications from catheterization	Pneumo-, hydro- and hemothorax
	Hydromediastinum
	Central venous thrombophlebitis
	Air embolism
	Catheter embolism
	Catheter misplacement
	Subclavion artery injury
Infection	Local infection
	Sepsis
Metabolic abnormalities	Hyperosmolar dehydration
	Hypercalcemia
	Hyponatremia or Hypenatremia
	Hypophosphatemia
	Hyperchloremic acidosis
	Hyperglycemia
	Hyperosmolar coma
Hepatic dysfunction	Liver function abnormalities
	Fatty metamorphosis of the liver

3 days earlier than the control patients (88). There was, however, no difference in the two groups' clinical outcomes; mortality, duration of hospital stay, incidences of sepsis, graft *vs* host disease and return of malignancy were equivalent; the findings consistent with adult data (44, 72).

In these studies it was demonstrated that parenteral nutrition could maintain body weight, but mostly with fat and water. A gain in protein or muscle mass has not been demonstrated. It appears protein malnutrition cannot be replaced with currently practiced parenteral nutritional support. Alternative approaches such as much longer durations of parenteral nutritional support have been advocated, but available data casts strong doubt that the present form of nutritional support would decrease therapy-related complications and increase survival of cancer patients in conjunction with radiotherapy and chemotherapy. Review papers on nutritional support during therapeutic intervention in cancer patients are available (1, 8, 11, 23, 40, 41, 47, 48, 55, 59, 61).

Review of available data on parenteral nutritional support of cancer patients led to the identification of patients who are in need of nutritional support. Selected patients with gastrointestinal cancer may benefit from preoperative nutritional support. Nutritional support is also indicated in patients with intestinal obstructions who have not been eating and have lost body weight and in whom response from therapeutic modalities is expected, e.g., ovarian carcinoma. Parenteral nutrition was also reported to be of value for faster improvements of radiation-induced enteritis (46). However, they constitute only a small percentage of the cancer population. Parenteral nutritional support was also reported to be of benefit in patients with advanced and terminal cancer (52); however, these cases should be regarded as exceptional. Parenteral nutritional support is an intensive clinical care requiring physicians, pharmacists, dieticians and experienced nurses who, as a team, have to make daily rounds to evaluate nutritional status and check complications. Complications from parenteral nutritional are multiple (Table 4). Among them the complications from infection are the most problematic when long term nutri-

tional support is utilized. In addition, the cost of nutrient solutions, prolonged hospitalization and/or frequent visits to special clinic/office are formidable financial burdens.

Lastly, psychological impact from parenteral support cannot be overlooked. A case was described in which parenteral nutritional support was given. When the patient did not respond he refused to have nutritional support stopped because of fear that if it was stopped, death would soon follow. The patient was on nutritional support for several months just to prolong misery without any therapeutic gain ("umbilicus cord syndrome") (58). For these reasons careful patient selection is essential before the start of parenteral nutritional support. Therapeutic complications as well as the financial and psychologic impact on the patient and his family cannot be justified if therapy has not shown clear-cut benefit.

REFERENCES

1. Apelgren KN, Wilmore DW: Parenteral nutrition: is it oncologically logical?: A response. *J Clin Oncol* 2: 539, 1984
2. Baile CA, Zinn WM, Mayer J: Effects of lactate and other metabolites on food intake of monkeys. *Am J Physiol* 219: 1606, 1970
3. Beutler B, Greenwald D, Hulmes JD, Chang M, Pam Y-CE, Mathison J, Ulevitch R, Cerami A: Identity of tumor necrosis factor and the macrophage-secreted factor cachectin. *Nature* 36: 552, 1985
4. Beutler B, Mahoney J, Le Trang N, Pekala P, Ceramit A: Purification of cachectin, a lipoprotein lipase-suppressing hormone secreted by endotoxin-induced RAW 264.7 cells. *J Exp Med* 161: 984, 1985
5. Bounous G, Le Bell EL, Shuster J, Gold P, Tahan WT, Bastin E: Dietary protection during radiation therapy. *Strahlentherapie* 149: 476, 1975
6. Bower RH, Talamini MA, Sax HC, Hamilton F, Fischer JE: Postoperative enteral vs parenteral nutrition. A randomized controlled trial. *Arch Surg* 121: 1040, 1986
7. Bozzetti F: Parenteral hyperalimentation in patients with gastrointestinal cancer. *Tumori* 64: 407, 1978
8. Brennan MF: Malnutrition in patients with gastrointestinal

malignancy. Significance and management. *Dig. Dis Sci* 31 (9 Suppl): 77S, 1986

9. Brister SJ, Chiu RC, Brown RA, Mulder DS: Clinical impact of intravenous hyperalimentation on esophageal carcinoma: is it worthwhile? *Ann Thorac Surg* 38: 617, 1984

10. Chandra RK: Nutrition, immunity and infection: present knowledge and future direction. *Lancet* I: 688, 1983

11. Chlebowski RT: Critical evaluation of the role of nutritional support with chemotherapy. *Cancer* 55: 268, 1985

12. Chlebowski RT, Heber D: Hypogonadism in male patients with metastatic cancer prior to treatment. *Cancer Res* 42: 2495, 1982

13. Chlebowski RT, Heber D, Richardson B, Block JB: Influence of hydrazine sulfate on abnormal carbohydrate metabolism in cancer patients with weight loss. *Cancer Res* 44: 857, 1984

14. Chlebowski RT, Herrold J, Richardson B, Block JB: Effects of decadurabolin in patients with advanced non-small cell lung cancer. *Clin Res* 23: 541, 1982

15. Clamon GH, Feld R, Evans WK, Weiner RS, Moran EM, Blum RH, Kramer BS, Makuch RW, Hoffman FA, DeWys WD: Effect of adjuvant central i.v. hyperalimentation on the survival and response to treatment of patients with small cell lung cancer: a randomized trial. *Cancer Treat Rep* 69: 167, 1985

16. Copeland EM, Daly JM, Dudrick SJ: Nutrition as an adjunct to cancer treatment in the adult. *Cancer Res* 37: 2451, 1977

17. Copeland EM, MacFadyen BV, Lanzotti VJ, Dudrick SJ: Intravenous hyperalimentation as an adjuvant to cancer chemotherapy. *Am J Surg* 129: 167, 1975

18. Copeland EM, Rodman CA, Dudrick SJ: Nutritional concepts of neoplastic disease. In: *Nutrition and Cancer*. Edited by J van Eys, MS Seelig and BL Nichols, New York, S.P. Medical and Scientific Books, pp. 133–156, 1979

19. Deitel M, Alexander M, Hew LR: Hyperalimentation and cancer. *Can J Surg* 23: 11, 1980

20. Deshpande PD, Harper AE, Elvehjem CA: Amino acid imbalance and nitrogen retention. *J Biol Chem* 230: 335, 1958

21. DeWys W: Abnormalities of taste sensation in cancer patients. *Cancer* 36: 1888, 1975

22. Dionigi R, Dominioni L: Perioperative nutritional support in cancer patients. *Bibl Nutr Diet* 35: 85, 1985

23. Donaldson SS: Nutritional support as an adjuvant to radiation therapy. *J Paren Ent Nutr* 18: 302, 1984

24. Donaldson SS, Wesley MN, Ghavimi F, Shils ME, Suskind RH, DeWys WD: A prospective randomized clinical trial of total parenteral nutrition in children with cancer. *Med Pediatr Oncol* 10: 129, 1982

25. Douglas HO Jr, Million S, Nava H, Erikson B, Thomas P, Novick A, Holyoke ED: Elemental diet as an adjuvant for patients with locally advanced gastrointestinal cancer receiving radiation therapy: A prospectively randomized study. *J Paren Ent Nutr* 2: 682, 1978

26. Edelstyn GA, MacRae KD, MacDonald FM: Improvement of life quality in cancer patients undergoing chemotherapy. *Clin Oncol* 5: 43, 1979

27. Ghavimi F, Shils ME, Scott BF, Brown M, Tamaroff M: Comparison of morbidity in children requiring abdominal radiation and chemotherapy, with and without total parenteral nutrition. *J Pediatr* 101: 530, 1982

28. Gold J: Cancer cachexia and gluconeogenesis. *Ann NY Acad Sci* 230: 14, 1974

29. Gold J: Use of hydrazine sulfate in terminal and pre-terminal cancer patients: Results of investigational new drug (IND) study in evaluable patients. *Oncol* 32: 1, 1975

30. Greenway B, Iqbal MJ, Johnson PJ, Williams RI: Low serum testosterone concentrations in patients with carcinoma of the pancreas. *Br Med J* 286: 93, 1983

31. Heatley RV, Williams RHP, Lewis MH: Preoperative intravenous feeding – a controlled trial. *Postgrad Med J* 55: 541, 1979

32. Holroyde CP, Gabuzda TG, Putnam RC, Paul P, Reichard GA: Altered glucose metabolism in metastatic carcinoma. *Cancer Res* 35: 3710, 1975

33. Holter AR, Fisher JE: The effects of perioperative hyperalimentation on complications in patients with carcinoma and weight loss. *J Surg Res* 23: 31, 1977

34. Hughes WT, Price RA, Sisko F, Havron S, Kafatos AG, Schonland M, Smythe PM: Protein-calorie malnutrition: A host determinant for pneumocystis carinii infection. *Am J Dis Child* 128: 44, 1974

35. Issell BF, Valdivieso M, Zaren HA, Dudrick SJ, Freireich EJ, Copeland EW, Bodey GP: Protection against chemotherapy toxicity by i.v. hyperalimentation. *Cancer Treat Rep* 62: 1139, 1978

36. Jensen S: Clinical effects of enteral and parenteral nutrition preceding cancer surgery. *Med Oncol Tumor Pharmacother* 2: 225, 1985

37. Jordan WM, Valdivieso M, Frankmann C, Gillespie M, Issell BF, Bodey GP, Freireich EJ: Treatment of advanced adenocarcinoma of the lung with ftoratur, doxorubicin, cyclophosphamide and cisplatin (FACP) and intensive IV hyperalimentation. *Cancer Treat Rep* 65: 197, 1981

38. Kansal V, Omura GA, Soong S: Prognosis in adult myelogenous leukemia related to performance status and other factors. *Cancer* 38: 329, 1976

39. Kinsella TJ, Malcolm AW, Bothe A, Valerio D, Blackburn GL: Prospective study of nutritional support during pelvic irradiation. *Int J Radiat Oncol Biol Phys* 7: 543, 1981

40. Klein S, Simes J, Blackburn GL: Total parenteral nutrition and cancer clinical trials. *Cancer* 58: 1378, 1986

41. Koretz RL: Parenteral nutrition: Is it oncologically logical? *J Clin Oncol* 2: 534, 1984

42. Kumta PS, Harper AE, Elvehjem CA: Amino acid imbalance and nitrogen retention in adult rats. *J Biol Chem* 233: 1505, 1958

43. Lerner HJ, Regelson W: Clinical trial of hydrazine sulfate in a solid tumor. *Cancer Treat Rep* 60: 959, 1976

44. Levine AS, Brennan MF, Ramu A, Fisher RI, Pizzo PA, Glaubiger DL: Controlled clinical trials of nutritional intervention as an adjunct to chemotherapy, with a comment on nutrition and drug resistance. *Cancer Res* 42: 774S, 1982

45. Lim STK, Choa RG, Lam KH, Wong J, Ong GB: Total parenteral nutrition versus gastrostomy in the preoperative preparation of patients with carcinoma of the esophagus. *Brit J Surg* 68: 69, 1981

46. Loiudice TA, Lang JA: Treatment of radiation enteritis: a comparison study. *Am J Gastroenterol* 78: 481, 1983

47. Mahaffey SM, Copeland EM 3d: Total parenteral nutrition in the cancer patient. *Adv Surg* 20: 47, 1987

48. Meguid MM, Megiud V: Preoperative identification of the surgical cancer patient in need of postoperative supportive total parenteral nutrition. *Cancer* 55: 258, 1985

49. Mider GB: Some tumor–host relationships. *Proc Canad Cancer Res Conf 1st Conf*, Honey Harbor, Ontario, 1954, pp. 120, 1955

50. Moertel CG, Schutt AJ, Hahn RG, Reitmeier FJ: Effects of patient selection on results of phase II chemotherapy trials in gastrointestinal cancer. *Cancer Chemotherap Rep* 58: 257, 1974

51. Moghissi K, Hornshaw J, Teasdale PR, Dawes EA: Parenteral nutrition in carcinoma of the oesophagus treated by surgery: nitrogen balance and clinical studies. *Br J Surg* 64: 125, 1977

52. Moley JF, August D, Norton JA, Sugarbaker PH: Home parenteral nutrition for patients with advanced intraperitoneal cancers and gastrointestinal dysfunction. *J Surg Oncol* 33: 186, 1986

53. Moreschi C: Beziehung zwischen Ernährung und Tumorwachstum. *Z Immunitaetsforsch* 2: 651, 1909

54. Muller JM, Brenner V, Dienst C, Pichlmaier H: Preoperative

parenteral feeding in patients with gastrointestinal carcinoma. *Lancet* i: 68, 1982

55. Nixon DW: The value of parenteral nutrition support. Chemotherapy and radiation treatment. *Cancer* 58(Suppl 8): 1902, 1986
56. Nixon DW, Moffitt S, Lawson DH, Ausley J, Lynn MJ, Kutner MH, Heymsfield SB, Wesley M, Chawla R, Rudman D: Total parenteral nutrition as an adjunct to chemotherapy of metastatic colorectal cancer. *Cancer Treat Rep* 65: (Suppl 5) 121, 1981
57. Ohnuma T: Systemic effects of cancer. In: *Cancer Medicine*. Edited by JF Holland, E Frei III. Lea & Febiger, Philadelphia, pp. 1220–1229, 1982
58. Ohnuma T: Cited in discussion on the paper by Trotter. In: *Nutrition and Metabolism in Cancer*. Edited by R Kluthe and G-W Lohr. Thieme-Stratton, New York, p. 34, 1981
59. Ohnuma T, Holland JF: Chemotherapy and immunotherapy and their consequences on nutritional status of the cancer patient. In: *Nutrition and Metabolism in Cancer*. Edited by R Kluthe and G-W Lohr. Thieme-Stratton, New York, pp. 17–30, 1981
60. Pareira MD, Conrad EJ, Hicks W, Elman R: Clinical response and changes in nitrogen balance, body weight, plasma proteins and hemoglobin following tube feeding in cancer cachexia. *Cancer* 8: 803, 1955
61. Pezner R, Archambeau JO: Critical evaluation of the role of nutritional support for radiation therapy patients. *Cancer* 55: 263, 1985
62. Popp MB, Fisher RI, Simon RM, Brennan MF: A prospective randomized study of adjuvant parenteral nutrition in the treatment of diffuse lymphoma: Effect of drug tolerance. *Cancer Treat Rep* 65: (Suppl 5) 129, 1981
63. Popp MB, Fisher RI, Wesley R, Aamodt R, Brennan MF: A prospective randomized study of adjuvant parenteral nutrition in the treatment of advanced diffuse lymphoma: Influence on survival. *Surgery* 90: 195, 1981
64. Rannot B: Malabsorption due to lymphomatous diseases. *Ann Rev Med* 22: 19, 1971
65. Ray PD, Hanson RI, Lardy HA: Inhibition by hydrazine gluconeogenesis in rat. *J Biol Chem* 245: 690, 1970
66. Recchione C, Galante E, Secreto G, Cavalleri A, Dan V: Abnormal serum hormone levels in lung cancer. *Tumori* 69: 293, 1983
67. Reichard GA, Moury NF, Hochella NJ, Patterson AL, Weinhouse S: Quantitative estimation of the Cori cycle in human. *J Biol Chem* 238: 495, 1963
68. Sako K, Lori JM, Kaufman S, Razuck MS, Bakamjian V, Reese P: Parenteral hyperalimentation in surgical patients with head and neck cancer: a randomized study. *J Surg Oncol* 16: 391, 1981
69. Salmon WD: The significance of amino acid imbalance on nutrition. *Am J Clin Nutr* 6: 487, 1958
70. Samuels ML, Selig DE, Ogden S, Grant S, Brown B: IV hyperalimentation and chemotherapy for stage III testicular cancer: A randomized study. *Cancer Treat Rep* 65: 615, 1981
71. Serrou B, Cupissol D, Plagne R, Boutin P, Chollet P, Cavcassonne T, Michel FB: Followup of a randomized trial for oal cell carcinoma evaluating the efficacy of peripheral intravenous nutrition (PIVN) as adjunct treatment. *Recent Results Cancer Res* 80: 246, 1982
72. Shamberger RC, Brennan MF, Goodgame JT Jr, Lowry SF, Maher MM, Wesley RA, Pizzo PA: A prospective randomized study of adjuvant parenteral nutrition in the treatment of sarcomas: results of metabolic and survival studies. *Surgery* 96: 1, 1984
73. Shamberger RC, Pizzo PA, Goodgame JT, Lowry SF, Maher MM, Wesley RA, Brennan MF: The effect of total parenteral nutrition on chemotherapy-induced myelosuppression. *Am J Med* 74: 40, 1983
74. Shils ME, Friedland IM, Fine AS, Shapiro DM: Quantitative biochemical differences between tumor and host as a basis for cancer chemotherapy. III Thiamine and coenzyme A. *Cancer Res* 16: 581, 1956
75. Silverman H: The role of preoperative parenteral nutrition in cancer patients. *Cancer* 55: (Suppl 2), 254, 1985
76. Solassol C, Joyeaux H, Dubois J-B: Total parenteral nutrition (TPN) with complete nutritive mixtures: An artificial gut in cancer patients. *Nutr Cancer* 1: 13, 1979
77. Spiers ASD, DeVita SF, Allar MJ, Richards S, Sedransk N: Beneficial effects of an anabolic steroid during cytostatic chemotherapy for metastatic cancer. *J Med* 12: 433, 1981
78. Spremulli E, Wampler GL, Regelson W: Clinical study of hydrazine sulfate in advanced cancer patients. *Cancer Chemotherap Pharm* 3: 121, 1979
79. Stevenson JAF, Box BM, Szlavko AJ: A fat mobilizing and anorectic substance in the urine of fasting rats. *Proc Soc Exp Biol Med* 116: 424, 1964
80. Sylven B, Holmberg B: On the structure and biological effects of a newly-discovered cytotoxic polypeptide in tumor fluid. *Europ J Cancer* 1: 199, 1965
81. Theologides A: The anorexia-cachexia syndrome: a new hypothesis. *Ann NY Acad Sci* 230: 14, 1974
82. Thompson BR, Julian TB, Stremple JF: Perioperative total parenteral nutrition in patients with gastrointestinal cancer. *J Surg Res* 30: 497, 1981
83. Uehara PS, Beaton JR: Note on the pituitary and the anorexigenic material isolated from urine. *Canad J Physiol Pharmacol* 48: 185, 1970
84. Valdivieso M, Bodey GP, Benjamin RS, Barkley HT, Freeman MB, Ertel M, Smith TL, Mountain CF: Role of intravenous hyperalimentation as an adjunct to intensive chemotherapy for small cell bronchogenic carcinoma. *Cancer Treat Rep* 65 (Suppl 5): 145, 1981
85. Valerio D, Overett L, Malcolm A, Blackburn GL: Nutritional support for cancer patients receiving abdominal and pelvic radiotherapy: A randomized prospective clinical experiment of intravenous versus oral feeding. *Surgical Forum* 29: 145, 1978
86. Van Eys J, Copeland EM, Cangir A, Taylor G, Teitell-Cohen B, Carter B, Ortiz C: A clinical trial of hyperalimentation in children with metastatic malignancies. *Med Pediatr Oncol* 8: 63, 1980
87. Weiner RS, Kramer BS, Clamon GH, Feld R, Evans W, Moran EM, Blum R, Weisenthal LM, Pee D, Hoffman FA, DeWys WD: The effects of intravenous hyperalimentation during treatment in patients with small cell lung cancer. *J Clin Oncol* 3: 949, 1985
88. Weisdorf S, Hofland C, Sharp HL, Teasley K, Schissel K, McGlace PB, Ramsay N, Kersey J: Total parenteral nutrition in bone marrow transplantation: a clinical evaluation. *J Pediat Gastroenterol Nutr* 3: 95, 1984
89. Yamada N, Koyama H, Hioki K, Yamada T, Yamamoto M: Effects of postoperative total parenteral nutrition (TPN) as an adjunct to gastrectomy for advanced gastric carcinoma. *Brit J Surg* 70: 267, 1983

PALLIATIVE CHEMOTHERAPY: CANCER CHEMOTHERAPY-INDUCED NAUSEA AND VOMITING

J. LASZLO and V.S. LUCAS, JR

Significant advances in the treatment of certain disseminated malignancies have been accompanied by increased awareness of the consequences of inadequate antiemetic therapy. In some patients, nausea and vomiting may lead to noncompliance with treatment regimens, and these complications commonly impose mental and physical suffering that diminishes the quality of life. The extent to which medical complications are associated with vomiting depends upon its severity and duration; these complications can include esophageal tears, bone fractures, malnutrition, and major fluid and electrolyte derangements.

Pharmacological management of chemotherapy-induced nausea and vomiting is influenced by the specific emetogenic agents available and their mechanism(s) of action, as well as by whether therapy takes place in the hospital or in an outpatient setting. No single antiemetic drug is successful in all cases. This chapter outlines general approaches in drug therapy of nausea and vomiting and points out factors that should be considered when planning antiemetic therapy.

Before planning antiemetic therapy for an individual patient, underlying conditions such as intestinal obstruction, peritonitis, or increased intracranial pressure should be evaluated and excluded. It is important not to assume that nausea and vomiting are ascribable to chemotherapy and thereby miss the opportunity of important alternative treatment. Explosive vomiting without nausea and excessively prolonged vomiting following a course of chemotherapy should at least raise the possibility of other medical or psychological causes (5).

A related concern in developing a program for a patient is whether the problem can be adequately managed in the outpatient clinic or whether the entire treatment should be dealt with during a brief period of hospitalization. Distance from the hospital and the extent of delay in the nausea and vomiting following chemotherapy are factors which, if they permit the patient to go home to a supportive environment, make it preferable for the problem to be dealt within that setting. At the same time, we must be aware that some patients may be so incapacitated by retching every 5—10 minutes that someone needs to stay with them, and if that is not possible at home, then it is preferable to hospitalize such patients. Fortunately that happens only rarely at the present time. For patients treated in the clinic, it is important to consider that most antiemetic agents produce sedation when given in the dosage needed to manage nausea and vomiting. Thus patients should be advised to refrain from driving vehicles or working with hazardous machinery while under the influence of some drugs.

When we consider the drugs that induce nausea and vomiting, we have a general sense of which ones are more potent than others, a rough estimate of these is given in Table 1. Clearly drugs such as cisplatin and cyclophosphamide have a high potential for inducing nausea, vomiting and retching, whereas vincristine and many antimetabolites are far less likely to do so. It is necessary to add that dosage considerations are extremely important because the nausea and vomiting produced by low doses of cisplatin may be handled by numerous antiemetics, whereas high doses of cisplatin respond poorly to most antiemetics. No single classification scheme of emetogenic agents can take into account all variables nor the fact that some antiemetics are more effective against one agent, whereas others may be preferable against a different agent (12). The latter discrepancies are undoubtedly related to the variable effects which emetogenic chemotherapeutic drugs can exert on the specialized receptor sites in the brain and gut. A number of reviews have been written about the pharmacologic management of chemotherapy-induced nausea and vomiting, such as those by Penta et al. (15, 16).

Turning first to the standard antiemetic agents, we should begin any such listing with the classic antiemetics – the phenothiazines (Table 2). Most of these are very familiar and a good deal has been written about them since they were introduced in the early 1950s. As a class the phenothiazines are the most widely used drugs in medical practice, being primarily employed in the management of patients with psychiatric disorders. However, phenothiazines are also useful for their antiemetic, antinausea, and antihistamine properties, as well as for their capacity to potentiate analgesics, sedatives and other central nervous system depressant agents (8, 21). Moertel and colleagues (9, 10) have studied emesis produced by anticancer agents, primarily 5-fluorouracil, for many years; they found that drugs such as prochlorperazine and thiopropazate were more effective than placebo in preventing 5-FU-induced nausea and vomiting.

Table 1. Emetogenic potency of chemotherapeutic drugs.*

Worst	Moderate	Least
Cisplatin	Nitrosoureas	Vincristine
DTIC	Procarbazine	Vinblastine
Nitrogen mustard	Mitomycin C	Bleomycin
Adriamycin		6-Mercaptopurine
Cyclophosphamide		Cytosine arabinoside

* Relationships based on usual doses.

P.V. Woolley (ed.), Cancer management in Man: Biological Response Modifiers, Chemotherapy, Antibiotics, Hyperthermia, Supporting Measures
© 1989, Kluwer Academic Publishers, Dordrecht.

Table 2. Antiemetic drugs.

1. Phenothiazines
   A. Chlorpromazine (Thorazine)
   B. Prochlorperazine (Compazine)
   C. Triethylperazine (Torecan)
   D. Promethazine (Phenergan)
   E. Triflupromazine (Vesprin)
   F. Perphenazine (Trilafon)

2. Antihistamines
   A. Hydroxyzine (Vistaril, Atarax)
   B. Cyclizine (Marizine)
   C. Meclizine (Antivert)
   D. Dimenhydrate (Dramamine)
   E. Buclizine (Bucladin)
   F. Diphenhydramine (Benadryl)

3. Miscellaneous
   A. Benzquinamide (Emete-Con)
   B. Haloperidol (Haldol)
   C. Droperidol (Inapsine)
   D. Metoclopramide (Reglan)
   E. Trimethobenzamide (Tigan)
   F. High-Dose Corticosteroids
   G. Lorazepam
   H. Domperidone
   I. Tetrahydrocannabinol (THC)
   J. Diphenidol (Vontrol)
   K. Scopolamine hydrobromide

More recent studies have compared various phenothiazones, mainly prochlorperazine, with several newer antiemetics such as tetrahydrocannabinol (THC) and nabilone, and in most (though not all) studies prochlorperazine was less effective than THC or nabilone (14, 18, 19). It seems to us that mild emetogenic programs such as 5-FU or radiation therapy may respond positively to phenothiazines; however, more potent drugs such as cisplatin, and combination chemotherapy with drugs such as doxorubicin and dacarbazine rarely respond satisfactorily (8). Furthermore, aggressive use of phenothiazines is associated with a considerable number of side effects, some of which are attributable to the actions of the drugs on the central and autonomic nervous systems while others are hypersensitivity reactions.

Antihistamines are often used as antinausea and antivomiting agents. Although extremely effective in motion sickness, they offer little protection against the nausea and vomiting produced by potent chemotherapeutic agents.

A variety of miscellaneous agents has been used in various situations in management of patients receiving cancer chemotherapy. Among these we might highlight the more potent drugs, including benzquinamide derivatives, butyrophenones such as haloperidol, and metoclopramide. For example, Neidhart *et al.* (12) found benzquinamide to completely eliminate vomiting in approximately 20% of patients who received doxorubicin, although it was rarely effective in entirely controlling cisplatin or nitrogen mustard-induced vomiting. They found that benzquinamide was occasionally effective even in patients who were unresponsive to prochlorperazine or haloperidol during prior therapies. Haloperidol is a major tranquilizer which appears to act as a membrane stabilizer blocking the action of dopamine at the post-synaptic membrane (4). The drug decreases apomor-phine-induced vomiting, suggesting its effectiveness at the chemoreceptor trigger zone (CTZ) as a major mechanism of action. In comparative studies against prochlorperazine or THC in patients receiving potent emetogenic chemotherapeutic agents, its overall efficacy was significantly better than prochlorperazine and about the same as THC (12, 13).

Metoclopramide has been highlighted recently by the elegant work of Gralla and associates at Memorial Sloan-Kettering Institute in New York; their controlled randomized double-blind studies showed marked effectiveness of high doses of this agent in management of cisplatin-induced nausea and vomiting (2). The drug has recently been marketed for cisplatin-induced nausea and vomiting and constitutes the most potent single antiemetic presently available for this problem.

There has been considerable interest in the use of several cannabinoids. Delta-9-tetrahydrocannabinol (THC), the most studied of these, can be extracted from marijuana plants or synthesized. The drug is difficult to formulate even in capsule form and its absorption is erratic; nonetheless, it is an effective antiemetic (6, 13, 14, 18, 19). Our studies using THC in 88 patients who had previously experienced severe nausea and vomiting despite the use of other antiemetics found 18% complete responses, 48% partial responses, and 34% who had less than a partial response; the response rate was improved even further with repeated courses of THC. A number of side effects have been reported, with the majority of patients experiencing somnolence, or high, or, to a lesser extent, other side effects, among which dysphoric reactions such as fear and anxiety are the most serious. Of note – THC is not particularly helpful in counteracting the emetogenic effects of cisplatin (6).

Nabilone was the first of the synthetic cannabinoid derivatives described; Herman and colleagues called it a significant advance in the management of cisplatin-induced nausea and vomiting which has now been amply confirmed (3, 20). Sallan and Laszlo have done Phase I–II studies on oral and parenteral levonantradol, another synthetic cannabinoid, and have found it to be an effective antiemetic agent by both of those routes (1, 7), an important attribute because of the flexibility provided by the parenteral route once the patient begins to vomit. (THC is now marketed, nabilone may be in the future and levonantradol apparently will not.) The unresolved question about the cannabinoids is whether their dysphoric properties can be eliminated by pharmacologic manipulation of the parent molecule or whether to do so would also eliminate the antiemetic effect.

No review of any pharmacologic program would be complete without mention of the high doses of corticosteroids which seem to be recommended for just about everything. In fact, there are a number of articles suggesting that high doses of steroids (methylprednisolone, dexamethasone), either alone or in combination with other antiemetics, are very effective (17, 22), and we agree.

In summary, the more recent and aggressive chemotherapeutic programs are also more emetogenic and, fortunately, major advances in counteracting this problem have also occurred. Oncologists recognize that inadequate management of nausea and vomiting is deleterious to the health and well-being of the patient and any delay in providing aggressive treatment merely aggravates the problem. When the pattern of nausea and vomiting becomes established or conditioned during a period of ineffective antiemetic therapy, then the anticipatory nausea and vomiting become extremely difficult to manage. The only current means of dealing with the anticipatory syndrome is the use of behavioral desensitization or relaxation (11).

REFERENCES

1. Cronin CM, Sallan SE, Gelber R, et al.: Antiemetic effect of intramuscular levonantradol in patients receiving cancer chemotherapy. *J Clin Pharmacol* 215:43, 1981
2. Gralla RJ, Itri LM, Pisko SE, et al.: Antiemetic efficacy of high-dose metoclopramide: randomized trials with placebo and prochlorperazine in patients with chemotherapy-induced nausea and vomiting. *N Engl J Med* 305:905, 1981
3. Herman TS, Einhorn LH, Jones E, Nagy C, Chester AB, Dean JC, Furnas B, Williams SD, Leigh SA, Dorr RJ, Moon TE: Superiority of nabilone over prochlorperazine as an antiemetic in patients receiving cancer chemotherapy. *N Engl J Med* 300:1295, 1979
4. Janssen PAJ: The pharmacology of haloperidol. *Int J Neuropsych* 3:10, 1967
5. Laszlo J: Emesis as limiting toxicity in cancer chemotherapy. In: *Antiemetics and Cancer Chemotherapy*. Edited by J Laszlo. Baltimore, Williams and Wilkins, 1983
6. Laszlo J, Lucas VS, Huang AT: Iatrogenic emesis model in cancer: Results of 120 patients treated with delta-9-tetrahydrocannabinol. In: *Treatment of Cancer Chemotherapy-Induced Nausea and Vomiting*. Edited by DS Poster, JS Penta, S Bruno, p. 61. Masson Publishing, New York, 1981
7. Laszlo J, Lucas VS, Hanson D, et al.: Levonantradol for chemotherapy-induced emesis: Phase I–II oral administration. *J Clin Pharmacol* 215:51, 1981
8. Lucas VS Jr: Phenothiazines as antiemetics. In: *Antiemetics and Cancer Chemotherapy*. Edited by J Laszlo. Baltimore, Williams & Wilkins, 1983
9. Moertel CEG, Reitemeier RJ: Controlled studies of metopimazine for the treatment of nausea and vomiting. *J Clin Pharmacol* 3:282, 1973
10. Moertel CG, Reitemeier RJ, Gage RP: A controlled clinical evaluation of antiemetic drugs. *JAMA* 186:116, 1963
11. Morrow GR, Morrell C: Behavioral treatment for anticipatory nausea and vomiting induced by cancer chemotherapy. *N Engl J Med* 307:1476, 1982
12. Neidhart JA, Gagen M, Young D, Wilson HE: Specific antiemetics for specific cancer chemotherapeutic agents: Haloperidol versus benzquinamide. *Cancer* 47:1439, 1981
13. Neidhart JA, Gagen MM, Wilson HE, Young DC: Comparative trial of the antiemetic effects of delta-9-THC and haloperidol. *J Clin Pharmacol* 215:38, 1981
14. Orr LE, McKernan JF, Lee P: Antiemetic effect of tetrahydrocannabinol. *Arch Intern Med* 140:1431, 1980
15. Penta JS, Poster D, Bruno S: The pharmacologic treatment of nausea and vomiting – a review. In: *Antiemetics and Cancer Chemotherapy*. Edited by J. Laszlo. Baltimore, Williams & Wilkins, 1983
16. Penta JS, Poster DS, Bruno S, Abraham D, Perinna K, MacDonald JS: Cancer chemotherapy-induced nausea and vomiting: a review. In: *Treatment of Cancer Chemotherapy-Induced Nausea and Vomiting*. Edited by DS Poster, JS Penta, S Bruno. New York, Masson Publishing, 1981
17. Rich WM, Abdulhayoglu G, DiSaia PJ: Methylprednisolone as an antiemetic during cancer chemotherapy. In: *Treatment of Cancer Chemotherapy-Induced Nausea and Vomiting*. Edited by DS Poster, JS Penta, S Bruno. New York, Masson Publishing, 1981
18. Sallan SE, Zinberg NE, Frei E III: Antiemetic effect of delta-9-tetrahydrocannabinol in patients receiving cancer chemotherapy. *N Engl J Med* 293:795, 1975
19. Sallan SE, Cronin C, Zelen M, Zinberg NE: Antiemetics in patients receiving chemotherapy for cancer. A randomized comparison of delta-9-tetrahydrocannabinol and prochlorperazine. *N Engl J Med* 302:135, 1980
20. Steele N, Gralla RJ, Braun DW, Young CW: Double-blind comparison of the antiemetic effects of nabilone and prochlorperazine on chemotherapy-induced emesis. *Cancer Treat Rep* 64:219, 1980
21. Wampler G: The pharmacology and clinical effectiveness of phenothiazines and related drugs for managing chemotherapy-induced emesis. *Drugs* 25(1):35, 1983
22. Winokur SH, Baker JJ, Lokey JL, et al.: Dexamethasone as an antiemetic during cancer chemotherapy. In: *Treatment of Cancer Chemotherapy-Induced Nausea and Vomiting*. Edited by DS Poster, JS Penta, S Bruno. New York, Masson Publishing, 1981

POSTSCRIPT

High dose metoclopramide and high dose steroids are among the most generally effective antiemetic agents. Indeed with newer programs, such as with these drugs plus droperidol and diphenhydramine it is possible to achieve complete control of nausea and vomiting in about 70% of patients.

POSTSCRIPT REFERENCE

Sridhar KS, Donnelly E: Combination antiemetics for cisplatin chemotherapy. *Cancer* 61:1508, 1988

21

CHRONIC PAIN MANAGEMENT

R.M. FRANK

Introduction

Pain is a perception and as such its form and content are dependent upon the subjective response of the patient who is experiencing it. All too often, the treatment of chronic pain depends upon the attitudes and mores of the health professionals rather than the patient's own perception (1). Generally speaking, pain progresses from an awareness to a discomfort, it may then intensify until it dominates the senses and finally explodes into agony (4). Pain at times can be debilitating as well as extremely unpleasant and is usually perceived as evidence of ill health. It evokes anxiety and fear of the unknown.

Pain and the cancer patient

The association of intractable pain with cancer is a misconception. The media have presented a picture of terminal cancer patients writhing in their beds, incapacitated with pain, but this picture is far from true. Up to half of all patients with terminal cancer have no pain or have minimal discomfort. A painful death from cancer is not inevitable (8). For those patients suffering with chronic pain, relief is available, if the health professionals have the will and the knowledge to treat it properly.

A study by Marks and Sacher (13) showed that three-quarters of medical inpatients who had received narcotic analgesics for severe pain continued to experience moderate to severe pain. A chart review showed that physicians prescribed narcotics at 50–67% of the dose required to relieve severe pain and that nurses then underadministered these drugs by another 33–50%. A follow-up survey showed that most house staff physicians underestimated the effective dose range and overestimated the duration of action and the potential for respiratory depression and addiction.

Chronic pain vs. acute pain

Chronic pain and acute pain are two different entities, and must be treated differently. A comparison shows the following:

Chronic pain	Acute pain
Usually a protracted course	Usually transient
Spectrum from mild to severe	Spectrum from mild to severe
Difficult to treat	Easier to treat
A noxious disease state in itself which can cause a complete alteration in the patient's perception of his/her life.	Represents a sensory system which may act as a warning signal alerting the body to a usually dangerous situation
A circular experience with no beginning and no end	A straight-line experience with a beginning and an end
A situation	An event
Can reduce the victim to a vegetative state	Stimulates body autonomic function

Chronic pain as a circular experience

Chronic pain has been characterized as a vicious circle with no set time limit. The fearful anticipation of its perpetuation leads to anxiety depression and insomnia which, in turn, accentuates the physical component of the pain (14). Chronic pain can be visualized as follows:

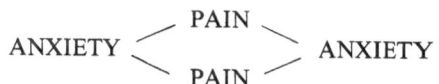

Meaninginglessness, helplessness and hopelessness are characteristics of the unreal nightmare world in which the patient with chronic pain lives every day. Chronic pain can become all consuming and the complete focus of the sufferer's life.

Aims of treatment (15)

The aims of treating chronic pain should include: Identifying the cause(s); preventing pain by anticipating rather than treating it; using carefully titrated scheduled doses: erasing pain memory, if anxious anticipation and memory of pain is lessened the treatment can be successful. An unclouded sensorium rescuing a patient from being trapped between perpetual pain and perpetual somnolence. The balance,

P.V. Woolley (ed.), Cancer management in Man: Biological Response Modifiers, Chemotherapy, Antibiotics, Hyperthermia, Supporting Measures
© 1989. Kluwer Academic Publishers, Dordrecht.

pain-free state without sedation can be achieved. Normal affect so that the patient can relate to his environment with neither an euphoric or depressed affect. Ease of administration so patient's independence and mobility are not impaired.

Diagnosing pain

Individuals have different pain thresholds. Two components make up pain, an unpleasant sensation and the emotional reaction to that sensation. The emotional component itself may contain depression, anxiety, fear of death and worries about finances and family. All these features must be dealt with in order to diagnose and treat chronic pain effectively.

The occurrence of pain may be the first symptom of disease or a sign of its spread. Pain may be the only symptom preventing a patient from leading a "normal" life and its successful treatment may lead to a great improvement in the patient's quality of life.

In order to diagnose chronic pain properly many factors should be evaluated. A complete physical, psychological, neurologic, orthopedic, radiologic and laboratory examination may be needed.

The cause of pain should be determined if possible. Is it the disease, the effects of the disease, the treatment of the disease or inactivity? Location: is the pain local or diffuse? Severity: is it mild or severe, aching, burning, sharp, dull, as judged by the patient and/or the health professionals? State of disease: is the patient potentially curable, will the patient be able to return home? Intensity as assessed by the patient's verbal description. Duration: is the pain continuous or periodic? Individual factors: age, mental status, physical status, reporting ability, family status and finances. Previous treatment: a comprehensive history of both drug and other modalities must be taken. Have other therapies been more adequate as to dose, administration and length of trial? Have any allergic reactions been noted?

The gate theory of pain (14)

Pain is the result of a complex pattern of interaction of fast and slow conducting nerve fibers and feedback from the brain impinging on the "gate". The gate consists of transmission nerve cells in the sensory (dorsal) horn of the spinal cord, the locus at which peripheral stimuli enter the cord. The larger fibers transmit impulses involving touch, while the smaller fibers transmit impulses involving pain. The smaller fibers conduct more slowly than the larger ones and both sets of nerves converge at the spinal cord. The gate allows nerve-borne messages to travel along the spinal cord to the brain, it widens or narrows depending on the sensation being transmitted. A moderate sensation keeps the gate partially open. If the sensation intensifies more small fibers become active and the pain becomes stronger. The gate can be closed by activity in the large fibers. Rubbing or scratching shuts the gate down. Emotional factors may influence the gate. Negative feelings such as anxiety, fear or sadness open it allowing more pain messages to reach the brain. One sensation cancels out the other, sometimes momentarily, sometimes longer. There is little doubt that pain perception and behavior is based upon complex anatomical, physiological and chemical factors, many of which are still poorly understood.

The chemical theory of pain (19)

This theory is based upon the discovery of opiate receptors in the human body and of the fact that we manufacture our own morphine-like substances which are intimately involved with analgesia. Pert & Snyder discovered receptors in the brain to which opiate derivatives attach themselves. These receptors apparently existed in the brains of vertebrate animals for millions of years before the discovery of opium. They theorized that there might be naturally occurring opiate-like substances which relieve pain. Hughes *et al.* reported the structure of a chemical from pig brain that resembled morphine and named it enkephalin. This chemical looked like and behaved like an opiate, binding receptor sites and producing pain suppression when injected. A variety of enkephalins have been isolated including endorphin, which is released by the pituitary and is 200 times as effective in pain relief as morphine. This implies that the body carried endogenous narcotics whose release can be triggered by certain stimuli such as acupuncture. Research is underway to synthesize these compounds and to produce the "ideal" analgesic, one which releaves pain without causing toxic effects. A lack of enkephalins or a deficiency in opiate receptors may explain why some people are extraordinarily sensitive to pain.

Treatment of chronic pain

A variety of modalities to treat pain exist: surgery, drugs, nerve block, electrical stimulation, hypnosis, acupuncture and biofeedback. Currently the most widely used method for the control of chronic pain is drug therapy.

Treatment of chronic pain: narcotic analgesics (2, 7)

The use of narcotic analgesics is still the most widely used method for the control of pain. It is possible that equianalgesic doses of narcotic analgesics will give the same degree of pain relief as well as similar toxic effects. Many compounds produce analgesia and other effects similar to morphine. None have proven clinically superior in relieving pain. Morphine is the standard against which all new analgesics are measured.

Narcotic analgesics: adverse effects (2, 7)

Narcotic analgesics exert their primary effect on the central nervous system (CNS) and the gastrointestinal (GI) tract. In terminal illness some adverse effects may help rather than hurt the patient (ex: euphoria, drowsiness).

CNS effects

Analgesics: these drugs may act on the sensory cortex of the frontal lobes and on the diencephalon of the brain; may interfere with pain conduction or the central response to pain; or may affect the patient's emotional response to pain. These drugs usually produce analgesia without loss of consciousness.

Drowsiness, sedation where the extremities feel heavy, the body is warm, the face may itch and the mouth may be dry. If conditions are favorable sleep may follow.

Change in mood, euphoria.

Respiratory depression: in part due to direct effect on the brain stem respiratory center. This involves a reduction in the responsiveness of the brain stem respiratory center to increases in carbon dioxide tension. Also depresses the centers involved with regulating respiratory rhythmicity and the responsiveness of the medullary respiratory center to electrical stimulation.

Cough suppression.

Mental clouding.

Nausea, vomiting by direct stimulation of the chemoreceptor trigger zone for emesis in the area posterior of the medulla. These effects are idiosyncratic.

Electroencephalologic changes.

GI effects

Gastric, biliary, and pancreatic sensations are decreased and the drugs may delay digestion.

Increased smooth muscle tone in the antral portion of the stomach, the small intestines, the large intestines and the sphincters.

Increase smooth muscle tone is the urinary tract.

Oliguria.

Constipation.

Cardiovascular effects

Little effect is seen on the patient when supine, orthostatic hypotension or fainting on arising may occur as a result of peripheral vasodilation.

Histamine release may lead to peripheral blood vessel dilation manifested by flushing, pruritis and sweating.

Large doses and/or rapid administration can lead to hypotension and bradycardia.

Blood pressure falls largely as a result of hypoxia. This dilates the vessels and decreases the capacity of the cardiovascular system to respond to gravitational shift.

Endocrinologic changes

Stimulates release of antidiuretic hormone (ADH). Inhibits release of ACTH and gonadotropin hormone from the pituitary. Inhibits release of thyroid stimulating hormone. Hyperglycemia. Decreases of basal metabolism rate.

Other effects

Ophthalmologic: miosis.

Rare anaphylactoid reactions have been noted.

Narcotic analgesics: contraindications

In patients with known hypersensitivity to the particular drug. Patients who are hypersensitive to one narcotic analgesic may be able to tolerate a different narcotic analgesic.

Narcotic analgesics: drug interactions

Depressant effects may be exaggerated and prolonged by phenothiazines, monoamine oxidase inhibitors and tricyclic antidepressants.

Narcotic analgesics: absorption, distribution, metabolism, excretion

Individual narcotic analgesics differ in onset and duration of action (see chart to follow). They are rapidly removed from the bloodstream, with approximately $\frac{1}{3}$ protein bound in the plasma.

They are distributed in the skeletal muscle, kidneys, liver, lungs, intestinal tract, spleen, and brain. They readily penetrate the placental barrier. They do not persist in the body and 24 hours after the last dose, tissue concentrations are usually very low. The plasma half life in young adults ranges from 2.5 to 3 hours, but may be considerably longer in older patients.

The drugs are primarily metabolized in the liver. The microsomes in the endoplasmic reticulum being the major site. To a lesser degree, metabolism takes place in the CNS, kidneys, lungs and placenta. The major pathway for detoxification is conjugation with glucouronic acid.

Excretion is primarily through the urine with 90% of the drug either unchanged or as metabolites eliminated in the first 24 hours. Elimination of the major metabolites is performed by glomerular filtration. Enterohepatic circulation occurs which probably accounts for the presence of small amounts of drug in the urine for several days. The feces account for 7–10% of excretion.

Narcotic analgesics: dosage

Doses must be carefully adjusted according to the severity of the pain and the response of the patient. If the initial dose is found to be ineffective and has not produced limiting adverse effects, then the dose should be increased before changing to another narcotic analgesic. The difference between morphine and its surrogates has been considerably overestimated. In equianalgesic doses (see chart to follow), most of these drugs produce approximately the same incidence and degree of unwanted side effects as well as approximately the same degree of analgesia.

Narcotic analgesics: mechanism of action

These drugs act as agonists which interact with binding sites or receptors which are widely but unevenly distributed through the central nervous system. The affinity of many narcotic analgesics for these binding sites correlate well with their potency as analgesics.

Narcotic analgesics: agonist–antagonist activity (5, 10)

Narcotic analgesics exhibit differences that are believed to be connected with complex interactions of these drugs with CNS opiate receptors. Morphine and pure morphine-like agonists (drugs that bind to opiate receptors) represent one such group. Another is a group that are pure antagonists (drugs that reverse or block the effects of morphine) while in between there are drugs that exhibit agonist–antagonist (mixed) properties.

Agonists	Mixed properties	Antagonists
Codeine	Butorphanol	Naloxone
Heroin	Nalbuphine	
Hydromorphone	Pentazocine	
Levorphanol		
Meperidine	*Partial agonists*	
Methadone	Buprenorphine	
Morphine		
Oxycodone		
Oxymorphone		
Propoxyphene		

Name of drug	Equianalgesic dose PO (mq)
Acetaminophen	650
Aspirin	650
Codeine	32
Meperidine	50
Oxycodone	2.5
Pentazocine	30
Propoxyphene	65

The agonist drugs may differ from morphine in relative potency, onset and duration of action but they all mimic morphine in desired and toxic effects. Mixed action drugs produce analgesia and other narcotic effects but may exhibit a lower liability for abuse, although this is still in question. Mixed action drugs in therapeutic doses may produce certain self-limiting psychotomimetic effects in some patients. Patients who have received repeated doses of a morphine-like drug to the point of physical dependency may experience withdrawal reactions when given a mixed action drug.

Narcotic analgesics: relative potency, and other pharmacologic parameters (2, 3, 7, 10)

The dosage and pharmacokinetic effects are based on acute, short-term use. Recent data suggest that chronic administration will significantly alter these parameters.

Name of drug	Equianalgesic dose (mg) (b)		Onset (min) (b)	Peak (hr) (b)	Duration (hr) (b)	Plasma half life (hr) (b)
Buprenorphine	Parenteral	0.4		$\frac{1}{2}$–1	4–6	
	Sublingual	0.8		2–3	5–6	
Butorphanol	Parenteral	2	5–15	$\frac{1}{2}$–1	3–6	3–4
Hydromorphone	Parenteral	1.5	15–30	$\frac{1}{2}$–1	4–5	2–3
	Oral	7.5	15–30	$1\frac{1}{2}$–2	4–7	2–3
Levorphanol	Parenteral	2	45–60	$\frac{1}{2}$–1	4–6	12–16
	Oral	4	45–60	$1\frac{1}{2}$–2	4–7	12–16
Meperidine	Parenteral	75	10–15	$\frac{1}{2}$–1	2–4	3–4
	Oral	300		$1\frac{1}{2}$–2	2–4	
Methadone	Parenteral	10	10–15	$\frac{1}{2}$–1	4–6	15–30
	Oral	20		$1\frac{1}{2}$–2	4–6	
Morphine	Parenteral	10	20–30	$\frac{1}{2}$–1	4–6	2–4
	Oral	20 (c)		$1\frac{1}{2}$–2	4–7	
Nalbuphine	Parenteral	10		$\frac{1}{2}$–1	4–6	5
Oxymorphone	Parenteral	1	5–10	$\frac{1}{2}$–1	4–6	2–3
Pentazocine	Parenteral	60		$\frac{1}{2}$–1	4–6	2–3
	Oral	180		$1\frac{1}{2}$–2	4–7	

(b) The dose and frequency of administration must be titrated to the individual patient.

(c) Clinical experience with Brompton and morphine sulfate solutions indicates the correct parenteral: Oral ratio for morphine should be 1:2 rather than 1:6 usually shown.

Relative potencies of oral analgesics expressed in terms of doses approximately equivalent in total effect to 650 mg of Aspirin (ASA).

Narcotic analgesics: suggested regimens

At this institution two suggested regimens of treatment for pain have been developed.

ORAL ADMINISTRATION

Acetaminophen or ASA	Acetaminophen or ASA + Codeine	Acetaminophen or ASA + Oxycodone	Hydromorphone	Morphine sulfate tablets
				Morphine sulfate oral solution
				Methadone
Mild		Moderate	Severe	

PARENTERAL ADMINISTRATION

	Meperidine	Hydromorphone	Morphine bolus
			Morphine infusion
			Methadone

Narcotic analgesics: dosing for the elderly (11)

Elderly patients are often very sensitive to these drugs. With respect to dose, particularly aged patients respond to morphine as though they had received 3–4 times the dose as compared to younger patients. This is primarily an increase in duration rather than an increase in peak analgesic effect, and is consistent with the suggestion that morphine is cleared from the body more slowly in the aged patient.

Narcotic analgesics: individual drug information (2, 5, 7)

The following statements contain information concerning individual drugs and will draw upon clinical experience, as noted, as well as the references cited.

Buprenophine
This drug is not available for clinical use in the United States. It can be used sublingually as well as by other traditional routes of administration.

Butorphanol
It is only available for parenteral administration and has not been widely used on a chronic basis. In contrast to morphine, it transiently increases urine output and decreases urine osmolality and sodium and potassium excretion in rats. These effects are due to inhibition of release of antidiuretic hormone from the hypothalamus.

Codeine
Useful as a first line analgesic in combination with 650 mg of Acetaminophen or ASA. We find a dose of 60 mg in combinations can be effective in treating mild chronic pain.

Heroin (17)
In equianalgesic doses compared to morphine its analgesic and mood-altering effects are similar. Onset of action is slightly faster but duration of action is shorter. Its toxic effects are similar to morphine. Clinical use of the drug in the United States is illegal. Recent studies indicate that heroin offers no special advantage compared with morphine.

Hydromorphone
Has a rapid onset of action which makes it particularly

useful on a when needed ("prn") basis. Because of its solubility large concentrations of drug can be given in small volumes, an advantage if subcutaneous or intramuscular route is to be used. As previously stated all narcotic analgesics are similar in desired and toxic effects when equianalgesic doses are given. This drug was included in both our oral and parenteral suggested regimens because many patients and their families equate the use of morphine with the end-stages of disease.

Levorphanol
Apparently produces more sedation and smooth muscle stimulation than morphine.

Meperidine
CNS hyperirritability has been reported including subtle changes in mood to more significant neurologic signs of tremors, multifocal myoclonus and seizures. This is secondary to accumulation of the active metabolite normeperidine. Systemic administration may cause corneal anesthesia which can abolish the corneal reflex. Excretion of the unchanged drug is enhanced by acidifying the urine. The drug has poor oral potency and in the doses usually administered (50–100 mg po q6h) it is not more effective than 650 mg of acetaminophen or ASA for treating chronic pain.

Methadone
A longer acting narcotic with good oral potency. While its half-life is 17–24 hours its duration of analgesic action seems to be 4–8 hours. Clinical experience indicates that the starting dose should be 20 mg every six hours, if the patient has failed other narcotic regimens. After pain has been controlled the frequency of administration may be cut back to every eight hours. It is firmly bound to tissue protein which may explain its cumulative effects and slow excretion.

Morphine
Experience with oral preparations has shown that this route is effective and well tolerated. Oral doses should be titrated to the patient's needs and are most effective if given on an around-the-clock schedule. Both oral sustained release tablets and liquid are available. The drug has been given intrathecally, (18) by continuous intravenous infusion (9) and

other parenteral routes. Experience at our institution shows that a starting dose of 40–80 mg/hour of morphine is needed when the continuous infusion method is administered. Often these doses can be reduced within a period of 24 hours. This is done only after consultation between the patient and the health professionals. We have maintained patients on continuous infusions of morphine sulfate for 2–3 months. Patients have remained lucid and ambulatory on doses in excess of 500 mg/hour for 1–2 days.

Nalbuphine

This drug is available for parenteral administration only. It may have less psychotomimetic effects than pentazocine but has not been widely used for chronic administration.

Naloxone

This is a narcotic antagonist. After administration there is an increase in respiration rate and minute volume, arterial PCO2 decreases toward normal and blood pressure returns to normal if depressed. Its duration of action is usually shorter than the narcotic. The precise mechanism of action is unknown but competitive inhibition seems to be important. Onset of action is 1–5 minutes with a duration of 45–90 minutes. It crosses the placental barrier and is the drug of choice when the nature of the depressant drug is not known since it will not cause further respiratory depression.

Oxycodone

A synthetic congener of morphine which is useful in combination with acetaminophen or ASA. The available combinations contain 5 mg of oxycodone and 325 mg of acetaminophen or ASA per tablet.

Oxymorphone

Useful as a rectal suppository. The onset of action rectally is 15 minutes with a duration of 3–6 hours.

Pentazocine

The introduction of pentazocine to a patient chronically receiving narcotic agonists, will precipitate an acute withdrawal state. Escalation of the dose is associated with psychotomimetic effects including hallucinations and unpleasant dreams. This limits the usefulness of this drug. In one study 50 mg of pentazocine NCl was not more effective than 650 mg of ASA. It is a mixed action drug with weak narcotic antagonist effects.

Propoxyphene

A weak narcotic analgesic. In some studies it could not be distinguished from placebo. Since it does not exhibit any antipyretic effects, it can be used for mild pain when masking of fever could present a problem. It passes into the cerebrospinal fluid.

Treatment of chronic pain: nonsteroidal anti-inflammatory drugs (2, 7, 12)

Nonsteroidal anti-inflammatory drugs (NSAIDS) control pain at the periphery where pain is engendered rather than the CNS. They reduce prostaglandin synthesis by interfering with the metabolizing enzymes. Some also modify the effects of kinins, complement and oxygen radicals.

NSAIDS: adverse effects (2, 7, 12)

Can cause upper gastrointestinal intolerance with nausea, vomiting and pyrosis; salt and water retention. Both these effects are due to a reduction of the prostaglandin produced locally in the stomach and kidney. Gastrointestinal effects can be minimized by administering with food or fluids.

Many of these drugs effect platelet aggregation and produce other hematological effects which may make these drugs unsuitable for cancer patients.

CNS effects including headache, somnolence, dizziness, tremors, confusion, insomnia, nervousness, asthenia, paresthesia, muscle weakness, fatigue, drowsiness, malaise, tinnitus, blurred vision with diplopia, and optic neuritis have been seen.

Renal effects with dysuria, cystitis, hematuria, nephrotic syndrome, renal failure, oliguria, anuria, azotemia, allergic nephritis, nephrosis, and papillary nephrosis have been noted.

Dermatologic effects with rash, pruritis, urticaria, increased sweating, dyspnea and anaphylaxis.

Hepatic effect including severe reactions including jaundice and cholestatic hepatitis, elevation of SGOT, SGPT, LDH and alkaline phosphatase.

Fenoprofen

The presence of food in the stomach retards absorption and lowers peak concentrations in plasma. The concomitant administration of antacids does not seem to alter concentrations.

Ibuprofen

Daily doses of 2400 mg in divided doses may be given, though doses up to 4200 mg per day have been reported. It may be possible to reduce the dose for maintenance purposes. The pediatric dose is 20 mg/kg but should not exceed 500 mg/day in children weighing less than 30 kg.

Indomethacin

The peak concentration in plasma is within 3 hours in the fasting subject but may be somewhat delayed when drug is taken after meals. Total plasma concentrations can be increased by concurrent use of probenecid. It antagonizes the natriuretic effect of furosemide. Severe frontal headache appears in 25–50% of patients who take the drug chronically. It can cause psychotomimetic effects possibly due to its serotonin-like chemical structure. The drug should be taken in divided doses with food or immediately after meals to lessen gastric distress.

Naproxen

Absorption may be accelerated by the concurrent administration of sodium bicarbonate or reduced by magnesium oxide or aluminum hydroxide. In children the half-life is probably shorter. The drug may be given with food to minimize gastric distress.

NSAIDS: metabolism, distribution

These drugs are primarily metabolized in the liver and excreted in the urine and feces. Most of these drugs bind firmly to plasma proteins and thus may displace other drugs from the binding sites.

NSAIDS

These drugs are contraindicated in patient with hypersensitivity to aspirin.

Combinations of NSAID's with opioids is rational since the former work in the periphery and the later centrally.

NSAIDS: individual drug information (2, 7, 12)

The following statements contain information concerning individual drugs and will draw upon clinical experience, as noted, as well as the references cited.

Acetylsalicyclic acid
This is the original NSAID and is the standard against which new mild analgesics are measured. The elimination of half-life becomes more prolonged with increased dose. Blood levels of $150 \, \mu m/ml$ is the minimum necessary for anti-inflammatory effect, levels greater than $300 \, \mu m/ml$ can cause a reversible tinnitus while higher blood levels can cause a metabolic acidosis with CNS effects. It has local toxic effect on the mucosa of the stomach, and has been administered with food or buffering agents to minimize this effect. The drug can effect platelet aggregation and thus may be unsuitable for use with cancer patients. Doses above 650 mg do not increase the effectiveness of ASA. High doses can interfere with prothrombin production. Overdosage is evidenced by hyperventilation, respiratory alkalosis and later metabolic acidosis.

Oxybutazone and phenylbutazone
These drugs can cause agranulocytosis and aplastic anemia. They cause significant retention of sodium and chloride accompanied by a reduction in urine volume, edema may result. This is a direct effect of the drugs on the renal tubules and is reversible. They reduce the uptake of iodine by the thyroid gland apparently secondary to inhibition of biosynthesis of organic iodine compounds. Significant concentrations may persist in the synovial spaces for up to three weeks. These drugs should be given only for short periods of time. Other anti-inflammatory, anticoagulant, hypoglycemic, sulfonamide, and other drugs may be displaced from binding to plasma proteins by these drugs.

NSAIDS and acetaminophen: usual dose, peak, duration and plasma half-life (2, 7)

Name of drug	Usual daily dose (mg)	Peak (hr)	Duration (hr)	Plasma-half-life (hr)
ASA	2600–3900	1½–2	4–6	2–3
Fenoprofen	2400–3000	2–4	4–6	4
Ibuprofen	1200–1600	1–2	4–6	2
Indomethacin	100–200	½–1	4–6	2–3
Naproxen	500	2–4	5–7	13–14
Oxybutazone/ Phenylbutazone	100–600	2–3	4–6	50–100
Acetaminophen	2600–3900	½–1	4–6	1–4

Acetaminophen (2, 7)

This drug has analgesic and antipyretic effects that do not differ significantly from ASA, however, it has only weak anti-inflammatory effects. It has no effect on platelet aggregation and can often be substituted for ASA in the treatment of pain for cancer patients. It produces its analgesic effect by a peripheral action.

Absorption, distribution, metabolism and elimination
When administered orally the drug is rapidly and completely absorbed. 25% is bound to plasma protein. It is metabolized by the liver microsomal enzyme system and is excreted primarily through the urine.

Adverse effects
Therapeutic doses have little effect on the cardiovascular and respiratory systems but toxic doses can cause circulatory failure and rapid shallow breathing. Acute overdosage can cause a fatal hepatic necrosis. Skin rash and occasional allergic reactions have been seen. Renal tubule necrosis and hypoglycemic coma may also occur.

Chronic pain management: treatment by non-drug modalities

A host of non-drug treatments for relief of chronic pain have been attempted. These include acupuncture, biofeedback, electrical stimulation, nerve block and surgery.

Acupuncture
This stimulates the small nerve fibers, sending impulses through the open gate that register in the brain as an acute pain of turning needles. When the signals reach the central biasing mechanism in the brain stem, they trigger counterimpulses that travel down the spinal cord and close the gate against the chronic pain. Acupuncture produces signals that may counteract pain by closing the spinal-cord gate or activating inhibitory fibers within the brain.

Biofeedback
This relies on the power of the mind. The significance of biofeedback is not the method but the message which is to put yourself in charge. By switching flashing lights on and off or by listening to beeps that vary in speed and light, subtle changes in body temperature pulse and other supposedly involuntary reactions can be registered. Patients can actually see and then learn to control what their environment does to their body.

Electrical stimulation
Transcutaneous Electrical Nerve Stimulation (TENS) uses electronic impulses to override pain. Electrodes powered by batteries are taped to the skin over any painful area. The stimulator is operated by the patient at will. Gentle electrical stimulation activates the large nerve fibers that close the gate. Stimulation of nerves to relieve pain may act by releasing enkephalins in the brain. Adverse effects include a sometimes annoying sensation similar to the tip of a needle touching the skin, irritation by the tape. This procedure does not work for all for reasons not yet elucidated.

Dorsal Skin Stimulation (DSS) in which fine wire electrodes are implanted directly in the spinal cord above the level of pain and attached to a receiver implanted beneath the skin of the back. A transmitter taped over the receiver sends electrical signals into the spine at the flick of a switch. This can be carried out whether or not the patient is in bed.

Nerve block

A local anesthetic, steroid or alcohol is injected into the area suspected of controlling the pain. The result is total numbness. The effects can last from hours to weeks or longer. There can be complications from the drugs or damage to muscle tissue.

Surgery

One of the oldest ways of dealing with chronic pain is surgery to cut the pain bearing nerve fibers. Cordotomy is used to relieve pain in the lower back and legs. The spinothalamic tract is cauterized above the area where the pain originates. There are risks of muscle weakness and paralysis. Frequently the effects wear off after several months.

Chronic pain management: successful treatment

The armamentarium against pain is vast, but the successful management of chronic pain depends on the will to treat on the part of the practitioners and the will to accept treatment by the patient and his/her family.

To be successful it is necessary to refocus the thinking about chronic pain management from the health professional's own attitudes and needs to those of the patient; and to develop a therapeutically rational approach to the control of chronic pain.

Some of the attitudes that we bring to the treatment of pain include

– a preference for stoic patients who are less demanding and easier to care for.

– the social conditioning about narcotics caused by stories in the media. We should not let drug abusers form our opinions about the proper use of narcotics, but often we do.

– the fear of addiction: a 1980 study by Porter & Jick (16) showed the incidence of addiction in hospitalized patients who had received narcotics, to be 1 per 4000.

It is possible to be physically dependent on drugs without being addicted (7). Cancer patients take narcotic analgesics for pain relief not for an altered state of mind.

Many family members wishing a patient to be adequately controlled for pain, have second thoughts when a patient becomes drowsy and lethargic even though this is usually a transient phenomenon and may reflect previous sleep deprivation due to the pain.

These attitudes and others conspire to cloud our vision when dealing with a patient in pain and lead us to what has been characterized as the 4-won't syndrome:

> The physician won't prescribe enough
> The pharmacist won't dispense enough
> The nurse/family won't administer enough
> The patient won't take enough medication to adequately treat chronic pain

To aid practitioners in understanding chronic pain and its appropriate treatment the following 10 principles of chronic pain management have been developed (6) at our institution.

The principles of chronic pain management

(1) The patient is the best judge of his/her pain. This is the most important concept and has to be accepted by all involved if proper management is to be achieved. Pain is what, and occurs when, the experiencing person says. We often erroneously assume that we must be able to identify the source of pain for the expression of pain to be valid. For many patients pain is the most feared manifestation of their disease. Cancer is what may eventually kill them, but pain is what makes them suffer.

(2) Placebos have no place in the treatment of chronic pain. If we are convinced of principle 1 then this is obvious. Using placebos reveals more about our own attitudes than the patient's comfort.

(3) All narcotic analgesics are equivalent if equivalent doses are given.

(4) All narcotic analgesics have similar adverse effects.

(5) Around-the-clock dosing is preferred over as-needed dosing. If chronic pain is thought of as a continuum, several problems exist when an analgesic is given on demand rather than on a regular schedule. It is discouraging to the patient when relief is not available until the pain recurs. Patients are often hesitant to ask for pain relief for a variety of reasons, including fear that complaining about pain is a sign of a weak or bothersome patient. Nurses or family may encourage patients to wait until pain becomes unbearable before giving a dose because they fear drug dependence. We have found excellent results when using morphine sulfate solution for chronic pain management on an around-the-clock schedule with the dose being titrated to the patient's needs. Perhaps any analgesic would work as well if administered in the same way.

(6) When changing from one narcotic analgesic to another, keep the old drug available on an as-needed basis for a short while. We have found it very comforting for the patient to keep the old analgesic available on an as-needed basis when a different drug is used on an around-the-clock schedule. Often within one to two days the call for the old drug ends, and the patient has adequate control of pain.

(7) Analgesic drugs should not be switched without an adequate trial. To treat chronic pain appropriately, it is necessary to have a treatment plan and follow it. Indiscriminate switching of drugs will only result in a diminution of trust on the part of the patient and the family since none of the drugs is given enough time to produce relief. When drugs must be switched, an equivalent dosing chart should be used.

(8) Think of analgesic orders in terms of daily equivalent doses. It would be useful for all health professionals dealing with chronic pain management to think of the equivalent daily doses of analgesic given to a patient.

(9) Dose and frequency of administration of narcotic analgesics should not generally be changed at the same time. A small change in the dose and frequency of administration can result in a substantial reduction in the daily dose of pain medication.

(10) Oral drugs are preferred over injectable drugs. Since the object is to treat chronic pain properly, it is hoped that many patients will then be able to return home. An oral regimen can facilitate this.

REFERENCES

1. Algos: *A Pain Forum* 1:1 March, 1976
2. American Hospital Formulary Service, ASHP Bethesda, Maryland, 1986
3. *Facts and Comparisons*: Lippincott Co, Philadelphia, PA, 1982
4. Fairley P: *The Conquest of Pain*. Charles Scribner's Sons, New York, 1978
5. Foley K: The practical use of narcotic analgesics. *The Medical Clinics of North America Symposium on Clinical Pharmacology of Symptom Control* 66:5, 1091, 1982
6. Frank RM: *Treating Chronic Pain*. ASHP Signal Sept/Oct:37, 1982
7. Goodman, Gilman: *The Pharmacological Basis of Therapeutics*, 6th ed. MacMillan Co Inc, New York, 1980
8. Gotz V: *Control of Cancer Related Pain*. Squibb CPE 1:2, 1980
9. Holmes AH: Morphine intravenous infusion for chronic pain. *Drug Intell Clin Pharm* 12:556, 1978
10. Inturrisi C: Narcotic drugs. *The Medical Clinics of North America Symposium on Clinical Pharmacology of Symptom Control*. 66:5, 1061, 1982
11. Kaiko RF et al: Narcotics in the elderly. *The Medical Clinics of North America Symposium on Clinical Pharmacology of Symptom Control*. 66:5, 1079, 1982
12. Kantor T: Control of pain by monsteroidal anti-inflammatory drugs. *The Medical Clinics of North America Symposium on Clinical Pharmacology of Symptom Control* 66:5, 1053, 1982
13. Marks RM et al: Undertreatment of medical inpatients with narcotic analgesics. *Ann Intern Med* 78:173, 1973
14. Melzack R, Wald PD: Pain mechanisms: a new theory. *Science* 150:971, 1965
15. Mount BM et al: Use of the Brompton mixture in treating the chronic pain of malignant disease. ND Summer. *Needs of the Cancer Patient*, 1977
16. Porter J, Jick H: Addiction rare in patients treated with narcotics. *NEJM* 302:123, 1980
17. Twycross RG: Heroin vs. morphine. *Pain* 3:93, 1977
18. Wang JK, Nauss CA, Thomas JE: Pain relief by intrathecally applied morphine in man. *Anesthesiology* 50:2, 149, 1979
19. Wolff B: Perceptions of pain. *The Sciences*. July/August 10–15, 1980

UPDATED REFERENCES

1. Abram SE (ed): *Cancer Pain*. Boston, Kluwer Academic Publishers, 1989
2. Kramer R: *Diagnosis and Management of Pain in Patients with Cancer*. Basel, S. Karger, 1988

22

CARE FOR THE TERMINALLY ILL: DEATH AND DYING

H.E. KAISER, D.B. BROCK, D.J. FOLEY, H. MAIER-GERBER and T.A. HODGSON

INTRODUCTION by H.E. Kaiser

The terminal phase of illness is the last stage of life. As such, it is also applicable to the neoplastic diseases. The terminal phase exhibits a varying appearance in different species and the terminal stage of neoplastic and related diseases is most complicated in man himself. When it occurs suddenly or unexpectedly, or in the case of lower organisms, death, may be met unconsciously. But it may also be a conscious event, even to the very end, even before a coma sets in. In man, the impact of approaching death may be experienced quite differently. Persons with greater acquiescence, or some form of hope, based upon religious convictions, better care or sound economic situations may lessen the burden incurred by the terminal phase. On the other hand, the situation, in addition to the sick individual, may pose serious problems on family, friends, community, state and even country.

The life span of an individual regardless of species, and the progression of particular phases of a given disease, are greatly influenced by the environment in which the individual lives. Man himself has remodeled his own environment in many physical and mental respects. It has been shown in Chapters 5 and 6 of the first volume, that the neoplastic diseases reach their highest phylogenetic development in the various species of mammals, especially man. The changing environmental factors which play a role in the well-being of an individual clearly indicate that the life span of each individual varies accordingly. This can be observed in mammals whether free-ranging, or in captivity. It is also noticeable in population groups or different nations. The terminal stage of the cancer patient is approached through various factors operating among the species. Natural, medical, therapeutic, educational, spiritual, perhaps even psychological and religious, as well as economic, factors may contribute to the formation of the terminal state of the individual. The basic factors influencing the terminal condition may differ clearly from those which are only of occasional importance. For example, unproven cancer therapies may exert, psychologically, a stimulating effect.

COMPARATIVE ASPECTS by H.E. Kaiser

The terminal phase of neoplastic diseases varies in members of the organismic kingdoms in accordance with the normal body plan and is reflected in neoplastic progression. The neoplasms or galls in the plectenchymata of fungi originating through the coalescence of cells offer a picture different from that of the tissues formed by the dividing cells of vascular plants. Plants, even as complex as the redwoods, may be considered less centralized organisms from the state of cells than a highly developed invertebrate, such as an insect, or highly developed vertebrates, as a mammal because the cellular state of the vascular plant lacks the nervous system. Malignant plant neoplasms are unable to metastasize or disseminate. Cell distribution from the primary malignant tumor, as it occurs in the animal, is comparatively impossible. A diseased plant portion may be discarded, a process comparable to the autolysis of larval structures in holometabolic insects or the regression of mammalian tumors. The terminal phase of plant malignancies differs from that of the animals because it has neither consciousness, nor dissemination.

In animals, especially mammals, metastases are common in the majority of tumors and they often terminate in general dissemination. This progression is realized by the highly developed nervous system; psychologically, it culminates in the mind of man. This fact must be borne in mind when, for example, mammalian neoplasms, and, particularly, their spreading, are compared to those of an invertebrate, such as the fruit fly *Drosophila melanogaster*. Primary tumors may be similar to a certain degree, but not secondary tumors and neither is their distribution, dissemination and the terminal phase.

CARE AND PSYCHOLOGY OF DYING by H.E. Kaiser

Some aspects of terminal care

The cancer patient is forced to accept the harsh reality of a relentless illness; family, or even a caring community, must hence assume very great responsibilities. The physician has the responsibility for providing palliative care for the incurable terminally ill patient. The financial pressures and emotional stress suffered by their families may well exceed their abilities to meet and overcome the challenge and must be considered an integral part of the social environment. With the exception of a number of very rapidly progressing malignancies, such as oat cell carcinoma of the lung, or cancer of the pancreas, these malignancies are diseases that progress slowly. Therapy can cure a few, but not the commonly occurring which can be included into the following categories: (1) rapidly progressing, and mainly fatal neoplasms (oat cell carcinoma of the lung); (2) treatable neoplasms of the young, where treatment may result in a second neoplasm

216

P.V. Woolley (ed.), Cancer management in Man: Biological Response Modifiers, Chemotherapy, Antibiotics, Hyperthermia, Supporting Measures
© 1989. Kluwer Academic Publishers, Dordrecht.

in later life, such as nephroblastoma, followed after 20 or more years by radiation-induced Hodgkin's disease; (3) the majority of slowly progressing neoplasms, such as the solid tumors (e.g., colon cancer), and certain types of Hodgkin's lymphoma; (4) certain treated neoplasms exhibiting a therapy-initiated, prolonged course, often with a second primary neoplasm. The terminal pathology may be neoplastic in character or the result of nonneoplastic diseases.

Palliative therapy tries to provide relief in patients, where cure or long-term survival is impossible due to the advanced stage of the disease. As in curative cancer therapy, surgery, chemotherapy, radiotherapy, immunotherapy, and other forms of therapy are used to cope with the functional impairment caused by the tumor itself or the damage that neoplastic disease has inflicted on the host organs and their proper function. Terminally ill patients, those with far advanced disease and generally in a rather weak condition require the physician to make decision with utmost care in order not to put an unnecessary burden on the enfeebled patient (Silberberg, 1982; Glick, 1982).

Suffering by the patient can be diminished by appropriate means. For example, morphine is hazardous for the healthy, but analgesics, both narcotic and nonnarcotic, are available and, if properly used, can provide effective relief of pain for most terminally ill (McGivney, 1984). Often, the physician, the relatives and the patient must consider the choice between death and a miserable existence. They should decide which option offers the best chance for a relative well-being of the patient. A prescription, for example, with strong side effects, may be used in the terminally ill, if it enables him or her to endure the last days (Lloyd, 1983).

The final stage as the end process of the disease is highly complex in man due to species specificity. The only appropriate comparison that can be made, with certain restrictions, is the terminal phase of neoplastic disease in animals under the care of a veterinarian. The substages of the terminal phase of life are characterized by increasing deterioration in the quality of life, which accelerates in the period between the third and last week or even the last day (Morris, 1986a; Brock, 1987) before death. Approximately 20% of patients, however, do not experience such an extremely low quality of life, even in the last week. There are variations with regard to the type of tumor, the primary, as well as of metastases, general dissemination, and the discomfort of the patient due to pain. Little has been published on dying as correlated to different types of neoplasms. The adjusted relative risk of cancer death was significantly greater in patients diagnosed from 1960 to 1969 as compared to those diagnosed from 1970 to 1974, in a study done in Hawaii (Hinds, 1983).

The disease process will affect the terminal stage of the patient differently, depending on the impairment of essential or nonessential body functions. A patient with terminal esophageal cancer with occlusion of the esophagus and inability to swallow even saliva must suffer more than another patient whose pain can be eliminated or alleviated by pain relievers. Pain was noted in 85% of primary bone tumor and 52% of breast cancer cases, compared to only 5% of cases involving leukemia (Foley KM, 1979). More than 80% of the patients who died reported some degree of pain during the course of the study, with increasing frequency and severity as death approached (McKegney,

1981). According to a study of 600 patients (Wilkes, 1974) pain was present in 82% of patients with cervical cancer, 75% with gastric cancer and 44–59% with cancer of the lung, rectum or breast. Patients in substantial pain were less likely to be fully conscious. As death approached, the percentage of the incidence of persistent pain increased, and at the final stage 18.2% of the patients were in persistent pain. The proportion of patients with severe pain increased dramatically within the last week of life, 25% of the 269 patients interviewed within 2 days of death were said to be in severe pain, while only 17% were in severe pain in the preceding 6 days. The percentage of patients who were "free of pain" remained fairly constant (Morris, 1986a). Prostate cancer and bone metastases were associated with more pain while patients with brain cancer or brain metastases were significantly more likely to be painfree. A significant relationship exists between age and pain insofar as patients over 75 years of age are more often free of pain or experience less existent pain. Due to its high percentage of bone metastases prostate cancer is characterized more often by severe pain whereas primary or secondary neoplasms of the brain are correlated with a painfree state which may be due to the decrease of the number of neurons in the brain cortex based on two facts: (1) decrease of the number of neurons during aging, based on their cell invariability; (2) further impairment of neurons by the neoplastic processes. Older patients obtain more pain relief than younger ones from the same dose of medication (Bellville, 1971). The relief of frequently undertreated pain (Krant, 1978) is a major problem in the provision of terminal care. There exists only little systematic research on the use of analgesics in terminal cancer patients (Goldberg, 1985). A chapter by R. Frank deals with chronic pain management. Chemotherapy induced nausea and vomiting is dealt with in a chapter by J. Laszlo and V.S. Lucas, Jr.

Various possibilities for patient care are available in the terminal phase. Recently, extensive studies were directed at the hospice and its capabilities. The terminal stage of any disease process, as the final one, has a particular impact on family, relatives, friends, health care personnel, and also involves particular choices of fiscal responsibility. The care for terminally ill patients varies dramatically from the needs of those who recover since the latter cannot be considered as being part of the final disease stage. The terminal cancer patient has the following options: (1) care in a hospital setting including intensive care units at the end of the final stage which supplies the most effective case in such measures including X-ray surveillance or pain control but hospital stay may be less convenient with regard to the quality of the patient's life; (2) the hospice, either with hospital-based care where the patient spends the last days of life or hospices without beds providing home care.

"Hospice" is both a philosophy and system of terminal care preparing people to experience dying as an inevitable, natural phase in the life cycle. It is a program of supportive services for terminally ill patients and their families, provided either at home or in designated inpatient besettings and resulting in lower cost than conventional terminal care stations. A review of cancer costs to the nation is provided in a later section of this chapter by T.A. Hodgson. It is the prerequisite to know what the quality of the dying process is really like. The character of life for the dying person assumes another shape: The direct environment may be limited to a single room, family and friends are seen differently and values of interest change. The emotional changes and social involvement remains important. Several concepts to measure the quality of life such as the Karnofsky performance and others have been used to investigate the characteristics of the terminal phase in neoplastic diseases (Morris, 1986a).

In a modal hospice 90% of patients have cancer, over 95% have a principal care person, all are over age 21, and over 90% require assistance with personal care at the time of hospice admission. In general, the length of life after admission was only 35 days (Goldberg, 1986). The average scores are relatively unchanged at 7 weeks: deterioration begins to become more pronounced between 5 and 3 weeks, and is most pronounced in the period between 3 and 1 week prior to death (Morris, 1986). The section by Brock and D. Foley enlarges on this topic.

Psychology of dying

Kuebler–Ross (1969) distinguishes five stages in the process of dying:
1. stage: Denial and isolation
2. stage: Anger
3. stage: Bargaining
4. stage: Depression
5. stage: Acceptance

The child dying of cancer

Very few investigations deal directly with the problems of the dying child. This is especially true of stages 1 through 5. Kuebler–Ross elaborates on this topic and Sandra Levy (1983/83) confirms that most of the literature deals with the dying adult. The time when the treatment of a terminally ill person should switch from a treatment aiming at cure/survival to a mainly palliative treatment of a child is a difficult decision to make (Chapman and Goodall, 1980). Important is pain control, pharmacologic or other methods for which dosage is not well enough known for children. The choices depend on the developmental condition, nutritional status, etc., of the child with terminal illness. The family contact more or less dictates the transmission of information to the siblings so that they are aware of the impending death of the ill child (Peck, 1980); see also OJ Sahler, 1978. It was advised keeping the dying child in the family as much as possible, but Peck has suggested that the parents be alone for a while with the child after death has occurred. Spinetta (1974) concluded that children from the age of 6 are aware of the terminal character of their illness.

The adult dying of cancer

Studies such as those by Kelly and Friesen (1950) or Kalish and Reynolds (1976) have indicated that more people wish to hear the truth if they are going to die of cancer, than not. Ethnic differences have been observed: 60% of the black patients, 49% of Japanese Americans, 37% of the Mexican

Americans, and 71% of the Anglos who responded, replied that they would tell a friend he had to die and more than 70% of each group, with the exception of 10% of Mexican Americans, wanted to be informed about their terminal condition (Kalish and Reynolds, 1976). Comparative aspects of this problem appeared not to be available regarding differences among various religious groups.

Kastenbaum (1977) and Gorer (1976) have described the cultural milieu within which Americans, in particular, succumb. Because of our increasing technology and perhaps our decreasing sense for the religious significance of events, until the late 1970s the experience of death itself had become intolerable and hence concealed within institutional walls. However, in 1979, Kastenbaum described the sources of a new quest for "healthy dying". That is, as the technology of our death industry has increased, a reaction to this dehumanizing process has set in. An image of a self-actualized death has begun to emerge.

Increasingly, the person with a life-threatening illness has some kind of positive conception of the death he or she wants to have. This is a distinct departure from the interpersonal climate that existed only a few years ago when death was not considered a fit topic of contemplation for either patient or caregiver.

Flynn and Stewart (1979) reviewed 55,288 death certificates in the state of Ohio, covering a period of 18 years. They found that for the total period, 65% of the patients died in acute and chronic care hospitals, 15% died in nursing homes, and 20% died at home. Trends over this period demonstrated a shift from patients dying at home to patients dying in nursing homes.

The elderly dying of cancer

Nursing care of the elderly patients with cancer has two aspects, namely meeting the basic biological, psychological and social needs and the oncologic care of the particular neoplastic disease. Intelligence, patience, attention to detail, love, gentleness, and hard work are required (Kersey-Cantril, 1986; see also Leventhal, 1986; Lyons, 1987, Woll, 1987; McCallum, 1987).* There have been no improvements as regards the electrical stimulation of the brain for relief of intractable pain due to cancer or the Denver type for peritoneovenous shunting of malignant ascites, or the isotonic methotrimeprazine by continuous infusion in terminal cancer care (Sykes, 1987).

Anthropologic variations

Anthropologic cultural variations will have an impact on the handling of cancer patients in population groups with variable civilizations which will be especially reflected on the terminal stages of the disease. The histology and anthropology of religions exhibit variations in the encounters with death (see Reynolds and Waugh, 1977) which may also have an influence on the psychology of the terminally ill in various ethnic population groups.

The British have been leaders in research on the psychol-

---

* See Brock and Foley.

ogy of dying for some time. A good example of this work is represented in the book *Life Before Death* (Cartwright, 1973), which reports results of a study of the lives and care of a random sample of adults who died in England in 1968–69. In addition to providing information on the psychological characteristics of the patients and their families, the study pointed out some deficiencies in level of services for dying patients. The book also stated the needs for additional research on common symptoms and conditions of the dying. Finally, the authors called for more resources to be devoted to the care of these individuals.

This book is supplemented by the American book, *Clinical Care of the Terminal Cancer Patient*, dealing directly with the cancer problem. Another addition in a certain sense is Lasclo's *Physicians Guide to Cancer Care* complications which contains also most relevant sections. Dr. Lasclo is also a coauthor in this section of the book.

REFERENCES

*Allbrook D: Dying of cancer. Home, hospice or hospital? *Med J Aust* 141(3):143, 1984

*Balber, P: Care of the dying patient. In: *Physician's Guide to Cancer Care Complications*, pp. 309–326. Edited by J Laszlo, Marcel Dekker, Inc, New York and Basel, 1986

*Bayer R, Callahan D, Fletcher J *et al*: The care of the terminally ill: morality and economics. *N Engl J Med* 309(24):1490, 1983

Bellville JW, Forrest WH, Miller E, Brown BW: Influence of age on pain relief from analgesics. *JAMA* 217:1835, 1971

Brock DB, Foley DJ, Losonczy KG: A survey of the last days of life: Overview and initial results. *Proc Amer Statistical Assn* (inn press), 1987

*Brooks CH, Smyth-Staruch K: Hospice home care cost savings to third-party insurers. *Med Care* 22(8):691, 1984

*Carson NE: How to succeed in practice by really trying. Guidelines for the care of dying patients. *Aust Fam Physician* 12(2):124, 1983

Cartwright A, Hockey L, Anderson JL: *Life Before Death*. Routledge and Kegan Paul, London/Boston, 1973

Cassileth BR, Cassileth PA (eds): *Clinical Care of the Terminal Cancer Patient*. Lea & Febiger, Philadelphia, 1982

Chapman JA, Goodall J: Helping a child to live whilst dying. *Lancet* 1(8171):753, 1980

*Davis LK, Wegman DH, Manson RR *et al*: Mortality experience of vermont granite workers. *Am J Ind Med* 4(6):705, 1983

Evans C, McCarthy M: Referral and survival of patients accepted by a terminal care support team. *J Epidemiol Comm Health* 38(4):310, 1984

Flynn A, Stewart D: Where do cancer patients die? A review of cancer deaths in Cuyahoga County, Ohio 1957–1974. *J Comm Health* 5(2):126, 1979

Foley KM: The management of pain of malignant origin. In: *Current Neurology*, Tyler HR, Dawson D (eds). Boston, Houghton Mifflin, Vol. 2, Chapter 18, 1979

Glick JH: Palliative chemotherapy: risk/benefit ratio. In: *Clinical Care of the Terminal Cancer Patient*, pp. 53–64. Edited by BR Cassileth, PA Cassileth. Lea & Febiger, Philadelphia, 1982

*Goldberg F: Personal observations of a therapist with a life-threatening illness. *Int J Group Psychother* 34(2):289, 1984

Goldberg RJ, Cullen LO: Factors important to psychosocial adjustment to cancer: a review of the evidence. *Soc Sci Med* 20(8):803, 1985

Goldberg RJ, Mor V, Wiemann M *et al*: Analgesic use in terminal cancer patients: report from the National Hospice Study. *J Chron Dis* 39(1):37, 1986

Gorer G: Death, Grief and Mourning. New York, Arno Press, 1976

*Greer DS, Mor V, Morris JN *et al*: An alternative in terminal care: results of the National Hospice Study. *J Chronic Dis* 39(1):9, 1986

Haid M, Fowler M, Nicklin O *et al*: People and dollars: the experience of one hospice. *South Med J* 77(4):470, 1984

Hinds MW, Nomura AM, Kolonel LN *et al*: A comparison of cancer survival by time period of diagnosis in Hawaii 1960–1974. *Cancer* 51(1):175, 1983

*Hurny C: The psyche and cancer. (Ger) *Schweiz Med Wochenschr* 114(49):1827, 1984

Jones DR, Goldblatt PO, Leon DA: Bereavement and cancer: some data on deaths of spouses from the longitudinal study of Office of Population Censuses and Surveys. *Br Med J (Clin Res)* 289(6443):461, 1984

Kalish RA, Reynolds DK, Farberow NL: Community attitudes toward suicide. *Community Ment Health J* 10(3):301, 1974

Kalish R, Reynolds D: Death and ethnicity. A psychocultural study. Los Angeles, University of Southern California Press, 1976

Kastenbaum RJ: *Death, Society and Human Experience*. St. Louis, Mosby, 1977

Kastenbaum R, Costa PT Jr: Psychological perspectives on death. *Annu Rev Psychol* 28:225, 1977

Kelly OE: *Make Today Count*. New York, Delacorte Press, 1975

Kelly W, Friesen S: Do cancer patients want to be told? *Surgery* 27:822, 1950

Kersey-Cantril CA: Nursing care of the elderly patient with cancer. The critical blend of science and art – back to basics. *Front Radiat Ther Oncol* 20:173, 1986

Kovar HG: The longitudinal study of aging: 1986 Re-interview Public Use File. In: *Proceedings of the 21st National Meeting of the Public Health Conference on Records and Statistics*, July, 1987

Krant MJ: Sounding board. The hospice movement. *N Engl J Med* 299(10):546, 1978

Kuebler-Ross E: *On Death and Dying*. MacMillan Publishing Co, Inc, New York, 1969

York, Laszlo J (ed): *Physician's Guide to Cancer Care Complications*. Marcel Dekker, Inc, New York and Basel, 1986

Leventhal EA: The dilemma of cancer in the elderly. *Front Radiat Ther Oncol* 20:1, 1986

Levy SM: Host differences in neoplastic risk: Behavioral and social contributors to disease. *Health Psychol* 2(1):21, 1983

Levy SM: The aging cancer patient: Behavioral research issues. In: *Perspectives on Prevention and Treatment of Cancer in the Elderly*. Edited by R Yancik *et al*. Raven Press, New York, 1983

Lloyd JW: Life and death. *Sangyo Ika Daigaku Zasshi* 5(1):127, 1983

Lubitz J: Use and costs of Medicare services in the last years of life. Presented at the Conference *Death on Your Balance Sheet: Costs and Choices in Terminal Care for the Elderly*. University of Hartford, Connecticut, November 14, 1986

Lyons JS, Silberman M, Hammer JS *et al*: Analysis of a hospital-based hospice program for terminally ill cancer patients: detailing patient needs to understand complex programs. *Am J Hosp Care* 4(1): 41, 1987

*Malden LT, Sutherland C, Tattersall MH *et al*: Dying of cancer. Factors influencing the place of death of patients. *Med J Aust* 141(3):147, 1984

*Martin J: Helping the dying to live – through hypnosis (news). *JAMA* 249(3):322, 1983

McCallum L, Carr-Gregg M: Adolescents with cancer. *Aust Nurses J* 16(7):39, 1987

*McCusker J: Where cancer patients die: an epidemiologic study. *Public Health Rep* 98(2):170, 1983

McGivney WT, Crooks GM: The care of patients with severe chronic pain in terminal illness. *JAMA* 251(9):1182, 1984

McKegney FP, Bailey L, Yates J: Prediction and management of pain in patients with advanced cancer. *Gen Hosp Psychist* 3:95, 1981

*Meister H: Prognosis disclosure to the dying patient (Ger). *Z Gesamte Inn Med* 39(22):555, 1984

_____

* References for additional reading

*Micetich KG, Steinecker PH, Thomas DC: Are intravenous fluids morally required for a dying patient? *Arch Intern Med* 143(5):975, 1983

*Moffat MJ (ed): *In the Midst of Winter*. Random House, New York, 1982

Moller TR: Cancer care programmes: the Swedish experience. *IARC Sci Publ* (66):109, 1985

Mor V, Hiris J: Determinants of site of death among hospice cancer patients. *J Health Soc Behav* 24(4):375, 1983

Morris JN, Mor V, Goldberg RJ *et al*: The effect of treatment setting and patient characteristics on pain in terminal cancer patients. A report from the National Hospice Study. *J Chron Dis* 39(1):27, 1986

Morris JN, Suissa S, Sherwood S *et al*: Last days: a study of the quality of life of terminally ill cancer patients. *J Chron Dis* 39(1):47, 1986a

*Morrow GR, Carpenter PJ, Hoagland AC: The role of social support in parental adjustment to pediatric cancer. *J Pediatr Psychol* 9(3):317, 1984

*Mulhern RK, Lauer ME, Hoffmann RG: Death of a child at home or in the hospital: subsequent psychological adjustment of the family. Pediatrics 71(5):743, 1983

*Nelson CC, Hertzberg BS, Klintworth GK: A histopathologic study of 716 unselected eyes in patients with cancer at the time of death. *Am J Ophthalmol* 95(6):788, 1983

*Nishikawa K: Psychology of cancer patients. The dying process. Kurinikaru Sutadi 4(3):321, 1984

*Norton B, Whalley LJ: Mortality of a lithium-treated population. *Br J Psychiatry* 145:277, 1984

On children dying well (editorial): *Lancet* 1(8331):966, 1983

Peck V: Death – The final relief. *Nurs Mirror* 15(9) XXXII, 1980

Reynolds FE, Waugh EH (eds): *Religious Encounters With Death*. The Pennsylvania State University Press, University Park and London, 198?

*Roussel JG, Kroon BB, Hart GA: The Denver type for peritoneovenous shunting of malignant ascites. *Surg Gynecol Obstet* 162(3):235, 1986

Sahler OJ (ed): The Child and Death. St. Louis, MO, CU Mosby, 1978

*Seeman I, Poe GS, Barbano J: Plans for the 1986 National Mortality Followback Survey. Presented at the *144th Annual Meeting of the American Statistical Association, Section on Survey Research Methods*, Philadelphia, Pennsylvania, August 14, 1984

*Seidman H, Mushinski MH, Gelb SK *et al*: Probabilities of eventually developing or dying of cancer – United States, 1985. *CA* 35(1):36, 1985

Shanfield SB: Some observations of a psychiatric consultant to a hospice. *Hillside J Clin Psychiatry* 5(1):31, 1983

Silberberg DH: Central nervous system manifestation. In: *Clinical Care of the Terminal Cancer Patient*, pp. 38–52. Edited by BR Cassileth, PA Cassileth. Lea & Febiger, Philadelphia, 1982

*Smith DK, Nehemkis AM, Charter RA: Fear of death, death attitudes, and religious conviction in the terminally ill. *Int J Psychiatry Med* 13(3):221, 1983–84

Summers D: Living with dying. 158(2):14, 1984

Sykes NP, Oliver DJ: Isotonic methotrimeprazine by continuous infusion in terminal cancer care (letter published erratum appears in *Lancet* 1 1987 Feb (8531):522). *Lancet* 1(8529):393, 1987

*Thiel R, Knispel J, Wallis H: Development, structure and initial evaluation of a comprehensive psychosocial care program for children with cancer and their families. *Monatsschr Kinderheilkd* 133(1):22, 1985

*Tsai SP, Wen CP: A quantitative evaluation of competing risks in occupational studies. *Ann Acad Med Singapore* 13(2 Suppl):321, 1984

Wilkes E: Some problems in cancer management. *Proc R Soc Med* 67:1001, 1974

Woll PJ: Who treats cancer? *J R Coll Physicians Lond* 21(1):61, 1987

*Wright MR, Nehemkis AM: Functional use of secondary cancer symptomatology. *Int J Psychiatry Med* 13(4):267, 1983–84

Young RF, Brechner T: Electrical stimulation of the brain for relief of intractable pain due to cancer. *Cancer* 57(6):1266, 1986

Young TK, Frank JW: Cancer surveillance in a remote Indian population in Northwestern Ontario. *Am J Public Health* 73(5):515, 1984

Zimmermann M, Drings P: Guidelines for therapy of pain in cancer patients. *Recent Results Cancer Res* 89:1, 1984

UPDATED REFERENCES

1. Goldberg RJ (ed.): Psychiatric Aspects of Cancer, Basel, S Karger 1988

2. Nathanson SN and Lerman D (ed.): Outpatient Cancer Centers. Implementation and Management. Chicago, American Hospital Publishing Inc. 1988

SURVEY OF THE LAST DAYS OF LIFE by D.B. Brock and D.J. Foley (1)

There exists a considerable amount of information on the quality of life before death in the terminally ill cancer patient but very little is known about life before death in the broader spectrum of disease-related mortality in the older age groups (9). About two-thirds of the 2 million deaths that occur annually in the United States are among those age 65 and over. The published underlying causes for national mortality for persons age 65 and over are: heart disease, 43 percent; cancer, 20 percent; stroke, 9 percent; pneumonia/influenza, 4 percent; and other, 24 percent (10). Further, the older population accounts for roughly one-third of this nation's health expenditures and much of this is consumed in the last year of life (3). Sound epidemiologic data on the circumstances in the last year of life and its implications for furthering biomedical research and shaping health policy are generally unavailable.

Only recently have large-scale studies been funded with the potential for providing information in this area including the National Long Term Care survey (7), the Longitudinal Study on Aging (5), the NHANES-I Epidemiologic Followup Survey (8), and the Established Populations for Epidemiologic Studies of the Elderly (4). Though these studies were designed to address a broader range of topics including the recovery from illness, and the need for long-term care support, a specific study of mortality was sponsored by the National Institute on Aging entitled "The Survey of the Last Days of Life". Data collection was recently completed on a sample of 1,200 decedents in Fairfield County, Connecticut through interviews with the decedents' next-of-kin on the lifetime history of conditions and circumstances surrounding death. Information from this study will provide a better understanding of the magnitude of sudden versus lingering death, the course of functional health (both mental and physical) prior to death, the presence of pain or discomfort, costs, and the trends in the quality of life before death in the older ages.

Preliminary data indicated that about 10 percent of the decedents died of cancer, though one-third had a lifetime history of a cancer-related diagnosis. Both the proportion with a lifetime diagnosis and the proportion dying of cancer decreased with advancing age. This trend was noted in another study of cancer mortality trends which implicated the role of selective survival in producing these trends (2). Furthermore, these data showed that unlike heart disease,

Proportion of Decedents With a Lifetime History of a Specific Diagnosis

(according to the history of a nursing home stay)

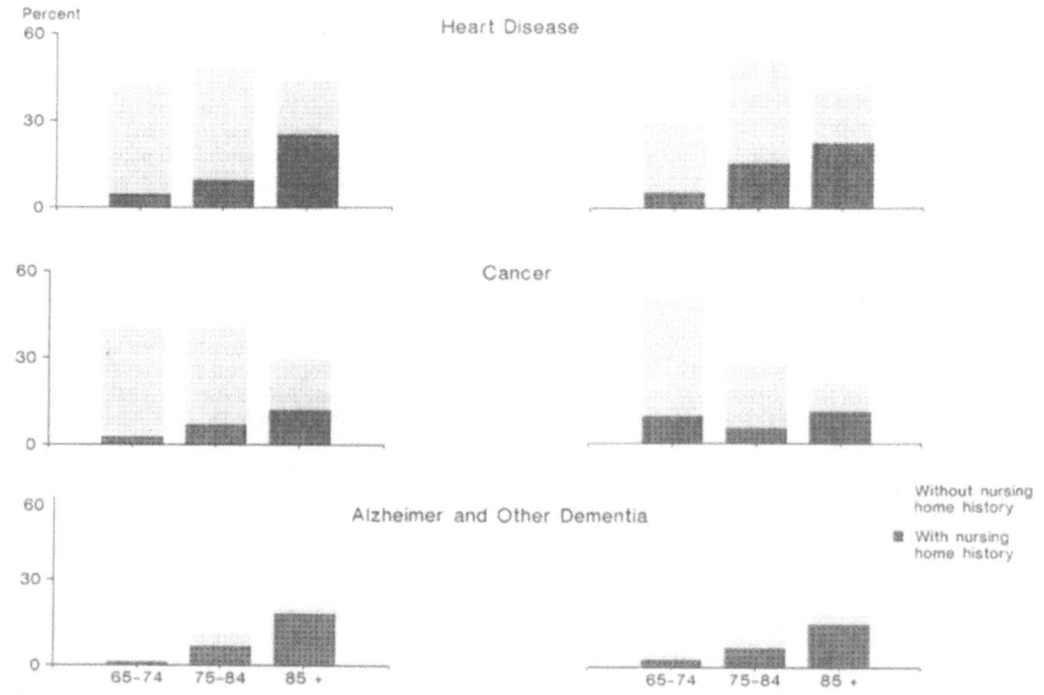

Figure 1.

Proportion of Decedents With a History of a Stroke or Hip Fracture

(according to the history of a nursing home stay)

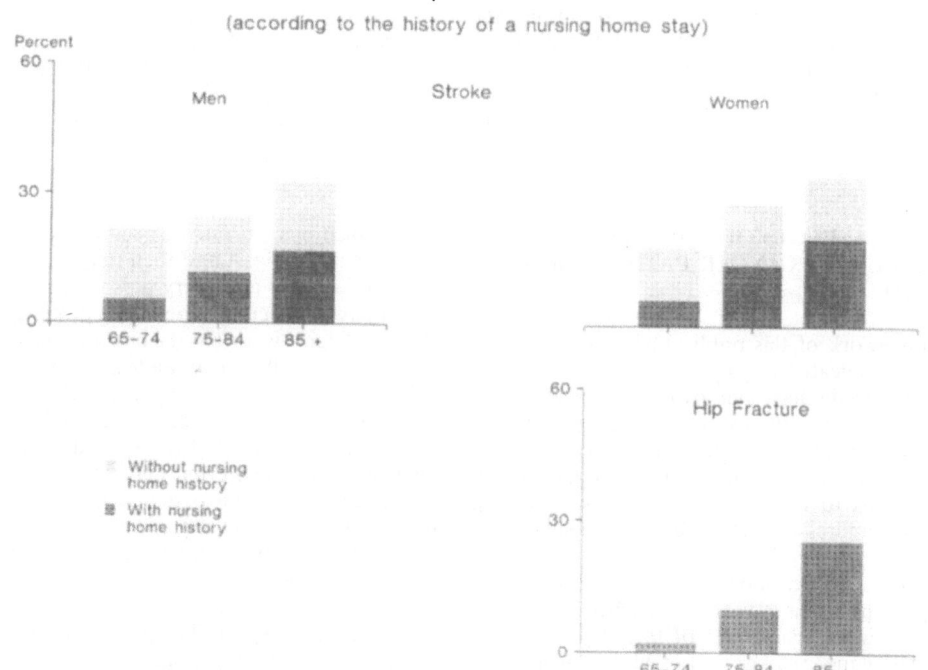

Figure 2.

stroke and the dementias, cancer-related deaths are not as highly associated with costly nursing home care in the last years of life (see Figs. 1 and 2).

Neoplasms exhibit many prognostic outcomes. Some are lingering diseases over many years and others take a fast and fatal course. A number of cancer types, especially the so-called solid tumors occur more commonly in the older ages. The most frequent neoplasms belong in this category, such as breast cancer in women, and prostate or colon/rectum cancers in men. In general, neoplastic diseases have shown an age-dependent increase in survival due to improvements in diagnoses, treatments and even cures over the years. But this varies according to the tumor type. These and the other data sources mentioned will allow for the study of neoplastic mortality in the framework of other cause-specific mortality in the older ages, such as cardiovascular disease, diabetes, dementia, and hip-fracture, to name a few.

The use and costs of medical care in the last year of life have been the focus of studies at the Health Care Financing Administration, which oversees the Federal Medicaid and Medicare reimbursement programs (6). Likewise, the National Center for Health Statistics has included this topic as a major content area in its 1986 National Mortality Followback Survey (10). Concern is growing over the use of life-sustaining technologies and the implications for unwanted aggressive medical treatment in the event of both catastrophic and lingering illness with a prognosis for terminal decline (12).

Knowledge about the last days of life will aid in informed decision-making and planning to ensure adequate care and avoid unnecessary suffering on the part of the patients and their families. Items such as changes in residence and household composition in the last months of life and questions regarding awareness of death, presence of pain, and the use of pain medication immediately before death are of importance because they characterize the onset, duration, and outcome of disease. We believe that these data will be extremely important in displacing fear with knowledge about death for those faced with the anxieties of terminal illness and to those who provide care to older persons during the last days of life.

REFERENCES

1. Brock DB, Foley DJ, Losonczy KG: A survey of the last days of life: overview and initial results. *Proceedings of the American Statistical Association, Social Statistics Section*, 306–311, 1987
2. Brody JA: Limited importance of cancer and of competing risk theories in aging. *Journal of Clinical and Experimental Gerontology* 5 (2):141–154, 1983
3. Fisher C: Differences by age groups in health care spending. *Health Care Financing Review* 1 (4), HCFA Pub. No. 03045. Health Care Financing Administration. Washington, DC, U.S. Government Printing Office, 1980, pp. 65–90
4. Huntley JC, Brock DB, Ostfeld AM, *et al*: Established populations for epidemiologic studies of the elderly. *NIH Publication No. 86-2443*. Washington, DC, U.S. Government Printing Office, 1986
5. Kovar MG, Harris T: Who will care for the Old? *Amer Demographics*, pp. 34–37, May 1988
6. Lubitz J, Prihoda R: Use and costs of medicare services in the last years of life. Health, United States, 1983. National Center for Health Statistics. *DHHS Pub. No. (PHS) 84-1232*. Public Health Service. Washington, DC, U.S. Government Printing Office, 71–77, 1983
7. Macken CL: A profile of functionally impaired elderly persons living in the community. *Health Care Financing Review*, Volume 7, No. 4, Summer, 33–49, 1986
8. Madans JH, Kleinman JC, Cox CS *et al*: Ten years after NHANES-I: Report of initial followup. *Public Health Reports*, Vol. 101, No. 5:465–473, 1986
9. Morris JN, Suissa S, Sherwood S *et al*: Last days: a study of the quality of life of terminally ill cancer patients. *Journal of Chronic Diseases*, Vol. 39, No. 1:47–62, 1986
10. National Center for Health Statistics: Advanced Report of Final Mortality Statistics, 1984. *Monthly Vital Statistics Report*, Vol. 35 (6), Supplement (2). DHHS Pub. No. (PHS) 86-1120. Public Health Service, Hyattsville, Maryland, 1986
11. Seeman I, Poe GS, Barbano J: Plans for the 1986 National Mortality Followback Survey. Presented at the *144th Annual Meeting of the American Statistical Association, Section on Survey Research Methods*, Philadelphia, Pennsylvania, 1984
12. United States Congress, Office of Technology Assessment: *Life-sustaining Technologies and the Elderly*. OTA-BA-306, Washington, DC, U.S. Government Printing Office, 1987

THEOLOGICAL ASPECTS OF THE TREATMENT OF TERMINALLY ILL CANCER PATIENTS by H. Maier-Gerber (1)

Within the framework of this publication, a theologically scientific treatise on death or dying should not be expected. We who are physicians have our own very practical and somewhat less than scientific form of theology. Since we must remain strictly scientific within our own field, the practice of medicine, we have more than enough of self-imposed limitations to observe; hence, in discussing the topic we are now addressing, let us for once speak in very personal terms.

When we physicians accompany the cancer patients we have known perhaps for many years as they move toward an evermore closely approaching end of their lives, we ourselves have in consequence taken part in this fateful journey. Through our close involvement with each patient's fate, we can achieve an ever-increasing spiritual maturity. For this reason we are already differentiated from those who pursue

other vocations. In our association with our patients, we must inwardly digest and then master every external situation and element and every personal inner experience if we wish to avoid reacting merely with professional detachment. But the latter is just what the patient very quickly notices; he becomes inwardly lonely and may form an attachment to others who are more warmly disposed toward him. Further, if the physician also wishes to lead his patients along this part of the way (and that he should), he is then himself challenged, he must bring himself into it and by word and action convey to the patient something of his own firm conviction and something of his own peace of mind. In this effort, psychological and psychotherapeutic insights may well be of assistance, but never be the source from which emanates the very essence of the physician, as it were, the radiation of his spirit. The power of his personality, however, and the convincing and so comfortingly unshakable assurance of his attitude toward the patient is derived directly from his own personal faith.

If, as a physician, I should already stand unshakable upon

this firm foundation of faith or as a new beginning were to accept these divine truths in true belief, I would then be able to meet my patients, especially those terminally ill, with a great sense of confidence to offer them much comfort and even support.

The question may be raised whether the bearing of such tidings to the patients is not the concern rather of the priest, pastor or other such spiritual advisor. If one of them with an equal faith is available, I gladly relinquish this mission to him. It is not unusual, however, for the patient to follow, and place his trust in the words of the attending physician – who knows his patient's true situation only too well – rather than in a man of the church who may put in an appearance only once or twice. In each instance, however, it is essential that through the warmth of the attending physician's handclasp and through his every word there glow that quiet and convincing confidence in a coming glory, and that there emanates from him an atmosphere of profound peace and joyous expectancy.

What I seek to express is the conviction that as physicians we cannot in good conscience accompany those in our care to the very limits of their biological existence without calling ourselves to account with respect to what is really transpiring here before us, to what is expected to follow thereafter, and to how we ourselves would respond in the same situation.

What do the words "dying with dignity" really signify? A little more attention and a more humanitarian treatment for those who, in their agony of dying, are helpless and without hope? It is not enough to provide the solution to their problem for which nearly all those who are about to pass on cry out. They yearn to know whether there is a life after this life and under what conditions they may anticipate forgiveness, sanctuary, and glory, or must they fear the approach of darkness and dread. They will not settle for less, and that is just as well.

REFERENCE

1. Maier-Gerber H: *Death – The Climax of Life*, 3rd edition, R. Brockhaus Pocketbook, Vol. 338. R. Brockhaus Publisher, Wuppertal, FRG, 1983

ECONOMIC ASPECTS OF NEOPLASTIC DISEASE IN THE UNITED STATES, 1987 by T.A. Hodgson (5)

Introduction

Illness and disease create a burden for the patient, his family and friends, and society. The individual's burden may include pain and suffering, reduced quality of life, premature mortality, and financial loss. Family and friends also may suffer emotional trauma, grief, and financial loss. Society must bear the negative impact on the social conscience created by distress of patients, families, and acquaintances and the costs of resources used for medical care and lost because of morbidity, disability, and premature mortality. The social and economic implication of disease for victims and the society at large are pain, suffering, disability, and death; millions of years of life lost; vast amounts of human and economic resources devoted to detection, diagnosis, and treatment; and billions of dollars of economic output forgone annually because of lost human resources.

Three categories of costs can be identified: direct costs, resulting from the use of resources; indirect costs, resulting from the loss of resources; and psychosocial costs, resulting from intangible impacts such as pain and suffering.

Direct costs

Direct costs include resources used for medical care in the prevention, diagnosis, and treatment of illness and disease and for the continuing care, rehabilitation, and terminal care of patients. In addition to medical care, other direct costs borne by patients and other individuals include costs of transportation to health providers, certain household expenditures, and costs of relocating such as moving expenses. Transportation costs could be incurred not only for local transportation to hospitals, clinics, physicians, and so on, but also for transportation out of state, and out-of-area living costs. Illness can force a family to incur numerous other expenses in caring and providing for the sick member of the family.

Financial costs include interest lost on withdrawal of savings to pay expenses, interest charges on funds borrowed to pay for illness-related expenses including interest on personal loans, mortgages, and loans against the cash value of life insurance.

Indirect costs

Indirect costs are the time and output lost or forgone by the patient, family, friends and others from employment, housekeeping, volunteer activities and leisure. The patient suffers a cessation or reduction of activity because of morbidity, disability or mortality associated with the illness.

Psychosocial costs

Disease may bring about personal catastrophes that are not reflected in direct and indirect economic costs. Illness and disease are responsible for a wide variety of deteriorations in the quality of life that are frequently referred to as psychosocial costs. Victims of illness and disease; children, spouses, and siblings of victims; friends of co-workers of victims; and those who render care may all be affected. A victim may

Table 1. Economic costs of cancer by type of cost: United States, 1985.

Type of cost	Amount (millions)	Percent distribution	Percent of all illnesses
Total	$72,494	100.00	10.7
Direct	18,104	25.0	4.9
Indirect	54,390	75.0	17.6
Morbidity	7,170	9.9	8.9
Mortality	47,220	65.1	20.8

Discounted at 4 percent.

suffer a loss of a body part or speech, disfigurement, disability, impending death, pain, and grief. The combination of financial strain and psychosocial problems can be especially devastating.

Economic costs of neoplasms

It is estimated that over five million Americans alive today have a history of cancer, two million of whom were diagnosed less than five years ago, and new cases are occurring at the rate of more than 900,000 per year (not counting 400,000 new cases of non-melanoma skin cancer) (1). Economic costs of cancer are estimated at $72.5 billion in 1985, of which $18.1 billion were health care expenditures, $7.2 billion were morbidity costs, and $47.2 billion were mortality costs (Table 1).

Personal health care expenditures

The Health Care Financing Administration annually estimates national health expenditures according to type of service and source of funds (13).

Health care expenditures for cancer were estimated at almost 4 billion dollars in 1976 by Cooper and Rice (4). This grew to over 13 billion dollars in 1980, and reached about 18 billion in 1985.

Most of the cost of medical care for cancer derives from the care received in short-stay hospitals by 1.9 million patients who required an average 8.9 days per stay for a total of 17 million days (5), and 20 million office visits to ambulatory care physicians for diagnosis and treatment (10). Hospital care of cancer patients accounted for $12.1 billion, or two-thirds of total medical care expenditures (Table 2). In contrast, hospital care spending for all illnesses comprised 45% of total medical spending in the United States. This relative difference is due to the higher rate of hospitalization and longer stays for cancer patients compared with many other illnesses. Physicians' services for cancer patients amounted to $4.1 billion (23% of total medical care expenditures for cancer), but considerably lesser amounts were spent for nursing home care ($919 million), drugs ($659 million), and other professional services ($326 million).

Morbidity losses

Illness due to cancer prevents people from leading their accustomed productive lives and keeping house. They may lose time from their activities, be forced out of the labor force, or become institutionalized. Morbidity costs of neoplasms are estimated for the currently employed, persons not in institutions who were unable to work, and women unable to keep house because of illness or disability. In addition, there may have been persons residing in institutions such as nursing homes and homes for the aged who were ill with cancer and unable to work or keep house. Morbidity and disability from cancer in the United States in 1985 resulted in $7.2 billion of lost output, representing 9.9% of the morbidity costs for all diseases. Cancer is high on the list of diseases causing morbidity and concomitant economic costs (12).

Mortality losses

Deaths from neoplasms represented 22% of all deaths, but the proportion varied markedly with age and sex. This proportion increased to 17% at 25–44 years of age, and to more than one-third of all deaths at ages 45–64 years, then decreased to about 20% of deaths at ages 65 years and over. Females 45–64 years of age had the highest proportion of deaths from neoplasms, 42% of the total in this group.

More than half of all cancer deaths were caused by malignant neoplasms of the digestive, respiratory, and intrathoracic organs (Table 3). Malignant neoplasms of the genitourinary organs were the third leading cause of cancer deaths and were responsible for 15% of the total. The contributions of specific sites were different for male and female mortality. The leading causes of cancer deaths among males were malignant neoplasms of the respiratory and intrathoracic, digestive, and genitourinary organs in that order with these three sites responsible for 75% of all male deaths from neoplasms. Among females, the leading sites were digestive organs, breast, respiratory and intrathoracic organs, and genitourinary organs which together accounted for 76% of cancer deaths of females.

Premature mortality from cancer is a significant drain on the productive capacity of the economy. Cancer deaths in

Table 2. Medical care expenditures for all conditions and cancer by type of medical service: United States, 1985.

Type of service	All conditions		Cancer	
	Amount (millions)	Percent distribution	Amount (millions)	Percent distribution
All services	$371,400	100.0	$18,104	100.0
Hospital care	166,700	44.9	12,118	66.9
Physicians' services	82,800	22.3	4,082	22.5
Nursing home care	35,200	9.5	919	5.1
Drugs	28,500	7.7	659	3.6
Other professional services	39,700	10.7	326	1.8
Other health services	18,500	5.0	a	a

a Not applicable.

1985 resulted in a loss of $47 billion. The cost per cancer death was $102 thousand. For males who died of cancer, an estimated 3.5 million person-years were lost (14 per death) at a cost of $26 billion. Females who died of cancer represented a loss of 3.7 million person-years (17 per death) and $21 billion. Males accounted for 53% of the productivity losses due to the higher earnings of males. Cancer was responsible for about one-fifth of all person-years lost and mortality costs.

Total indirect costs

Morbidity and mortality from neoplasms in 1985 deprived the Nation of more than seven million person-years of productive activity at an estimated value of $54 billion. This grew from 12 billion in 1972 (4).

Summary of economic costs

Total economic costs of neoplasms, including direct and indirect costs, were estimated at $72.5 billion in 1985. While medical care expenditures have caused concern for some years now, our analysis shows that indirect costs of neoplasms in 1985 were 3 times direct costs. Personal health care expenditures for neoplasms were almost one-fourth of total costs, morbidity losses acounted for 10%, and mortality losses were 65% of all costs. Chronic diseases characterized by morbidity, disability and mortality generate high indirect costs relative to medical care expenditures. This is also the case for heart disease for which indirect costs were even a larger percent of the total. For all conditions together, total costs were more evenly distributed among direct and indirect costs. This reflects the influence in the costs of all diseases of acute illnesses for which mortality is low but medical care is required and time is lost from work and other activities when people are sick.

Medical care expenditures were a larger proportion of disease costs for females than for males. This results not so much because personal health care expenditures were higher for females (which they were) but because morbidity and mortality losses were so much lower for females. Indirect costs are determined both by the time lost from productive activities and the value of that time. Total person-years lost for all diseases were higher for males, but females had higher years lost for some conditions. However, the lower values of earnings and housekeeping services for females compared to males usually outweighed any differences in person-years lost and resulted in higher indirect costs for males for most conditions. It is only at ages 65 and over, when labor force participation declines sharply among men while women continue keeping house, that the expected value of earnings and housekeeping services lost for a woman ill with disease exceeds that for a man who becomes ill. Rice (11) and Hodgson (7) discuss these relationships in some detail and address the issue of a methodology that is based on earnings patterns and tends to give greater weight to working-age men compared to women, the young, and older persons.

Neoplasms accounted for 11% of economic costs of all diseases in 1985. Mortality losses are a large share of total economic costs, one-third for all conditions, and almost two-thirds of the total estimated for neoplasms. Indirect losses are especially important for chronic conditions that cause morbidity and disability and conditions that result in death, especially at relatively young ages. It is important, therefore, to consider both direct and indirect costs in order to more fully account for the burden of illness and more accurately compare costs of several diseases.

Conclusion

Our understanding of the economic aspects of neoplastic diseases would benefit if greater specificity could be introduced and we were able: (a) to distribute costs among

Table 3. Number of deaths, person-years lost, and mortality costs, according to cancer site: United States, 1985.

Cancer site	Number of deaths	Person-years lost		Mortality costs[a]	
		Total (thousands)	Per death	Total (millions)	per death (thousands)
Total	461,563	7,210	15.6	$47,220	$102
Lip, oral cavity, and pharynx	8,290	136	16.4	1,045	126
Digestive organs and peritoneum	116,609	1,614	13.8	9,418	81
Respiratory and intrathoracic organs	127,311	1,951	15.3	12,869	101
Breast	40,383	793	19.6	5,165	128
Genital organs	49,690	687	13.8	3,607	73
Urinary organs	18,897	251	13.3	1,450	77
Leukemia	17,319	327	18.9	2,511	145
Lymphatic and hematopoietic tissues	25,159	416	16.5	3,097	123
Other and unspecified sites	57,905	1,035	17.9	8,057	139

Source: Number of deaths from National Center for Health Statistics (1987); person-years lost and costs calculated by the author.
[a] Discounted a 4 percent.

diagnosis, treatment, rehabilitation, and continuing care; (b) estimate non-health sector costs such as those for transportation, special diets, equipment, clothing, vocational, social, and family counseling, and indirect losses to family members; (c) relate functional health status and costs; (d) estimate costs according to significant attributes of disease, such as tumor site, stage of disease at diagnosis, and treatment modality; (e) estimate costs per person with the disease or per case. Included in this would be ascertaining the medical care used, expenditures incurred, disability, morbidity and mortality suffered from onset of a condition until death or cure, thus facilitating the calculation of incidence-based costs.

In conclusion, there are limitations to the costs of illness estimated in this chapter and not all relevant costs can be measured. Nevertheless, the methodology and data employed provide estimates of certain economic aspects of the burden of disease on society.

REFERENCES

1. American Cancer Society: *Cancer Facts and Figures*. New York, American Cancer Society, 1986
2. Anderson LG, Settle RF: *Benefit–Cost Analysis: A Practical Guide*. D.C. Lexington, Mass, Health, 1975
3. Collins JG: Physician visits: volume and interval since last visit, United States, 1980. Data from the National Health Survey Series 10, No. 144. *DHHS Pub. No. (PHS) 83-1572*. Washington, U.S. Government Printing Office, 1983
4. Cooper BS, Rice DR: The economic cost of illness revisited. *Social Security Bulletin*. 39 no. 2:21, 1976
5. Graves EJ: Utilization of short-stay hospitals, United States, 1985. *Vital and Health Statistics*, Series 13, No. 91, DHHS Pub. No. (PHS) 87-1752. Washington D.C., U.S. Government Printing Office, 1987
6. Hodgson TA, Meiners MR: Cost-of-illness methodology: a guide to current practices and procedures. *Milbank Memorial Fund Quarterly*. 60, no. 3:429, 1982
7. Hodgson TA: The state of the art of cost-of-illness estimates. In: *Advances in Health Economics and Health Services Research*, vol. 4, pp. 129–164. Edited by RM Scheffler, IF Rossiter. Greenwich, Conn, JAI Press, 1983
8. Levit KR, Lazenby H, Waldo DR, Davidoff LM: National Health Expenditures, 1984. *Health Care Financing Review* 7, No. 1:1, 1985
9. National Center for Health Statistics: Advance report of final mortality statistics, 1985. *Monthly Vital Statistics Report*. 36, No. 5 (Suppl), DHHS Pub. No. (PHS) 87-1120, Washington, D.C., U.S. Government Printing Office, 1987
10. Nelson C, McLemore T: The national ambulatory medical care survey, United States, 1975–81. *Vital and Health Statistics*, Series 13, No. 93, DHHS Pub. No. (PHS) 88-1754, Washington D.C., U.S. Government Printing Office, 1988
11. Rice DP: Sex differences in mortality and morbidity: some aspects of the economic burden. In: *Sex Differences in Mortality*, pp. 335–369. Edited by AD Lopez, LT Ruzicka. Canberra, Australian National University, 1983
12. Rice DP, Hodgson TA, Kopstein AN: The economic cost of illness – a replication and update. *Health Care Financing Review*, 7, No. 1:61, 1985
13. Waldo DR, Levit KR, Lazenby H: National Health Expenditures, 1985. *Health Care Financing Review*, 8(1):1, Fall, 1986

INDEX

POSTSCRIPT TO CHAPTER 4. ANTIFOLATES BY M. G. NAIR

Like folate and methotrexate, PDDF (CB3717) is also metabolized to polygamma glutamates in tumor cells (73) and animal tissues (102). These metabolites were chemically synthesized (103) and evaluated as inhibitors of thymidylate synthase derived from several species (103, 122). The di-, tri-, and tetraglutamates of PDDF were equipotent with 5-fluorodeoxyuridylate as inhibitors of thymidylate synthesis in permeabilized L1210 cells, and they were shown to be the most potent antifolate inhibitors of *L. casei* and L1210 thymidylate synthases yet described. Unfortunately in preclinical toxicology studies with mice, precipitation of PDDF in the nephron and subsequent renal failure was observed. Due to its unacceptable nephrotoxicity CB 3717 has been withdrawn from further clinical trials. In an attempt to develop PDDF analogues with more favorable therapeutic indices, analogues 15, 16 and 17 were synthesized (103); but all of them were weaker inhibitors of TS than the parent compound. Quite recently two groups (66, 109) have independently synthesized a PDDF analogue (DMPDDF), in which the 2-amino group of PDDF was replaced with a methyl group. Although 2-desamino-2-methyl-N^{10}-propargyl-5,8-dideazafolic acid (DMPDDF) was a waeker inhibitor of TS than PDDF, it exhibited excellent antitumor activity against selected tumor cells in culture. The replacement of the 2-amino group of PDDF with a methyl group resulted in enhancement of transport (109) and accumulation in tumor cells. The inhibitory activities of DMPDDF were 43 and 65-fold greater than that of PDDF in Manca human lymphoid leukemia and H35 hepatoma cells in culture (109). Transport studies *in vitro* established that DMPDDF

effectively inhibits MTX influx in to H35 hepatoma cells whereas PDDF has no effect on MTX transport in this cell line (109). These data suggest that the greater activity of DMPDDF relative to PDDF is due to the ability of the former to be transported and metabolized to polyglutamates more efficiently in tumor cells than PDDF. The polyglutamyl derivatives of DMPDDF were substantially better inhibitors of TS than the monoglutamate form (67).

5,8-Dideaza-5,6,7,8-tetrahydrofolate (DDATHF) which is a specific inhibitor of glycinamide ribonucleotide transformylase (GAR-transformylase) has been synthesized and evaluated as an antitumor agent by Taylor and co-workers (137). DDATHF exhibited a wide spectrum of antitumor activity both *in vitro* and *in vivo*. For example it was a potent inhibitor of the growth of L1210 murine and CCRF-CEM human leukemia cells with IC_{50} values ranging from 20-50 nM. DDATHF was not cross resistant to a subline of CCRF-CEM cells that are resistant to MTX by virtue of overproduction of dihydrofolate reductase. When screened against a variety of murine solid tumor models *in vivo*, DDATHF exhibited a broad spectrum of activity.

A related analogue of DDATHF, 11-deazatetrahydrohomofolic acid was found to be (104) a potent inhibitor of *L. casei* GAR-transformylase. However, it was not a good inhibitor of the L1210 enzyme. The polyglutamyl derivatives of tetrahydrohomofolate also showed inhibition of GAR transformylase indicating that the antitumor activity of tetrahydrohomofolate may be due to inhibition of *de novo* purine biosynthesis.

243

P.V. Woolley (ed.), Cancer management in Man: Biological Response Modifiers, Chemotherapy, Antibiotics, Hyperthermia, Supporting Measures
© 1989. Kluwer Academic Publishers, Dordrecht.

POSTSCRIPT TO CHAPTER 5. PURINE ANTIMETABOLITES BY W. SADEE AND B. NGUYEN

Synergistic toxicity of methotrexate and 6-mercaptopurine was shown to result from interactions among purine *de novo* synthesis and purine salvage pathways in malignant lymphoblasts (3). This interaction is an example of potentially useful combinations of antipurine drugs. Some enzymes, such as ADA, PNP, and 5NT of the purine degradative pathway are important in diagnosis and treatment of lymphomas and lymphocytic leukemia (5). The clinical use of the ADA inhibitor deoxycoformycin is of particular interest (2). In a patient with T-cell lymphoma, deoxycoformycin exhibited highly specific toxicity against immature lymphoblasts (1): Among the IMP-dehydrogenase inhibitors, tiazofurin is a novel C-nucleoside with significant antitumor activity against murine tumor models (4).

REFERENCES

1. de Korte D, Haverkort WA, van Leeuwen EF et al: Biochemical consequences of 2'deoxycoformycin treatment in a patient with T-cell lymphoma. Some unusual findings. *Cancer* 60(4):750, 1987
2. Ho AD, Ganeshaguru K: Enzymes of purine metabolism in lymphoid neoplasms, clinical relevance for treatment with enzyme inhibitors. *Klin Wochenschr* 66(11):467, 1988
3. Lazarow PB: The role of peroxisomes in mammalian cellular metabolism. *J. Inherited Metab Dis* 10 Suppl 1:11, 1987
4. Roberts JD, Stewart JA, McCormack JJ et al: Phase I trial of tiazofurin administered by i.v. bolus daily for 5 days, with pharmacokinetic evaluation. *Cancer Treat Rep* 71(2):141, 1987
5. Stoeckler JD, Ealick SE, Bugg CE, Parks RE Jr: Design of purine nucleoside phosphorylase inhibitors. *Fed Proc* 45(12):2773, 1986

P.V. Woolley (ed.), Cancer management in Man: Biological Response Modifiers, Chemotherapy, Antibiotics, Hyperthermia, Supporting Measures
© 1989. Kluwer Academic Publishers, Dordrecht.

POSTSCRIPT TO CHAPTER 7. PLATINUM COMPOUNDS BY C. L. LITTERST AND E. REED

One new area of research has undergone substantive development since the writing of the initial draft of this chapter; defining the role of platinum-DNA adducts in the biology of cancer drug therapy. Such studies have employed the use of immunochemical methodologies to explore the pharmacology of cisplatin-DNA binding in human cancer patients, as well as in animal models.

Several cohorts of patients have been studied by Reed and Poirier for platinum-DNA adduct formation in normal and malignant tissues (5,8 - 13). In initial studies which focused on the pharmacology of adduct formation in peripheral blood leukocyte DNA, measurable levels of adduct were shown to occur in some patients but not in others. Those patients receiving single agent therapy with either cisplatin or carboplatin who did not form measurable levels of adduct in leukocyte DNA did not respond to therapy. Even in patients receiving cisplatin-based combination chemotherapy, formation of adduct correlated well with disease response. The measured level of adduct was independent of the leukocyte differential of the patient, appeared to increase with successive cycles of treatment, had an apparent half-life of no less than 28 days, and for an individual patient was not simply a direct reflection of total drug exposure as measured by the product of plasma drug concentration and time [area-under-the-curve].

For groups of patients, however, there did appear to be a general direct relationship between adduct level and the dose of cisplatin or carboplatin administered. These studies showed that the level of adduct formed in leukocyte DNA strongly correlated with disease response in ovarian cancer patients and in testicular cancer patients. Further, adduct levels measured in bone marrow specimens obtained at autopsy closely approximated adduct levels measured in tumor tissues (10, 12). These studies imply that biochemical factors such as rates of drug inactivation of DNA repair, may be common to both tumor and some normal tissues, and thus possibly determined by the host genome of the individual and not uniquely by the tumor.

Fichtinger-Schepman and colleagues showed that using their assay, a patient's adduct levels in leukocytes *in vivo* from therapy could be predicted by measuring the adduct level after exposing that individual's leukocytes to cisplatin *in vitro* (1). They also showed that in cisplatin treated patients, adduct is removed from leukocyte DNA in a biphasic fashion, and more than 90% of DNA adduct is removed in the first 16 to 24 hours (2). Although a different

ELISA was used in the Fichtinger-Schepman studies as compared to the studies of Reed and Poirier, the range of adduct values observed in patients in the respective studies showed substantive overlap.

Studies done in rodent animal models have resulted in several observations that shed light on similar observations made in the human studies. In rats, adduct persistence was studied in kidney and gonadal tissues of male and female animals. Following a single parenteral exposure of cisplatin, adduct removal from kidney and gonadal tissues followed a biphasic pattern where the initial half-life of removal was 2 to 3 days, followed by a plateau phase of no less than 7 days (3,6). Further, by administering sequential drug exposures in small doses seven days apart, one could obtain greater adduct levels in kidney tissues than if the animal was given an equivalent dose as a single exposure (3,6). Thus, the persistence of adduct in kidney and gonadal tissues of male and female rats contributes to the total adduct level formed following a series of cisplating exposures. It is clear that in human tissues, adduct persistence plays a major role in determining the adduct level measured after a series of drug treatments (4, 13).

In rats, gender plays an important role in the determination of adduct level following a cisplatin drug exposure. When male and female animals are treated concurrently from the same solution of cisplating, adduct levels in kidney and gonadal tissues are far greater in males than in females (7). Castration studies show that this gender difference appears not to be related to testosterone or estrogen levels, but is inversely related to progesterone level suggesting that progesterone may exert a "protective" effect for the DNA. In human patients, males with testicular cancer appear to form adduct in peripheral blood cell DNA more readily that females with ovarian cancer (4), paralleling the observation made in rats.

It is possible that as technological advances allow more precise and sensitive measurement of the DNA binding of this class of compounds, plasma pharmacokinetics of drug may be correlated with DNA binding effects. Pharmacokinetic models could in principle be extended to include the compartments of DNA-bound drug and specific drug-DNA lesions. However, it is also possible that DNA binding and cytotoxicity may be determined more by the ability of cells to inactivate platinum complexes and/or to repair adducts, and to a lesser extent by pharmacokinetics.

P.V. Woolley (ed.), Cancer management in Man: Biological Response Modifiers, Chemotherapy, Antibiotics, Hyperthermia, Supporting Measures
© 1989. Kluwer Academic Publishers, Dordrecht.

REFERENCES

1. Fichtinger-Schepman AMJ, et al. (1987) Interindividual human variation in cisplatinum sensitivity, predictable in an *in vitro* assay? *Mutat Res* 190:59–62.

2. Fichtinger-Schepman AMJ, et al. (1987) cis-Diamminedichloroplatinum (II)-induced DNA adducts in peripheral leukocytes from seven cancer patients: quantitative immunochemical detection of the adduct induction and removal after a single dose of cis-diamminedichloroplatinum (II). *Cancer Res* 47:3000–3004

3. Litterst CL, Poirier MC, Reed E. (1988) Factors influencing the formation and persistence of platinum-DNA adducts in tissues of rats treated with cisplatin. *In* MP Hacker, JS Lazo, and TR Tritton (eds) *Organ Directed Toxicities of Anticancer Drugs.* Martinus Nijhoff Publishing, Boston, pp 159–171

4. Poirier MC, Reed E, Ozols RF, Yuspa SH (1986) DNA adduct formation and removal in human cancer patients. *In* C Harris (ed) Biochemical and Molecular Epidemiology of Cancer (Abbott Laboratories-UCLA Symposia on Molecular and Cellular Biology New Series, vol. 35), Alan R. Liss, Inc., New York, pp 303–311.

5. Reed E, et al. Poirier MC (1988) Platinum-DNA adduct levels in malignant and non-malignant tissues of cancer patients correlate with disease response. *Clinical Res* 36:499A.

6. Reed E, et al. (1987) Persistence of platinum-DNA adducts in renal and gonadal tissues of male and female rats Proc AACR 28:450, Abst # 1784.

7. Reed E, et al. (1987) cis-Diamminedichloroplatinum (II)-DNA adduct formation in renal, gonadal, and tumor tissues of male and female rats. *Cancer Res* 47:718–722

8. Reed E, et al. (1988) High dose cisplatin in hypertonic saline: Toxicity versus therapeutic benefit. *In* MP Hacker, JS Lazo, and TR Tritton (eds) Organ Directed Toxicities of Anti-Cancer Drugs. Martinus Nijhoff Publishers, Boston, pp 203–213.

9. Reed E, et al. (1986) Biomonitoring of cisplatin-DNA adducts in cancer patients receiving cisplatin chemotherapy. *Prog Clin Biol Res* 209B:247–252.

10. Reed E, et al. (1987) Platinum-DNA adducts in leukocyte DNA correlate with disease response in ovarian cancer patients receiving platinum-based chemotherapy. *Proc Natl Acad Sci* USA 84:5024–5028.

11. Reed E, et al. (1988) The measurement of cisplatin-DNA adduct levels in testicular cancer patients. *Carcinogenesis* 9:1909–1911.

12. Reed E, Sauerhoff S, and Porier MC (1988) Quantitation of platinum-DNA binding in human tissues following therapeutic levels of drug exposure. *Atomic Spectroscopy* 9:93–95.

13. Reed E, et al. (1986) Quantitation of cisplatin-DNA intrastrand adducts in testicular and ovarian cancer patients receiving cisplatin chemotherapy. *J Clin Invest* 77:545–550.

POSTSCRIPT TO CHAPTER 15. HYPERTHERMIA BY M. W. DEWHIRST

A number of new developments have occured in the field of hyperthermia since this chapter was first written. Many of these have the potential to contribute significantly to the field and are thus highlighted below.

Biology

Early reports from *in vitro* experiments indicated that acute pH shifts to pH's below 7.0 would dramatically increase the thermal sensitivity of cells. Thus, it was felt that since low pH conditions exist in human tumors that the use of hyperthermia might be particularly advantageous in those regions of tumor which resided at low pH. However, more recent studies by Hahn and Shiu have shown that cells that are adapted to grow in low pH conditions are no more sensitive to heat than their normal counterparts (5). In addition, they are able to develop thermotolerance at the same rate as non-chronically pH adapted cells at normal pH. These results indicate that it may be necessary to acutely drop pH to take advantage of pH sensitization from hyperthermia. Hyperglycemia has been investigated as a technique to drive down tumor pH (22). Thistlethwaite *et al.* (18) utilized oral glucose administration in human patients with superficially accessible tumors in which they could measure tumor pH. The regimen reduced pH 0.1 to 0.3 units in some patients, which would be sufficient to overcome the chronic pH conditioning effect based on results obtained *in vitro* (5). High energy phosphorus metabolites have been shown to play a role in hyperthermic sensitivity in that concomitant depletion of oxygen and glucose depletes intracellular PCr and ATP levels, which is highly correlated with increased thermal sensitivity (4). Considerable interpatient variability has been seen in magnetic resonance spectroscopy (MRS) studies of human tumors, with some cases indicative of low energy status (11, 16). It is possible that tumors of this type might be preferentially sensitive to hyperthermia therapy.

Recent reports by Herman and co-workers have served to highlight the potential role of heat, radiation, and chemotherapy in the management of locally advanced malignancies (6). Of particular interest are drugs such as cisplatin and mitomycin C, which demonstrate selective cytotoxicity under hypoxic and low pH conditions and are potentiated with hyperthermia. Another potentially exciting related area is in the development of drugs which are selectively more cytotoxic at elevated temperatures than their parent compounds, such as platinum-dye complexes (7). In addition, platinum resistant sublines have been shown not to be cross-resistant to platinum dye complexes, especially at elevated temperatures. Kano et al have recently reported that heat plus bleomycin overcomes bleomycin resistance seen at 37° C (9).

Physics

It has been recognized for some time that one of the major limitations to the effective use of hyperthermia is the general inability to heat tumors in a predictable and uniform fashion. Largely in response to these constraints, a number of new and improved hyperthermic devices are currently under development. One emphasis has been on development of microwave devices which have phase and amplitude control, such that the pattern of maximum power deposition can be moved to different parts of the heated region (19, 20). Another innovation is the scanning spiral microwave array, which can be used to heat large body surface areas as might be needed for chest wall lesions from recurrent carcinoma of the breast (14). Scanned, focused ultrasound, pioneered by Lele, has undergone continued development. Newer devices are capable of focusing ultrasound to heat tumor masses located deep within the abdomen, pelvis, and brain (10, 8).

A major limitation to the evaluation and improvement of hyperthermia efficacy has been the inability to completely measure the temperature field (3). Work has continued in the development of heat transfer models which could be used to calculate temperature distributions based on a few invasive temperature measurements. While considerable work still needs to be done to develop these models, especially into the three-dimensional realm, they have the potential to truly modernize the utilization of hyperthermia clinically (2).

Another significant advance has been the recent development of relatively strict guidelines for quality assurance and data standards in hyperthermia trials (15, 17). These efforts have contributed to the development of closely controlled multi-institutional studies which are necessary for the ultimate development and proof of the efficacy of hyperthermia.

Clinical results

In 1984 the results summarized by Overgaard from paired

P.V. Woolley (ed.), Cancer management in Man: Biological Response Modifiers, Chemotherapy, Antibiotics, Hyperthermia, Supporting Measures
© 1989. Kluwer Academic Publishers, Dordrecht.

lesion studies provided the strongest rationale for continuing work in the clinical applications of hyperthermia (13). Since that time, however, a number of the long-term follow-up data are now available (21). Prognostic variables which have consistently been shown to be important include tumor size, radiation dose, and descriptors of the temperature distribution (3, 12). Of particular importance is the observation that complete responses generally last for a considerable length of time. These results lend credence to the notion that adjuvant hyperthermia may be of value in improving local control rates over that achievable with radiotherapy alone. The relationship between complete response rate and radiation dose for groups of patients receiving radiation alone and compared with radiation plus heat has been recently examined. In these retrospective analyses involving advanced neck nodes, malignant melanoma, and brest carcinoma, enhancement ratios in the range of 1.4 to 2.0 have been consistently obtained, which indicate that significant improvements in local control rates may be achievable for a variety of tumor types (1).

Summary

There are a number of exciting new areas of ongoing research in the biologic, physical, and clinical aspects of hyperthermia. Some biologic studies are aimed at trying to increase the effectiveness of hyperthermia through pharmacologic manipulation of tumor physiology and the addition of chemotherapeutic drugs to target cells that might be resistant to heat and/or radiation. Improvements in hyperthermia devices continue. Further, methods for quality assurance have matured. Development of heat transfer models may significantly improve utilization of hyperthermia because of more accurate assessment of the efficacy of treatment. Finally, and possibly most signifcantly, the more recent clinical results further support the strong rationale for continued efforts in further refining the scope of usefulness of this modality in the treatment of human malignancies.

REFERENCES

1. Arcangeli G. Overgaard, J. Gonzale DG, Shrivastava PN: Hyperthermia trials. *Int J Radiation Oncology Biol Phys* 14(suppl. 1):S93-S110, 1988
2. Clegg ST, Roemer, RB, Cetas TC: Estimation of complete temperature fields from measured transient temperatures. *Int J Hyperthermia* 1:265-286, 1985
3. Dewhirst MW, et al.: Clinical application of thermal isoeffect dose. *Int J Hyperthermia* 3:307-310, 1987
4. Gerweck LE, Dhalberg WK, Epstein LF, Shimm DS: Influence of nutrient in energy deprivation on cellular response to single and fractionated heat treatments. *Rad Res* 99:573-581, 1984
5. Hahn GC, Shiu EC: Adaptation to low pH modifies thermal and thermochemical responses of mammalian cells. *Int J Hyperthermia* 2:379-388, 1986

6. Herman TS, et al.: Rationale for use of local hyperthermia with radiation therapy and selected anti-cancer drugs in locally advanced human malignancies. *Int J Hyperthermia* 4:143-158, 1988
7. Herman TS, et al.: The effect of hyperthermia on *cis*-diamminedichloroplatinum (II) (rhodamine 1,2,3)$_2$ [tetrachloroplatinum (II)] in human squamous cell carcinoma line and a *cis*-diammine-dichloroplatinum (II)-resistant subline. *Cancer Res* 48:5101-5105, 1988
8. Hynynen K, et al.: A scanned, focussed, multiple transducer ultrasonic system for localized hyperthermia treatments. *Int J Hyperthermia* 3:21-25. 1987
9. Kano E, et al.: Sensitivities of bleomycin resistant variant cells enhanced by 40° C hyperthermia *in vitro*. *Int J Hyperthermia* 4:547-553, 1988
10. Lele PP: Physical aspects and clinical studies with ultrasonic hyperthermia. In: *Hyperthermia in Cancer Therapy*. Edited by FK Storm. GK Hall Medical Publishers, Boston, pp. 333-367, 1983
11. Oberhaensli RD, et al.: Biochemical investigation of human tumours *in vivo* with phosphorous-31 magnetic resonance spectroscopy. *The Lancet* 2:8-11, 1986
12. Oleson JR, et al.: Tumor temperature distributions predict hyperthermia effect, *Int J Radiation Oncology Biol Phys* 16:559-570, 1989
13. Overgaard J: Rationale and problems in the design of clinical studies. In: *Hyperthermia Oncology, Vol. 2.* Edited by J Overgaard. Taylor and Francis, London, pp 325-338, 1984
14. Samulski TV, et al. Spiral microstrip hyperthermia applicators: Technical design and clinical performance. *Int J Radiation Oncology Biol Phys,* in press, 1989
15. Sapareto SA, Corry PM: A proposed standard data file format for hyperthermia treatments. *Int J Radiation Oncology Biol Phys* 16:613-627, 1988
16. Semmler W, et al.: Monitoring human tumor response to therapy by means of P-31 MR spectroscopy. *Radialogy* 166:533-539, 1988
17. Shrivastava P, et al.: Hyperthermia quality assurance guidelines. *Int J Radiation Oncology Biol Phys* 16:559-570, 1989
18. Thistlethwaite AJ, et al. Modification of human tumor pH by elevation of blood glucose, *Int J Radiation Oncology Biol Phys* 13:603-610, 1987
19. Trembly BS, et al.: Control of the SAR pattern within an interstitial microwave array through variation of antenna driving phase. *IEEE MT* 34:560-567, 1986
20. Turner PF, Kumar L: Computer solutions for applicator heating patterns. *IEEE MTT* 34:508-513, 1986
21. Valdagni R, Liu FF, Kapp DS: Important prognostic factors influencing outcome of combined radiation and hyperthermia. *Int J Radiation Oncology Biol Phys* 15:959-972, 1988
22. Ward-Hartley KA, Jain RK: Effect of glucose and galactose on microcirculatory flow in normal and neoplastic tissues in rabbits. *Cancer Res* 47:371-377, 1987